Critical Care of the Pediatric Immunocompromised Hematology/Oncology Patient

Christine N. Duncan
Julie-An M. Talano • Jennifer A. McArthur
Editors

Critical Care of the Pediatric Immunocompromised Hematology/Oncology Patient

An Evidence-Based Guide

Springer

Editors
Christine N. Duncan
Pediatric Hematology-Oncology
Dana-Farber Cancer Institute
Boston, MA
USA

Jennifer A. McArthur
Department of Pediatric Medicine
St. Jude Children's Research Hospital
Memphis, TN
USA

Julie-An M. Talano
Children's Hospital of
Wisconsin-Milwaukee
Medical College of Wisconsin
Milwaukee, WI
USA

ISBN 978-3-030-01321-9 ISBN 978-3-030-01322-6 (eBook)
https://doi.org/10.1007/978-3-030-01322-6

Library of Congress Control Number: 2018965743

This Springer imprint is published by the registered company Springer Nature Switzerland AG
The registered company address is: Gewerbestrasse 11, 6330 Cham, Switzerland

To families of children with cancer and hematological disorders that we have cared for in our ICUs

Contents

Contributors

Asya Agulnik, MD, MPH Department of Global Pediatric Medicine, Division of Critical Care, St. Jude Children's Research Hospital, Memphis, TN, USA

Stacey Albuquerque Boston Children's Pharmacy Department, Dana Farber/ Boston Children's Cancer and Blood Disorders Center, Boston, MA, USA

Fayhan Alroqi Department of Pediatric, King Abdullah Specialized Children's Hospital, Riyadh, Saudi Arabia

King Saud bin Abdulaziz University for Health Sciences, Riyadh, Saudi Arabia

King Abdullah International Medical Research Center, Riyadh, Saudi Arabia

Abdulrahman Alsultan Department of Pediatric, King Abdullah Specialized Children's Hospital, Riyadh, Saudi Arabia

Department of Pediatric, College of Medicine, King Saud University, Riyadh, Saudi Arabia

Joseph Angelo, MD Department of Pediatrics, Renal Section, Texas Children's Hospital/Baylor College of Medicine, Houston, TX, USA

Natasha Archer, MD, MPH Department of Pediatric Hematology and Oncology, Dana-Farber Boston Children's Cancer and Blood Disorders Center, Harvard Medical School, Boston, MA, USA

Ayse A. Arikan, MD Renal Section, Critical Care Section, Texas Children's Hospital/Baylor College of Medicine, Houston, TX, USA

Rajinder Bajwa, MD Nationwide Children's Hospital, Columbus, OH, USA

Neel Bhatt, MD Department of Pediatrics, Division of Pediatric Hematology/ Oncology, Medical College of Wisconsin, Children's Hospital of Wisconsin, Milwaukee, WI, USA

Michael Burke, MD Division of Hematology/Oncology/Blood and Marrow Transplant, Department of Pediatrics, Medical College of Wisconsin and Children's Hospital of Wisconsin, Milwaukee, WI, USA

Candice Chow, PhD Department of Psychosocial Oncology and Palliative Care, Dana-Farber Boston Children's Cancer and Blood Disorders Center, Harvard Medical School, Boston, MA, USA

Jessica Clymer, MD Pediatric Neuro-oncology, Dana-Farber/Boston Children's Cancer and Blood Disorders Center, Boston, MA, USA

Barbara Cuccovia Pediatric Stem Cell Transplant Unit, Boston Children's Hospital, Boston, MA, USA

Christine N. Duncan, MD Pediatric Hematology-Oncology, Dana-Farber Cancer Institute, Boston, MA, USA

Mohammed Essa Department of Pediatric, King Abdullah Specialized Children's Hospital, Riyadh, Saudi Arabia

King Saud bin Abdulaziz University for Health Sciences, Riyadh, Saudi Arabia

Jorge Ricardo Galvez Silva, MD Nicklaus Children's Hospital, Miami Children's Health System, Miami, FL, USA

Saad Ghafoor, MD Department of Pediatrics, Division of Critical Care Medicine, St. Jude Children's Research Hospital, Memphis, TN, USA

Jason Goldberg, MD Pediatric Cardiomyopathy and Heart Transplantation, University of Tennessee School of Health Sciences, Memphis, TN, USA

Department of Pediatrics, Division of Critical Care Medicine, St. Jude Children's Research Hospital, Memphis, TN, USA

Melissa Hines, MD Department of Pediatric Medicine, Division of Critical Care, St. Jude Children's Research Hospital, Memphis, TN, USA

Caitlin Hurley, MD Division of Critical Care Medicine and Department of Bone Marrow Transplantation, St. Jude Children's Research Hospital, Memphis, TN, USA

Marshay James, DNP, MSNEd, CNE Department of Pediatrics, Division of Critical Care Medicine, St. Jude Children's Research Hospital, Memphis, TN, USA

Vanderbilt University School of Nursing, Nashville, TN, USA

Sajad Khazal, MD The University of Texas MD Anderson Cancer Center, Houston, TX, USA

James S. Killinger, MD, F.C.C.M. Memorial Sloan Kettering Cancer Center, New York, NY, USA

Whitney Kopp, M.D. Division of Pediatric Critical Care Medicine, Medical College of Wisconsin/Children's Hospital of Wisconsin, Milwaukee, WI, USA

Brienne Leary Pediatric Medical-Surgical Intensive Care Unit, Boston Children's Hospital, Boston, MA, USA

Leslie E. Lehmann, MD Department of Pediatric Oncology, Dana-Farber Cancer Institute/Boston Children's Hospital, Boston, MA, USA

Kris M. Mahadeo, MD University of Texas MD Anderson Cancer Center, Houston, TX, USA

Peter E. Manley, MD Pediatric Neuro-oncology, Dana-Farber/Boston Children's Cancer and Blood Disorders Center, Boston, MA, USA

David Margolis, MD Children's Hospital of Wisconsin, Milwaukee, WI, USA

Steven Margossian, MD, PhD Harvard Medical School, Department of Pediatric Oncology, Dana Farber Cancer Institute, Boston Children's Hospital, Boston, MA, USA

Jennifer A. McArthur, DO Department of Pediatrics, Division of Critical Care Medicine, St. Jude Children's Research Hospital, Memphis, TN, USA

Medical College of Wisconsin, Milwaukee, WI, USA

David McCall, MD University of Texas MD Anderson Cancer Center, Houston, TX, USA

Jerelyn Moffet, PNP Duke Children's Hospital, Durham, NC, USA

Robert A. Niebler, MD Department of Pediatrics, Section of Critical Care, Medical College of Wisconsin, Milwaukee, WI, USA

Colleen Nixon Pediatric Hematology/Oncology Unit, Boston Children's Hospital, Boston, MA, USA

Lauren Pommert, MD Division of Hematology/Oncology/Blood and Marrow Transplant, Department of Pediatrics, Medical College of Wisconsin and Children's Hospital of Wisconsin, Milwaukee, WI, USA

Prakadeshwari Rajapreyar, M.D. Division of Pediatric Critical Care Medicine, Medical College of Wisconsin/Children's Hospital of Wisconsin, Milwaukee, WI, USA

Adrienne Randolph, M.D., M.Sc Division of Critical Care Medicine, Department of Anesthesia, Critical Care and Pain Medicine, Boston Children's Hospital, Boston, MA, USA

Departments of Anesthesia and Pediatrics, Harvard Medical School, Boston, MA, USA

Tolulope Rosanwo Case Western Reserve University School of Medicine, Cleveland, OH, USA

Hilary C. Schreiber, MD Memorial Sloan Kettering Cancer Center, New York, NY, USA

Julie-An M. Talano, MD Department of Pediatrics, Division of Pediatric Hematology/Oncology, Medical College of Wisconsin, Children's Hospital of Wisconsin, Milwaukee, WI, USA

Agne Taraseviciute, MD, PhD Children's Hospital Los Angeles, University of Southern California, Los Angeles, CA, USA

Sarah Tarquini, PhD Department of Psychosocial Oncology and Palliative Care, Dana-Farber Boston Children's Cancer and Blood Disorders Center, Harvard Medical School, Boston, MA, USA

Priti Tewari, MD University of Texas MD Anderson Cancer Center, Houston, TX, USA

Monica Thakar, MD Children's Hospital of Wisconsin, Milwaukee, WI, USA

Chani Traube Department of Pediatrics, Division of Pediatric Critical Care Medicine, Weill Cornell Medical College, New York, NY, USA

Christina Ullrich, MD, MPH Department of Pediatric Oncology; Department of Psychosocial Oncology and Palliative Care, Dana-Farber Cancer Institute and Boston Children's Hospital, Harvard Medical School, Boston, MA, USA

Matt Zinter, MD Department of Pediatrics, Division of Critical Care Medicine, UCSF Benioff Children's Hospitals, University of California, San Francisco, San Francisco, CA, USA

Part I
Predisposing Diseases and Specific Considerations in Critical Illness

Chapter 1
The Changing Landscape of the Critical Care of Pediatric Immunocompromised Hematology and Oncology Patients

Christine N. Duncan

Immunocompromised children and adolescent patients who have hematologic or oncologic diseases represent a small percentage of patients treated in pediatric intensive care units (PICUs) but have a disproportionately high mortality rate. A single-center study of 1278 patients admitted to a pediatric hematology-oncology service over an 11-year period found an admission rate of 4.2% with an overall PICU mortality rate of 38.9% [1]. Risk factors for PICU admission included older age, diagnosis of nonmalignant disease, and treatment with HCT. A more recent retrospective multicenter cohort analysis of almost 250,000 consecutive PICU admissions using the Virtual PICU Systems database identified 10,365 patients diagnosed with a malignancy who were admitted to PICUs for reasons other than perioperative admissions during the study period [2]. Children with cancer accounted for 11.4% of all PICU deaths and had mortality of 6.8% (43% in those who were mechanically ventilated) compared to 2.4% in patients without malignancy.

Outcome data regarding patients admitted to PICUs who have nonmalignant hematologic or immunologic diseases is limited, with the exception of those treated with hematopoietic cell transplantation (HCT). Far more is known about patients with oncologic diagnoses, and the literature is most robust regarding those treated with HCT. The survival of children with hematologic and oncologic diseases has improved in recent years despite remaining higher than those of other patients treated in the PICU (Table 1.1). A meta-analysis of mortality trends of children treated in the PICU after HCT over time showed a significant decrease in mortality associated with the year of inclusion as did a large single-center study comparing outcomes over time [3, 4]. However, interpreting comparisons of mortality across multiple

C. N. Duncan (✉)
Pediatric Hematology-Oncology, Dana-Farber Cancer Institute, Boston, MA, USA
e-mail: christine_duncan@dfci.harvard.edu

C. N. Duncan et al. (eds.), *Critical Care of the Pediatric Immunocompromised Hematology/Oncology Patient*, https://doi.org/10.1007/978-3-030-01322-6_1

Table 1.1 Published mortality of hematology, oncology, and HCT patients over time

Reference	Study period	Population	Number of PICU patients	PICU mortality (%)
Hayes et al. [5]	1987–1997	HCT	39	73
Hallahan et al. [6]	1987–1996	Oncology and HCT	150	27
Diaz De Heredia et al. [7]	1991–1995	HCT	31	45
Lamas et al. [8]	1991–2000	HCT	44	70
Kache et al. [9]	1992–2004	HCT	81	82 (1992–1999) 41 (2000–2004)
Cheuk et al. [10]	1992–2002	HCT	19	84
Diaz et al. [11]	1993–2001	HCT	42	69
Jacobe et al. [12]	1994–1998	HCT	40	44
Heying et al. [13]	1995–1999	Oncology (no HCT)	48	25
Tamburro et al. [4]	1996–2004	Oncology and HCT	329	41
Tomaske et al. [14]	1998–2001	HCT	26	58
Gonzalez-Vincent et al. [15]	1998–2002	HCT	36	53
Hassan et al. [16]	1998–2008	HCT	19	17
Faraci et al. [1]	1999–2010	Hematology/ oncology	54	39
Asperberro et al. [17]	2000–2006	HCT	53	51
Bartram et al. [18]	2000–2008	Sickle cell disease	46	7
Chima et al. [19]	2004–2010	HCT	155	37
Duncan et al. [20]	2005–2006	HCT	129	38
Zinter et al. [21]	2009–2012	HCT	1102	16.2
Zinter et al. [2]	2009–2012	Oncology	10,365	6.8
Rowan et al. [22]	2009–2014	HCT	222	60

HCT hematopoietic cell transplantation

studies must be done with caution. The published literature is comprised almost exclusively of retrospective studies, and the inclusion criteria are not consistent across studies. Some studies include only those felt to be at highest risk for worst outcome, specifically HCT patients supported with mechanical ventilation, whereas others include patients with all oncology diagnoses and admitted to the PICU for all indications. There are multiple reasons for the improved outcomes including scientific advances in critical care, hematology, oncology, and HCT. Equally important have been advances in supportive care and infectious disease management.

The severity of illness of immunocompromised hematology and oncology patients admitted to PICUs is broad including planned postoperative admissions, semi-urgent admissions of patients with worsening illness, and the emergent transfer of rapidly decompensating children. Equally broad are the reasons for critical illness in this diverse population including infection, organ compromise, and complications of the primary disease. The management of critically ill immunocompromised children and adolescents must be guided by the primary disease and patient's treatment. General principles of the initial management and stabilization of critically ill hematology and oncology patients, in most cases, can follow practices applied to other children. Thereafter, the management is strongly influenced not only by the reason for the need for critical care, but by the unique features of the underlying disease as well. For example, the early care of a child with sickle cell anemia experiencing acute respiratory dysfunction may mirror that of a patient with acute lymphoblastic leukemia or one with severe combined immune deficiency. After the primary stabilization of the patient, an understanding of the underlying disease is key to the next steps of diagnosis and management. In the example, one may consider acute chest syndrome as the cause of the respiratory distress in the patient with sickle cell anemia. Clearly this would not be on the list of potential etiologies in a child with leukemia in whom infection may be a chief concern. The therapy that the child receives to treat the primary disease is important as the critical illness may be a direct result or influenced heavily by the treatment. A clear example is that of children undergoing HCT who may have organ compromise, bleeding, infection, graft-versus-host disease, and other toxicities related to the recent and past therapy in addition to underlying comorbidities.

A goal of this textbook is to provide an understanding of the specific aspects of different diagnoses and therapies that impact the critical care of immunocompromised hematology and oncology patients. It is unrealistic to expect PICU providers to have a comprehensive understanding of all the diseases and therapies used in this population and for hematologists-oncologists to fully understand advances in ICU care. This is particularly true given the rapidly changing landscape of pediatric hematologic and oncologic care. Recent years have seen the development and expanded use of molecularly targeted medications, chimeric antigen receptor T-cell (CAR-T) therapy, and gene therapy. Each of these and other emerging therapies carry unique risks. Because of the complexity of diagnoses and treatment, a collaborative relationship between the PICU and the disease-specific teams is important to the care of these patients. Different models for cooperative care are addressed later in this text.

Multiple research consortia including the Pediatric Acute Lung Injury and Sepsis Investigators and Pediatric Blood and Marrow Transplant Consortium have focused on the care of immunocompromised hematology and oncology patients. The work of these and other groups is important as the community works to improve the survival of these vulnerable patients.

References

1. Faraci M, Bagnasco F, Giardino S, Conte M, Micalizzi C, Castagnola E, et al. Intensive care unit admission in children with malignant or nonmalignant disease: incidence, outcome, and prognostic factors: a single-center experience. J Pediatr Hematol Oncol. 2014;36(7):e403–9. https://doi.org/10.1097/MPH.0000000000000048.

2. Zinter MS, DuBois SG, Spicer A, Matthay K, Sapru A. Pediatric cancer type predicts infection rate, need for critical care intervention, and mortality in the pediatric intensive care unit. Intensive Care Med. 2014;40(10):1536–44. https://doi.org/10.1007/s00134-014-3389-2.
3. van Gestel JP, Bollen CW, van der Tweel I, Boelens JJ, van Vught AJ. Intensive care unit mortality trends in children after hematopoietic stem cell transplantation: a meta-regression analysis. Crit Care Med. 2008;36(10):2898–904. https://doi.org/10.1097/CCM.0b013e318186a34a.
4. Tamburro RF, Barfield RC, Shaffer ML, Rajasekaran S, Woodard P, Morrison RR, et al. Changes in outcomes (1996–2004) for pediatric oncology and hematopoietic stem cell transplant patients requiring invasive mechanical ventilation. Pediatr Crit Care Med. 2008;9(3):270–7. https://doi.org/10.1097/PCC.0b013e31816c7260.
5. Hayes C, Lush RJ, Cornish JM, Foot AM, Henderson J, Jenkins I, et al. The outcome of children requiring admission to an intensive care unit following bone marrow transplantation. Br J Haematol. 1998;102(3):666–70.
6. Hallahan AR, Shaw PJ, Rowell G, O'Connell A, Schell D, Gillis J. Improved outcomes of children with malignancy admitted to a pediatric intensive care unit. Crit Care Med. 2000;28(11):3718–21.
7. Diaz de Heredia C, Moreno A, Olive T, Iglesias J, Ortega JJ. Role of the intensive care unit in children undergoing bone marrow transplantation with life-threatening complications. Bone Marrow Transplant. 1999;24(2):163–8. https://doi.org/10.1038/sj.bmt.1701874.
8. Lamas A, Otheo E, Ros P, Vazquez JL, Maldonado MS, Munoz A, et al. Prognosis of child recipients of hematopoietic stem cell transplantation requiring intensive care. Intensive Care Med. 2003;29(1):91–6. https://doi.org/10.1007/s00134-002-1549-2.
9. Kache S, Weiss IK, Moore TB. Changing outcomes for children requiring intensive care following hematopoietic stem cell transplantation. Pediatr Transplant. 2006;10(3):299–303. https://doi.org/10.1111/j.1399-3046.2005.00453.x.
10. Cheuk DK, Ha SY, Lee SL, Chan GC, Tsoi NS, Lau YL. Prognostic factors in children requiring admission to an intensive care unit after hematopoietic stem cell transplant. Hematol Oncol. 2004;22(1):1–9. https://doi.org/10.1002/hon.724.
11. Diaz MA, Vicent MG, Prudencio M, Rodriguez F, Marin C, Serrano A, et al. Predicting factors for admission to an intensive care unit and clinical outcome in pediatric patients receiving hematopoietic stem cell transplantation. Haematologica. 2002;87(3):292–8.
12. Jacobe SJ, Hassan A, Veys P, Mok Q. Outcome of children requiring admission to an intensive care unit after bone marrow transplantation. Crit Care Med. 2003;31(5):1299–305. https://doi.org/10.1097/01.CCM.0000060011.88230.C8.
13. Heying R, Schneider DT, Korholz D, Stannigel H, Lemburg P, Gobel U. Efficacy and outcome of intensive care in pediatric oncologic patients. Crit Care Med. 2001;29(12):2276–80.
14. Tomaske M, Bosk A, Eyrich M, Bader P, Niethammer D. Risks of mortality in children admitted to the paediatric intensive care unit after haematopoietic stem cell transplantation. Br J Haematol. 2003;121(6):886–91.
15. Gonzalez-Vicent M, Marin C, Madero L, Sevilla J, Diaz MA. Risk score for pediatric intensive care unit admission in children undergoing hematopoietic stem cell transplantation and analysis of predictive factors for survival. J Pediatr Hematol Oncol. 2005;27(10):526–31.
16. Hassan NE, Mageed AS, Sanfilippo DJ, Reischman D, Duffner UA, Rajasekaran S. Risk factors associated with pediatric intensive care unit admission and mortality after pediatric stem cell transplant: possible role of renal involvement. World J Pediatr. 2013;9(2):140–5. https://doi.org/10.1007/s12519-012-0391-z.
17. Aspesberro F, Guthrie KA, Woolfrey AE, Brogan TV, Roberts JS. Outcome of pediatric hematopoietic stem cell transplant recipients requiring mechanical ventilation. J Intensive Care Med. 2014;29(1):31–7. https://doi.org/10.1177/0885066612457343.
18. Bartram JL, Thein SL, Gardner K, Egberongbe Y, D'Silva P, Height SE, et al. Outcome of children with sickle cell disease admitted to intensive care – a single institution experience. Br J Haematol. 2010;150(5):614–7. https://doi.org/10.1111/j.1365-2141.2010.08272.x.

19. Chima RS, Daniels RC, Kim MO, Li D, Wheeler DS, Davies SM, et al. Improved outcomes for stem cell transplant recipients requiring pediatric intensive care. Pediatric Crit Care Med. 2012;13(6):e336–42. https://doi.org/10.1097/PCC.0b013e318253c945.
20. Duncan CN, Lehmann LE, Cheifetz IM, Greathouse K, Haight AE, Hall MW, et al. Clinical outcomes of children receiving intensive cardiopulmonary support during hematopoietic stem cell transplant. Pediatr Crit Care Med. 2013;14(3):261–7. https://doi.org/10.1097/PCC.0b013e3182720601.
21. Zinter MS, Dvorak CC, Spicer A, Cowan MJ, Sapru A. New insights into multicenter PICU mortality among pediatric hematopoietic stem cell transplant patients. Crit Care Med. 2015;43(9):1986–94. https://doi.org/10.1097/CCM.0000000000001085.
22. Rowan CM, Gertz SJ, McArthur J, Fitzgerald JC, Nitu ME, Loomis A, et al. Invasive mechanical ventilation and mortality in pediatric hematopoietic stem cell transplantation: a multicenter study. Pediatr Crit Care Med. 2016;17(4):294–302. https://doi.org/10.1097/PCC.0000000000000673.

Chapter 2
Diagnosis and Treatment-Related Complications of Acute Leukemia

Lauren Pommert, Steven Margossian, and Michael Burke

Introduction

Acute leukemia remains the most common malignancy in children and accounts for one third of all pediatric cancer diagnoses, with 75% of those being acute lymphoblastic leukemia (ALL) [1]. In the United States, there are approximately 3,100 children and adolescents under 20 years of age who are diagnosed with ALL each year and 750 who are diagnosed with acute myeloid leukemia (AML) [2]. Significant progress has been made in the treatment of pediatric leukemias over the past 70 years with current long-term survival rates above 90% for ALL and 60–70% for AML, compared to virtually 0% survival in the 1950s [3, 4]. This improvement has been attributed to the introduction of prophylactic intrathecal therapy; intensification of multi-agent chemotherapy; refined treatment stratification based on somatic mutations and early treatment response measured by minimal residual disease; introduction of targeted chemotherapeutic agents; and overall advances in supportive care [3, 5]. Most of these developments have been accomplished through randomized clinical trials performed by major international cooperative study groups [3]. Recent research has been directed toward risk stratification and response-based prognostic factors to allow for intensification of treatment for high-risk patients and decreasing acute toxicities and long-term sequelae through targeted novel agents, leukemia signal pathway inhibitors, immunotherapy, and cellular therapy [6].

L. Pommert (✉) · M. Burke
Division of Hematology/Oncology/Blood and Marrow Transplant, Department of Pediatrics, Medical College of Wisconsin and Children's Hospital of Wisconsin, Milwaukee, WI, USA
e-mail: lpommert@mcw.edu

S. Margossian
Harvard Medical School, Department of Pediatric Oncology, Dana Farber Cancer Institute, Boston Children's Hospital, Boston, MA, USA

C. N. Duncan et al. (eds.), *Critical Care of the Pediatric Immunocompromised Hematology/Oncology Patient*, https://doi.org/10.1007/978-3-030-01322-6_2

Despite our advances in treatment and improvements in survival, 2–4% of patients with leukemia still experience treatment-related deaths [7]. These are most often attributable to infections; bleeding or thrombosis; tumor burden complications such as superior vena cava syndrome, hyperleukocytosis, leukostasis, and tumor lysis syndrome; and therapy-induced organ toxicities [7]. Here, we will review some of the most common toxicities and oncologic emergencies associated with the diagnosis and treatment of childhood acute leukemia that may require management in the pediatric intensive care unit (PICU).

Tumor Lysis Syndrome

Tumor lysis syndrome (TLS) is characterized by metabolic abnormalities resulting from the rapid release of intracellular contents from malignant cells into the bloodstream. This process can overwhelm the patient's normal physiologic mechanisms of maintaining homeostasis and result in life-threatening hyperkalemia, hyperuricemia, hyperphosphatemia, hypocalcemia, and/or uremia. Both uric acid and calcium phosphate, when serum levels become high enough, can precipitate in the renal tubules leading to acute renal failure, worsened electrolyte abnormalities, and even death [6, 8]. TLS may occur spontaneously related to high tumor burden and increased cell turnover but is most commonly observed 12–72 h after the initiation of chemotherapy secondary to leukemic cell death and cell lysis [6, 8, 9]. The incidence of TLS in AML is 3.4% compared to 5.2% for ALL [10]. Risk factors for developing TLS in ALL and AML include high presenting white blood cell count (hyperleukocytosis) and pre-existing kidney injury (dehydration, oliguria, anuria, renal insufficiency or failure) [8, 9, 11]. Patients have a higher risk for developing TLS (defined as >5%) when the white blood count (WBC) is >50,000 for AML compared to >100,000 for ALL. Likewise, intermediate risk for developing TLS (1–5%) is seen with a WBC between 10,000–50,000 for AML and 50,000–100,000 in ALL. Patients are at a lower risk for developing TLS (<1%) when WBC is <10,000 in AML and <50,000 in ALL [8, 11].

TLS Classification and Grading

A classification system was previously developed to differentiate clinical tumor lysis syndrome (CTLS) and laboratory tumor lysis syndrome (LTLS) to help identify which patients may require immediate therapeutic intervention [3]. LTLS is present if patients have either serum levels above the high end of normal or a 25% change from baseline in two or more of the following lab values: uric acid, potassium, phosphate, and calcium within 3 days before or 7 days after starting chemotherapy. CTLS is defined by the presence of LTLS plus one or more of the three most significant clinical complications associated with TLS: renal insufficiency, cardiac arrhythmias/sudden death, and/or seizures. Clinical signs of TLS may include nausea, vomiting, lethargy, edema, fluid overload, cardiac dysrhythmias, seizures, muscle cramps, tetany, syncope, altered mental status, and/or death secondary to electrolyte abnormalities [6, 8, 9]. At diagnosis and during induction or re-induction chemotherapy, while patients are at greatest risk of developing TLS, vigilant electrolyte monitoring of serum uric acid, phosphate, potassium, creatinine, calcium, and lactate dehydrogenase (LDH) should be performed in addition to strict fluid management and monitoring total fluid input and urine output. Laboratory evaluations for TLS should begin every 4–6 h or more frequently based on the clinical condition and/or laboratory results in patients at risk for this oncologic complication [8, 11].

TLS Management

Aggressive hydration and diuresis are the main treatments of TLS to improve a patient's intravascular volume, maintain renal perfusion, and increase urinary flow. This enhances glomerular filtration and urinary excretion of uric acid and phosphate with the goal to decrease crystal formation [6, 8, 9]. Patients should receive 2–4 times of their daily fluid maintenance (3 L/m^2/d or 200 mL/kg/d if <10 kg) without the addition of potassium, calcium, or phosphate. Urine output should be maintained at >100 mL/m^2/h (>3 mL/kg/h if <10 kg) with a urine-specific gravity <1.010 [6, 9]. Diuretics may be required to maintain adequate urine output but are contraindicated in patients with hypovolemia or obstructive uropathy [8]. Although urine alkalinization was historically part of TLS management, it is no longer recommended as it can lead to metabolic alkalosis and worsen obstructive uropathies during the treatment of hyperuricemia [8, 9]. Below we will discuss each of the electrolyte derangements and treatment strategies which are also summarized in Table 2.1.

Hyperuricemia

After the release of intracellular nucleic acids into the bloodstream, adenine and guanine are metabolized to xanthine, which is then broken down to uric acid by the enzyme xanthine oxidase which results in hyperuricemia [12]. Hyperuricemia is defined as serum uric acid >476 µmol/L or 8 mg/dL [8, 9]. In the presence of an acidic urine, uric acid can crystallize in the renal tubules causing obstruction, which can lead to acute obstructive neuropathy and renal dysfunction [9].

There are multiple medications available for treatment of hyperuricemia in addition to aggressive IV hydration to help improve renal excretion. The most commonly used medication, allopurinol, inhibits xanthine oxidase and prevents formation of new uric acid; however it does not reduce elevated levels of pre-existing

Table 2.1 Electrolyte derangements associated with TLS and their management

Fluid management		Aggressive IV hydration (without K^+, phosphate or Ca^{+2}) at 2–4x maintenance rate (3 L/m²/d or 200 mL/kg/d if ≤10 kg)
		Maintain urine output at ≥100 mL/m²/h. (≥3 mL/kg/h if ≤10 kg) with a urine specific gravity ≤1.010
		Diuretics can be used to maintain urine output (furosemide 0.5–1.0 mg/kg) but are contraindicated in patients with hypovolemia or obstructive uropathy
Electrolyte abnormalities		Monitor serum uric acid, phosphate, potassium, creatinine, calcium, and LDH every 4–6 h
Hyperuricemia	≥476 μmol/L or 8 mg/dL or 25% increase from baseline	Allopurinol: 50–100 mg/m²/dose PO every 8 h – maximum 300 mg/m²/d or 10 mg/kg/d divided every 8 h – maximum dose 800 mg/d. Can be given IV 200–400 mg/m²/day IV in 1–3 divided doses – maximum 600 mg/d
		Urate oxidase (rasburicase): 0.2 mg/kg IV daily to BID
Hyperkalemia	>6.0 mmol/L or > 6.0 mg/L or 25% increase from baseline	Asymptomatic: sodium polystyrene sulfonate (1 g/kg with 50% sorbitol)
		Symptomatic: insulin (0.1 units/kg IV) and glucose infusion (25% dextrose 2 mL/kg) or sodium bicarbonate (1 to 2 mEq/kg IV push)
		Arrhythmias: calcium gluconate (100 to 200 mg/kg/dose) by slow IV infusion (not through the same line as sodium bicarbonate due to the risk of precipitation)
		Dialysis if severe
Hyperphosphatemia	>2.1 mmol/L or 25% increase from baseline	Phosphate binders such as aluminum hydroxide (50–150 mg/kg/day PO or NG q6hr)
		Dialysis if severe
Hypocalcemia	≤1.75 mmol/L or 25% decrease from baseline	Symptomatic: calcium gluconate 50–100 mg/kg IV
Dialysis		Renal dysfunction
		Volume overload
		Persistent electrolyte derangements which do not respond to medical management
		Acidosis
		Uremia

uric acid [8, 9, 13]. Dosing for allopurinol ranges 50–100 mg/m²/dose PO every 8 h (maximum 300 mg/m²/d) or 10 mg/kg/d divided every 8 h (maximum dose 800 mg/d). In addition, allopurinol can be given 200–400 mg/m²/day IV in one to three divided doses (maximum 600 mg/d) [8, 9]. When used prophylactically in pediatric patients with a variety of cancers including acute leukemia at high risk for developing TLS, it prevented hyperuricemia in 92% of patients [14]. Allopurinol can be started prophylactically 12–24 h prior to the start of chemotherapy and continued for 3–7 days or until uric acid levels and other TLS labs have normalized and risk for ongoing TLS has decreased [8]. Limitations to the use of allopurinol include its inability to break down preformed uric acid; the associated increase in levels of xanthine and hypoxanthine, both of which have lower solubility in urine and can precipitate in the renal tubules; its interference with renal clearance of other purine chemotherapies (i.e., 6-mercaptopurine); and its renal excretion which requires a dose reduction in patients with renal failure [8, 9, 15, 16].

In patients with acute leukemia found to have hyperuricemia at diagnosis, treatment with recombinant urate oxidase (rasburicase) is indicated and allows for rapid breakdown of the pre-existing uric acid to allantoin which is renally excreted without precipitation [9, 15, 17]. Rasburicase (0.2 mg/kg) is administered IV once daily in 50 mL normal saline over 30 min and can be repeated daily or twice daily as needed. Clinical judgment should be used for duration of therapy based on response and subsequent uric acid levels [6, 8, 16]. Once rasburicase is given, blood samples to measure uric acid levels should be immediately placed on ice and run within 4 h of collection [8].

Rasburicase is more potent and faster-acting than allopurinol [16, 17]. Goldman et al. [16] performed a randomized study in children with acute leukemia and lymphoma comparing oral allopurinol to IV rasburicase which found that 4 h after the first dose, patients randomized to rasburicase had an 86% decrease in uric acid levels compared to a 12% decrease in the allopurinol group ($p < 0.0001$). In a retrospective review by Cairo et al. [13] comparing pediatric and adult patients with TLS treated with either allopurinol or rasburicase, the rasburicase group had more effective treatment of their hyperuricemia which was associated with significantly shorter ICU stays, overall hospital stays, and lower total inpatient costs. Rasburicase is contraindicated in patients with G6PD deficiency which can result in a hemolytic crisis when given.

Hyperkalemia

Hyperkalemia is defined as a serum potassium >6.0 mmol/L and results from massive cellular degradation and release of intracellular potassium [9]. Supplemental oral and IV potassium should be eliminated in patients at risk for TLS, and continuous cardiac monitoring should be used for patients who develop hyperkalemia. Immediate intervention may be required if levels are greater than 7.0–7.5 mmol/L or there is ECG evidence of widening QRS complexes or peaked T waves. Asymptomatic patients can be treated with sodium polystyrene sulfonate (1 g/kg with 50% sorbitol). Symptomatic patients can be treated with rapid-acting insulin (0.1 units/kg IV) and glucose infusion (25% dextrose 2 mL/kg) or sodium bicarbonate (1–2 mEq/kg IV push) to induce the influx of potassium into the cells. In patients with arrhythmias, calcium gluconate (100–200 mg/kg/dose) by slow IV infusion can be given, but not through the same line as sodium bicarbonate due to the risk of precipitation [6, 8, 11].

Hyperphosphatemia

Hyperphosphatemia secondary to release of intracellular phosphate can result in tissue precipitation after binding to calcium (calcium phosphate) which can lead to hypocalcemia, acute obstructive uropathy, and renal failure. Phosphorus levels >2.1 mmol/L should be treated with aggressive hydration and phosphate binders such as aluminum hydroxide 50–150 mg/kg/day enterally given every 6 h. If hyperphosphatemia is severe, patients should receive hemodialysis or continuous veno-venous hemofiltration (CVVH) [6, 8, 11].

Hypocalcemia

Hypocalcemia occurs due to precipitation of calcium with phosphate in the setting of hyperphosphatemia and is defined as serum calcium <1.75 mmol/L [8, 9]. In general, treatment of asymptomatic hypocalcemia is not recommended due to the risk of increased precipitation with phosphate and worsening acute kidney injury. Typically, the hypocalcemia resolves without treatment as TLS improves. For patients who have symptomatic hypocalcemia causing muscular, cardiovascular, or neurologic complications, calcium gluconate (50–100 mg/kg IV) can be used for treatment; however, this will increase the risk of calcium phosphate precipitation and acute kidney injury such that the risks/benefits should be weighed for each patient [8, 9].

Indications for Dialysis

Although rasburicase has dramatically decreased the need for dialysis in patients with moderate/severe TLS, about 1.5% of pediatric patients still require this for renal insufficiency, volume overload, acidosis, persistent electrolyte derangements, and/or uremia which are not responsive to medical management [6, 9, 15]. Hemodialysis is the preferred modality for rapid clearance of potassium and uric acid in the setting of life-threatening hyperkalemia or hyperuricemia [9, 12, 18]. Otherwise, continuous renal replacement (CRRT) (such as continuous veno-venous hemodialysis (CVVHD), CVVH, continuous arteriovenous hemofiltration (CAVHD), or continuous arteriovenous hemodialysis (CAVHD)) is preferred at high dialysate flow rates (3–4 L/h) to decrease the rate of rebound hyperkalemia and hyperphosphatemia [12, 18, 19]. CRRT is the preferred modality for hyperphosphatemia because clearance is time dependent [12, 19]. Peritoneal dialysis is generally not recommended in children with TLS due to its poor uric acid clearance [9, 12].

Hyperleukocytosis and Leukostasis

Hyperleukocytosis is defined as a WBC count greater than $100,000/mm^3$ [20]. Symptoms and complications from hyperleukocytosis are secondary to leukostasis which is the accumulation of peripheral leukemic blasts in the vasculature resulting in increased blood viscosity, microvascular obstruction, and/or tissue hypoxia [20–22]. Interactions between blasts and endothelial cells which result in the secretion of cytokines and adhesion receptors are also thought to play a role in further blast recruitment and endothelial damage leading to leukostasis [20, 22, 23]. Although hyperleukocytosis is more common in ALL than AML, hyperviscosity and leukostasis occur at lower WBC counts in patients with AML (100,000/μL compared to >400,000/μL in ALL) resulting in higher rates of clinical symptoms and early death (9–16% for AML compared to 2–6% in ALL) [20–25]. This difference is likely secondary to the larger mean cell volume of myeloblasts (particularly FAB subtypes M4 and M5) which are twice as large as lymphoblasts and therefore cause a higher fractional volume of leukocytes and increased viscosity at a lower total WBC count [20, 22, 23]. For patients with AML, the following features have been associated with hyperleukocytosis: infants less than 1 year of age; FAB subtypes M1, M4, or M5; chromosomal rearrangements in 11q23; inversion chromosome 16; or having FLT3-ITD [20, 25]. For ALL, patients are at greater risk of developing hyperleukocytosis if they have infant ALL, T-cell ALL with a mediastinal mass, or if their leukemias have chromosomal rearrangements involving 11q23 or translocations of t(4:11), t(1:19), and t(9:22) or loss of p16 [20, 22].

The higher rates of early morbidity and mortality seen in patients with hyperleukocytosis are attributed to intraparenchymal brain hemorrhage, pulmonary leukostasis syndrome (defined as infiltrates on chest x-ray, tachypnea, and hypoxia), severe TLS, and/or disseminated intravascular coagulopathy (DIC) [20–22]. Due to this risk of early mortality, children presenting with WBC counts over 100,000/μL should be evaluated for symptoms of hyperleukocytosis and leukostasis including respiratory distress, hypoxemia, diffuse interstitial or alveolar infiltrates, altered mental status, headache, dizziness, visual field changes, seizures, signs of right ventricular overload, myocardial ischemia, priapism, acute limb ischemia, bowel infarctions, and renal vein thrombosis [20, 22].

Treatment of hyperleukocytosis focuses on aggressive hyperhydration (2–4 times maintenance fluids), treatment of any underlying TLS, and prompt cytoreduction of the leukemia which can be achieved with leukapheresis, hydroxyurea, and/or induction chemotherapy [6, 20, 22, 23, 25]. One particular problem in hyperleukocytosis is that if the WBC count is not reduced prior to the start of induction chemotherapy, leukostasis, TLS, and DIC can be further worsened with treatment [22]. In this setting, hydroxyurea can be very efficient in reducing the WBC count, often by 50–80% within 24–48 hours, and can be given orally at doses of 50–100 mg/kg/day [20]. Leukapheresis can be a life-saving procedure in which WBCs are rapidly removed from the peripheral circulation and plasma, while the

RBCs and platelets are returned to the patient through a closed-circuit cell apheresis [22, 23]. The main indication for this is evidence of leukostasis-related complications [22]. The use of leukapheresis in asymptomatic hyperleukocytosis is controversial, and there has been no general consensus regarding its prophylactic use for the prevention of leukostasis in pediatric leukemia. Additionally, leukapheresis is not recommended for treatment of patients with acute promyelocytic leukemia (APL) due to its association with worsening of the coagulopathy and increased risk of death [6, 23].

To date, there have been no randomized trials evaluating the benefits of leukapheresis, and there are currently no guidelines for when or how long to use it once it has been initiated in pediatrics [20, 23]. One study that examined the early complications in hyperleukocytosis and leukapheresis in patients with pediatric leukemia demonstrated that leukapheresis resulted in an average WBC count reduction of 53%, and there was no significant difference in responses to induction treatment in patients who underwent leukapheresis compared to those who did not [23]. Another recent Children's Oncology Group (COG) study of patients with AML demonstrated that leukapheresis did not reduce induction mortality [25]. Potential disadvantages of leukapheresis include requiring placement of a large bore central venous catheter which may require anesthesia and can predispose patients to bleeding or thrombosis at the catheter site; limited availability for apheresis at the pediatric center; patient blood loss; fragmentation of the WBCs leading to possible DIC and early death; requiring citrate as the anticoagulant in the apheresis circuit which can lead to hypocalcemia; and/or the potential delay of induction chemotherapy while awaiting apheresis [20, 23]. Additionally, packed red blood cell (PRBC) transfusions and high hemoglobin concentrations in patients with hyperleukocytosis can result in increased blood viscosity and have been associated with worsening leukostasis and increased morbidity and mortality [6, 20–23, 25]. Therefore, PRBCs should be transfused cautiously, and only after treatment for hyperleukocytosis is initiated as long as the patient is hemodynamically stable. Because severe thrombocytopenia is a known risk factor for central nervous system (CNS) hemorrhage in patients with hyperleukocytosis [26] and platelets do not significantly add to blood viscosity [6], platelets should be transfused liberally for the treatment of thrombocytopenia [25] to maintain a platelet goal of >50,000 in the setting of hyperleukocytosis.

Mediastinal Masses and Superior Vena Cava Syndrome

Anterior mediastinal masses are characteristic of T-cell ALL and estimated to occur in 53–64% of newly diagnosed pediatric patients [27]. These masses, caused by thymic enlargement, can result in compression of the trachea and/or mediastinal vessels and heart, leading to superior vena cava syndrome (SVCS) and cardiorespiratory compromise [27, 28]. The superior vena cava carries blood from the head, arms, and upper torso to the heart, supplying one third of the body's venous return [29]. Compression of this vessel can cause increased venous pressure in the upper body resulting in edema of the head, neck, and arms, often with cyanosis, plethora, and distended superficial vessels leading to thrombosis, cerebral edema, and/or hemodynamic instability secondary to decreased venous return [29]. As the trachea and the right mainstem bronchus are more compressible in children, especially in infants and toddlers compared to adults, respiratory symptoms can be more pronounced [29]. Common clinical signs of a mediastinal mass include shortness of breath, cough, stridor, respiratory distress, orthopnea, dyspnea, chest pain, syncope, hoarseness, and dysphagia, all of which may be worsened by the supine position [30–33].

As part of the work-up for newly diagnosed patients with acute leukemia, posterior-anterior and lateral chest x-rays should be performed to evaluate for the presence of a mediastinal mass. In patients who are found to have mediastinal widening or cardiorespiratory symptoms, chest computed tomography (CT) with contrast and echocardiogram can be performed (as long as the patient is clinically stable) in order to assess the severity of cardiopulmonary compression (Fig. 2.1) [28, 30]. The CT can be performed in the prone position if the supine position exacerbates symptoms [6]. Anterior mediastinal masses can be due to other malignancies as well including Hodgkin and non-Hodgkin lymphoma and less frequently neuroblastoma, germ cell tumors, or other sarcomas [2].

Children with anterior mediastinal masses may be at significant risk of life-threatening complications from general anesthesia, including death from airway obstruction and cardiovascular collapse which is estimated to occur in 15% of cases [30, 34, 35]. This is primarily due to direct airway compression, decreased lung volumes and compliance, loss of normal bronchial smooth muscle tone, and loss of normal negative pressure on the trachea with inspiration. In addition, there is the

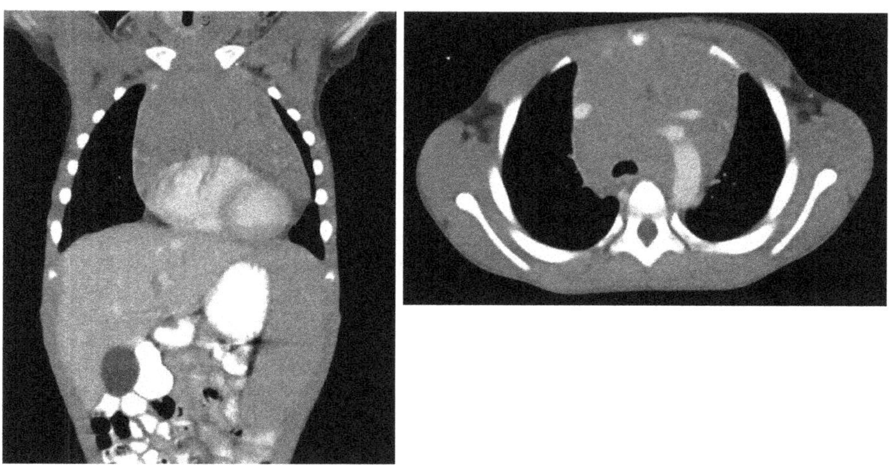

Fig. 2.1 CT images of patient with T-cell ALL demonstrate a large anterior mediastinal mass measuring approximately 8.8 cm × 3.3 cm and causing narrowing and mass effect on the SVC, brachiocephalic veins, and trachea

potential for cardiac compression, decreased venous return, and decreased cardiac output [28, 34, 36]. Conscious sedation and anti-anxiolytics may also be contraindicated as they can decrease respiratory drive and dilate peripheral vessels which can lead to decreased venous return [6]. Children are at greater risk of anesthetic complications if their mediastinal mass is >45% of the chest diameter; they have orthopnea or acute respiratory distress, have compression of the mainstem bronchus, and/or have a tracheal cross-sectional area <50% predicted or evidence of SVCS [28, 31, 33, 34]. Management of airway collapse in these patients can be extremely difficult as masses at or below the level of the carina may cause an inability to ventilate or oxygenate despite endotracheal intubation [28]. Recommendations for children with mediastinal masses who are undergoing general anesthesia include maintenance of spontaneous ventilation, avoidance of muscle relaxants, immediate availability of airway manipulation tools (reinforced tracheal tubes, mainstem bronchus intubation, rigid bronchoscopy), and the availability of heliox and cardiopulmonary bypass [31]. Arterial extracorporeal membrane oxygenation (ECMO) has been successfully used to support a patient through diagnosis and treatment of their mediastinal mass [37].

Management of SVCS and airway compression caused by a leukemic mediastinal mass involves treatment of the underlying malignancy with chemotherapy which results in the mass rapidly shrinking over a period of days to weeks [29, 33, 34]. Intravenous corticosteroids (methylprednisolone or dexamethasone 1 mg/kg every 6 hours) should be given empirically to patients who have respiratory or cardiovascular compromise [32, 33, 36]. In addition, tumor lysis syndrome precautions should be initiated when steroid treatment is started [6]. Supportive care management includes elevation of the head of the bed to decrease hydrostatic pressure, supplemental oxygen, and anticoagulation for any thrombosis-related SVC obstruction [32].

CNS Emergencies

Patients with acute leukemia may be at increased risk for CNS complications either from the leukemia itself or the therapy required to treat it. These can range from arterial/venous thrombosis, intracranial hemorrhage (ICH), CNS leukemia (often in the setting of hyperleukocytosis), chemotherapy-related toxicities effecting the CNS, cranial irradiation, and leukemia-associated coagulopathies or infection [6].

In regard to ICH, patients at greatest risk include those with acute promyelocytic leukemia (APL) as a result of the significant coagulopathy associated with this form of AML and patients with hyperleukocytosis (WBC >400,000 × 10^9/L in ALL [21]; WBC >100,000 × 10^9/L in AML [20]), secondary to hyperviscosity and subsequent leukostasis [6, 38]. Patients with ICH typically present with altered mental status, acute motor and/or speech impairments, headache, vomiting, and/or seizures [6]. Treatment in both of these cases is primarily supportive with platelets and plasma to correct the coagulopathy and minimize further bleeding with the potential for leukapheresis to decrease blood viscosity in cases of hyperleukocytosis [6]. In cases where the CNS event escalates to increased intracranial pressure and the risk of herniation exists, emergent neurosurgical intervention may be necessary.

Systemic and intrathecal chemotherapy as well as CNS irradiation can result in arterial ischemic strokes and/or venous thromboembolism [6]. Venous thromboembolism can be relatively common in patients with acute leukemia and is discussed in further detail in the thrombosis section of this chapter. In patients who experience an arterial ischemic stroke, treatment is often supportive and aimed at maximizing cerebral perfusion. Typically, patients are maintained in the supine position for 48 hours and kept normothermic, normoglycemic, and normotensive or minimally hypertensive with adequate circulating blood volumes to minimize morbidities and potential mortality [6]. Data supporting the safety and efficacy of thrombolytic therapy in pediatric patients with arterial thrombosis is lacking and therefore has not been routinely recommended.

Methotrexate, an antimetabolite which inhibits folate synthesis, is associated with a 3–15% incidence of neurotoxicity in patients with leukemia which includes subacute leukoencephalopathy [38]. The mechanism is thought to be disruption of CNS folate homeostasis and/or direct neuronal damage from the cytotoxic agents [39]. Patients can present with transient stroke-like hemiparesis and/or weakness, encephalopathy, seizures, aphasia, and emotional liability that can wax and wane and typically develops 2–14 days after receiving methotrexate either intravenously or intrathecally [38, 39]. If MRI of the brain is performed, it typically demonstrates characteristic white matter hyperintensities on T2-weighted and fluid-attenuated inversion recovery consistent with cytotoxic edema in the white matter tracts [38, 39]. The CSF is typically normal, and electroencephalogram (EEG), when performed, shows nonspecific diffuse or focal slowing [38]. Most neurologic symptoms will resolve within 7 days including MRI findings returning to normal. Additionally, patients typically will tolerate subsequent methotrexate treatment without recurrence of similar CNS symptoms [38, 39].

Cytarabine, a pyrimidine nucleoside analogue, commonly given in high systemic doses or intrathecally for patients with AML, can also cause an acute encephalopathy characterized by cerebellar dysfunction with dysarthria, nystagmus, gait ataxia, confusion, and/or somnolence 2–5 days after treatment. MRI of the brain may demonstrate white matter changes in the cerebellum, and CSF studies are typically normal [38]. Symptoms tend to improve over the course of weeks; however, complete resolution of symptoms is seen in only 30% of patients, and further cytarabine treatment is often excluded [38]. Intrathecal chemotherapy, in general, can cause an aseptic meningitis or chemical arachnoiditis which affects up to 10% of patients with leukemia. Patients typically present with headache, meningismus, nausea, vomiting, fever, and/or altered mental status where the CSF analysis shows a pleocytosis with negative cultures. Clinical care is again predominantly supportive, and patients can typically go on to receive further intrathecal chemotherapy without additional complications [38].

Nelarabine, a purine analogue used in the treatment of T-cell ALL, has been associated with acute neurotoxicity characterized by Guillain-Barre-like demyelinating ascending neuropathy which occurred in 1.3% of pediatric patients during the early phase trials [40–42]. When this occurs, care is supportive, and symptoms generally seem to be reversible after discontinuation of this medication; however, reports of death do exist [40].

Posterior reversible encephalopathy (PRES) can also be seen in patients undergoing leukemia treatment. This reversible neurologic complication is characterized by headache, altered mental status, seizure, vision changes, and brain MRI white matter changes in the bilateral parieto-occipital lobes [38, 43, 44]. The underlying mechanism is not fully understood but is proposed to be related to sudden elevations in blood pressure and medication-induced vascular endothelial damage resulting in capillary leakage and vasogenic edema [38, 43]. Patients are at greater risk of PRES if they have hypertension and renal impairment or are on specific immunosuppressive medications such as calcineurin inhibitors in patients treated with hematopoietic cell transplantation [38, 43]. This complication occurs most commonly during induction therapy where high-dose steroids are given but has been associated with other chemotherapeutic medications including vincristine, intrathecal methotrexate, cytarabine, and asparaginase [38, 43]. This condition is reversible when recognized promptly and is highly treatable with antihypertensive and antiepileptic medications [38, 43]. In most cases, PRES resolves in about 48 hours with the brain MRI findings resolving over 3–6 months [44].

Other causes for seizures in patient with leukemia which have not already been discussed include electrolyte disturbances (e.g., hyponatremia secondary to vincristine-induced SIADH), CNS leukemia, and primary CNS infections. The evaluation of patients presenting with seizures should include at a minimum, a CBC, electrolyte, creatinine, BUN, hepatic function panel, and coagulation profile in addition to CNS imaging and an EEG once the patient has been stabilized. Electrolyte derangements should be corrected, anticonvulsant therapy should be used, and antibiotics and antifungal medications are indicated in patients with fevers and meningeal signs and those in whom infection is a concern [6].

Spinal cord compression secondary to epidural involvement of leukemia (most often with chloromas) is a very rare presentation of acute leukemia or relapsed disease and is more commonly seen in patients with AML; however, case reports in ALL exist [45–47]. Spinal hematomas resulting in cord compression can be a complication of lumbar punctures, particularly in patients who have profound thrombocytopenia and/or coagulopathy [48]. Symptoms of spinal cord compression can include back pain, extremity weakness, sensory abnormalities, paralysis, and urinary or fecal incontinence/retention [6]. Early symptom recognition is critical and essential to achieve better outcomes of spinal cord compression-related symptoms [46]. MRI of the spine remains the gold standard for diagnosis [6]. Initial treatment includes dexamethasone to decrease vasogenic cord edema (pediatric dosing of 1–2 mg/kg followed by 0.25–0.5 mg/kg every 6 hours has been suggested) followed by chemotherapy, radiation, and/or surgery to reduce or remove the mass [6, 45, 46].

Thrombosis

Venous thrombosis (VT) can be a relatively common complication of treatment in children with acute leukemia. A meta-analysis of 1,752 pediatric patients with acute leukemia from 17 prospective trials demonstrated an incidence of 5.2% for symptomatic thrombosis [49]. Risk factors for thrombosis include the underlying leukemia burden, presence of central venous catheters (CVL), chemotherapy-induced coagulation defects, and/or pro-thrombotic hereditary risk factors [49, 50]. The most common sites of thrombosis include central venous catheters (usually in the upper extremities) and the cerebral venous sinuses [49, 51]. Line-associated thromboses typically present with upper extremity pain or swelling and CVL dysfunction, whereas sinus venous thromboses present with headache, seizure, and/or acute neurologic changes [50]. The risk for thrombosis development is greatest during induction therapy for ALL when patients have their highest leukemia burden while undergoing cytolysis from the chemotherapy which includes asparaginase and glucocorticoids, both known to raise the risk VT [49, 51]. Glucocorticoids increase pro-clotting factor VIII and von Willebrand factor and decrease plasminogen and alpha-2 plasmin, both of which have fibrinolytic effects [52]. Asparaginase depletes several hemostatic proteins including plasminogen, antithrombin, and fibrinogen which increase the risk of thrombosis [53]. Reexposure to asparaginase is feasible and safe in patients who have previously developed an asparaginase-associated VT and is typically given in conjunction with anticoagulation once the previous thrombosis has resolved [50, 51].

The pediatric CHEST guidelines suggest that anticoagulation for thrombosis should be with either (1) low-molecular-weight heparin (LMWH) or (2) unfractionated heparin (UFH) followed by LMWH for a minimum of 3 months until the precipitating factor has resolved (e.g., use of asparaginase) [54]. But therapy must be tailored to the individual patient. Therapeutic LMWH heparin is typically started at 1 mg/kg/dose every 12 h and should be monitored to target anti-Xa activity (range, 0.5–1.0 units/mL) in a serum sample taken 4–6 hours after subcutaneous injection (>3rd dose) [54]. As the mechanism of heparin anticoagulation involves antithrombin III (AT), some centers periodically monitor AT levels during anticoagulation and replete when levels fall below 50–75% [2]. Thrombolysis therapy should be used only for life- or limb-threatening thrombosis [54]. Because a CVL generally remains in place in these patients, prophylactic LMWH anticoagulation is often continued until the line is removed; however, the risk-benefit ratio for treatment of VT should be evaluated on an individual basis in this complex patient population [54]. The risk of bleeding complications in pediatric patients with leukemia on anticoagulation is relatively low at 2%, and thus often the benefit of preventing further thrombosis may outweigh the potential risk of bleeding [49].

Typhlitis

Typhlitis, also known as neutropenic enterocolitis, is an important gastrointestinal complication observed in patients with acute leukemia characterized by abdominal pain, fever, and neutropenia [6, 55, 56]. Abdominal distension, diarrhea, nausea, vomiting, and GI bleeding can also occur, and symptoms typically improve rapidly upon neutrophil recovery [6, 55, 57, 58]. The incidence is estimated to be ~10% in pediatric patients with leukemia and is seen more frequently in patients with AML compared to those with ALL. It is important to note that typhlitis is associated with a 5–20% mortality rate, most often from sepsis [55–57, 59].

The pathogenesis of typhlitis is thought to be multifactorial. The most common associations include chemotherapy, underlying immunosuppression, mucositis, impaired vascular blood flow to the intestines, and/or bacterial overgrowth and translocation leading to bowel wall edema, mucosal ulceration, and necrosis. This pathology most often affects the cecum and transverse colon, although other areas of the colon and the rectum can be involved [6, 55–57]. Symptoms can be diagnosed clinically or by imaging with abdominal CT or ultrasound which can demonstrate bowel wall edema and, in advanced stages, pneumatosis and/or abdominal free air [6, 56]. Bacteremia and sepsis are common complications of typhlitis with the most likely causative organisms being *Pseudomonas* species, *Escherichia coli*, *Clostridium* species, *Staphylococcus* species, *Streptococcus* species, and *Enterococcus* species [6]. Fungal pathogens as the causative organism in typhlitis, including *Candida* and *Aspergillus* species, are less common but have been reported [6].

Overall outcomes for typhlitis tend to be good with conservative medical management alone which includes bowel rest, parenteral nutrition, abdominal decompression, and broad-spectrum antibiotics to cover gram-negative organisms, anaerobes, and fungi, with the occasional use of granulocyte colony-stimulating factor (G-CSF) to improve neutrophil recovery [6, 55–58]. Surgical intervention is required in 4–8% of cases due to clinical deterioration despite conservative management, the presence of bowel necrosis, complete bowel obstruction, intestinal perforation, and/or abdominal abscess requiring drainage [6, 56, 58, 60].

A retrospective chart review of a large pediatric center in the United Kingdom identified 40 oncology patients who developed typhlitis during a 5-year period, 67% of whom had a diagnosis of acute leukemia [56]. One hundred percent of these patients presented with abdominal pain, and 78% presented with the typical triad of fever, abdominal pain, and neutropenia. Thirty-seven patients (92.5%) were treated with conservative medical management, and three patients required surgery (bowel necrosis ($n = 1$) and bowel perforation ($n = 2$)). One child died within 24 h of the diagnosis of typhlitis in the conservatively treated group due to *Pseudomonas aeruginosa* septicemia. A second retrospective chart review of children with acute leukemia over a 3-year period at a single pediatric institution identified a 4.5% incidence of typhlitis (10 patients) in patients who were admitted with neutropenic fever, 7.4% of patients with ALL, and 28.5% of patients with AML [57]. Again, 100% of patients presented with abdominal pain and 90% had fever and nausea. The median duration of symptoms was 6 days (range, 2–11 days), and median period of neutropenia was 14 days (range, 3–25 days). All patients in this cohort were treated conservatively with medical management. Three patients developed bacteremia with *Candida* species (1), *E. coli* (1), and *viridans* group strep (1), and two died of sepsis with multi-organ failure. Overall, typhlitis in a child with acute leukemia can be successfully treated with conservative management; however, early diagnosis and treatment remain critical to mitigate potential mortality.

Pancreatitis

Between 2 and 18% of patients treated with asparaginase, an essential chemotherapeutic agent in the treatment of ALL, develop acute pancreatitis, which is a cause of substantial morbidity [6, 61–64]. Asparaginase, available in three commercial formulations (native *E. coli* L-asparaginase, pegylated-asparaginase, and *Erwinia* L-asparaginase), works by reducing plasma concentrations of asparagine by metabolizing it into aspartic acid and ammonia. This asparagine depletion results in the deprivation of this amino acid in the leukemic blasts resulting in cell death [61, 63]. The use of asparaginase in multi-agent chemotherapy regimens has improved survival in ALL, and early discontinuation of this therapy, most commonly the result of hypersensitivity or pancreatitis, has been associated with inferior outcomes [63, 65, 66].

Pancreatitis typically occurs within 2 weeks of asparaginase exposure where patients present with a constellation of symptoms that can include abdominal pain, nausea, vomiting, fever, back pain, hypotension, elevated serum amylase and lipase (at least three times the upper limit of normal), and/or characteristic findings of pancreatitis on abdominal imaging [62, 64]. In severe cases, acute pancreatitis can lead to a systemic inflammatory response (SIRS) resulting in pancreatic hemorrhage, necrosis, intestinal perforation, and/or sepsis and carries a 2% overall mortality rate [62]. Late complications of asparaginase-associated pancreatitis include the development of pancreatic pseudocysts, insulin-dependent diabetes, and chronic/relapsing pancreatitis or abdominal pain [62, 64]. Treatment of acute pancreatitis is predominantly supportive management with fluid resuscitation, broad-spectrum antibiotics to cover gram-negative and anaerobic organisms (at least until an infection can be ruled out), complete bowel rest, parenteral nutrition, IV narcotics for pain control, and close clinical monitoring for further complications [6, 64]. Fortunately, most cases of asparaginase-associated pancreatitis are self-limited and can be treated medically; however, surgical drainage of pancreatic abscesses, pseudocyst, or necrotizing pancreatitis may be required based on the patient's clinical course, presence of obstruction, and/or severe abdominal pain [6]. Further treatment with asparaginase should be discontinued in cases of severe grade 3–4 pancreatitis, as there is an almost 50% risk of subsequent pancreatitis with asparaginase reexposure [62, 64].

Acute Promyelocytic Leukemia and Differentiation Syndrome

Acute promyelocytic leukemia (APL) is a subtype of AML occurring in 5–10% of children with de novo AML, characterized by a block in differentiation at the promyelocytic stage of hematopoiesis caused by a reciprocal translocation between the promyelocytic (PML) gene on chromosome 15 and the retinoic receptor α (RAR-α) gene on chromosome 17 [67, 68]. APL is considered a medical emergency and, in pediatrics, can be associated with a 7.4% risk of death during induction therapy due to profound disseminated intravascular coagulopathy (DIC) and differentiation syndrome [67, 69–71]. Treatment for the coagulopathy is early initiation of chemotherapy and aggressive replacement of coagulation factors with fresh frozen plasma, fibrinogen, and/or cryoprecipitate in addition to platelet transfusions to maintain fibrinogen concentration above 100–150 mg/dL, platelets above >50 × 10^9/L, and PT/PTT near-normal range [68–70]. Leukapheresis must be avoided in this patient population due to increased risk of fatal hemorrhage secondary to the overwhelming release of anticoagulant factors from leukemic cells during the pheresis procedure [69].

All-trans retinoic acid (ATRA) and arsenic (ATO) therapy have become the standard of care in standard-risk APL patients to differentiate the leukemic promyelocytes into mature granulocytes [68, 70]. In high-risk patients, ATRA in combination with anthracycline-based chemotherapy has led to significantly improved outcomes for this disease with 10-year overall survival of 89% and event-free survival of 76% [72]. ATRA should be started at the first suspicion of APL at a pediatric dose of 25 mg/m^2 divided twice a day [68, 72].

Differentiation syndrome (DS), formerly known as retinoic acid syndrome, is a relatively common and serious complication occurring in 10–20% of pediatric patients with APL who are receiving induction therapy with ATRA and/or ATO and is associated with a 4% risk of death [70]. It is clinically characterized by unexplained fever, weight gain, peripheral edema, dyspnea with interstitial pulmonary infiltrates, pleuro-pericardial effusions, hypotension, and/or renal failure [6, 69, 70, 73]. These symptoms can occur at any time within days to weeks of starting ATRA or ATO, with most frequent occurrences in the first and third weeks of treatment [73]. Patients with a WBC >10,000/μL (considered high risk) are at increased risk of this complication [68, 73]. The pathogenesis of DS is not fully understood but is thought that ATRA/ATO therapy may lead to a systemic inflammatory response syndrome (SIRS), endothelial damage with capillary leak and occlusion of the microcirculation, and tissue infiltration, resulting in the DS phenotype [73]. At the earliest clinical suspicion of DS, dexamethasone 0.5–1 mg/kg (max 10 mg per dose) IV every 12 h should be started to help mitigate the syndrome [69]. ATRA, ATO, and other chemotherapy should only be stopped if symptoms are life-threatening and should be resumed when symptoms resolve [69, 73]. Prophylactic use of steroids in patients with APL and an elevated WBC count has been associated with decreased morbidity from DS in adults with APL, but due to a lack of data in pediatrics, this practice remains controversial in children [6, 70].

Conclusion

Due to large collaborative and international randomized clinical trials conducted by the COG and other pediatric consortia over the past 50 years, survival rates of children with acute leukemia have significantly improved. However, these patients continue to suffer from disease-related and treatment-related complications associated with a 2–4% death rate, often requiring ICU management. To further decrease these toxicities and risk of death, research has been aimed at identifying potential genetic risk factors and certain phenotypic patient subsets that might predispose one to develop certain acute organ toxicities and/or disease-related complications. If discoveries could be made, such as identifying a genetic polymorphism to a specific chemotherapeutic agent predicting increased toxicity, guidelines could be developed for treatment adaptation to decrease treatment-related toxicities and long-term organ effects which would improve the overall quality of life for these patients. Leukemia treatment in the next decade will incorporate cellular-based therapies including chimeric antigen receptor therapies. This treatment modality has a unique set of toxicities which will be reviewed elsewhere in this textbook.

In summary, a myriad of possible serious disease and/or treatment-related complications exist for children and young adults with acute leukemia, many of which may necessitate ICU management. This chapter outlined the diagnosis and management of these oncologic emergencies, most of which can be successfully treated through a team-based approach incorporating both oncology and ICU care.

References

1. Siegel RL, Miller KD, Jemal A. Cancer statistics, 2018. CA Cancer J Clin. 2018;68(1):7–30.
2. Ward E, DeSantis C, Robbins A, Kohler B, Jemal A. Childhood and adolescent cancer statistics, 2014. CA Cancer J Clin. 2014;64(2):83–103. https://doi.org/10.3322/caac.21219.
3. Pui CH, et al. Childhood acute lymphoblastic leukemia: progress through collaboration. J Clin Oncol. 2015;33(27):2938–48.
4. Gamis AS, et al. Children's Oncology Group's 2013 blueprint for research: acute myeloid leukemia. Pediatr Blood Cancer. 2013;60(6):964–71.
5. Stary J, Hrusak O. Recent advances in the management of pediatric acute lymphoblastic leukemia. F1000Res. 2016;5:2635.
6. Freedman JL, Rheingold SR, Fisher MJ. Oncologic emergencies. In: Pizzo P, Poplack D, editors. Principles and practice of pediatric oncology. Philadelphia: Wolters Kluwer; 2016. p. 967–91.
7. Lund B, et al. Risk factors for treatment related mortality in childhood acute lymphoblastic leukaemia. Pediatr Blood Cancer. 2011;56(4):551–9.
8. Coiffier B, et al. Guidelines for the management of pediatric and adult tumor lysis syndrome: an evidence-based review. J Clin Oncol. 2008;26(16):2767–78.
9. Cairo MS, Bishop M. Tumour lysis syndrome: new therapeutic strategies and classification. Br J Haematol. 2004;127(1):3–11.
10. Annemans L, et al. Incidence, medical resource utilisation and costs of hyperuricemia and tumour lysis syndrome in patients with acute leukaemia and non-Hodgkin's lymphoma in four European countries. Leuk Lymphoma. 2003;44(1):77–83.

11. Cairo MS, et al. Recommendations for the evaluation of risk and prophylaxis of tumour lysis syndrome (TLS) in adults and children with malignant diseases: an expert TLS panel consensus. Br J Haematol. 2010;149(4):578–86.
12. Wilson FP, Berns JS. Onco-nephrology: tumor lysis syndrome. Clin J Am Soc Nephrol. 2012;7(10):1730–9.
13. Cairo MS, et al. A clinical and economic comparison of rasburicase and allopurinol in the treatment of patients with clinical or laboratory tumor lysis syndrome. Clin Lymphoma Myeloma Leuk. 2017;17(3):173–8.
14. Smalley RV, et al. Allopurinol: intravenous use for prevention and treatment of hyperuricemia. J Clin Oncol. 2000;18(8):1758–63.
15. Jeha S, et al. Efficacy and safety of rasburicase, a recombinant urate oxidase (Elitek), in the management of malignancy-associated hyperuricemia in pediatric and adult patients: final results of a multicenter compassionate use trial. Leukemia. 2005;19(1):34–8.
16. Goldman SC, et al. A randomized comparison between rasburicase and allopurinol in children with lymphoma or leukemia at high risk for tumor lysis. Blood. 2001;97(10):2998–3003.
17. Kikuchi A, et al. A study of rasburicase for the management of hyperuricemia in pediatric patients with newly diagnosed hematologic malignancies at high risk for tumor lysis syndrome. Int J Hematol. 2009;90(4):492–500.
18. Wilson FP, Berns JS. Tumor lysis syndrome: new challenges and recent advances. Adv Chronic Kidney Dis. 2014;21(1):18–26.
19. Agha-Razii M, et al. Continuous veno-venous hemodiafiltration for the treatment of spontaneous tumor lysis syndrome complicated by acute renal failure and severe hyperuricemia. Clin Nephrol. 2000;54(1):59–63.
20. Porcu P, et al. Hyperleukocytic leukemias and leukostasis: a review of pathophysiology, clinical presentation and management. Leuk Lymphoma. 2000;39(1–2):1–18.
21. Lowe EJ, et al. Early complications in children with acute lymphoblastic leukemia presenting with hyperleukocytosis. Pediatr Blood Cancer. 2005;45(1):10–5.
22. Ganzel C, et al. Hyperleukocytosis, leukostasis and leukapheresis: practice management. Blood Rev. 2012;26(3):117–22.
23. Abla O, et al. Early complications of hyperleukocytosis and leukapheresis in childhood acute leukemias. J Pediatr Hematol Oncol. 2016;38(2):111–7.
24. Nguyen R, et al. The role of leukapheresis in the current management of hyperleukocytosis in newly diagnosed childhood acute lymphoblastic leukemia. Pediatr Blood Cancer. 2016;63(9):1546–51.
25. Sung L, et al. Predictors and short-term outcomes of hyperleukocytosis in children with acute myeloid leukemia: a report from the Children's Oncology Group. Haematologica. 2012;97(11):1770–2.
26. Nowacki P, et al. Co-existence of thrombocytopenia and hyperleukocytosis ('critical period') as a risk factor of haemorrhage into the central nervous system in patients with acute leukaemias. Haematologia (Budap). 2002;31(4):347–55.
27. Attarbaschi A, et al. Mediastinal mass in childhood T-cell acute lymphoblastic leukemia: significance and therapy response. Med Pediatr Oncol. 2002;39(6):558–65.
28. Pearson JK, Tan GM. Pediatric anterior mediastinal mass: a review article. Semin Cardiothorac Vasc Anesth. 2015;19(3):248–54.
29. Wilson LD, Detterbeck FC, Yahalom J. Clinical practice. Superior vena cava syndrome with malignant causes. N Engl J Med. 2007;356(18):1862–9.
30. Acker SN, et al. A multidisciplinary approach to the management of anterior mediastinal masses in children. J Pediatr Surg. 2015;50(5):875–8.
31. Anghelescu DL, et al. Clinical and diagnostic imaging findings predict anesthetic complications in children presenting with malignant mediastinal masses. Paediatr Anaesth. 2007;17(11):1090–8.
32. McCurdy MT, Shanholtz CB. Oncologic emergencies. Crit Care Med. 2012;40(7):2212–22.
33. Perger L, Lee EY, Shamberger RC. Management of children and adolescents with a critical airway due to compression by an anterior mediastinal mass. J Pediatr Surg. 2008;43(11):1990–7.

34. Garey CL, et al. Management of anterior mediastinal masses in children. Eur J Pediatr Surg. 2011;21(5):310–3.
35. Ng A, et al. Anaesthetic outcome and predictive risk factors in children with mediastinal tumours. Pediatr Blood Cancer. 2007;48(2):160–4.
36. Hack HA, Wright NB, Wynn RF. The anaesthetic management of children with anterior mediastinal masses. Anaesthesia. 2008;63(8):837–46.
37. Frey TK, et al. A child with anterior mediastinal mass supported with veno-arterial extracorporeal membrane oxygenation. Pediatr Crit Care Med. 2006;7(5):479–81.
38. Vagace JM, et al. Central nervous system chemotoxicity during treatment of pediatric acute lymphoblastic leukemia/lymphoma. Crit Rev Oncol Hematol. 2012;84(2):274–86.
39. Bhojwani D, et al. Methotrexate-induced neurotoxicity and leukoencephalopathy in childhood acute lymphoblastic leukemia. J Clin Oncol. 2014;32(9):949–59.
40. Zwaan CM, et al. Safety and efficacy of nelarabine in children and young adults with relapsed or refractory T-lineage acute lymphoblastic leukaemia or T-lineage lymphoblastic lymphoma: results of a phase 4 study. Br J Haematol. 2017;179(2):284–93.
41. Berg SL, et al. Phase II study of nelarabine (compound 506U78) in children and young adults with refractory T-cell malignancies: a report from the Children's Oncology Group. J Clin Oncol. 2005;23(15):3376–82.
42. Dunsmore KP, et al. Pilot study of nelarabine in combination with intensive chemotherapy in high-risk T-cell acute lymphoblastic leukemia: a report from the Children's Oncology Group. J Clin Oncol. 2012;30(22):2753–9.
43. Tang JH, et al. Study of posterior reversible encephalopathy syndrome in children with acute lymphoblastic leukemia after induction chemotherapy. J Child Neurol. 2016;31(3):279–84.
44. Kwon S, Koo J, Lee S. Clinical spectrum of reversible posterior leukoencephalopathy syndrome. Pediatr Neurol. 2001;24(5):361–4.
45. Meltzer JA, Jubinsky PT. Acute myeloid leukemia presenting as spinal cord compression. Pediatr Emerg Care. 2005;21(10):670–2.
46. Isome K, et al. Spinal cord compression by epidural involvement over 21 vertebral levels in acute lymphoblastic leukemia. J Pediatr Hematol Oncol. 2011;33(2):153–7.
47. Mantadakis E, et al. Spinal cord compression in an adolescent with relapsed B-precursor acute lymphoblastic leukemia and mental neuropathy. Int J Hematol. 2008;88(3):294–8.
48. van Veen JJ, Nokes TJ, Makris M. The risk of spinal haematoma following neuraxial anaesthesia or lumbar puncture in thrombocytopenic individuals. Br J Haematol. 2010;148(1):15–25.
49. Caruso V, et al. Thrombotic complications in childhood acute lymphoblastic leukemia: a meta-analysis of 17 prospective studies comprising 1752 pediatric patients. Blood. 2006;108(7):2216–22.
50. Grace RF, et al. The frequency and management of asparaginase-related thrombosis in paediatric and adult patients with acute lymphoblastic leukaemia treated on Dana-Farber Cancer Institute consortium protocols. Br J Haematol. 2011;152(4):452–9.
51. Qureshi A, et al. Asparaginase-related venous thrombosis in UKALL 2003- re-exposure to asparaginase is feasible and safe. Br J Haematol. 2010;149(3):410–3.
52. Appel IM, et al. Influence of two different regimens of concomitant treatment with asparaginase and dexamethasone on hemostasis in childhood acute lymphoblastic leukemia. Leukemia. 2007;21(11):2377–80.
53. Hunault-Berger M, et al. Changes in antithrombin and fibrinogen levels during induction chemotherapy with L-asparaginase in adult patients with acute lymphoblastic leukemia or lymphoblastic lymphoma. Use of supportive coagulation therapy and clinical outcome: the CAPELAL study. Haematologica. 2008;93(10):1488–94.
54. Monagle P, et al. Antithrombotic therapy in neonates and children: antithrombotic therapy and prevention of thrombosis, 9th ed: American College of Chest Physicians evidence-based clinical practice guidelines. Chest. 2012;141(2 Suppl):e737S–801S.
55. Shafey A, et al. Incidence, risk factors, and outcomes of enteritis, typhlitis, and colitis in children with acute leukemia. J Pediatr Hematol Oncol. 2013;35(7):514–7.

56. Mullassery D, et al. Diagnosis, incidence, and outcomes of suspected typhlitis in oncology patients – experience in a tertiary pediatric surgical center in the United Kingdom. J Pediatr Surg. 2009;44(2):381–5.
57. Altinel E, et al. Typhlitis in acute childhood leukemia. Med Princ Pract. 2012;21(1):36–9.
58. Gray TL, et al. Gastrointestinal complications in children with acute myeloid leukemia. Leuk Lymphoma. 2010;51(5):768–77.
59. Fike FB, et al. Neutropenic colitis in children. J Surg Res. 2011;170(1):73–6.
60. McCarville MB, et al. Typhlitis in childhood cancer. Cancer. 2005;104(2):380–7.
61. Hijiya N, van der Sluis IM. Asparaginase-associated toxicity in children with acute lymphoblastic leukemia. Leuk Lymphoma. 2016;57(4):748–57.
62. Wolthers BO, et al. Asparaginase-associated pancreatitis in childhood acute lymphoblastic leukaemia: an observational Ponte di Legno Toxicity Working Group study. Lancet Oncol. 2017;18(9):1238–48.
63. Oparaji JA, et al. Risk factors for Asparaginase-associated pancreatitis: a systematic review. J Clin Gastroenterol. 2017;51(10):907–13.
64. Schmiegelow K, et al. Non-infectious chemotherapy-associated acute toxicities during childhood acute lymphoblastic leukemia therapy. F1000Res. 2017;6:444.
65. Silverman LB, et al. Improved outcome for children with acute lymphoblastic leukemia: results of Dana-Farber Consortium Protocol 91-01. Blood. 2001;97(5):1211–8.
66. Pession A, et al. Long-term results of a randomized trial on extended use of high dose L-asparaginase for standard risk childhood acute lymphoblastic leukemia. J Clin Oncol. 2005;23(28):7161–7.
67. Stein EM, Tallman MS. Acute promyelocytic leukemia in children and adolescents. Acta Haematol. 2014;132(3–4):307–12.
68. Gregory J, Feusner J. Acute promyelocytic leukemia in childhood. Curr Oncol Rep. 2009;11(6):439–45.
69. Sanz MA, et al. Management of acute promyelocytic leukemia: recommendations from an expert panel on behalf of the European LeukemiaNet. Blood. 2009;113(9):1875–91.
70. Kutny MA, Gregory J Jr, Feusner JH. Treatment of paediatric APL: how does the therapeutic approach differ from adults? Best Pract Res Clin Haematol. 2014;27(1):69–78.
71. Fisher BT, et al. Induction mortality, ATRA administration, and resource utilization in a nationally representative cohort of children with acute promyelocytic leukemia in the United States from 1999 to 2009. Pediatr Blood Cancer. 2014;61(1):68–73.
72. Testi AM, et al. GIMEMA-AIEOPAIDA protocol for the treatment of newly diagnosed acute promyelocytic leukemia (APL) in children. Blood. 2005;106(2):447–53.
73. Sanz MA, Montesinos P. How we prevent and treat differentiation syndrome in patients with acute promyelocytic leukemia. Blood. 2014;123(18):2777–82.

Chapter 3
Neuro-oncologic Emergencies

Jessica Clymer and Peter E. Manley

Introduction

Primary central nervous system (CNS) tumors are the second most common pediatric cancer diagnosed in the United States each year. Comprising approximately 22% of new cases of pediatric cancer per year, CNS tumors are second only to pediatric leukemia in incidence. Brain and CNS tumors are the most common solid tumor in children with an annual age-adjusted incidence rate of 5.47 per 100,000 population [1, 2]. While brain and CNS tumors are the second most common pediatric cancer, they account for the majority of cancer-related mortality in children [3].

However, survival of pediatric patients with primary brain tumors has increased over the years, but the treatment of brain tumors has the potential for significant and life-threatening neurologic complications. It is imperative that critical care professionals recognize and appropriately treat common neurologic emergencies associated with these tumors. These emergencies can be the result of direct effects of the CNS tumor (increased intracranial pressure, seizures, spinal cord compression), indirect effects (CNS infection), or complications of various treatment strategies (chemotherapy toxicity, radiation necrosis, pituitary damage). Prompt diagnosis and treatment of these emergencies may not only be lifesaving but can preserve neurologic function both in the short term and have long-lasting effects on overall quality of life.

J. Clymer · P. E. Manley (✉)
Pediatric Neuro-oncology, Dana-Farber/Boston Children's Cancer and Blood Disorders Center, Boston, MA, USA
e-mail: Peter_Manley@dfci.harvard.edu

C. N. Duncan et al. (eds.), *Critical Care of the Pediatric Immunocompromised Hematology/Oncology Patient*, https://doi.org/10.1007/978-3-030-01322-6_3

Increased Intracranial Pressure/Hydrocephalus/Herniation

In children with primary CNS tumors, a frequent emergency that develops is increased intracranial pressure (ICP). This can arise because of hydrocephalus, vasogenic edema, or combination of the two. If not addressed adequately, increased intracranial pressure can progress to irreversible neurologic deficits, herniation, and death.

The Monro-Kellie doctrine serves as the basis of understanding the pathophysiology of increased intracranial pressure. The intracranial volume ranges from 1400 to 1700 mL. The brain constitutes roughly 80% of that volume, with blood and cerebrospinal fluid (CSF) each comprising an additional 10% [4]. Given the fixed volume of the cranial vault, owing to the rigid skull surrounding it, the Monro-Kellie doctrine states that an increase in volume of the brain, blood, or CSF must trigger a decrease in one or both of the other components. When the system fails to compensate appropriately, there is a resultant increase in intracranial pressure.

One cause of increased ICP commonly encountered in children with primary CNS tumors is hydrocephalus. This occurs due to obstruction of the CSF outflow system. For example, pineal tumors may block CSF outflow from the 3rd ventricle resulting in dilatation of the lateral ventricles, or posterior fossa tumors can obstruct the 4th ventricle resulting in dilatation of the entire ventricular system. As CSF cannot drain adequately, its volume within the cranial vault increases and therefore results in increased ICP.

A common symptom of elevated intracranial pressure is headache. The classic description of headache associated with elevated ICP is one that is most severe in the morning due to nocturnal hypercarbia causing vasodilatation and supine posture [5]. However, this dogma has been challenged, and some report that morning headache occurs in a minority of patients presenting with increased ICP [6]. Other presenting symptoms of elevated intracranial pressure include vomiting, diplopia from abducens nerve palsy, and papilledema. When unchecked, elevated intracranial pressure may result in brainstem compression manifested by Cushing's triad of hypertension, bradycardia, and irregular breathing, which heralds impending herniation.

With imminent herniation, patients with elevated ICP often become stuporous; therefore management often starts with securing an airway. Sedation and intubation have the added benefit of being means of lowering elevated ICP. Sedation lowers intracranial pressure, though at the expense of a reliable neurologic examination. Intubation allows for hyperventilation to a pCO2 of 26–30 mm Hg which causes vasoconstriction and decreased cerebral blood flow quickly albeit transiently [7].

Following these short-term interventions, osmotherapy is the mainstay of medical treatment of increased ICP. Hyperosmolar agents such as hypertonic saline and mannitol are used to create an osmotic gradient across the blood-brain barrier and shift fluid out of the brain thereby lowering ICP [8, 9]. Neither of these agents can be continued indefinitely as repeated doses without time for clearance between doses can lead to a rebound increase in ICP. Additionally, corticosteroids, specifically dexamethasone, play a critical role in alleviating vasogenic edema associated with brain tumors, by decreasing vascular permeability of the blood-brain barrier, leading to decreased ICP. Finally, following these temporizing interventions, one must quickly determine if surgical interventions are necessary and/or appropriate for management of hydrocephalus, particularly in the case of obstructive hydrocephalus. Neurosurgical interventions include insertion of an extraventricular drain to alleviate pressure, endoscopic third ventriculostomy, or insertion of a ventriculoperitoneal shunt.

Seizures/Status Epilepticus

Another complication of primary brain tumors are seizures. Brain tumors are structural abnormalities that can cause cortical irritability and subsequent seizures. Prophylaxis with antiepileptic drugs is not commonly recommended, as a subset of patients with brain tumors never experience seizures [10]. Tumors located in epileptogenic areas such as the cortex, mesial temporal lobe, and insula are more likely to cause seizures. Low-grade gliomas are more epileptogenic than high-grade gliomas [11]. Of patients with low-grade gliomas, those with oligodendroglioma are more likely to develop seizures than those with astrocytoma likely owing to their cortical location and white matter involvement [12, 13].

Specific seizure semiology often reflects the tumor's location. Brain tumor patients generally have localization-related epilepsy with subtypes including simple partial seizures, complex partial seizures, and focal seizures with secondary generalization [13]. Status epilepticus can occur at any stage of a tumor's course – at presentation, progression, or during periods of stability [14]. In addition to seizure location, seizures can be triggered in those with CNS tumors as a complication of treatment whether due to electrolyte abnormalities, treatment-related posterior reversible encephalopathy, or by medications, which lower the seizure threshold commonly used as supportive care in cancer patients.

After recognition of status epilepticus, treatment according to standard management algorithms is vital. First-line treatment of status epilepticus starts with prompt administration of a benzodiazepine (IV lorazepam or IM midazolam if IV access cannot be obtained) followed by phenytoin if needed. Third-line treatments include phenobarbital, valproic acid, lacosamide, and levetiracetam [15]. Choosing ongoing antiepileptic drug therapy in children with brain tumors are challenging due in large part to the potential interactions between antiepileptic drugs and chemotherapy. Levetiracetam is often recommended as initial maintenance monotherapy given its efficacy, tolerability, and pharmacokinetic properties when used in combination with chemotherapy [16].

Spinal Cord Compression

Spinal cord compression from an epidural mass is a somewhat common complication in specific pediatric cancers such as soft tissue sarcoma, neuroblastoma, medulloblastoma, atypical teratoid rhabdoid tumors (AT/RT), and lymphoma [17, 18]. It constitutes a neuro-oncologic emergency as favorable neurologic outcome depends on early recognition and management.

Prior to spinal cord compression, those with spinal tumors may report pain, particularly in the case of extradural masses arising from the bone. Another source of pain is Lhermitte's sign, an electrical sensation spreading from the spine to the arms or legs following neck flexion. This pain is due to irritation or compression of the dorsal columns. While Lhermitte's sign suggests cord dysfunction, other classic signs include weakness, loss of sensation, and bowel or bladder dysfunction. If compression occurs in the cervical or high thoracic region, patients can develop autonomic dysreflexia with bradycardia and hypertension, which can be triggered by constipation or an excessively full bladder.

A bolus of dexamethasone is the first-line treatment when cord compression is recognized. Steroids should be continued at a maintenance dosing schedule until definitive treatment can be achieved. Definitive treatment may include surgery, radiation therapy, or both. Small studies in adult patients have shown that those patients with acute onset (<48 h) of paraplegia and radiographically proven cord compression were more likely to regain the ability to walk and had improved pain control with treated with surgery followed by radiation compared to radiation alone [19]. Surgery can be avoided in patients with radiosensitive/chemosensitive tumors. Thus, multidisciplinary evaluation by neurosurgery, radiation oncology, and oncology is vital in the management of acute spinal cord compression.

Encephalopathy with Chemotherapy

Certain cytotoxic and biologic agents can produce neurotoxicity (Table 3.1). The severity depends on the treatment dose, duration, and concomitant use of other neurotoxic therapies.

Within days of administration, high-dose methotrexate, ifosfamide, high-dose cytarabine, and procarbazine can all cause acute encephalopathy including confusion, hallucination, drowsiness, and seizures. Additionally, high doses of cytarabine can cause cerebellar syndromes including progressive and potentially permanent ataxia [20, 21]. Intrathecal chemotherapies including methotrexate or cytarabine can cause aseptic meningitis with symptoms including neck pain, headache, fever, nausea, and vomiting. These intrathecal agents can also cause transverse myelopathy with paraplegia, leg pain, sensory level, and even neurogenic bladder dysfunction [22]. Unfortunately, treatment for most of these neurotoxic side effects is drug cessation and supportive care, with the exception of ifosfamide encephalopathy, which responds to treatment with methylene blue. (50 mg Q4 hours until resolution of symptoms or 1 mg/kg for children under 50 kg.)

Newer biologic agents can cause neurologic side effects as well. Bevacizumab, an anti-VEGF monoclonal antibody, can be associated with thromboembolic stroke, intracranial hemorrhage, and has been associated with PRES. Cessation of therapy and supportive care are the mainstays of treatment with bevacizumab toxicity. Ipilimumab, an anti-CTLA-4 monoclonal antibody, has been associated with acute inflammatory reaction including myopathy, aseptic meningitis, temporal arteritis,

Table 3.1 Chemotherapy neurologic toxicities and their treatments

Complication	Agents	Treatment
Encephalopathy	Ifosfamide, HD-MTX, HD-cytarabine, procarbazine, vincristine	Methylene blue (for Ifosfamide induced only), discontinue drugs
Aseptic meningitis	IT-MTX, cytarabine Cetuximab Ipilimumab	Discontinue/reduce drugs Discontinue drug Discontinue drug, IV corticosteroids, IVIG, plasmapheresis
Cerebellar syndromes	HD-cytarabine	Discontinue drugs
Seizures	Cisplatin, cytarabine, cyclophosphamide, ifosfamide, vincristine	Discontinue drugs
Stroke	Bevacizumab	Discontinue drugs
PRES	Cisplatin, cyclophosphamide, gemcitabine, bevacizumab	Discontinue drugs
Myelopathy	IT-MTX and cytarabine	Discontinue drugs
Guillen-Barre syndrome	Ipilimumab	Discontinue drugs, IV corticosteroids, IVIG, plasmapheresis
Acute sensory dysesthesia	Ifosfamide, cytarabine (rare)	Discontinue/reduce drugs, anti-epileptics (carbamazepine, lamotrigine, gabapentin), tricyclic antidepressants, SSRIs

and Guillain-Barre syndrome. These neurologic complications are often immune mediated and therefore are treated with immune modulating therapies such as corticosteroids or IVIG.

Endocrinopathies

Endocrine dysfunction and disruption of water regulation are common findings of patients with intracranial neoplasms, particularly those arising from the sella and parasellar regions. Tumors that commonly arise in this area include craniopharyngioma, germ-cell tumors, astrocytomas, or pituitary adenomas and may present with endocrinopathies. Additionally, endocrinopathies and disordered water metabolism may result from surgical resection or manipulation of these lesions.

Disordered water regulation can be associated with anatomic injury to the hypothalamus, pituitary stalk, or posterior pituitary gland before or during surgery for sella or parasellar neoplasms. This damage changes water metabolism controlled by the antidiuretic hormone (ADH). ADH is produced by neurons of the paraventricular and supraoptic nuclei. It is then transported along the axons of the hypothalamic neurons and stored in the posterior pituitary. ADH is then released in response to two major stimuli: a raise in plasma osmolality and a decrease in blood pressure/circulating blood volume. After ADH is released, it acts on the kidneys and blood vessels resulting in water reabsorption at the renal collecting duct and stimulating vasoconstriction respectively [23]. Disorders of water metabolism can occur due to a decrease in ADH release resulting in central diabetes insipidus, or excess ADH release resulting in water retention, and the syndrome of inappropriate ADH secretion (SIADH). Additionally, an ADH-independent condition, cerebral salt wasting syndrome (CSWS) can occur after neurosurgical interventions.

Diabetes insipidus (DI) is defined as the presence of inappropriate hypotonic polyuria in the presence of high or normal serum sodium [24]. While the presence of serum hyperosmolality and hypernatremia are suggestive of DI, these findings may be absent if the patient is conscious, with an intact thirst mechanism and access to free water. Thus, to screen for potential development of postoperative DI, close measurement of urine output and fluid intake, urine specific gravity, and serum sodium are vital. Treatment includes replacement of urine/fluid losses as well as administration and titration of vasopressin or desmopressin (the former having a shorter duration of action and thus easier to titrate if water metabolism continues to evolve). While DI can be transient or permanent, the risk of permanent DI is higher in younger patients, males, those with large intrasellar masses [25], in those with a preoperative diagnosis of DI, and following surgery for craniopharyngioma [26].

While DI is the predominate process resulting in hypernatremia, intracranial neoplasms and their treatment can also result in hyponatremia. In fact, hyponatremia occurs in 10–15% of pediatric patients following intracranial tumor surgery [27, 28]. Postoperative hyponatremia is commonly associated with two conditions: the syndrome of inappropriate antidiuretic hormone (SIADH) and CSWS. Unfortunately, clinical distinction between the two can be challenging; however, it is vitally important as their treatment is divergent (Table 3.2).

SIADH is a syndrome of hypoosmolar hyponatremic euvolemia. It is characterized by an even fluid balance/euvolemia, hyponatremia, hypoosmolality, increased urine osmolality, and elevated urine sodium concentration in an individual with normal salt and water intake [29]. These symptoms are a result of excessive ADH release and therefore increased water reabsorption from the glomerular filtrate at the distal nephron. This produces inappropriately concentrated urine despite serum hypoosmolality. The key feature distinguishing SIADH from CSWS is volume status as SIADH is a state of euvolemia, while CSWS is one of hypovolemia. Thus, patients with SIADH will be unlikely to have changes in blood pressure, body weight, heart rate, or other signs associated with volume loss. Once the diagnosis of SIADH has been established, it is treated with fluid restriction and possible administration of diuretics such as furosemide.

On the other hand, CSWS is a syndrome marked by hypovolemia and/or net negative fluid balance, hyponatremia and serum hypoosmolality, and an elevated urine osmolality and elevated urine sodium [29]. CSWS is caused by excessive renal sodium and water excretion and is often associated with an increase in urine output [30]. The sodium excretion is higher than that of water, and therefore the urine is inappropriately concentrated. Again, accurate assessment of volume status

Table 3.2 Differentiation of sodium abnormalities

	DI: Diabetes insipidus	SIADH: Syndrome of inappropriate antidiuretic hormone	CSW: Cerebral salt wasting
Disorder	ADH Deficit Decreased reabsorption of water by the distal tubules of the kidney Loss of free water in the urine	ADH Excess Inappropriate secretion of ADH Increased permeability of renal distal tubules and increased water reabsorption	Renal sodium loss Decreased renal sodium reabsorption Free water loss
Volume status	Decreased, hypovolemia	Increased; fluid overload	Decreased, hypovolemia
CVP	Decreased	Normal or increased	Decreased
Weight	Decreased	Normal or increased	Decreased
Salt balance	Variable	Variable	Negative
Serum sodium	Increased	Decreased	Decreased
Urine sodium	Decreased or normal	Increased	Markedly increased
Serum osmolality	Increased	Decreased	Increased or normal
Urine osmolality	Decreased	Increased	Increased
Urine spec gravity	Decreased	Increased	Normal or slightly increased
Signs/ symptoms	Polyuria, hypoosmolar urine (clear), hyperosmolar plasma, hypernatremia, thirst, polydipsia, dehydration, shock, fatigue, mental status changes, seizure, irritability, lethargy, tachycardia, poor perfusion	Decreased concentrated urine, hyponatremia, hypertension, mental status changes, seizures, lethargy, nausea, vomiting	Differentiate from SIADH with confirmed hypovolemia Anorexia, nausea, vomiting, weakness, hypotension, tachycardia, poor skin turgor, syncope
Treatment	Evaluate and replace fluid/ urine loss frequently Administer and titrate vasopression (IV or DDAVP) for UO M 2 mL/ kg/h. Prevent overtreatment, hypernatremia correction should be about 2 mEq/L/h	Restrict fluids and consider giving furosemide Correct hyponatremia with 3% NaCL infusion for goal sodium of >/= 125 mEq/L. Replaced deficit over 24–48 h. Observe for water intoxication and cerebral edema due to rapid overcorrection of hypernatremia	Isotonic saline volume loss replacement Enteral sodium replacement Use of 3% saline is restricted to sodium levels <125 mEq/L and is done over 24 h

is vital to distinguishing SIADH from CSWS. Classic signs of hypovolemia include hypotension, weight loss, increased heart rate, increased capillary refill time, and loss of skin turgor. Once the diagnosis of CSWS has been established, the mainstay of treatment includes the replacement of the sodium and water lost as a result of pathologic natriuresis and diuresis. Initial management includes administration of isotonic fluids (often normal saline) with the goal of restoring intravascular volume. Once euvolemia is achieved, if hyponatremia persists, management can then be directed at correcting hyponatremia. This can be achieved through oral sodium replacements, hypertonic saline administration, or mineralocorticoid use [29]. Generally speaking, the serum sodium concentration should be corrected slowly with an average increase no more than 0.5 mEq/L/h [31].

Not only do intracranial neoplasms and their treatments cause abnormalities in water metabolism, they can also be associated with endocrinopathies. Such hormone deficiencies are often due to injury of the hypothalamus and/or pituitary (either through direct surgical injury or a delayed effect of radiation therapy). Such injuries can cause partial or total hypopituitarism. The risk of postoperative hypopituitarism varies according to case series and tumor type; however, it peaks at 75% for craniopharyngioma [32]. Pituitary hormone deficiencies can include decreased levels of ACTH, TSH, GH, LH, and FSH.

Adrenal insufficiency (AI) is a potentially life-threatening endocrinopathy. It can present as central AI following neurosurgical intervention (oftentimes pituitary surgery) or as secondary AI due to persistent corticosteroid use. In either case, it must be promptly recognized and treated with glucocorticoid replacement. Additionally, it is vital that patients and families understand the importance of recognizing an adrenal crisis and receive instruction on steroid replacement in times of stress, such as with surgeries or acute illnesses.

Additional endocrinopathies may not be readily apparent postoperatively or immediately following treatment of brain tumors but rather may develop over time. Their deficiencies are often not life-threatening or urgent; however, their normalization can significantly alter a patient's quality of life. One can monitor TSH/T4 for thyroid axis function. Sex hormone monitoring can be done with morning serum testosterone in males or with LH, FSH, and menses history in premenopausal females. The growth hormone axis can be monitored by serum insulin-like growth factor-1 (IGF-1) though if low is often confirmed with a GH stimulation test.

Radiation Injury and Radiation Necrosis

The nervous system is vulnerable to the effects of radiation, and thus its use in the treatment of brain tumors can be associated with tissue injury at various time points during and after radiation therapy. Acute injury (during or less than 1 month after radiation therapy) is associated with capillary injury with associated leak and edema. Neurologic symptoms can include somnolence, headache, nausea, vomiting, and exacerbation of baseline neurologic deficits and are often responsive to corticosteroids. Early-delayed injury (1–6 months post radiation therapy) complications are often due to edema and demyelination. Patients may present with somnolence syndrome (increased drowsiness, fatigue, anorexia, irritability), and MRI may demonstrate increased edema and contrast enhancement concerning tumor progression, termed pseudo-progression. Again, symptoms are often responsive to corticosteroids. Late injury (more than 6 months after radiation therapy) is hypothesized to be due to small- to medium-sized vessel injury as well as demyelination and is often referred to as radiation necrosis.

Radiation necrosis is a well-characterized toxicity of brain tumor treatment, which refers to necrotic degradation of brain tissue following intracranial radiation. MRI findings include white matter contrast enhancement, soap-bubble/swiss-cheese enhancement, along with edema and mass effect early followed by volume loss later [33]. These imaging findings may or may not be associated with new neurologic findings such as confusion, seizures, or focal neurologic deficits. Retrospective studies of children report widely varying rates of radiation necrosis of 3–26%. Radiation necrosis poses a challenge as it can occur at any time during and after radiation therapy – from acute (during and immediately after radiation therapy) to late-delayed (months to years after radiation therapy) though most often is a late stage complication of radiation therapy. One meta-analysis found that children treated with proton radiation therapy who presented with radiation necrosis were younger and had shorter time to development of radiation necrosis [34]. Additionally, they found that younger children tended to present with ataxia and older children with headache when diagnosed with radiation necrosis, though this may be due to tumor location (infratentorial vs. supratentorial) in the two age groups. Thus, when a child who has received radiation therapy in the past presents with new MRI changes and/or new neurologic findings, one must consider radiation necrosis as a potential etiology.

Radiation necrosis is thought to occur as a result of cerebral vascular injury. It begins as acute cellular injury with endothelial cell death; this causes platelet aggregation, thrombus formation, and occlusion of microvasculature [35]. Vascular endothelial growth factor (VEGF) is released by the dysfunctional endothelial cells, which results in capillary leakage, brain edema, neuronal demyelination, and damage of the blood-brain barrier. It is hypothesized that radiation leads to cellular injury and vascular damage, which in turn leads to tissues hypoxia. This results in degradation of collagen, disruption of the blood-brain barrier [36], release of VEGF, capillary leakage [37], perivascular inflammation, and edema. This process can occur throughout the white matter or focally. Total radiation dose, volume of irradiated area, as well as fractionation regimen are predictive of risk of radiation necrosis [38].

Once recognized, there are typically three modalities of treatment for radiation necrosis – corticosteroids, bevacizumab, and hyperbaric oxygen therapy. These can be used alone or in combination [34]. While corticosteroids are often the mainstay of early treatment of radiation necrosis due to their potent anti-inflammatory effects, they are associated with a significant adverse effect profile, making them less likely to be used long term. Bevacizumab is humanized monoclonal antibody that blocks

VEGF, an important mediator of capillary leakage and brain edema [38]. Hyperbaric oxygen is thought to improve tissue oxygenation, which leads to a reduction of inflammation and neovascularization.

CNS Infection

Central nervous system (CNS) infections are an important cause of neurologic morbidity and mortality in patients with cancer. While the risk of general CNS infections is greatest in those patients with significant and prolonged immunosuppression, patients with CNS tumors pose a unique risk group. Having disrupted the blood-brain barrier with cranial surgery, frequent need for ventricular shunt placement, and skin breakdown from radiation therapy, patients with brain tumors are at risk for cutaneous skin flora infections. Such pathogens include *Staphylococcus aureus*, *Staphylococcus epidermidis*, *Propionibacterium acnes*, and *Candida* species [39, 40]. These patients may or may not manifest typical signs/symptoms of CNS infection, such as fever, headache, nuchal rigidity, if in the midst of chemotherapy, and therefore immunodeficiency [41]. Instead, altered mental status may be the only indication of a CNS infection. Early recognition and diagnosis of CNS infections with prompt initiation of antimicrobials is vital.

Conclusions

Children with CNS tumors are at risk for a variety of life-threatening and/or neurologic function compromising complications due to their tumors, treatment of their tumors, or indirect effects of their tumors. Prompt recognition and management of these complications has the potential to preserve neurologic function already at risk.

References

1. Ostrom QT, et al. CBTRUS statistical report: primary brain and other central nervous system tumors diagnosed in the United States in 2009–2013. Neuro-Oncology. 2016;18(suppl_5):v1–v75.
2. Ostrom QT, et al. Alex's lemonade stand foundation infant and childhood primary brain and central nervous system tumors diagnosed in the United States in 2007–2011. Neuro-Oncology. 2015;16(Suppl 10):x1–x36.
3. de Blank PM, et al. Years of life lived with disease and years of potential life lost in children who die of cancer in the United States, 2009. Cancer Med. 2015;4(4):608–19.
4. Smith ER, Madsen JR. Cerebral pathophysiology and critical care neurology: basic hemodynamic principles, cerebral perfusion, and intracranial pressure. Semin Pediatr Neurol. 2004;11(2):89–104.

5. Lin AL, Avila EK. Neurologic emergencies in the patients with cancer. J Intensive Care Med. 2017;32(2):99–115.
6. Forsyth PA, Posner JB. Headaches in patients with brain tumors: a study of 111 patients. Neurology. 1993;43(9):1678–83.
7. Stocchetti N, et al. Hyperventilation in head injury: a review. Chest. 2005;127(5):1812–27.
8. Damek DM. Cerebral edema, altered mental status, seizures, acute stroke, leptomeningeal metastases, and paraneoplastic syndrome. Emerg Med Clin North Am. 2009;27(2):209–29.
9. Pater K, Puskulluoglu M, Zygulska AL. Oncological emergencies: increased intracranial pressure in solid tumours' metastatic brain disease. Przegl Lek. 2014;71(2):91–4.
10. Glantz MJ, et al. Practice parameter: anticonvulsant prophylaxis in patients with newly diagnosed brain tumors. Report of the quality standards subcommittee of the American Academy of Neurology. Neurology. 2000;54(10):1886–93.
11. Kerkhof M, Vecht CJ. Seizure characteristics and prognostic factors of gliomas. Epilepsia. 2013;54(Suppl 9):12–7.
12. Ruda R, et al. Seizures in low-grade gliomas: natural history, pathogenesis, and outcome after treatments. Neuro-Oncology. 2012;14(Suppl 4):iv55–64.
13. Vecht CJ, Kerkhof M, Duran-Pena A. Seizure prognosis in brain tumors: new insights and evidence-based management. Oncologist. 2014;19(7):751–9.
14. Cavaliere R, Farace E, Schiff D. Clinical implications of status epilepticus in patients with neoplasms. Arch Neurol. 2006;63(12):1746–9.
15. Brophy GM, et al. Guidelines for the evaluation and management of status epilepticus. Neurocrit Care. 2012;17(1):3–23.
16. Rossetti AO, et al. Levetiracetam and pregabalin for antiepileptic monotherapy in patients with primary brain tumors. A phase II randomized study. Neuro-Oncology. 2014;16(4):584–8.
17. Pollono D, et al. Spinal cord compression: a review of 70 pediatric patients. Pediatr Hematol Oncol. 2003;20(6):457–66.
18. Lewis DW, et al. Incidence, presentation, and outcome of spinal cord disease in children with systemic cancer. Pediatrics. 1986;78(3):438–43.
19. Patchell RA, et al. Direct decompressive surgical resection in the treatment of spinal cord compression caused by metastatic cancer: a randomised trial. Lancet. 2005;366(9486):643–8.
20. Sylvester RK, Fisher AJ, Lobell M. Cytarabine-induced cerebellar syndrome: case report and literature review. Drug Intell Clin Pharm. 1987;21(2):177–80.
21. Herzig RH, et al. Cerebellar toxicity with high-dose cytosine arabinoside. J Clin Oncol. 1987;5(6):927–32.
22. Kwong YL, Yeung DY, Chan JC. Intrathecal chemotherapy for hematologic malignancies: drugs and toxicities. Ann Hematol. 2009;88(3):193–201.
23. Prete A, Corsello SM, Salvatori R. Current best practice in the management of patients after pituitary surgery. Ther Adv Endocrinol Metab. 2017;8(3):33–48.
24. Fenske W, Allolio B. Clinical review: current state and future perspectives in the diagnosis of diabetes insipidus: a clinical review. J Clin Endocrinol Metab. 2012;97(10):3426–37.
25. Loh JA, Verbalis JG. Diabetes insipidus as a complication after pituitary surgery. Nat Clin Pract Endocrinol Metab. 2007;3(6):489–94.
26. Mortini P, et al. Neurosurgical treatment of craniopharyngioma in adults and children: early and long-term results in a large case series. J Neurosurg. 2011;114(5):1350–9.
27. Williams C, et al. Hyponatremia with intracranial malignant tumor resection in children. J Neurosurg Pediatr. 2012;9(5):524–9.
28. Williams CN, et al. The incidence of postoperative hyponatremia and associated neurological sequelae in children with intracranial neoplasms. J Neurosurg Pediatr. 2014;13(3):283–90.
29. Yee AH, Burns JD, Wijdicks EF. Cerebral salt wasting: pathophysiology, diagnosis, and treatment. Neurosurg Clin N Am. 2010;21(2):339–52.
30. Hardesty DA, Kilbaugh TJ, Storm PB. Cerebral salt wasting syndrome in post-operative pediatric brain tumor patients. Neurocrit Care. 2012;17(3):382–7.
31. Adrogue HJ, Madias NE. Hyponatremia. N Engl J Med. 2000;342(21):1581–9.

32. Lo AC, et al. Long-term outcomes and complications in patients with craniopharyngioma: the British Columbia Cancer Agency experience. Int J Radiat Oncol Biol Phys. 2014;88(5):1011–8.
33. Rogers LR, et al. Morphologic magnetic resonance imaging features of therapy-induced cerebral necrosis. J Neuro-Oncol. 2011;101(1):25–32.
34. Drezner N, et al. Treatment of pediatric cerebral radiation necrosis: a systematic review. J Neuro-Oncol. 2016;130(1):141–8.
35. Sundgren PC, Cao Y. Brain irradiation: effects on normal brain parenchyma and radiation injury. Neuroimaging Clin N Am. 2009;19(4):657–68.
36. Greene-Schloesser D, et al. Radiation-induced brain injury: a review. Front Oncol. 2012;2:73.
37. Sadraei NH, et al. Treatment of cerebral radiation necrosis with bevacizumab: the cleveland clinic experience. Am J Clin Oncol. 2015;38(3):304–10.
38. Delishaj D, et al. Bevacizumab for the treatment of radiation-induced cerebral necrosis: a systematic review of the literature. J Clin Med Res. 2017;9(4):273–80.
39. Pruitt AA. Central nervous system infections in cancer patients. Semin Neurol. 2004;24(4):435–52.
40. Pruitt AA. CNS infections in patients with cancer. Continuum (Minneap Minn). 2012;18(2):384–405.
41. Baldwin KJ, Zivkovic SA, Lieberman FS. Neurologic emergencies in patients who have cancer: diagnosis and management. Neurol Clin. 2012;30(1):101–28. viii

Chapter 4
Solid Tumors Outside of the Central Nervous System

Hilary C. Schreiber and James S. Killinger

Solid tumors which occur outside of the central nervous system (CNS) have some similar, relevant characteristics important in the pediatric intensive care unit (PICU). In addition to tumors which arise in the anterior mediastinum, there are other disease-specific complications documented in this section. Many of the critical care issues focus on the postsurgical care of children after having (often) large tumors removed from the chest, the abdomen, or the pelvis. In this chapter, three distinct solid tumors will be discussed, highlighting these critical care issues. Furthermore, focus on the emerging "fast-track" or early recovery after surgery (ERAS) concepts in the perioperative period for children appears to improve surgical outcomes in some patient populations.

Anterior Mediastinal Masses

Anterior mediastinal masses present a unique clinical dilemma for surgeons, oncologists, interventional radiologists, anesthesiologists, and intensivists. With a new mass in the anterior mediastinum, a biopsy is often needed for the definitive diagnosis, to initiate appropriate therapy. However, depending on the size and location of the mass, the anesthesia risk of obtaining a tissue biopsy may outweigh the benefit of obtaining tissue prior to initiating a potential therapy. Because of this unusual risk-benefit analysis, the approach to anterior mediastinal masses requires a thoughtful, multidisciplinary approach.

H. C. Schreiber · J. S. Killinger (✉)
Memorial Sloan Kettering Cancer Center, New York, NY, USA
e-mail: killingj@mskcc.org

C. N. Duncan et al. (eds.), *Critical Care of the Pediatric Immunocompromised Hematology/Oncology Patient*, https://doi.org/10.1007/978-3-030-01322-6_4

In children, the leading causes of anterior mediastinal mass are lymphoma (Hodgkin's and non-Hodgkin's), leukemia, thymoma, histiocytosis, and neuroblastoma, all with varying treatment strategies [1–3]. Typically, the sedation and anesthesia needed for obtaining appropriate tissue for diagnosis are done in an operating room or interventional radiology suite. However, it is important for the pediatric intensivist to understand the rationale for sedation and anesthesia, as complications will impact the post-biopsy course in the PICU.

Airway and Cardiovascular Compromise

Symptomatic tracheal compression is a significant concern to anesthesia providers and is thought to be an increased risk of airway compromise intraoperatively. It has been demonstrated that children with >50% decrease in tracheal cross-sectional area are more likely to be symptomatic [4] and are at highest risk of developing intraoperative airway complications [5, 6]. Conversely, children with <50% decrease in the cross-sectional area of the trachea are less likely to have intraoperative airway compromise [7, 8].

From a physiologic standpoint, anterior mediastinal masses grow and develop in the same space with not only the trachea and main stem bronchi but also major components of the cardiovascular system. Thin-walled structures that are more responsive to changes in intrapleural pressures are particularly at risk: superior vena cava, right atrium, and pulmonary artery. With this in mind, maintaining a spontaneously breathing patient with negative intrapleural pressures is important, as the inspiratory muscle tone, elastic recoil of the chest wall, and displacement of the diaphragm serve to maintain functional residual capacity [9].

Developing the anesthesia plan in a multidisciplinary fashion serves to best address the diagnostic needs and the anesthesia risks of getting tissue. To that end, patients with anterior mediastinal masses can be divided into three broad categories for anesthesia [9]:

- *Low risk*: Asymptomatic of mildly symptomatic, without postural symptoms or radiographic evidence of significant compression of structures
- *Intermediate risk*: Mild to moderate postural symptoms, tracheal compression <50%
- *High risk*: Severe postural symptoms, stridor, cyanosis, tracheal compression >50% or tracheal compression with associated bronchial compression, pericardial effusion or SVC syndrome

With each incremental increase of risk, increased attention needs to be paid to both the possible increased risks and the potential risk mitigation strategies:

- *Awake intubation*: For patients requiring general anesthesia with an anterior mediastinal mass, the preferred method to secure the airway is via awake, fiberoptic bronchoscopy [10]. Attention is to be paid to minimize laryngospasm with topical anesthetics and with rescue plan in case of airway loss or hemodynamic collapse during or after intubation.

- *Reinforced endotracheal tube*: For patients with both tracheal and bronchial compression from an anterior mediastinal mass, a reinforced endotracheal tube may be passed beyond the obstruction in order to ventilate the patient [9]. However, reinforced endotracheal tubes may have unusual complications should the patient bite down on the tube or the reinforcement dissect into the lumen of the tube [11–13].
- *Rigid bronchoscopy*: Like the use of the reinforced endotracheal tube, the rigid bronchoscopy can be useful in patients with both tracheal and bronchial obstruction from an anterior mediastinal mass [14]. A rigid bronchoscope may be a particularly useful temporizing method to maintain oxygenation and ventilation should the need for emergent cardiopulmonary bypass arise.
- *Cardiopulmonary bypass*: In addition to the rescue availability of cardiopulmonary bypass (CPB), CPB has been used prophylactically in select patients thought to be at greatest risk of cardiovascular collapse following induction of anesthesia with an anterior mediastinal mass [15–17]. This may be particularly true in adults, who are less responsive to changes in positioning compared to pediatric patients [16].
- *Prone positioning*: This may be more useful in children than in adolescents and adults with anterior mediastinal mass. As older patients have a more ossified thoracic cage compared to children, the impact of prone positioning may not have the same effect in either the intubated or the extubated patient [14].
- *Heliox*: Heliox is a mixture of helium with oxygen at 70/30 and may be a useful adjuvant for use during a procedure both to obtain tissue from an anterior mediastinal mass [18] and to facilitate the extubation of a patient with an anterior mediastinal mass [19].
- In a long-standing mass, which may lead to some degree of laryngomalacia, the laminar flow from the heliox mixture may aid in delivering flows to the distal airways, beyond the residual obstruction.

Neuroblastoma

Neuroblastoma is the most common extracranial solid tumor in children, with approximately 650 new cases per year and an incidence of 10.5 cases/million/year for children younger than 15 years of age [20, 21]. It is most predominantly seen in children younger than 5 years of age. Derived from neural crest cells, neuroblastoma involves organs of the sympathetic nervous system, with the adrenal glands being the most common primary site.

Prognosis is highly variable based on risk group. Patients are stratified to low risk, intermediate risk, and high risk based on tumor stage, age at diagnosis, presence of the oncogene, MYC-N amplification, histology, tumor differentiation, DNA ploidy, and 11q aberration. High-risk features include age greater than 18 months at the time of diagnosis, MYC-N amplification, and metastatic disease. Patients with low- and intermediate-risk disease have an overall survival rate greater than 90%, while those with high-risk disease have an overall survival rate of less than 50% [20, 22].

Neuroblastoma treatment depends heavily on the risk group of the patient. In patients with low-risk disease, surgical resection, if possible, is often curative, with no need for systemic chemotherapy. Infants younger than 12 months with localized disease, Stage 4S, may also have spontaneous regression of disease without need for surgery or chemotherapy. These patients can be observed alone with overall survival rate of approximately 100% at 3 years. Intermediate-risk patients are treated with multiagent chemotherapy and surgical resection if possible [21].

High-risk patients, who represent about 50% of all patients with neuroblastoma, are difficult to treat and have much lower long-term survival compared to low- and intermediate-risk patients [20]. Regimens to treat these patients consist of induction, local control, consolidation, and maintenance therapy. Children's Oncology Group (COG) induction consists of alternating cycles of chemotherapy with multiple agents, including topotecan, cyclophosphamide, vincristine, doxorubicin, cisplatin, and etoposide. Local control includes surgical resection and/or radiation therapy. Consolidation often consists of high-dose, myeloablative chemotherapy with autologous stem cell rescue [23]. Maintenance therapy is designed to prevent relapse after patients achieve a clinical remission. In recent years, immunotherapy has been used either alone or with isotretinoin as maintenance therapy for patients in remission. Immunotherapy consists of anti-GD2 monoclonal antibodies such as humanized 3F8 (Hu3F8) and chimeric 14.18 (dinutuximab) [22]. These antibodies have become an important component of treatment for neuroblastoma.

Immunotherapy for Neuroblastoma

A major new component to neuroblastoma therapy, in addition to chemotherapy, surgery, and radiation, is immunotherapy. Several different antibodies exist to target ganglioside GD2, which is expressed on the surface of neuroblastoma cells [24]. These immunotherapies have been incorporated into neuroblastoma treatment as an important component of maintenance therapy but require careful monitoring during and following infusion due to their side-effect profile. Dinutuximab is a commercially available chimeric human-murine monoclonal antibody to GD2. A similar monoclonal antibody, Hu3F8, is used at Memorial Sloan Kettering Cancer Center (MSKCC). These antibodies are associated with infusion-related side effects that are important for pediatric critical care practitioners. Dinutuximab is infused in the inpatient setting, sometimes in the PICU, with infusions from 10 to 20 hours for 4 consecutive days. Hu3F8 is given in the outpatient setting over 30 minutes every other day for a total of three doses per cycle.

During the infusion, pain is the most common adverse event, with grades 3–4 pain in the abdomen, back, and extremities occurring in about 50% of patients [25]. GD2 is expressed on neuroblastoma cells, but also on peripheral nerve cells, leading to severe pain during infusion often requiring high doses of opioids for management. Respiratory depression requiring reversal of narcotics with naloxone can occur due to the opioid doses needed to achieve adequate pain control. In some cases, adequate pain control can only be achieved with continuous infusions of analgesics such as opioids with dexmedetomidine, lidocaine, or ketamine, each of which has adverse effects of which the critical care physician should be aware. Opioids with dexmedetomidine can lead to hypotension and bradycardia [26]. Continuous lidocaine infusion is generally safe but has a narrow therapeutic window, with toxicity leading to CNS depression [27]. Ketamine infusions are well tolerated without hallucinations or respiratory compromise but can lead to dysphoria and nystagmus [28, 29]. These alternative or adjuvant analgesics improve pain control and may also decrease opioid use.

These antibodies are also immunogenic and can generate anaphylactic-like hypersensitivity responses, bronchospasm, urticaria, hypotension, hypertension, and capillary leak [25]. Anaphylaxis and anaphylactoid reactions can be treated with epinephrine. Bronchospasm responds to short-acting beta-agonists such as albuterol. Rash and urticaria are managed with antihistamines. Hypotension and capillary leak respond to fluid resuscitation. In patients receiving both antihistamines and opioids, the hypotension can be more profound, requiring multiple fluid boluses, although patients generally tolerate the periods of hypotension and maintain perfusion and mentation while receiving fluids.

Hypertension is seen acutely with pain but can also be a later effect with Hu3F8 and has been linked to posterior reversible encephalopathy syndrome (PRES) [30]. PRES can present with headache, altered mental status, visual disturbances, and seizure. It is diagnosed based on clinical and radiographic findings. Patients with PRES frequently require management in the PICU for close neurological monitoring. Treatment involves blood pressure control, optimization of electrolytes, and antiepileptic medications as needed for seizures [31].

Spinal Cord Compression

Neuroblastoma can extend from the sympathetic chain into the spinal canal and cause peripheral nerve root or spinal cord compression. Additionally, leptomeningeal disease or osseous metastases can lead to spinal cord compression. Spinal cord compression in neuroblastoma is seen in about 10–15% of cases, most frequently in progressive, terminal disease, but it can be a presenting symptom in 1–4% on cases [32]. Spinal cord compression requires rapid treatment to prevent permanent neurologic sequelae, although even with treatment up to 50% of patients have residual neurologic deficits [33]. Treatment modalities include neurosurgical decompression, radiation therapy, high-dose systemic glucocorticoids, and chemotherapy. The best treatment modality to prevent long-term neurologic sequelae remains unclear, and each treatment modality is associated with short- and long-term complications.

Chemotherapy can be used for treatment of intraspinal neuroblastoma, but does not provide immediate relief of spinal cord compression symptoms. Neurosurgical decompression provides the most immediate relief of symptoms, but it is not clear if there is any difference in long-term outcomes in these patients. Radiation can also provide rapid relief of symptoms but is associated with long-term side effects, especially in young, developing children. For patients who have disease progression and subsequent spinal cord compression despite chemotherapy, neurosurgery or radiation therapy is an appropriate treatment [33]. Glucocorticoids can reduce edema and provide rapid relief of symptoms but also have not necessarily been shown to impact long-term outcomes [33]. Treatment of these patients often involves multidisciplinary teams including the PICU, neurosurgery, and oncology to determine the best approach for each patient.

Surgery and Surgical Complications

Surgical resection is an important component of neuroblastoma treatment. The surgeries are often long, technically difficult cases that involve dissection of tissue in the thorax, abdomen, and sometimes the spine. Average operative time is around 8.5 hours, and average estimated blood loss is around 30 cc/kg [34]. These procedures involve retroperitoneal lymph node dissection, hepatic lobe biopsy, and dissection of the tumor from major surrounding vasculature including the renal arteries, mesenteric arteries, and the aorta. Additionally, most of the surgeries are done via a thoracoabdominal approach leading to placement of a thoracostomy tube and manipulation of the diaphragm. Fluid shifts following surgery can result in hemodynamic instability (hypotension, decreased urine output, and poor perfusion). Patients often require multiple fluid boluses in the first 24–48 hours postoperatively, and around 33% of patients require vasoactive medications for fluid refractory hemodynamic instability. Patients may remain intubated following surgery for 1–4 days (average 1.5 days). In a minority of patients, around 3%, the best surgical procedure requires nephrectomy. Additional surgical complications include small bowel obstruction (3%), systemic or local infection postoperatively (3%), and clinically significant intraoperative bleeding (6%) [34].

Metastatic Osteosarcoma

Osteogenic sarcoma is the most common bone tumor in children and young adults [35]. Though the overall survival in osteosarcoma is roughly 75% [36], metastatic disease to the lung can occur within the first 12 months after initiation of treatment

[37]. Relapse of osteosarcoma in the lung occurs in greater than 30% of patients [38]. The survival in children with metastatic disease to the lung has as low as a 40% and 22% 3-year and 5-year survival, respectively [39]. As a result, children with metastatic disease to the lung are in need of complete resection in order to maximize survival benefit. Systemic therapies are not as reliable a treatment modality for improving survival, as the ability to achieve complete resection is the most relevant prognostic factor for long-term survival [40]. Children undergoing open thoracotomy for metastatic disease resection represent an important patient population for many PICUs. While not solely a PICU issue, the comprehensive care from preoperative planning through discharge provides an important framework for discussion of the multidisciplinary, comprehensive care plan which can be so effective for children undergoing major surgery, both in the chest and in the abdomen.

Surgical Approach

The surgical approach to patients with pulmonary metastatic disease varies based on several clinical factors. While the majority of patients presenting with pulmonary metastatic disease have bilateral pulmonary disease, there may be between 24% and 40% of patients who present with unilateral disease [38]. For those presenting with bilateral pulmonary disease, it remains controversial as to approach this as a single-stage operation via median sternotomy or staged thoracotomies [38, 39].

The most common approach to either unilateral or bilateral metastatic disease is via thoracotomy. Postoperative complications from thoracotomy surgery include pleural pain, bleeding, respiratory failure, and need for mechanical ventilation [39]. Management of these predictable issues often falls to the multidisciplinary team caring for the patient in the PICU or acute care ward. For patients undergoing thoracotomy surgery, thoracic epidural pain management has proven to be a safe and effective mode of nonsystemic pain relief [41, 42]. Avoidance of systemic narcotics and sedatives has significant advantages in the "fast-track" surgical approach to perioperative care (discussed below) and at reducing the risk for oversedation and the development of delirium in the postoperative period [43]. While the majority of patients undergoing thoracotomy do not have other significant postoperative issues beyond pain, those who have intraoperative bleeding complications may continue to have significant bleeding postoperatively requiring frequent blood transfusion or even re-exploration to stop active bleeding [39].

Desmoplastic Round Blue Cell Tumor

Desmoplastic round blue cell tumors (DSRCT) represent a very small percentage of solid tumors in children. In fact, a recent publication found a total of 450 cases in the literature since its discovery in 1989 [44]. However, the novel approach to this rare tumor gives insight into the future of multimodality treatment of solid tumors which may be relevant to those who care for critically ill children.

Sharing some biological similarities to both Ewing sarcoma and Wilms tumor, DSRCT is thought to originate in the peritoneum and spread locally to the intraperitoneal organs. Without surgical debulking, it is universally fatal [45]. The most generally accepted treatment regimens involve Ewing-like regimen involving cyclophosphamide or ifosfamide, doxorubicin, and vincristine, surgical cytoreduction, and radiotherapy [44–46]. The surgical cytoreduction can be a big surgery. As the tumors can be as large as 40 cm, and invading multiple intraperitoneal organs, the cases can be quite long (up to 12 hours), with complications consistent with other long surgeries that have significant fluid shifts [45, 47, 48]. Surgery entails resection of tumor implants commonly found on the omentum, diaphragm, spleen, Morrison's pouch, abdominal wall peritoneum, small bowel mesentery, and pelvis [47, 48]. Pain, fluid shifts, systemic inflammatory response, wound dehiscence, and surgical site infections are all possible following this surgery [48].

In addition to the standard regimen of systemic chemotherapy, cytoreduction therapy, and radiation, there have been a variety of studies aimed at addressing the residual intraperitoneal nodules [44, 47, 48]. The use of hyperthermic intraperitoneal chemotherapy (HIPEC) in some uterine cancers has shown some efficacy [49, 50]. The same approach has been explored in the use of hyperthermic cisplatin or oxaliplatin +/− mitomycin and/or irinotecan in DSRCT [51, 52]. The data as of yet are inconclusive, and the use of HIPEC is best used in the framework of a clinical trial. The early studies of the use of HIPEC had clinically relevant side effects to the pediatric intensivist with renal failure and urinary tract infection complications [48]. Another potential therapy targeting residual intraperitoneal tumor in DSRCT is the use of immunotherapy remote from the tumor debulking surgery. The efficacy of intraperitoneal ^{131}I-8H9, which targets surface cell antigen 4Ig-B7H3 expressed in DSRCT, is currently being evaluated. In this protocol, an intraperitoneal catheter is placed during the debulking surgery, and intraperitoneal 8H9 is instilled via surgically placed intraperitoneal catheter as an adjunct to the systemic chemotherapy, cytoreductive surgery, and radiotherapy (Abstract presented at Connective Tissue Oncology Society Annual Meeting, 2016).

Enhanced Recovery After Surgery

Enhanced recovery after surgery (ERAS) programs are designed to utilize a multidisciplinary team to optimize recovery for postoperative patients, leading to increased patient (and caregiver) satisfaction, efficient use of hospital resources, and reduced hospital length of stay without increasing the rate of readmission [53]. The concepts for ERAS derive from the experience of adult patients undergoing elective colonic surgery [54], elective rectal and pelvic surgery [55], and pancreaticoduodenectomy [56]. The elements of the adult-derived ERAS programs highlight the surgical experience in totality, from preadmission counseling through maximization of intraoperative pain management with mid-thoracic epidural anesthesia/analgesia and short-acting anesthetic agents, careful use of intraoperative fluids, postoperative mobilization plan, nonnarcotic pain management, prevention of nausea and vomiting, minimizing drains and catheters, and stimulation of gut motility [57]. These principles have been documented in children undergoing large abdominal surgeries for inflammatory bowel disease [53] and can be applied to our patients undergoing surgery for metastatic osteosarcoma, neuroblastoma, and DSRCT as well as other common thoracic and abdominal surgeries performed on children with solid tumors.

Applying these concepts to children has been retrospectively documented for relatively common surgical procedures such as appendectomy [58], renal surgery [59, 60], and even cardiac surgery [61]. Furthermore, these concepts have also been evaluated in prospective studies in ambulatory surgeries [62], as well as in pediatric colorectal surgery specifically [53].

Though there may be institution-dependent variation, our experience at MSKCC has been positive, with all elective surgeries now being screened for participation in ERAS. Areas of focus include preoperative, intraoperative, and postoperative, although there are several elements of ERAS that span the entirety of the perioperative period, from preadmission screening to follow-up after discharge. Several elements are critical for success:

- Active patient involvement
- Audit of compliance and outcomes
- Multidisciplinary team involvement

Preoperative

ERAS is intended to encompass the entirety of the surgical experience for patients and their families. The elements in the preoperative arena are:

- Targeted patient and parent education and selective bowel preparation
- Reduced fasting duration
- Carbohydrate "preload" drinks
- After admission and before the initiation of surgery, non-opioid analgesia and regional anesthesia barring any contraindications
- Active patient and parent involvement
- Appropriate management of expectations from the multidisciplinary team.

Intraoperative

Intraoperatively, the surgical and anesthesiology teams work together to improve the perioperative experience. Important aspects of the intraoperative experience include:

- Actively warming of the patients to maintain normothermia.
  - The use of Bair Hugger and warmed intravenous fluids as necessary
- Goal-directed fluid therapy to minimize water and sodium overload.
- Maximizing regional anesthesia so as to decrease opioid use.
- Alternatively, non-opioid infusions can be used with anesthetic inhalational agents to provide appropriate sedation and analgesia for the case.
- Postoperative nausea and vomiting protocols that include dexamethasone and ondansetron.
- Close attention to the need (or lack of need) for postoperative drains to remain in place, including nasogastric tubes.

Postoperative

Postoperative care focuses on return of normal function. The multidisciplinary team works together to achieve the goal of timely, appropriate discharge while meeting the postoperative needs of the patient. The important elements include:

- Minimizing intravenous fluids
- Initiating early oral nutrition when appropriate
- Early indwelling urinary catheter removal
- Early ambulation to aid in reducing postoperative ileus and delirium

Throughout the perioperative period, there is also a focus on active patient involvement (including clear discharge criteria), active multidisciplinary team involvement, and continued auditing of compliance and outcomes for quality improvement. This comprehensive team approach involves representation from hospital administration, nursing, advanced practice providers, anesthesia, surgery, pediatrics, child life, physical and occupational therapy, nutrition, and the pediatric ERAS coordinator. In studies in routine pediatric surgery, length of stay was reduced, as well as reduced post-discharge convalescence [53, 62]. Whether these results are reproducible in a pediatric oncology population is a question actively being investigated.

References

1. Acker SN, Linton J, Tan GM, Garrington TP, Bruny J, Hilden JM, et al. A multidisciplinary approach to the management of anterior mediastinal masses in children. J Pediatr Surg. 2015;50(5):875–8. https://doi.org/10.1016/j.jpedsurg.2014.09.054.
2. Carter BW, Marom EM, Detterbeck FC. Approaching the patient with an anterior mediastinal mass: a guide for clinicians. J Thorac Oncol. 2014;9(9 Suppl 2):S102–9. https://doi.org/10.1097/jto.0000000000000294.

3. Priola AM, Priola SM, Cardinale L, Cataldi A, Fava C. The anterior mediastinum: diseases. Radiol Med. 2006;111(3):312–42. https://doi.org/10.1007/s11547-006-0032-5.
4. Shamberger RC, Holzman RS, Griscom NT, Tarbell NJ, Weinstein HJ. CT quantitation of tracheal cross-sectional area as a guide to the surgical and anesthetic management of children with anterior mediastinal masses. J Pediatr Surg. 1991;26(2):138–42.
5. Bechard P, Letourneau L, Lacasse Y, Cote D, Bussieres JS. Perioperative cardiorespiratory complications in adults with mediastinal mass: incidence and risk factors. Anesthesiology. 2004;100(4):826–34. discussion 5A.
6. Stricker PA, Gurnaney HG, Litman RS. Anesthetic management of children with an anterior mediastinal mass. J Clin Anesth. 2010;22(3):159–63. https://doi.org/10.1016/j.jclinane.2009.10.004.
7. Shamberger RC. Preanesthetic evaluation of children with anterior mediastinal masses. Semin Pediatr Surg. 1999;8(2):61–8.
8. Shamberger RC, Holzman RS, Griscom NT, Tarbell NJ, Weinstein HJ, Wohl ME. Prospective evaluation by computed tomography and pulmonary function tests of children with mediastinal masses. Surgery. 1995;118(3):468–71.
9. Blank RS, de Souza DG. Anesthetic management of patients with an anterior mediastinal mass: continuing professional development. Can J Anaesth. 2011;58(9):853. https://doi.org/10.1007/s12630-011-9539-x.
10. Erdos G, Kunde M, Tzanova I, Werner C. Anaesthesiological management of mediastinal tumors. Anaesthesist. 2005;54(12):1215–28. https://doi.org/10.1007/s00101-005-0895-1.
11. Choi YH, Lee DH. A rare airway obstruction caused by dissection of a reinforced endotracheal tube. J Emerg Med. 2018. https://doi.org/10.1016/j.jemermed.2017.12.043.
12. Kim SH, Park AY, Cho HB, Yoo JH, Park SY, Chung JW, et al. A rare case of nonresterilized reinforced ETT obstruction caused by a structural defect: a case report. Medicine. 2017;96(48):e8886. https://doi.org/10.1097/md.0000000000008886.
13. Shim SM, Park JH, Hyun DM, Lee HM. Airway obstruction by dissection of the inner layer of a reinforced endotracheal tube in a patient with Ludwig's angina: a case report. J Dent Anesth Pain Med. 2017;17(2):135–8. https://doi.org/10.17245/jdapm.2017.17.2.135.
14. Gardner JC, Royster RL. Airway collapse with an anterior mediastinal mass despite spontaneous ventilation in an adult. Anesth Analg. 2011;113(2):239–42. https://doi.org/10.1213/ANE.0b013e31821f9c95.
15. Asai T. Emergency cardiopulmonary bypass in a patient with a mediastinal mass. Anaesthesia. 2007;62(8):859–60. https://doi.org/10.1111/j.1365-2044.2007.05210.x.
16. Said SM, Telesz BJ, Makdisi G, Quevedo FJ, Suri RM, Allen MS, et al. Awake cardiopulmonary bypass to prevent hemodynamic collapse and loss of airway in a severely symptomatic patient with a mediastinal mass. Ann Thorac Surg. 2014;98(4):e87–90. https://doi.org/10.1016/j.athoracsur.2014.06.104.
17. Sendasgupta C, Sengupta G, Ghosh K, Munshi A, Goswami A. Femoro-femoral cardiopulmonary bypass for the resection of an anterior mediastinal mass. Indian J Anaesth. 2010;54(6):565–8. https://doi.org/10.4103/0019-5049.72649.
18. Polaner DM. The use of heliox and the laryngeal mask airway in a child with an anterior mediastinal mass. Anesth Analg. 1996;82(1):208–10.
19. Bigham MT, Nowak JE, Wheeler DS. Therapeutic application of helium-oxygen and mechanical ventilation in a child with acute myelogenous leukemia and airway obstruction. Pediatr Emerg Care. 2009;25(7):469–72. https://doi.org/10.1097/PEC.0b013e3181aba7de.
20. Whittle SB, Smith V, Doherty E, Zhao SB, McCarty S, Zage PE. Overview and recent advances in the treatment of neuroblastoma. Expert Rev Anticancer Ther. 2017;17(4):369–86. https://doi.org/10.1080/14737140.2017.1285230.
21. Matthay KK, Maris JM, Schleiermacher G, Nakagawara A, Mackall CL, Diller L, et al. Neuroblastoma. Nat Rev Dis Primers. 2016;2:21. https://doi.org/10.1038/nrdp.2016.78.
22. Sait S, Modak S. Anti-GD2 immunotherapy for neuroblastoma. Expert Rev Anticancer Ther. 2017;17(10):889–904. https://doi.org/10.1080/14737140.2017.1364995.

23. Matthay KK, Villablanca JG, Seeger RC, Stram DO, Harris RE, Ramsay NK, et al. Treatment of high-risk neuroblastoma with intensive chemotherapy, radiotherapy, autologous bone marrow transplantation, and 13-cis-retinoic acid. N Engl J Med. 1999;341(16):1165–73. https://doi.org/10.1056/nejm199910143411601.
24. Cheung NKV, Kushner BH, Yeh SDJ, Larson SM. 3F8 monoclonal antibody treatment of patients with stage 4 neuroblastoma: a phase II study. Int J Oncol. 1998;12(6):1299–306.
25. Yu AL, Gilman AL, Ozkaynak MF, London WB, Kreissman SG, Chen HX, et al. Anti-GD2 antibody with GM-CSF, interleukin-2, and isotretinoin for neuroblastoma. N Engl J Med. 2010;363(14):1324–34. https://doi.org/10.1056/NEJMoa0911123.
26. Gorges M, West N, Deyell R, Winton P, Cheung W, Lauder G. Dexmedetomidine and hydromorphone: a novel pain management strategy for the oncology ward setting during anti-GD2 immunotherapy for high-risk neuroblastoma in children. Pediatr Blood Cancer. 2015;62(1):29–34. https://doi.org/10.1002/pbc.25197.
27. Wallace MS, Lee J, Sorkin L, Dunn JS, Yaksh T, Yu A. Intravenous lidocaine: effects on controlling pain after anti-GD(2) antibody therapy in children with neuroblastoma – a report of a series. Anesth Analg. 1997;85(4):794–6. https://doi.org/10.1097/00000539-199710000-00014.
28. Zempsky WT, Loiselle KA, Corsi JM, Hagstrom JN. Use of low-dose ketamine infusion for pediatric patients with sickle cell disease-related pain a case series. Clin J Pain. 2010;26(2):163–7. https://doi.org/10.1097/AJP.0b013e3181b511ab.
29. Bredlau AL, Thakur R, Korones DN, Dworkin RH. Ketamine for pain in adults and children with cancer: a systematic review and synthesis of the literature. Pain Med. 2013;14(10):1505–17. https://doi.org/10.1111/pme.12182.
30. Kushner BH, Modak S, Basu EM, Roberts SS, Kramer K, Cheung NKV. Posterior reversible encephalopathy syndrome in neuroblastoma patients receiving anti-G(D2) 3F8 monoclonal antibody. Cancer. 2013;119(15):2789–95. https://doi.org/10.1002/cncr.28137.
31. Neil EC, Hanmantgad S, Khakoo Y. Neurological complications of pediatric cancer. J Child Neurol. 2016;31(12):1412–20. https://doi.org/10.1177/0883073815620673.
32. Punt J, Pritchard J, Pincott JR, Till K. Neuro-blastoma – a review of 21 cases presenting with spinal-cord compression. Cancer. 1980;45(12):3095–101. https://doi.org/10.1002/1097-0142(19800615)45:12<3095::aid-cncr2820451236>3.0.co;2-y.
33. Kraal K, Blom T, van Noesel M, Kremer L, Caron H, Tytgat G, et al. Treatment and outcome of neuroblastoma with intraspinal extension: a systematic review. Pediatr Blood Cancer. 2017;64(8):12. https://doi.org/10.1002/pbc.26451.
34. Ross SLP, Greenwald BM, Howell JD, Pon S, Rutigliano DN, Spicyn N, et al. Outcomes following thoracoabdominal resection of neuroblastoma. Pediatr Crit Care Med. 2009;10(6):681–6. https://doi.org/10.1097/PCC.0b013e3181a708c1.
35. Dorfman HD, Czerniak B. Bone cancers. Cancer. 1995;75(1 Suppl):203–10.
36. Meyers PA, Schwartz CL, Krailo MD, Healey JH, Bernstein ML, Betcher D, et al. Osteosarcoma: the addition of muramyl tripeptide to chemotherapy improves overall survival – a report from the Children's Oncology Group. J Clin Oncol. 2008;26(4):633–8. https://doi.org/10.1200/jco.2008.14.0095.
37. Chi SN, Conklin LS, Qin J, Meyers PA, Huvos AG, Healey JH, et al. The patterns of relapse in osteosarcoma: the Memorial Sloan-Kettering experience. Pediatr Blood Cancer. 2004;42(1):46–51. https://doi.org/10.1002/pbc.10420.
38. Su WT, Chewning J, Abramson S, Rosen N, Gholizadeh M, Healey J, et al. Surgical management and outcome of osteosarcoma patients with unilateral pulmonary metastases. J Pediatr Surg. 2004;39(3):418–23. https://doi.org/10.1016/j.jpedsurg.2003.11.030.
39. Harting MT, Blakely ML, Jaffe N, Cox CS Jr, Hayes-Jordan A, Benjamin RS, et al. Long-term survival after aggressive resection of pulmonary metastases among children and adolescents with osteosarcoma. J Pediatr Surg. 2006;41(1):194–9. https://doi.org/10.1016/j.jpedsurg.2005.10.089.

40. Heaton TE, Hammond WJ, Farber BA, Pallos V, Meyers PA, Chou AJ, et al. A 20-year retrospective analysis of CT-based pre-operative identification of pulmonary metastases in patients with osteosarcoma: a single-center review. J Pediatr Surg. 2017;52(1):115–9. https://doi.org/10.1016/j.jpedsurg.2016.10.034.
41. Chou J, Chan CW, Chalkiadis GA. Post-thoracotomy pain in children and adolescence: a retrospective cross-sectional study. Pain Med (Malden, Mass). 2014;15(3):452–9.
42. Soliman IE, Apuya JS, Fertal KM, Simpson PM, Tobias JD. Intravenous versus epidural analgesia after surgical repair of pectus excavatum. Am J Ther. 2009;16(5):398–403. https://doi.org/10.1097/MJT.0b013e318187de3e.
43. Traube C, Augenstein J, Greenwald B, LaQuaglia M, Silver G. Neuroblastoma and pediatric delirium: a case series. Pediatr Blood Cancer. 2014;61(6):1121–3. https://doi.org/10.1002/pbc.24917.
44. Honore C, Amroun K, Vilcot L, Mir O, Domont J, Terrier P, et al. Abdominal desmoplastic small round cell tumor: multimodal treatment combining chemotherapy, surgery, and radiotherapy is the best option. Ann Surg Oncol. 2015;22(4):1073–9. https://doi.org/10.1245/s10434-014-4123-6.
45. Lal DR, Su WT, Wolden SL, Loh KC, Modak S, La Quaglia MP. Results of multimodal treatment for desmoplastic small round cell tumors. J Pediatr Surg. 2005;40(1):251–5. https://doi.org/10.1016/j.jpedsurg.2004.09.046.
46. Kushner BH, LaQuaglia MP, Wollner N, Meyers PA, Lindsley KL, Ghavimi F, et al. Desmoplastic small round-cell tumor: prolonged progression-free survival with aggressive multimodality therapy. J Clin Oncol. 1996;14(5):1526–31. https://doi.org/10.1200/jco.1996.14.5.1526.
47. Hayes-Jordan A, LaQuaglia MP, Modak S. Management of desmoplastic small round cell tumor. Semin Pediatr Surg. 2016;25(5):299–304. https://doi.org/10.1053/j.sempedsurg.2016.09.005.
48. Zmora O, Hayes-Jordan A, Nissan A, Kventsel I, Newmann Y, Itskovsky K, et al. Cytoreductive surgery (CRS) and hyperthermic intraperitoneal chemotherapy (HIPEC) for disseminated intraabdominal malignancies in children-a single-institution experience. J Pediatr Surg. 2017. https://doi.org/10.1016/j.jpedsurg.2017.09.014.
49. Stirrups R. HIPEC improves survival in stage III epithelial ovarian cancer. Lancet Oncol. 2018. https://doi.org/10.1016/s1470-2045(18)30065-2.
50. van Driel WJ, Koole SN, Sikorska K, Schagen van Leeuwen JH, HWR S, RHM H, et al. Hyperthermic intraperitoneal chemotherapy in ovarian cancer. N Engl J Med. 2018;378(3):230–40. https://doi.org/10.1056/NEJMoa1708618.
51. Hayes-Jordan AA, Coakley BA, Green HL, Xiao L, Fournier KF, Herzog CE, et al. Desmoplastic small round cell tumor treated with cytoreductive surgery and hyperthermic intraperitoneal chemotherapy: results of a phase 2 trial. Ann Surg Oncol. 2018. https://doi.org/10.1245/s10434-018-6333-9.
52. Honore C, Atallah V, Mir O, Orbach D, Ferron G, LePechoux C, et al. Abdominal desmoplastic small round cell tumor without extraperitoneal metastases: is there a benefit for HIPEC after macroscopically complete cytoreductive surgery? PLoS One. 2017;12(2):e0171639. https://doi.org/10.1371/journal.pone.0171639.
53. West MA, Horwood JF, Staves S, Jones C, Goulden MR, Minford J, et al. Potential benefits of fast-track concepts in paediatric colorectal surgery. J Pediatr Surg. 2013;48(9):1924–30. https://doi.org/10.1016/j.jpedsurg.2013.02.063.
54. Gustafsson UO, Scott MJ, Schwenk W, Demartines N, Roulin D, Francis N, et al. Guidelines for perioperative care in elective colonic surgery: Enhanced Recovery After Surgery (ERAS(R)) Society recommendations. Clin Nutr (Edinburgh, Scotland). 2012;31(6):783–800. https://doi.org/10.1016/j.clnu.2012.08.013.
55. Nygren J, Thacker J, Carli F, Fearon KC, Norderval S, Lobo DN, et al. Guidelines for perioperative care in elective rectal/pelvic surgery: Enhanced Recovery After Surgery (ERAS(R))

Society recommendations. Clin Nutr (Edinburgh, Scotland). 2012;31(6):801–16. https://doi.org/10.1016/j.clnu.2012.08.012.
56. Lassen K, Coolsen MM, Slim K, Carli F, de Aguilar-Nascimento JE, Schafer M, et al. Guidelines for perioperative care for pancreaticoduodenectomy: Enhanced Recovery After Surgery (ERAS(R)) Society recommendations. Clin Nutr (Edinburgh, Scotland). 2012;31(6):817–30. https://doi.org/10.1016/j.clnu.2012.08.011.
57. Fearon KC, Ljungqvist O, Von Meyenfeldt M, Revhaug A, Dejong CH, Lassen K, et al. Enhanced recovery after surgery: a consensus review of clinical care for patients undergoing colonic resection. Clin Nutr (Edinburgh, Scotland). 2005;24(3):466–77. https://doi.org/10.1016/j.clnu.2005.02.002.
58. Grewal H, Sweat J, Vazquez WD. Laparoscopic appendectomy in children can be done as a fast-track or same-day surgery. JSLS. 2004;8(2):151–4.
59. Mohamed M, Hollins G, Eissa M. Experience in performing pyelolithotomy and pyeloplasty in children on day-surgery basis. Urology. 2004;64(6):1220–2 discussion 2–3. https://doi.org/10.1016/j.urology.2004.08.065.
60. Mulholland TL, Kropp BP, Wong C. Laparoscopic renal surgery in infants 10 kg or less. J Endourol. 2005;19(3):397–400. https://doi.org/10.1089/end.2005.19.397.
61. Vricella LA, Dearani JA, Gundry SR, Razzouk AJ, Brauer SD, Bailey LL. Ultra fast track in elective congenital cardiac surgery. Ann Thorac Surg. 2000;69(3):865–71.
62. Reismann M, Dingemann J, Wolters M, Laupichler B, Suempelmann R, Ure BM. Fast-track concepts in routine pediatric surgery: a prospective study in 436 infants and children. Langenbeck's Arch Surg. 2009;394(3):529–33. https://doi.org/10.1007/s00423-008-0440-1.

Chapter 5
Primary Immunodeficiency Diseases

Fayhan Alroqi, Abdulrahman Alsultan, and Mohammed Essa

Introduction

The immune system has a fundamental role in protection from infection. One manner of protection is mediated by innate immunity through blocking the entry of microbes and mediating inflammation and subsequent direct microbial killing [1]. Another mode of defense is necessary for the elimination of those pathogens that resist innate immunity. For that reason, adaptive immunity ensured by T and B lymphocytes is important to maintain proper protection [2]. Several studies have shown high rate of infections in patients who have deleterious genetic mutations that affect immune system and lead to primary immunodeficiency diseases (PIDs). The International Union of Immunological Societies listed in their recent report more than 350 PIDs. PIDs are classified according to the primary defective component of

F. Alroqi (✉)
Department of Pediatric, King Abdullah Specialized Children's Hospital, Riyadh, Saudi Arabia

King Saud bin Abdulaziz University for Health Sciences, Riyadh, Saudi Arabia

King Abdullah International Medical Research Center, Riyadh, Saudi Arabia

A. Alsultan
Department of Pediatric, King Abdullah Specialized Children's Hospital, Riyadh, Saudi Arabia

Department of Pediatric, College of Medicine, King Saud University, Riyadh, Saudi Arabia

M. Essa
Department of Pediatric, King Abdullah Specialized Children's Hospital, Riyadh, Saudi Arabia

King Saud bin Abdulaziz University for Health Sciences, Riyadh, Saudi Arabia

C. N. Duncan et al. (eds.), *Critical Care of the Pediatric Immunocompromised Hematology/Oncology Patient*, https://doi.org/10.1007/978-3-030-01322-6_5

the immune system. Defects of innate immunity include congenital defects of phagocyte number or function, Toll-like receptors (TLR) signaling pathway deficiency, and complement deficiencies. On the other hand, PIDs due to defect in adaptive immunity include severe combined immunodeficiencies (SCIDs), combined immunodeficiencies (CIDs) with or without syndromic features, antibody deficiencies, and immune dysregulation [3].

Patients with PID are most often present with recurrent infections that range from mild infection to severe sepsis with multi-organ failure. They can also present with other manifestations including allergy, autoimmunity, persistent inflammation, lymphoproliferation, and cancers [4]. Therapeutic options for PID patients range from starting antimicrobial agents and immunoglobulin replacement therapy to the advanced treatments like hematopoietic cell transplantation and gene therapy. This group of patients requires an urgent management to decrease disease-associated morbidity and mortality. However, a significant number of those patients need critical care management because of life-threatening complications.

The aim of this review is to highlight the defining features of PIDs as well as their classification and phenotypes with particular emphasis on the management of these serious disorders.

Normal Immune System

The immune system is a very complex system that has a crucial role in protecting our body from dangerous invaders. These invaders can elicit immune responses and include a wide range of infectious and noninfectious antigens. Therefore, the immune system must be able to defend against different types of microbial antigens. This protective measure explains the high frequency of the infectious complications in those patients with immune system defects. It is also important for this system to recognize the harmful noninfectious antigens such as foreign macromolecules, tumor cells, and transplanted organs or tissues. Our immune system has the capability to differentiate between self- and nonself antigens to avoid attacking the body's own tissue. Failure of this fundamental property, self-tolerance, results in immune dysregulation and autoimmunity. In this section, we will outline the normal functions of innate and adaptive immunity.

Innate Immunity

Innate or naïve immunity is the first line of defense that provides a nonspecific and immediate protection against a wide variety of organisms. It is a mature system that does not require previous exposure to the pathogen to work effectively. This immune response is important in preventing and controlling infections by promoting inflammation and antiviral defense as well as stimulating the adaptive immune system to respond to the invading antigens. It provides protection through multiple defensive mechanisms including (1) physical and chemical barriers such as the skin, mucous membranes, low stomach pH, lysozymes, and others; (2) proteins that include complements, C-reactive protein, and cytokines; and (3) numerous cells such as granulocytes, macrophages, dendritic cells, natural killer cells, and other innate lymphoid cells. This part of the immune system uses molecules and receptors such as Toll-like receptors and NOD-like receptors to recognize invaders by identifying the common shared structures between classes of microbes (pathogen-associated molecular patterns) or some molecules released from damaged cells (damaged-associated molecular patterns) [5].

Adaptive Immunity

There are two types of adaptive or acquired immunity: cellular and humoral immunity. The main cellular components of humoral immunity are B lymphocytes, while the T lymphocytes are the main component of cellular immunity. Both lymphocytes, B and T, developed from bone marrow stem cells that give rise to the common lymphoid progenitors. B lymphocytes continue steps of differentiation in the bone marrow starting from the stage of pro-B cells to the mature B cells that subsequently move to the secondary lymphoid organs. These mature B cells proliferate on exposure to foreign antigens and differentiate into plasma cells that secrete antibodies. Those antibodies are vital for protection against extracellular organisms as they neutralize toxins, prevent the entry of pathogens, and activate the complement system to enhance microbial phagocytosis. On the other hand, T lymphocytes differentiate into mature T cells and get trained to recognize self- and nonself antigens in thymus. Subsequently, they move on from thymus to the blood and lymphoid organs as variable cell subsets including T-helper cells (CD4), T-cytotoxic cells (CD8), and T-regulatory cells. Cell-mediated immunity is important for protection against intracellular organisms like some bacteria, viruses, fungi, and parasites. The T-cell response starts with microbial phagocytosis by antigen-presenting cells like macrophages, which process and present the antigen on their cell surface. T-helper cells recognize the presented antigen and initiate activation and proliferation of multiple cells including phagocytes, B cells, cytotoxic T cells, and other cells to promote an effective destruction of the microbe. For subsequent exposures, cellular immunity is important in the development of memory T and B cells that is needed to mount future immune responses against previous antigens. Finally, both innate and adaptive immunity need to have good collaboration to provide effective defense against invaders [6].

Primary Immunodeficiency Diseases

Defects in innate or adaptive immunity can lead to serious disorders known as immunodeficiency disorders. These immune defects are classified into primary (congenital) and secondary (acquired) immunodeficiencies. PIDs are a heterogeneous group of genetic disorders that lead to increased susceptibility to infections, tumors, and/or autoimmunity. Secondary immunodeficiency disorders are not inherited like PIDs but acquired during life as a consequence of other causes, such as severe malnutrition, immunosuppressive medications, or infections. In this section, we will focus on the classification and the clinical manifestations of PIDs [7].

Classification

PIDs are classified according to the clinical features and the primary component of the immune system that is affected. Innate immunity disorders include congenital phagocytic disorders, complement deficiencies, Toll-like receptor (TLR) pathway defects, and interleukin-12/interferon-gamma (IL-12/INF-γ) pathway defects. Adaptive immunity disorders include humoral immune defects like hypogammaglobulinemia and cellular immune defects such as DiGeorge syndrome. Most of the defects in cellular immunity lead to combined immunodeficiencies (CIDs) or even severe combined immunodeficiencies (SCIDs) which highlights the importance of cellular immunity in providing effective B-cell-mediated antibody production and class switching [3].

Clinical Manifestations

The clinical manifestations of PIDs are variable according to the component of the immune system that is primarily disrupted (Table 5.1).

Innate Immunodeficiencies

Phagocytes: Microbial phagocytosis by macrophages and neutrophils is one of the most important mechanisms of innate immunity. The phagocytic defects range from defects in phagocytic number like neutropenia to defects in migration or intracellular killing like leukocyte adhesion defects (LAD) and chronic granulomatous disease (CGD). Patients with phagocytic defects suffer from recurrent chest infections, lymphadenitis, deep-seated abscesses, and oral stomatitis. Those infections are usually due to bacterial (catalase positive bacteria), fungal (*Candida and Aspergillus*), and mycobacterial infections [8, 9].

Complements: The complement system is an essential part of innate immunity as it promotes inflammation (C3a, C5a), opsonization (C3b), and microbial killing (membrane attack complex). It consists of three pathways: classical, alternative, and lectin pathway. Early classical pathway defects (C1q, C1r, C1s, C4, C2, C3) lead to autoimmunity and increased risk of infections due to encapsulated organisms, while late classical pathway defects (C5–C9) as well as alternative pathway

Table 5.1 Classification and clinical presentations of primary immunodeficiency diseases

Classification	Examples	Clinical manifestations
Immunodeficiencies affecting cellular and humoral immunity	Severe combined immunodeficiencies	Respiratory and gastrointestinal infections. Oral thrush and disseminated BCGitis
	Combined immunodeficiencies	Respiratory and gastrointestinal infections and liver/biliary tract disease
Combined immunodeficiencies with associated or syndromic features	Wiskott-Aldrich syndrome	Thrombocytopenia with small platelets, recurrent bacterial and viral infections, bloody diarrhea, eczema, lymphoma, and autoimmune disease
	Ataxia-telangiectasia	Ataxia, telangiectasia, pulmonary infections, lymphoreticular and other malignancies, increased alpha fetoprotein, increased radiosensitivity, and chromosomal instability
Predominantly antibody deficiencies	Agammaglobulinemia	Severe bacterial infections with absent B cells
	Common variable immunodeficiency	Clinical phenotypes vary: most have recurrent infections, some have polyclonal lymphoproliferation, autoimmune cytopenias, and/or granulomatous disease
Diseases of immune dysregulation	IPEX (immune dysregulation, polyendocrinopathy, enteropathy X-linked)	Autoimmune enteropathy, early-onset diabetes, thyroiditis, hemolytic anemia, thrombocytopenia, eczema, elevated IgE, and IgA.
	Familial hemophagocytic lymphohistiocytosis (HLH)	Fever, hepatosplenomegaly HLH, and cytopenias
Congenital defects of phagocyte number or function	Leukocyte adhesion deficiency	Delayed cord separation, skin ulcers, periodontitis, leukocytosis
	Chronic granulomatous disease	Infections with deep-seated abscesses, autoinflammatory, and IBD phenotype
Defects in intrinsic and innate immunity	Mendelian susceptibility to mycobacterial disease (MSMD)	Susceptibility to mycobacteria and salmonella
	TLR signaling pathway deficiency with bacterial susceptibility	Pyogenic bacterial infections
Complement deficiencies	Deficiency in early complement pathway components (C1q, C1r, C2, C4)	Systemic lupus erythematosus, multiple autoimmune diseases and infections with encapsulated organisms
	Deficiency in late complement pathway components (C5, C6, C7, C8, C9)	Neisserial infections

defects (factor D, properdin) are associated with recurrent meningitis caused by *Neisseria* species [10].

Toll-Like receptors: TLRs, pattern recognition receptors, are important in recognizing different microbes and dying cells. Defects in TLRs lead to a wide range of infections. TLR3 pathway defects increase the risk for herpes simplex encephalitis, while defects in myeloid differentiation primary response 88 (MyD88) and interleukin-1 receptor-associated kinase 4 (IRAK4) are associated with increased susceptibility to pyogenic bacterial infections that cause meningitis or other invasive infections.

IL-12/INF-γ pathway: Patients with disseminated mycobacterial disease and recurrent infections with *Salmonella* species or herpesviruses should be screened for defects in IL-12/INF-γ pathway. Genetic defects in this pathway lead to Mendelian susceptibility to mycobacterial disease (MSMD). These defects include mutations in INF-γ receptor 1/2, IL-12 p40, IL-12 receptor B1, signal transducer and activator of transcription1 (*STAT1*), interferon-stimulated gene15 (*ISG15*), and interferon regulatory factor 8 (*IRF8*). In addition to IL-12/INF-γ pathway defects, the risk for disseminated mycobacterial diseases is increased in other disorders that involve NF-κB pathway like NF-κB essential modulator (NEMO) deficiency [11].

Humoral Immunodeficiencies

Humoral immune defects are the most common type of PIDs. Patients with antibody deficiency, due to defective B-cell development, maturation, and/or function, present with recurrent sinopulmonary infections and chronic suppurative otitis media. The most common isolated organisms are extracellular microbes like *Streptococcus pneumoniae*, *Haemophilus influenzae*, and *Moraxella catarrhalis*. Defects in humoral immunity might lead to other clinical manifestations including skin abscesses, viral meningitis, intestinal giardiasis, lung lymphocytic infiltration, and autoimmunity [12].

Cellular Immunodeficiencies

SCIDs are the most serious form of cellular immunodeficiencies in which there is a profound defect in lymphocyte-dependent adaptive immunity. Patients with SCID usually start to acquire life-threatening infections early in life and typically die in infancy if untreated. These infections include pneumonia, meningitis, chronic diarrhea, and disseminated viral, bacterial, and mycobacterial diseases. The most common isolated organisms are the intracellular pathogens that include *Candida albicans*, *Pneumocystis jirovecii*, *Cryptosporidium*, *Mycobacterium* species, and herpesviruses. There is also an increased susceptibility to extracellular organisms in patients with SCID due to defective antibody response that might be attributed to intrinsic B-cell defect or lack of T-cell help. Physical examination reveals failure to thrive, oral thrush, skin rash, lack of palpable lymphoid tissue, and absence of thymic shadow in chest imaging. SCIDs are classified according to the peripheral lymphocytic profile to four general categories including $T^-/B^+/NK^+$, $T^-/B^+/NK^-$, $T^-/B^-/NK^+$, and $T^-/B^-/NK^-$ [13]. CIDs and leaky SCIDs like Omenn syndrome might present like the classical SCID, but they are usually less severe due to the presence of residual T-lymphocyte number and/or function [14].

Immune Dysregulation

Some forms of PID are associated with significant autoimmunity and lymphoproliferation due to defective immune tolerance. Central immune tolerance for cellular immunity is achieved in thymic tissue by clonal deletion or successful inactivation of the autoreactive T-cell clones that recognize self-antigens with high affinity [15]. Compelling evidence has shown high rates of autoimmunity in genetic disorders that affect thymic central tolerance like the observed profound immune dysregulatory manifestations in autoimmune polyendocrinopathy-candidiasis-ectodermal dystrophy syndrome due to *AIRE* gene mutation [16]. Peripheral immune tolerance is important for the autoreactive T cells that escaped thymic tissue to the periphery. This kind of tolerance is usually obtained by the suppressive function of the T-regulatory cells [17]. Defects that affect T-regulatory cell number and/or function, like the immunodysregulation, polyendocrinopathy, enteropathy, and X-linked inheritance syndrome (IPEX) and IPEX-like disorders, present with autoimmunity, lymphoproliferation with lymphocytic infiltration in multiple organs, and allergic disorders [18]. Immune homeostasis in the periphery is also achieved by apoptosis of these autoreactive lymphocytes. Autoimmune lymphoproliferative syndrome (ALPS) is an example of immune dysregulation due to defect in apoptosis [19].

Diagnosis

The diagnosis of PID is readily entertained when a patient presents with unexplained frequent or invasive infections. A detailed history including family history and physical examination are important to delineate the possible underlying defect of the immune system that leads to high microbial susceptibility and other immune complications. The laboratory evaluation is essential for the diagnosis of primary immunodeficiency and also for providing early effective treatment that leads to reduced patient morbidity and mortality (Table 5.2) [20].

Investigation of patients with putative phagocytic defect includes absolute neutrophilic count (ANC) and peripheral blood smear for congenital neutropenia, serial ANCs for cyclic neutropenia, oxidative burst test for CGD and CD18 expression for LAD1. Patients who have sinopulmonary infections and or autoimmunity should be screened for suspected complement deficiency by measuring C3 and C4 levels as well as testing the total hemolytic complement activity (CH50) and alternative pathway hemolytic activity (AP50). Regarding TLRs, it can be tested independently by measuring IL-1β, IL-6, TNF-α, and CXCL10 productions after the stimulation of peripheral blood mononuclear cells with TLR-specific ligands.

Evaluation of humoral immunodeficiency involves B lymphocyte enumeration by flow cytometry, measurement of serum immunoglobulins (IgA, IgM, IgG, and IgE), and specific antibody titers in response to protein and polysaccharide antigens. It is important to compare serum immunoglobulin levels with the age-adjusted normal values. If any specific antibody titer is below normal range, it is recommended

Table 5.2 Laboratory tests of immune function

Immune function	Screening tests
Humoral immunity	Serum immunoglobulin levels Serum-specific antibody titers Flow cytometry to enumerate B-cell subsets
Cellular immunity	T-cell receptor excision circles (TREC) newborn screening Flow cytometry to enumerate T-cell subsets and NK cells In vitro proliferative response to mitogens and antigens
Phagocytic cells	Blood cell count with differential Neutrophil staining, morphology on a peripheral blood smear Dihydrorhodamine (DHR) reduction or nitro blue tetrazolium Flow cytometry for adhesion molecules
Complement	CH50 assay (total hemolytic complement activity) AH50 assay (alternative pathway hemolytic activity) Level or function of individual complement components Lectin pathway function

to revaccinate the patient with killed vaccine and to assess the titer 4–6 weeks after vaccination.

The initial evaluation for patients with an underlying cellular immune defect is obtained by calculating the absolute lymphocyte count (ALC). It is important to exclude HIV infection in patients with low lymphocytic count before entertaining the diagnosis of PID due to cellular immune defect. Lymphocyte enumeration, naive/memory T-cell flow cytometry, and T-lymphocyte proliferations after both antigen and mitogen stimulation are helpful in confirming a diagnosis of SCID or CID.

Genetic testing is widely available nowadays. Knowing the genetic defect is important not only for confirming diagnosis but also essential for anticipating prognosis and family counseling [21].

Complications

Patients with PID are prone to multiple complications that need urgent diagnosis and appropriate management. Some of these complications are attributed to progression of the disease, while others are secondary to the offered therapy like Hematopoietic cell transplantation (HCT). In this section, we will discuss some of the complications related to the disease progression.

Infectious Complications

The knowledge of the type of immunodeficiency is crucial to guide us for the best empirical antimicrobial treatment as the early administration and appropriateness of antimicrobials are major prognostic factors in treating sepsis in PID patients [22]. The main infections for antibody and complement deficiencies are sinopulmonary infections due to extracellular encapsulated organisms. Infections due to

Table 5.3 Type of organisms associated with PIDs

Immune defect	Type of organisms
Antibody deficiencies	Enteroviruses
	Encapsulated organisms (*Streptococcus pneumoniae*, *Haemophilus influenzae*, *Moraxella catarrhalis*, and *Staphylococcus aureus*). *Pseudomonas aeruginosa*, *Mycoplasma*
	Giardia lamblia
SCIDs/CIDs	CMV, EBV, RSV, and other viruses
	Encapsulated organisms and other organisms like *Listeria monocytogenes* and gram-negative organisms
	Atypical mycobacterium, including BCGitis
	Candida species, *Aspergillus* species, and other fungal infections
	Pneumocystis jirovecii, *Toxoplasma gondii*, *Cryptosporidium parvum*
Phagocytic defects	Catalase-positive organisms (*Staphylococcus aureus*, *Pseudomonas*, *Burkholderia*, and *Serratia*)
	Atypical mycobacterium
	Candida, *Aspergillus*, and *Nocardia*
Complement deficiencies	Encapsulated organisms (*Streptococcus pneumoniae* and *Neisseria*)

intracellular organisms like Gram-negative bacteria, fungal, and mycobacterium are more prominent in cellular and phagocytic immune defects. Chest infection attributed to *Pneumocystis jirovecii* is classically described in patients with severe CD4 lymphopenia like those patients with SCID. Viral infections and other opportunistic infections are likely to occur early in SCID patients but usually later in CID. The main observed viruses in humeral immunodeficiency are enteroviruses while in cellular immunodeficiency they are herpesviruses (CMV, HSV, VZV, HHV6) and respiratory viruses such as influenza, RSV, and adenovirus (Table 5.3).

Noninfectious Complications

Pulmonary complications: Pulmonary complications are very common in patients with PID. Most of these complications are attributed to the infection of either upper airway leading to sinusitis and otitis media or lower airway and lung parenchyma causing bronchiolitis, bronchitis, pneumonia, and lung abscesses. Noninfectious pulmonary complications also have been reported among patients with PID. Chronic bronchiectasis is a major pulmonary complication in humoral and combined immunodeficiencies. Chest high-resolution computed tomography (HRCT) should be considered for all immunodeficient patients with chronic chest symptoms to monitor their disease progression. High-dose immunoglobulin replacement therapy, aggressive antibiotic treatment, and physiotherapy are the most important preventive measures. Interstitial lung disease (ILD) is another noninfectious complication especially in those with humoral immunodeficiency. ILD includes lymphocytic interstitial pneumonia, follicular bronchiolitis, granulomatous lung disease, and organizing pneumonia. Granulomatous-lymphocytic interstitial lung disease (GLILD) is the most common form of ILD that is associated with poor clinical outcomes, and using immunosuppressive therapies like rituximab and azathioprine can lead to clinical improvement. Patients with PID may also present with hilar and/or mediastinal adenopathies either due to infections, lymphoproliferative disorders, or malignancy. Organizing pneumonia (OP), known as bronchiolitis obliterans, is a relatively rare complication in PID patients. It is recommended to do inspiratory and expiratory HRCT to show the characteristic air trapping, alveolar opacities, and ground-glass consolidation. Lung biopsy might be considered to confirm the diagnosis. There are other rare complications that should be considered in PID patients including pulmonary alveolar proteinosis in patients with SCID due to adenosine deaminase deficiency and pulmonary dysgenesis in patients with DiGeorge syndrome [23–25].

Hemophagocytic lymphohistiocytosis (HLH) in PIDs: HLH is a life-threatening syndrome that should be considered in any critically ill child who has history of persistent fever, hepatosplenomegaly, and pancytopenia. It is caused by hyperstimulated but inefficient immune system that results in hyperinflammatory response and cytokine storm [26]. Diagnosis is based on fulfillment of HLH-2004 diagnostic criteria [27]. HLH is a known complication of some PIDs such as SCID, CID, and CGD. Most cases of HLH in PID are associated with infections. Viral infections due to EBV, CMV, and adenovirus are frequently observed with HLH in SCID and CID patients, while bacterial, fungal, and Leishmanial infections are more associated with HLH in CGD patients [28]. Although an etoposide-based regimen (HLH-94) is the standard treatment protocol in patients with familial HLH and XLP, there is no consistent approach to treat HLH in patients with PID [29]. Steroids and IVIG are important components of therapy; however, the use of etoposide might be harmful in some patients [28]. The addition of rituximab should be considered in EBV-induced HLH [30]. The definitive therapy for PID patients who presents with HLH is HCT.

Autoimmunity: Autoimmunity is a significant manifestation of PID that presents with antibody-mediated inflammation and lymphoproliferation [31]. The most common autoimmune disorders in PID patients are immune thrombocytopenic purpura (ITP) and autoimmune hemolytic anemia (AIHA). IVIG, steroids, rituximab, sirolimus, abatacept, and ultimately HCT are examples of treatment strategies to manage autoimmunity in PID [32].

Inflammation and autoimmunity in Omenn syndrome (OS): Oligoclonal autoreactive T cells in Omenn syndrome can trigger a severe inflammatory reaction that affects multiple organs causing generalized skin erythroderma, hepatosplenomegaly, lymphadenopathy, and other autoimmune manifestations. OS is associated with hypereosinophilia, high IgE, and high memory cells in the absence of maternal engraftment [14]. It is important to diagnose OS promptly to start immunosuppressive therapies such as steroids and cyclosporine to suppress the autoreactive T-cell clones and to ameliorate the autoimmune manifestations prior to HCT [33].

Graft-versus-host disease (GVHD) secondary to transplacental maternal engraftment (TME): The immune system in normal newborns eliminates maternal T cells that pass through the placenta. However, typical SCID patients might not be able to reject transplacental maternal T cells leading to persistent TME [34]. TME in SCID patients might be uneventful; however, some patients will have features of GVHD, mostly in the skin and liver, that could be severe and resemble OS [35]. In addition, TME increases the risk of GVHD and possibility of graft rejection posttransplant in SCID patients [34, 36]. It is imperative that all SCID patients receive irradiated blood products to prevent transfusion-associated GVHD that could be fatal and it occurs secondary to engraftment and proliferation of transfused T cells [37].

Management

General Medical Management

PID patient needs urgent medical treatment to eliminate disease-associated complications [7]. Treatment of the innate immunity disorders depends on the type of defect. Phagocytic defects are primarily managed by supportive therapy that includes antibiotic such as cotrimoxazole and antifungal such as itraconazole prophylaxis. INF-γ-replacement therapy was reported to be beneficial in patients with CGD. Subcutaneous recombinant granulocyte colony-stimulating factor has been used successfully to increase ANC in severe congenital neutropenia.

Immunoglobulin G (Ig) replacement therapy is the mainstay of therapy in antibody deficiency. It comes in different preparations that can be given through intravenous access (IVIG) or subcutaneously (SCIG). The usual dose of IVIG is 400–600 mg/kg/month, while the usual dose of SCIG is 100 mg/kg/week. Providing higher doses of Ig has been reported to be effective in treating some complications of hypogammaglobinemia like bronchiectasis, viral meningoencephalitis, and autoimmunity. Prophylactic antibiotic such as amoxicillin might be beneficial in those patients who are continuing to have persistent sinopulmonary infections despite optimal Ig replacement therapy.

Patients with SCID or CID require aggressive management with Ig replacement therapy and prophylactic antibiotic (cotrimoxazole) to decrease infection-related morbidity and mortality. Antifungal and antiviral prophylactic therapies are usually recommended for high-risk patients. Infections should be treated aggressively with parenteral broad-spectrum antibiotics that will be narrowed subsequently based on the results of cultures. Positive pressure isolation and meticulous skin and mucosal hygienic care are necessary to avoid infections. Good nutritional support is recommended for those patients with diarrhea and failure to thrive. Blood products must be irradiated and lymphocyte depleted to prevent fatal (GVHD). Patients should avoid all live virus vaccines as they could develop disease from attenuated viruses and may even die after exposure to these vaccines. Babies with SCID should avoid breastfeeding from CMV-seropositive mothers. Enzyme replacement therapy with polyethylene glycol-modified bovine adenosine deaminase (PEG-ADA) is recommended for the management of SCID patients due to adenosine deaminase deficiency before HCT [21]. Immunosuppressive medications might be used to control autoimmunity in PID patients and also to control the persistent inflammation that associated with maternal engraftment or autoreactive leaky SCID like Omenn syndrome [38].

Critical Care Management
Patients with PID are at high risk for morbidity and mortality due to their underlying compromised immune systems. The most common reason for admission to pediatric intensive care unit (PICU) is infectious pulmonary complications that require assessed ventilation. Avoiding intubation and mechanical ventilation if possible is a major goal in the management of respiratory failure in PID patients as the mortality risk is higher in those patients requiring ventilation support [39]. Severe infections that need broad-spectrum antibiotics and inotropic support are important indications for critical care management. Sepsis and pneumonia were reported to be the most common causes of death in PID patients. For that reason, infections in this group of patients need urgent intervention to avoid major complications [40]. Empirical broad-spectrum antimicrobial treatment should be initiated as soon as possible in any event of fever or more severe symptoms. It is very important to monitor central line devices and to consider antibiotic locks if needed. Persistent positive blood culture may require central line removal.

Other complications that necessitate PICU management include bleeding, acute kidney injury (AKI), cardiac, and liver dysfunction. Early diagnosis and appropriate interventions that include inotropic support and renal replacement therapy might be life-saving in critically ill PID patients.

There are several risk factors that predict poor outcome in PID patients including requirement of mechanical ventilation, the use of inotropes and renal replacement therapy, presence of organ failures, higher pediatric logistic organ dysfunction (PELOD) score, and prolonged length of PICU stay [39]. Previous studies showed that the overall mortality rate of PID patients was 1.99% [41]. The highest rate was seen in younger children less than 5 years of age due to the early in life presentation of SCID and other severe forms of PID. Mortality rate varied considerably between patients affected by different PID categories. The death rate was highest among patients with combined T- and B-cell immunodeficiency, familial HLH, and neutrophil dysfunction [40].

Hematopoietic Cell Transplantation
Allogeneic (HCT) is the treatment of choice in many immunodeficiency disorders including SCIDs, CIDs and phagocytic disorders [42]. The purpose of transplantation in PIDs is to replace the defective immune cells, i.e., restoring the immune system with a functional lymphocytes or neutrophils. However, if the defect is in trafficking at the thymus level, HCT may not solve the problem such as DiGeorge syndrome. HCTs include transplantation from matched or mismatched related and unrelated donors, cord blood transplantation, and haploidentical transplantation.

Since SCID is fatal, HCT should be initiated as soon as possible. Using stem cells from an (HLA)-matched sibling, it provides good immune recovery and excellent long-term outcome. Encouraging results have been reported among patients with SCID who underwent HCT at the age of 3.5 months or younger regardless of donor type [43]. However, the outcome of HCT is less satisfactory in older patients except for those who have no active infections at the time of transplantation. Patients with some types of SCID can receive stem cells without conditioning therapy – this will correct T cells, but B cells may take longer time to recover. Many experts consider giving conditioning or immunosuppressive therapy in Omenn syndrome with autoreactive T cells or SCID with maternal engraftment. The rate of complications is higher in patients with radiation-sensitive SCID and Omenn syndrome who do not have HLA-matched sibling donors [44].

Recently, many patients with combined immunodeficiencies have been identified and offered HCT with conditioning therapy as a potentially curative treatment option. The intensity of the regimen depends on the underlying genetic defect, patient factors such as the presence of active infection, and the source of stem cells. HCT from a matched sibling donor provides curative treatment for patients with Wiskott-Aldrich syndrome [45]. Results from matched unrelated donors are also good, but mixed chimerism and autoimmune cytopenia are common posttransplantations.

Although, patients with immune dysregulation and autoimmunity benefit from immunosuppressive therapies, alternative strategies can be considered depending on the severity of the underlying defect. In particular, HCT is highly recommended for patients with IPEX and IPEX-like disorders [46].

Cellular therapy is the treatment of choice for phagocytic defects like CGD and LAD who have HLA-matched family donors. Overall survival in patients with CGD is currently around 93% after using reduced intensity regimen with no obvious difference between transplants from related and unrelated donors [47].

HCT should be considered without delay in patients with X-linked lymphoproliferative disease (XLP) and Chediak-Higashi syndrome (CHS). Immunosuppressive treatment is required to treat the accelerated phase in XLP. HCT can cure the hematological and immunological manifestations of CHS, but it does not prevent progressive neurological deterioration [48].

Gene Therapy

Gene therapy involves introducing normal genetic material into patient's cells to compensate for the abnormal gene. It is currently being investigated in patients with certain SCIDs, such as X-linked SCID and ADA deficiency, especially if no available matched sibling donor [49]. Prospective studies are required to follow the duration of immune reconstitution status post-gene therapy and to document the long-term safety of these gene-transduced cells in human.

Conclusions

The immune system is essential for protection from infectious and noninfectious invaders. This protection is achieved by collaboration between innate and adaptive immunity. Congenital defect in innate or adaptive immunity leads to PID. There are more than 350 PIDs that are classified according to the defective component of the immune system. Although the most common presentation of PID is recurrent infections, other manifestations are common including allergic disorders, autoimmunity, lymphoproliferation, and cancers. PID patients are at high risk for morbidity and mortality due to the underlying immune defect and the presence of complications. Pulmonary complications and sepsis are the most common indications for PICU care. The management of PIDs varies from medical treatment with IVIG and prophylactic antibiotic to advanced therapies like HCT and gene therapy.

Conflict of Interest The authors declare that they have no conflict of interest.

References

1. Medzhitov R, Janeway C Jr. Innate immune recognition: mechanisms and pathways. Immunol Rev. 2000;173:89–97.
2. Cooper MD, Alder MN. The evolution of adaptive immune systems. Cell. 2006;124(4):815–22.
3. Picard C, et al. International union of immunological societies: 2017 primary immunodeficiency diseases committee report on inborn errors of immunity. J Clin Immunol. 2018;38(1):96–128.
4. Bousfiha A, et al. Primary immunodeficiencies of protective immunity to primary infections. Clin Immunol. 2010;135(2):204–9.
5. Turvey SE, Broide DH. Innate immunity. J Allergy Clin Immunol. 2010;125(2 Suppl 2):S24–32.
6. Bonilla FA, Oettgen HC. Adaptive immunity. J Allergy Clin Immunol. 2010;125(2 Suppl 2):S33–40.
7. Notarangelo LD. Primary immunodeficiencies. J Allergy Clin Immunol. 2010;125(2 Suppl 2):S182–94.
8. Leiding JW, Holland SM. Chronic granulomatous disease. In: Adam MP, et al., editors. GeneReviews((R)). Seattle: University of Washington; 1993.
9. Etzioni A. Defects in the leukocyte adhesion cascade. Clin Rev Allergy Immunol. 2010;38(1):54–60.
10. Frank MM. Complement deficiencies. Pediatr Clin N Am. 2000;47(6):1339–54.
11. Al-Muhsen S, Casanova JL. The genetic heterogeneity of mendelian susceptibility to mycobacterial diseases. J Allergy Clin Immunol. 2008;122(6):1043–51. quiz 1052–3.
12. Conley ME, et al. Primary B cell immunodeficiencies: comparisons and contrasts. Annu Rev Immunol. 2009;27:199–227.
13. Fischer A, et al. Severe combined immunodeficiencies and related disorders. Nat Rev Dis Primers. 2015;1:15061.
14. Shearer WT, et al. Establishing diagnostic criteria for severe combined immunodeficiency disease (SCID), leaky SCID, and Omenn syndrome: the Primary Immune Deficiency Treatment Consortium experience. J Allergy Clin Immunol. 2014;133(4):1092–8.
15. Ohashi PS. Negative selection and autoimmunity. Curr Opin Immunol. 2003;15(6):668–76.
16. Peterson P, et al. APECED: a monogenic autoimmune disease providing new clues to self-tolerance. Immunol Today. 1998;19(9):384–6.
17. Sakaguchi S, et al. Pillars article: immunologic self-tolerance maintained by activated T cells expressing IL-2 receptor alpha-chains (CD25). Breakdown of a single mechanism of self-tolerance causes various autoimmune diseases. J Immunol. 1995. J Immunol. 2011;186(7):3808–21.
18. Alroqi FJ, Chatila TA. T regulatory cell biology in health and disease. Curr Allergy Asthma Rep. 2016;16(4):27.
19. Rieux-Laucat F. Inherited and acquired death receptor defects in human Autoimmune Lymphoproliferative Syndrome. Curr Dir Autoimmun. 2006;9:18–36.

20. Oliveira JB, Fleisher TA. Laboratory evaluation of primary immunodeficiencies. J Allergy Clin Immunol. 2010;125(2 Suppl 2):S297–305.
21. Bonilla FA, et al. Practice parameter for the diagnosis and management of primary immunodeficiency. J Allergy Clin Immunol. 2015;136(5):1186–205.e1–78.
22. Aguilar C, et al. Prevention of infections during primary immunodeficiency. Clin Infect Dis. 2014;59(10):1462–70.
23. Buckley RH. Pulmonary complications of primary immunodeficiencies. Paediatr Respir Rev. 2004;5(Suppl A):S225–33.
24. Yazdani R, et al. Infectious and noninfectious pulmonary complications in patients with primary immunodeficiency disorders. J Investig Allergol Clin Immunol. 2017;27(4):213–24.
25. Chase NM, et al. Use of combination chemotherapy for treatment of granulomatous and lymphocytic interstitial lung disease (GLILD) in patients with common variable immunodeficiency (CVID). J Clin Immunol. 2013;33(1):30–9.
26. Janka GE, Lehmberg K. Hemophagocytic syndromes – an update. Blood Rev. 2014;28(4):135–42.
27. Henter JI, et al. HLH-2004: diagnostic and therapeutic guidelines for hemophagocytic lymphohistiocytosis. Pediatr Blood Cancer. 2007;48(2):124–31.
28. Bode SF, et al. The syndrome of hemophagocytic lymphohistiocytosis in primary immunodeficiencies: implications for differential diagnosis and pathogenesis. Haematologica. 2015;100(7):978–88.
29. Bergsten E, et al. Confirmed efficacy of etoposide and dexamethasone in HLH treatment: long-term results of the cooperative HLH-2004 study. Blood. 2017;130(25):2728–38.
30. Vadyvaloo V, et al. Transit through the flea vector induces a pretransmission innate immunity resistance phenotype in Yersinia pestis. PLoS Pathog. 2010;6(2):e1000783.
31. Rae W, et al. Autoimmunity/inflammation in a monogenic primary immunodeficiency cohort. Clin Transl Immunol. 2017;6(9):e155.
32. Vignesh P, Rawat A, Singh S. An update on the use of immunomodulators in primary immunodeficiencies. Clin Rev Allergy Immunol. 2017;52(2):287–303.
33. Villa A, Notarangelo LD, Roifman CM. Omenn syndrome: inflammation in leaky severe combined immunodeficiency. J Allergy Clin Immunol. 2008;122(6):1082–6.
34. Wahlstrom J, et al. Transplacental maternal engraftment and posttransplantation graft-versus-host disease in children with severe combined immunodeficiency. J Allergy Clin Immunol. 2017;139(2):628–633.e10.
35. Muller SM, et al. Transplacentally acquired maternal T lymphocytes in severe combined immunodeficiency: a study of 121 patients. Blood. 2001;98(6):1847–51.
36. Palmer K, et al. Unusual clinical and immunologic manifestations of transplacentally acquired maternal T cells in severe combined immunodeficiency. J Allergy Clin Immunol. 2007;120(2):423–8.
37. Sebnem Kilic S, Kavurt S, Balaban Adim S. Transfusion-associated graft-versus-host disease in severe combined immunodeficiency. J Investig Allergol Clin Immunol. 2010;20(2):153–6.
38. Walter JE, et al. Mechanism-based strategies for the management of autoimmunity and immune dysregulation in primary immunodeficiencies. J Allergy Clin Immunol Pract. 2016;4(6):1089–100.
39. Odek C, et al. Patients with primary immunodeficiencies in pediatric intensive care unit: outcomes and mortality-related risk factors. J Clin Immunol. 2014;34(3):309–15.
40. Al-Herz W, Moussa MA. Survival and predictors of death among primary immunodeficient patients: a registry-based study. J Clin Immunol. 2012;32(3):467–73.
41. Rubin Z, et al. Prevalence and outcomes of primary immunodeficiency in hospitalized children in the United States. J Allergy Clin Immunol Pract. 2018;6(5):1705–10.
42. Antoine C, et al. Long-term survival and transplantation of haemopoietic stem cells for immunodeficiencies: report of the European experience 1968–99. Lancet. 2003;361(9357):553–60.
43. Buckley RH. Molecular defects in human severe combined immunodeficiency and approaches to immune reconstitution. Annu Rev Immunol. 2004;22:625–55.

44. Pai SY, et al. Transplantation outcomes for severe combined immunodeficiency, 2000–2009. N Engl J Med. 2014;371(5):434–46.
45. Shin CR, et al. Outcomes following hematopoietic cell transplantation for Wiskott-Aldrich syndrome. Bone Marrow Transplant. 2012;47(11):1428–35.
46. Barzaghi F, et al. Long-term follow-up of IPEX syndrome patients after different therapeutic strategies: an international multicenter retrospective study. J Allergy Clin Immunol. 2018;141(3):1036–1049.e5.
47. Gungor T, et al. Reduced-intensity conditioning and HLA-matched haemopoietic stem-cell transplantation in patients with chronic granulomatous disease: a prospective multicentre study. Lancet. 2014;383(9915):436–48.
48. Seo JJ. Hematopoietic cell transplantation for hemophagocytic lymphohistiocytosis: recent advances and controversies. Blood Res. 2015;50(3):131–9.
49. Fischer A, Cavazzana-Calvo M. Gene therapy of inherited diseases. Lancet. 2008;371(9629): 2044–7.

Chapter 6
Care of the Critically Ill Pediatric Sickle Cell Patient

Tolulope Rosanwo, Jennifer A. McArthur, and Natasha Archer

Introduction and Chapter Overview

Sickle cell disease (SCD) is the most common inherited genetic disease in the United States with 1 in 13 Americans of African descent found to be carriers (sickle cell trait) and an estimated 100,000 individuals living with the disease. The incidence of SCD in West and Central Africa is even more pervasive as 1000 babies with SCD are born daily, and 1 in 4 Africans in the regions with the highest incidence of SCD have the trait [1].

Sickle hemoglobin (Hb S) within the red blood cell (RBC) polymerizes under hypoxic conditions. Hb S polymerization distorts the cell's biconcave shape and characteristic flexibility, providing the main pathological bases of this disease, hemolysis and vaso-occlusion (Fig. 6.1). Occluded and damaged vasculature contributes to pan-organ damage impacting the cardiovascular, hepatic, splenic, musculoskeletal, neurological, renal, and pulmonary systems predominantly.

T. Rosanwo
Case Western Reserve University School of Medicine,
Cleveland, OH, USA

J. A. McArthur
Department of Pediatrics, Division of Critical Care Medicine,
St. Jude Children's Research Hospital, Memphis, TN, USA

Medical College of Wisconsin, Milwaukee, WI, USA
e-mail: jennifer.mcarthur@stjude.org

N. Archer (✉)
Department of Pediatric Hematology and Oncology,
Dana-Farber Boston Children's Cancer and Blood Disorders Center,
Harvard Medical School, Boston, MA, USA
e-mail: Natasha.Archer@childrens.harvard.edu

C. N. Duncan et al. (eds.), *Critical Care of the Pediatric Immunocompromised Hematology/Oncology Patient*, https://doi.org/10.1007/978-3-030-01322-6_6

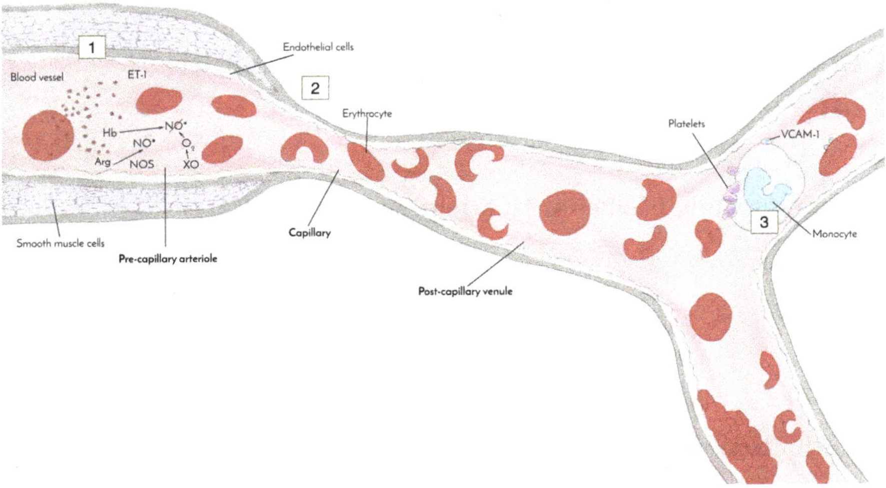

Fig. 6.1 The pathology of sickle cell disease. (1) Intracellular sickle hemoglobin (Hb S) polymerization contributes to the hallmark red cell deformation seen in SCD. Intravascular hemolysis releases hemoglobin, activating endothelin-1 (ET-1). ET-1 inactivates the production of nitric oxide (NO) from arginine, exacerbating vasoconstriction. (2) Inflexible sickled cells vaso-occlude capillaries resulting in ischemia and infarction. (3) SCD is an inflammatory state. Red cells adhere to platelet-monocyte aggregations *via* adhesion molecules like vascular cell adhesion protein 1 (VCAM-1) in vaso-occlusive episodes. Hydroxyurea, one of the two FDA-approved pharmacological treatments for pediatric sickle cell disease, reduces sickling via the upregulation of fetal hemoglobin production and the reduction of circulating leukocytes, reducing inflammation and vaso-occlusion)

SCD is a debilitating disorder, and all patients are at high risk of both sudden and deadly vaso-occlusive complications. The most common indication for intensive care unit (ICU) admission is acute chest syndrome (ACS) [1]. Shock, stroke, and multiple organ failure are also potential causes of critical illness (Fig. 6.2) [2, 3]. In the United States and Great Britain, pediatric SCD patients account for roughly 2% of pediatric ICU (PICU) admissions. Eight percent of SCD patients will require at least one ICU admission within an 8-year follow-up [4], and 13% of patients with ACS will require ICU admission and mechanical ventilation [5]. Even more alarming, the mortality of SCD patients admitted to the ICU can be as high as 44% [6]. Timely admission to the ICU facilitates better outcomes for patients, and it is imperative for physicians to regard even apparently uncomplicated vaso-occlusive episodes as potentially life threatening.

This chapter will highlight the impact of SCD-related organ damage in a critically ill pediatric patient and outline evidenced-based strategies for management in the intensive care setting.

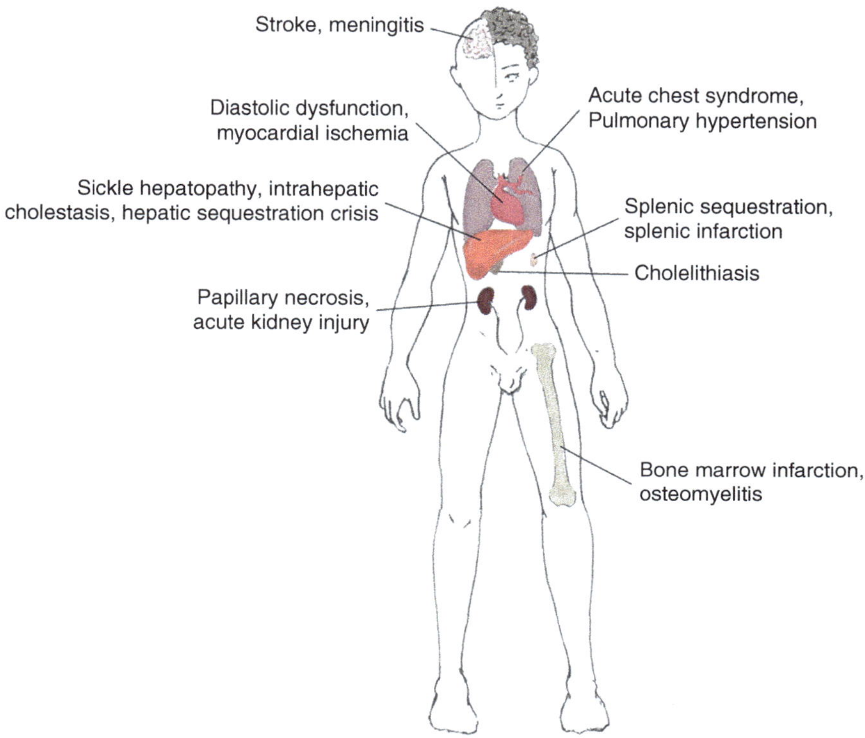

Fig. 6.2 Acute complications of sickle cell disease (Acute complications of SCD can impact nearly every organ system. Acute chest syndrome and stroke are leading causes of ICU admission. Each acute complication will be addressed in the chapter sections below)

Cardiovascular Concerns

23.4% of SCD adult death at home or in the hospital is sudden [7]. This figure is not known in children, although pediatric patients with sickle cell trait alone have a 21-fold higher risk of sudden cardiac death than those with completely normal hemoglobin [8]. The cardiac concerns discussed below, particularly cardiomegaly, left ventricular dysfunction, arrhythmias, and pulmonary hypertension (PH), contribute to sudden cardiac death [9]. Appropriate management of the cardiac consequences of SCD will reduce this risk in the critical SCD ICU patient.

Baseline Cardiovascular Pathology in SCD

Cardiomegaly and Left Ventricular Dysfunction

The SCD patient's underlying anemia reduces their oxygen-carrying capacity despite increased baseline cardiac output [10]. Severe anemia correlates with ventricular dilation leading to both compensatory hypertrophy and increased left ventricular (LV) mass. The sustained elevated cardiac output contributes to the cardiomegaly seen in most sickle cell patients after 3 years of age [11]. Enlarged hearts despite usually normal coronary vasculature put children with lower hemoglobin levels at risk for induced ischemic ECG changes [12]. It is also to be noted that children with LV hypertrophy have lower average sleep and waking oxygen saturation. Sleep studies are informative predictors of cardiomegaly risk. An ACE inhibitor like enalapril can reduce cardiac remodeling in advanced cases. SCD patients are also prone to LV dysfunction although the link between vaso-occlusion and reduced ventricular contractility is not apparent.

Cardiac Consequences of Iron Overload

Twenty percent of children with SCA are regularly transfused to reduce their stroke and ACS risk. The regular supply of RBCs, "bags" of iron-containing hemoglobin can push patients into an iron-overloaded state with cardiac consequences. Free iron fuels the formation of reactive oxidative species (ROS), leading to lipid, protein, and DNA abnormalities. In this toxic state during which transferrin is fully bound to iron, non-transferrin bound iron (NTBI) enters cardiomyocytes as ferrous iron via L-type Ca^{2+}(voltage-dependent) channels. Iron accumulates in the epicardium, ventricular septum, papillary muscles, and ventricular wall.

Iron deposition begins first in the ventricular myocardium and then the atrial myocardium [10]. The accumulation clinically manifests as progressive cardiac dysfunction beginning with diastolic dysfunction followed by systolic dysfunction and heart failure [13]. First-degree heart block and supraventricular arrhythmias are also lethal consequences of cardiac iron toxicity [14].

Diagnosis via signs of cardiotoxicity measured by ECG, echocardiogram, and radionucleotide angiography are not suggested as these are not apparent until late/severe stages of iron overload. T2* magnetic resonance for cardiac iron, however, is a noninvasive way to detect iron deposition in subclinical patients.

ICU Concerns

High-output cardiac failure and high-grade diastolic dysfunction and PH are the most common cardiac concerns in the ICU in adult patients but are usually less severe in pediatric patients.

Diastolic Dysfunction

Both diastolic dysfunction and PH are poor prognostic indicators for SCD ICU patients. In a cohort of 107 patients between 3 and 18 years of age, 11.2% had PH, a lower percentage than found in adults (32%), and grade I diastolic dysfunction was seen in the majority of patients [11, 15]. Like cardiomegaly, diastolic dysfunction in children is elevated in patients with lower sleeping and waking oxygen desaturation [16]. Non-transfused patients often have a larger LV mass than transfused patients. LV end-diastolic diameter, end-systolic diameter, and late-diastolic mitral flow are also increased.

Pulmonary Hypertension

Pulmonary hypertension (PH) is a major cause of early mortality in SCD. Those diagnosed have been seen to have a tenfold greater risk of death [15]. Intravascular hemolysis, a hallmark of SCD, releases hemoglobin and arginase into the plasma, and these proteins are taken up by nitric oxide (NO) and L-arginine, its precursor. Subsequent reduced bioavailability of NO exacerbates baseline vaso-occlusion in the pulmonary vasculature, as capillaries fail to dilate. Endothelin-1, a vasoconstrictor, is also elevated in SCD patients during vaso-occlusive episodes and may contribute to PH severity.

Patients particularly at risk of PH have high rates of chronic intravascular hemolysis evidenced by low steady-state hemoglobin levels, elevated lactic dehydrogenase (LDH), bilirubin, and reticulocyte counts.

PH evaluation and diagnosis via echocardiogram has low sensitivity with a positive predictive value of about 25% (21). This finding might contribute to the underreporting of PH in SCD patients. To improve noninvasive diagnosis, measuring the N-terminal fragment of brain natriuretic peptide (NT-proBNP) has been encouraged [17]. NT-proBNP is a cardiac ventricular prohormone made in response to myocyte stretch. BNP, the downstream hormone, facilitates systemic vasodilation. NT-proBNP levels are elevated in PH and are also an independent predictor of mortality. In pediatric patients, NT-proBNP is strongly correlated with high reticulocyte count [17].

Hydroxyurea and chronic exchange transfusion are long-term management treatments for pulmonary hypertension [18]. However, in the acute setting of right ventricular heart failure, exchange transfusion should also be initiated. In addition, case reports have noted that some patients have responded to nitric oxide, endothelin receptor antagonists, or prostanoids [19].

Myocardial Ischemia

Autopsy reports indicate that myocardial infarction (MI) is often underdiagnosed in patients with SCD [20]. MI must be considered in any patient presenting with chest pain as it may be clinically indistinguishable from more common causes of chest pain such as acute chest syndrome, rib infarction, or epigastric pain [10].

MI is underdiagnosed perhaps because the mechanism of MI in SCD is not well understood. Reduced oxygen content due to underlying anemia and abnormal myocardial microvasculature both could contribute to fibromuscular dysplasia of small vessels and ischemic changes. Abnormal platelets seen in SCD may also release thromboxane resulting in vasospasm, infarct, and necrosis.

The nonspecific ST-T wave changes existing in some SCA patients make ECG often unhelpful in MI diagnosis. However, in one study, a useful pediatric scoring system for MI which used ECG in early detection of MI was found to be helpful [21]. Cardiac enzymes may also be low in patients with SCD having an MI due to cardiomyocyte death secondary to apoptosis instead of necrosis. Given the lack of sensitivity of the traditional MI workup in patients with SCA, cardiac magnetic resonance has been proposed to detect microvascular disease in symptomatic patients. However, it seems more practical to use echocardiogram to look for regional wall motion abnormalities as they are often normal at baseline in SCD patients even in patients that have a baseline abnormal EKG [22].

MI management must reduce ischemia via standard medical approaches and implement reperfusion of myocardium via thrombolysis or mechanical revascularization. In addition, exchange transfusion has also had a positive effect in MI cases in patients with SCD [23, 24]. Keeping in mind that a higher hemoglobin transfusion threshold may be beneficial in all MI patients, simple transfusion may be not only faster but clinically more helpful. In the setting of right heart failure, inhaled nitric oxide (NO) may be useful as a vasodilator and inhibitor of platelet activation; however, there is no clinical data to support this.

Hepatic and Biliary Concerns

Sickle cell-associated hepatic and biliary complications are numerous and can be significant (Table 6.1). Complications secondary to sickling as well as coexisting conditions will be addressed in this section.

Hepatobiliary Clinical Syndromes Secondary to Sickling

Acute Sickle Hepatic Crisis

One in ten SCD patients will have an acute sickle hepatic crisis. Vaso-occlusive obstruction of liver sinusoids results in ischemia, which presents clinically with right upper quadrant (RUQ) pain, fever, nausea, jaundice, and hepatomegaly [25]. A patient's alanine transaminase (ALT) and/or aspartate amino transferase (AST) levels may be elevated but not in every case [25]. Patients should be well hydrated with intravenous fluids and treated with analgesia if needed.

Table 6.1 Hepatic and biliary complications of sickle cell disease

	Secondary to sickling versus coexisting condition	Etiology	Presentation	Management
Acute hepatic crisis	Secondary	Vaso-occlusion of liver sinusoids	RUQ pain, fever, nausea, jaundice, ↑ALT/AST	Hydration, analgesia
Intrahepatic cholestasis	Secondary	Sickled cells adherence to hepatic endothelium	RUQ pain, low-grade fever, tender hepatomegaly, jaundice ↑ bilirubin	PRBC transfusion
Hepatic sequestration crisis	Secondary	Sickled cells trapped in liver vasculature	RUQ pain, hepatomegaly, ↓ hematocrit	Simple transfusion
Hepatic Iron overload	Coexisting	Transfusion		Iron chelation
Viral hepatitis	Coexisting	Hep A, B, C, E		
Acute cholecystitis	Coexisting	Hemolysis	Asymptomatic, RUQ	Exchange transfusion
Pyogenic liver abscess	Coexisting	↓ GI integrity, ↑enteric microorganisms	Fever, jaundice, tender hepatomegaly	Drain abscess, broad-spectrum antibiotics, analgesia, hydration
Autoimmune hepatitis	Coexisting	Unknown	↑ALT/AST, jaundice	Prednisolone, azathioprine, ursodeoxycholic acid
Focal nodular hyperplasia	Coexisting	Vascular anomaly + vaso-occlusion	Distended abdomen, tender hepatomegaly	Surgical resection

Intrahepatic Cholestasis

Intrahepatic cholestasis is a severe variation of hepatic crisis. The pathological mechanism underlying this condition is largely unknown, but it is suspected that sickled cells adhere to the hepatic endothelium, facilitating the vaso-occlusive state, tissue infarction, and then liver dysfunction [26]. The hypoxic damage that occurs as a result leads to both hepatocyte ballooning and intracanalicular cholestasis.

The presentation of intrahepatic cholestasis is nonspecific with acute RUQ pain, low-grade fever, hepatomegaly tender with palpation, jaundice, and icteric sclera. Upon further investigation, patients will have high bilirubin levels (direct > indirect) and, in the progression to hepatic failure, coagulopathy.

Other potential causes with a similar clinical presentation such as biliary obstruction, sequestration crisis, viral hepatitis, medication-induced toxicity, autoimmune disease, and iron overload must be excluded. Diagnosis via ultrasound should reveal an enlarged liver with thickened gallbladder wall and no gallstones. Magnetic resonance cholangiopancreatography (MCRP) should detect periportal thickening in the absence of intra- and extrahepatic biliary duct dilation.

Liver biopsy is associated with serious complications in SCD patients and should be avoided [27]. Histology would reveal sickle thrombin in liver sinusoids, Kupffer cell hypertrophy, centrilobular necrosis, and bile stasis.

Packed red blood cell (PRBC) transfusion followed by manual exchange transfusion should be initiated at the onset of treatment with the goal to reduce sickle hemoglobin to below 30% [28]. Liver transplantation is indicated in patients with fulminate failure [29] although recurrence of sickle cell hepatopathy is possible [27]. Fresh frozen plasma can also be used to correct coagulopathy [25]. Coagulopathy is common and worsens as the liver undergoes necrosis. The data on whether bilirubin can be used to predict outcomes is inconclusive [30, 31]. Progression to severe liver disease is possible even if not found on presentation. Therefore patients should be monitored closely until bilirubin levels begin to decrease.

Hepatic Sequestration Crisis

Hepatic sequestration crisis is a deadly hepatic pathology in SCD patients. When sickled RBCs are trapped or "sequestered" in the liver vasculature, the reduced levels in circulation exacerbate the anemic state. Patients present with RUQ pain, increasing hepatomegaly, and rapidly declining hematocrit levels. Of note that liver function enzymes may be at baseline levels.

The main goal of management is to replenish the blood volume to treat hypovolemia and prevent shock [32]. Treatment typically begins with simple transfusion to the absolute minimum levels to treat symptomatic anemia (5 cc/kg for children).

"Autotransfusion" or "reverse sequestration" is a phenomenon when sequestered blood cells re-enter the circulation causing hyperviscosity syndrome. Death secondary to hyperviscosity syndrome is a result of hypervolemia, hypertension, heart failure, and/or intracerebral hemorrhage [33]. Therefore, it is critically important to closely monitor hemoglobin levels in hepatic sequestration patients. If the hemoglobin concentration rises above 11 g/dl, phlebotomy should be considered.

Hepatobiliary Dysfunction Secondary to Coexisting Conditions

Hepatic Consequences of Iron Overload

Steady-state ferritin levels that are comparatively very low (less than 1000 ng/ml) or very high (greater than 3000 ng/ml) can be used to estimate the severity of iron overload [34]. Excess iron in chronically transfused patients is deposited in the reticuloendothelial cells and is visually determined via T2 magnetic resonance for hepatic iron. In these instances, iron chelation increases excretion of iron. When left untreated, iron accumulation in the liver parenchyma results in hemochromatosis and cirrhosis.

Viral Hepatitis

The incidence of hepatitis A, B, and E is low in the sickle cell population. Hepatitis C had been increased in comparison to the general population especially in chronically transfused patients, but that has declined with blood donor screening for the virus [35, 36].

Acute Cholecystitis

Hemolysis, a key component of SCD pathology, necessitates the removal of bilirubin from circulation. As a result, almost half of all patients with SCA will have developed calcium bilirubinate gallstones by their 18th birthday [37]. Data suggests that most SCD patients with cholelithiasis, even those that are asymptomatic, should undergo cholecystectomy. Emergent procedures are associated with a higher risk of mortality [38]. Increasing the hemoglobin to a goal of 10 g/dl as opposed to more aggressive transfusion to reduce Hb S to less than 30%, is recommended [39].

Pyogenic Liver Abscess

Hepatic infarction is common in SCD as it is detected in 34% of autopsies of patients with the disease [40]. Pyogenic liver abscess, a potential consequence of infarct, arises after the infarcted tissue facilitates mucosal capillary thrombosis. Gastrointestinal integrity is compromised, and commensal enteric microorganisms overgrow [41]. Other causes of increased risk of pyogenic liver abscess are secondary to functional asplenia or impaired opsonin phagocytic function seen in complement pathways [41].

Patients appear very ill, presenting with fever, jaundice, and tender hepatomegaly. Abdominal radiograph (elevation of the right diaphragmatic cupola) as well as ultrasound (abscess in the right hepatic lobe) is useful for diagnosis. To avoid sepsis and rapid decline, the abscess must be drained carefully with broad-spectrum antibiotics administered. IV fluids as well as appropriate analgesics are also necessary in management [42].

Autoimmune Hepatitis

In a single study from 1999 to 2015, 17% of pediatric SCD patients with hepatic dysfunction were diagnosed with autoimmune liver disease [43]. These patients, often female, presented with increased liver enzymes and progressive jaundice.

Patients can also present with acute hepatitis and acute liver failure. Autoimmune hepatitis is difficult to diagnose but is suspected in patients with elevated ALT/AST, positive autoantibodies, hypergammaglobulinemia, and interface hepatitis with histological evidence of portal plasma cell infiltrates without evidence of other disease. Young patients have achieved full remission with treatment including prednisone, azathioprine, and ursodeoxycholic acid [43].

Focal Nodular Hyperplasia

Although the etiology is unclear, it is suspected that SCD patients with an underlying vascular anomaly such as an arteriovenous malformation in combination with vaso-occlusion are at risk for focal hyperplasia of the liver as the ischemic tissue regenerates [44]. These patients present with distended abdomens and tender hepatomegaly. Diagnosis can be made via liver radionuclide scans in which a significant defect in liver filling is apparent. Ultrasound can detect the mass, while selective arteriography can detect both a mass and its blood supply.

If the mass is providing symptomatic pressure on internal organs and there is internal bleeding caused by abdominal trauma or significant discomfort, surgical resection is an appropriate treatment. Uncontrollable bleeding and blood loss resulting in death is a risk of this intervention [44].

Hemodynamic Concerns

Thromboembolism in Sickle Cell Disease

SCD is a hypercoagulative state [45]. The prevalence of pulmonary embolism (PE) in hospitalized patients is more than three times higher than in racially matched controls [46]. PE, normally presenting in middle-aged to older adults (average age 57 years), can also occur in younger (average age 28 years) SCD patients [46].

Risk Factors Secondary to Sickling

SCD is a disease of both RBC and endothelial dysfunction, key drivers of the hypercoagulable state. Structural changes in the sickled RBC membranes expose phosphatidylserine, which degrades lipids, inactivates coagulation proteins, and creates oxidative stress. Antiphospholipid antibodies are common in SCD patients, increasing their risk of thrombotic events [47].

Risk Factors Secondary to Traditional Causes

Venous thromboembolism, which is more common in severe disease, is associated with increased mortality [48]. Deep vein thrombosis prophylaxis is recommended in adult hospitalized patients, but there is no standard practice for children. Pediatric SCD patients who have higher risk of venous thromboembolism (VTE) may undergo prophylactic pharmacologic therapies especially if in a critical care setting, mechanically ventilated, hospitalized for 5 days or more (particularly if postpubertal), fighting systemic infection, using oral contraception, and immobile [49–52]. Low molecular weight heparin may be advantageous in this patient population as the response is highly predictable, does not require IV access (as this may be difficult in SCD patients), and does not cross the placenta (if the patient is pregnant).

Splenic Concerns

The spleen's involvement in SCD pathology has been closely studied. The spleen is often rendered afunctional in SCD patients by 10 years of age, if not earlier, secondary to splenic infarction [37]. Patients with homozygous hemoglobin SS disease are at the greatest risk of functional asplenia, while half of compound heterozygotes maintain splenic function. As the patient becomes functionally asplenic, the risk of infection by encapsulated organisms such as *Haemophilus influenzae* and *Streptococcus pneumoniae* increases. In much of the resource-limited countries of the world impacted by SCD, the leading cause of death in children is infection. Splenic concerns of particular note in the pediatric SCD ICU patient are sepsis as a result of serious bacterial infection and splenic sequestration crisis.

Splenic Sequestration Crisis

Splenic sequestration is a consequence of vaso-occlusion in the spleen in one third of young children with hemoglobin SS disease usually between 6 months to 2 years of age [53, 54]. This crisis requires blood flow to the spleen, putting young children with hemoglobin SS disease at higher risk than adults. RBCs pool in occluded blood vessels resulting in a systemic drop in hemoglobin and blood volume. Shock and death occur as a result.

Patients at risk include those with auto-infarcted spleens to the point of fibrosis. The risk is also elevated in patients with past parvovirus B19 infection [55]. Upon examination, patients present with a rapidly enlarging spleen, decreased hemoglobin count, and reticulocytosis [56].

Transfusion of packed RBCs is necessary to raise hemoglobin to previous steady-state level and decrease Hb S so that blood begins to flow again resulting in auto-transfusion of trapped splenic blood. Avoid saline infusion or the expansion of plasma before blood is available, as this is likely to lead to heart failure. Ten to fifteen percent of patients die as a result of splenic sequestration, often prior to transfusion [53, 54]. Therefore, timely transfusion following diagnosis is paramount. Although mortality risk is the greatest for a patient during their first sequestration crisis, up to 50% of patients not splenectomized will have a repeated crisis [54]. Therefore, most clinicians will recommend splenectomy once the patient is stable and if they are already 5 years of age.

Sepsis

Fever in any child with SCD is a cause for concern and may be the only presenting symptom in sepsis. While viral causes are common, functional asplenia puts children with SCD at increased risk of bacteremia and sepsis. Pneumonia is the most common infection leading to sepsis in children with SCD; other serious causes include urinary tract infection, osteomyelitis, and meningitis [57, 58]. Broad-spectrum antibiotics such as ceftriaxone or cefotaxime should be used in febrile patients. Vancomycin must be added if bacterial organisms are found in CSF fluid.

Musculoskeletal Concerns

Infarcts within the bone marrow are a major cause of pathology of SCD and classic precipitant of pain crisis. Poor blood supply increases the risk of avascular necrosis and joint damage in adult patients. Osteomyelitis, secondary to bacterial infection, is less common in adults and more common in children. Additionally, in younger patients and adults, fat embolism syndrome (FES) can be a serious complication of bone marrow necrosis.

Fat Embolism Syndrome

In patients without infection, FES contributes to 9% of acute chest syndrome (ACS) cases in children and adolescents with previously "mild" disease [59]. Necrotic bone marrow precipitates the release of fat globules into venous circulation. Patients often present with a history of mild disease with a seemingly uncomplicated vaso-occlusive crisis (VOC) and at times thrombocytopenia. This is then followed by a rapid decline resulting to respiratory failure, altered mental status, and/or coma. Exchange transfusion should be implemented as soon as fat embolism syndrome is suspected as more than half of diagnoses occur at autopsy [59].

Neurological Concerns

Cerebrovascular incidents occur in up to 11% of SCD patients under 20 years of age – particularly those with hemoglobin SS disease and those that have not been screened with transcranial Doppler [60]. In most pediatric cases, ischemic stroke predominates over hemorrhagic stroke, although hemorrhagic stroke risk begins to increase in the late teens [60]. The key challenge in managing stroke in this population is in discerning stroke from other cerebrovascular manifestations of SCD – mainly migraines, meningitis, cerebral malaria, and seizure disorder.

Initial Management of Possible Stroke

The initial treatment of a possible cerebrovascular incident is guided by presenting symptoms. When suspecting acute ischemic stroke, instead of a hemorrhagic event, simple and/or exchange transfusion should be implemented [61]. If a patient presents with fever and acute neurologic findings, treatment for bacterial infection is essential until meningitis is ruled out via differential diagnosis. Patients with bacterial meningitis often present with septic features. It is of note that fever can be a presenting symptom of stroke.

Diagnosis

Standard clinical and neuroimaging are usually satisfactory in the diagnosis of stroke. CT scan is adequate in children to diagnose ischemic stroke, but MRI is more sensitive in that it excludes other diagnoses of cerebrovascular manifestations. Children under 8 years of age may require sedation for MRI imaging. Magnetic resonance angiography (MRA) or CT angiography can be used to determine the existence of large vessel arteriopathy to exclude aneurysm [62]. If cerebral venous sinus thrombosis is suspected, MRI with magnetic resonance venography (MRV) is sensitive [63].

Baseline laboratory testing is critical in the diagnosis and management of a cerebrovascular manifestation of SCD. A complete blood count, reticulocyte count, as well as sickle hemoglobin percentage are informative. Blood cross-matching is needed for transfusion therapy. Coagulation studies as well as a basal metabolic panel are necessary to rule out other clinical phenotypes such as hypoglycemia.

Ischemic Stroke

While managing a patient with ischemic stroke, it is important to protect the airway from aspiration and maintain oxygen saturation at 95% [64]. It is important to keep patients calm and comfortable. Further cerebral ischemia occurs via vasoconstriction in hyperventilating and crying patients. Similar to management of traumatic brain injury, cerebral perfusion pressure should be maintained by ensuring adequate blood pressure, normoglycemia should be the goal, and fever should be avoided. Normal carbon dioxide levels should be maintained to avoid decreased cerebral perfusion seen with hyperventilation or increased intracranial pressure seen with hypercarbia. Patients should be hydrated with isotonic saline (1.25–1.5 normal rate). Hypotonic saline will exacerbate cytotoxic cerebral edema and should be avoided [64].

Simple transfusion to the patient's baseline should be done carefully to avoid hyperviscosity syndrome and transitioned to exchange transfusion [64]. To date, there are no randomized clinical trials comparing transfusion to other interventions. However, it is suspected that transfusion reduces the Hb S and hypoxemia facilitating the vaso-occlusive state. It has been found that recurrent strokes are reduced in children receiving exchange transfusion as opposed to only simple transfusion [65].

Anticoagulation is generally not recommended in treatment of ischemic stroke. However, as SCD is a hypercoagulable state, prophylactic anticoagulation may be appropriate in the event of arterial dissection, cerebral sinus thrombosis, or thromboembolism following a hemorrhagic episode [64].

Hemorrhagic Stroke

Hemorrhagic stroke, more commonly seen in adult patients, impacts 3% of patients with SCD, patients under 20 years of age [60]. In the event of a hemorrhagic stroke, management is dependent on the etiology whether it be ischemic transformation, subarachnoid hemorrhage secondary to aneurysm, or intraventricular hemorrhage.

Ischemic Transformation

Ischemic transformation should be managed similarly to the typical intracerebral hemorrhage. Anticoagulation must be terminated. Platelet transfusion should be implemented if needed to keep platelet counts above 100,000 cells per microliter.

Subarachnoid Hemorrhage

Subarachnoid hemorrhage is often secondary to aneurysm. Management should focus on maintaining blood pressure at normal values and providing the appropriate analgesia. If intracranial pressure is too great and ventriculostomy is scheduled, transfusion is recommended prior to the procedure [66].

Intraventricular Hemorrhage

The patients at risk of intraventricular hemorrhage are those who present with a subarachnoid hemorrhage which spreads into the ventricles [67] or previously had an ischemic stroke, months to years prior to this event [68]. Hemorrhage into the third ventricle or cerebral aqueduct is often detected late in its course. Ventricular drainage may be warranted.

Renal Concerns

Sickle cell nephropathy (SCN) begins in childhood and can eventually progress into renal failure [69]. Before a patient reaches 10 years of age, glomerular changes are apparent in even asymptomatic children with SCD.

Baseline Renal Pathology in SCD

The kidney's natural hyperosmolar, acidotic, and hypoxic environment is a prime site of further complication in SCD – particularly in the vasa recta capillaries. There, microthrombotic infarction and extravasation of blood into the renal medulla can occur. The natural history of SCN is often progressive. The repetitive infarction of the renal medulla first leads to hyposthenuria (secretion of dilute urine with a low specific gravity in comparison to blood plasma) in infancy to isosthenuria (excretion of urine with specific gravity equivalent to blood plasma) by adolescence. Papillary infarcts are responsible for renal papillary necrosis, which presents with painless hematuria (Fig. 6.3).

Acute Kidney Injury

Acute kidney injury (AKI) is common in hospitalized SCD patients. In one cohort of patients admitted with ACS, AKI occurred in 8% children [70]. In another cohort of children admitted with vaso-occlusive crisis, 50% developed AKI [69]. Three quarters of vaso-occlusive episodes are compounded by acute multiorgan failure, and hemodialysis is a necessary treatment in 19% of these episodes [2].

Risk factors for AKI depend on the type of kidney injury: prerenal, intrinsic, or postrenal. In children, prerenal and intrinsic causes are most common as repeated bouts of vaso-occlusive crisis; volume depletion secondary to hyposthenuria and the use of NSAIDs contribute to AKI [71].

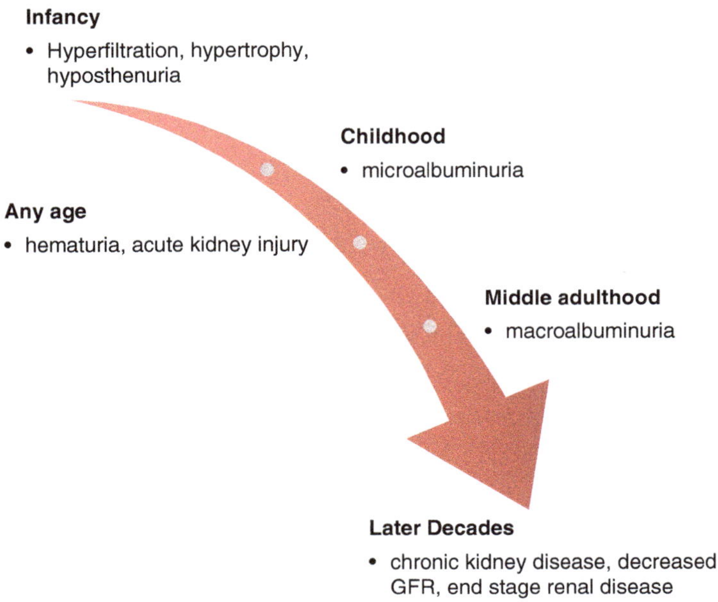

Fig. 6.3 Natural history of sickle cell nephropathy (SCN) (Sickle cell nephropathy (SCN) begins in childhood and progresses in severity to adulthood. While hematuria and acute kidney injury can occur at any age, hyperfiltration is seen in early life, while chronic kidney disease and end-stage renal disease are typically seen in the later decades of life)

Prerenal AKI

Hyposthenuria, which begins often in infancy, results in intravascular volume depletion facilitating prerenal injury.

Intrinsic AKI

Direct damage to the kidney via rhabdomyolysis, infection, NSAID use, sepsis, drug-induced nephrotoxicity (see "Iatrogenic Concerns" section), renal vein thrombosis, and hepatorenal syndrome results in intrinsic kidney disease.

Postrenal AKI

Papillary necrosis is a rare but possible cause of postrenal AKI. Thrombi, blocking the urinary tract, is a risk factor for this phenomenon.

Pulmonary Concerns

Since the introduction of the pneumococcal conjugate vaccine in 2000, pediatric SCD-related mortality in the United States has shifted from predominantly infection to mortality risks seen in adult patients such as acute chest syndrome (ACS) and stroke [72]. ACS is the most common cause of ICU admission and death with mortality rates ranging from 1.8% to 25%. Pulmonary hypertension (PH), asthma, and restrictive lung disease are additional compounding factors leading to poor ICU outcomes in SCD patients. In this section, ACS, the most severe pulmonary concern, will be discussed in detail.

Precipitating Factors

Isolated and seemingly uncomplicated vaso-occlusive crisis is a key precipitating factor of ACS in hospitalized sickle cell patients [5]. Infection, pulmonary vascular obstruction by pulmonary arterial thrombi and fat emboli, and chest wall pain crisis precipitating alveolar hypoventilation also contribute to ACS onset. However, in 40% of cases the precipitating cause is known [5].

Diagnosis

Chest radiograph or CT scan revealing alveolar consolidation in lower zones is often indicative of ACS in addition to one or more of these signs symptoms: chest pain, fever, increased work of breathing, or hypoxemia relative to baseline [5, 73]. Children with severe disease should undergo echocardiogram to assess for intervenable PH and/or cor pulmonale.

Complications and Severity

Severe ACS cases are complicated by acute respiratory distress syndrome (ARDS). This syndrome often presents with PH, right ventricular dilation, and cor pulmonale in the most severe cases.

Increased right ventricular afterload as a result of in situ thrombi, fat embolism, pulmonary vasoconstriction, hemolysis, or worsening anemia is a major complication of ACS leading to poor outcomes. In a pediatric study of ACS, pulmonary embolism was the most common cause of death in ACS. As pediatricians commonly do not prescribe anticoagulants in ACS, there may be a danger of under-prescribing these medications in comparison to adult patients [74].

Markers of severe ACS include high LDH, a dramatic and sustained drop in hemoglobin, thrombocytopenia, elevated respiratory rate, extensive lobar involvement on lung imaging, PH, and AKI.

Catastrophic Sickle Cell Disease Syndrome

SCD-related multiorgan failure (SMOF) or "catastrophic SCD syndrome" has been defined as the sudden onset of organ failures involving the lungs (severe ACS), liver, and/or kidneys [2, 75]. Clinical signs of this syndrome include a swift reduction in hemoglobin level and platelet count and shock (the most common cause of death in this syndrome) in the absence of a history of severe disease [2]. SMOF often overlaps with fat embolism and thrombotic microangiopathy syndromes, particularly in patients with a worsening presentation despite aggressive transfusion [76, 77].

Respiratory Support

The mode of respiratory support is critical in ACS cases. Mechanical ventilation is correlated with a high mortality rate during acute complications of SCD [75, 78]. Instead, a protective ventilator strategy is suggested to protect the right ventricle as high mean airway pressures can worsen pulmonary hypertension which is commonly seen in ACS [79]. Guiding principles include limiting plateau and driving pressures with a low tidal volume and prone position and limiting positive end-expiratory pressure (PEEP) as much as possible [80, 81].

Early Intervention Prevention

While early transfusion shortens the duration and improves oxygenation in established ACS [82] and may even prevent ACS during VOC, delayed hemolytic transfusion reactions are particularly hazardous in a critical patient with ACS; therefore careful blood matching and indication for transfusion are required. This is explained further in the "Iatrogenic Concerns" section.

Iatrogenic Concerns

When a patient is deteriorating despite seemingly appropriate management, it is important to consider iatrogenic causes of worsening presentation. Reactions to particular medications and blood products can be catastrophic.

Toxic Side-Effects to Medications

Opioid overdose in the critical care setting is possible during management of painful VOC. High doses of inconsistent levels of these drugs increase the risk of this outcome [83]. In cases of AKI, close attention to nephrotoxic drugs and antibiotics such as gentamicin is imperative. It is recommended to avoid antibiotics known to cause acute tubular necrosis of the kidney. Other antibiotics such as piperacillin/tazobactam may cause drug-induced cardiac toxicity such as bradycardia [84]. Fluoroquinolones, ketolides, and macrolides predispose patients to a myriad cardiac toxicities including ventricular tachycardia and QTc prolongation [85].

Delayed Hemolytic Transfusion Reaction (DHTR)

DHTR arises when alloimmunization to RBC antigens or human leukocyte antigens occurs following transfusion. Patients of an older age, female sex, and clinical history of frequent transfusion and acute transfusion elevate the risk of this reaction [86–89].

The onset is variable often beginning 24 h to 21 days following a transfusion, and the presentation is insidious, often mimicking acute VOC [89]. Patients present with an acute drop in hemoglobin – a particular fall in HbA levels (evidence of donor RBC destruction), increased LDH, hemoglobinuria (a result of intravascular hemolysis), and relative or absolute reticulocytopenia. Diagnosis is often inconsistent. New RBC antibodies or a positive direct antiglobulin test are suggestive in combination with the clinical picture above [89].

Hyperhemolysis syndrome is a further complication of DHTR where the hemoglobin falls below the pre-transfusion level. Patients undergoing this reaction should not be transfused unless the anemia is life-threatening. An erythropoiesis-stimulating agent and intravenous iron may be helpful as well as an immunomodulatory therapy [89, 90].

Conclusion

The intensive care unit is the site of half of SCD-related deaths [91]. The high risk of mortality in this vulnerable population is often underappreciated by clinicians. Careful attention to detail and meticulous evidenced-based management of this unique population in the critical care setting have potential to improve outcomes.

References

1. Al Khawaja SA, Ateya ZM, Al Hammam RA. Predictors of mortality in adults with sickle cell disease admitted to intensive care unit in Bahrain. J Crit Care. 2017;42:238–42.
2. Hassell KL, Eckman JR, Lane PA. Acute multiorgan failure syndrome: a potentially catastrophic complication of severe sickle cell pain episodes. Am J Med. 1994;96(2):155–62.

3. Platt OS, Brambilla DJ, Rosse WF, et al. Mortality in sickle cell disease. Life expectancy and risk factors for early death. N Engl J Med. 1994;330(23):1639–44.
4. Gardner K, Bell C, Bartram JL, et al. Outcome of adults with sickle cell disease admitted to critical care – experience of a single institution in the UK. Br J Haematol. 2010;150(5):610–3.
5. Vichinsky EP, Neumayr LD, Earles AN, et al. Causes and outcomes of the acute chest syndrome in sickle cell disease. National Acute Chest Syndrome Study Group. N Engl J Med. 2000;342(25):1855–65.
6. Jacobe SJ, Hassan A, Veys P, Mok Q. Outcome of children requiring admission to an intensive care unit after bone marrow transplantation. Crit Care Med. 2003;31(5):1299–305.
7. Darbari DS, Kple-Faget P, Kwagyan J, Rana S, Gordeuk VR, Castro O. Circumstances of death in adult sickle cell disease patients. Am J Hematol. 2006;81(11):858–63.
8. Berger S, Utech L, Fran HM. Sudden death in children and adolescents. Pediatr Clin N Am. 2004;51(6):1653–77. ix–x.
9. James TN, Riddick L, Massing GK. Sickle cells and sudden death: morphologic abnormalities of the cardiac conduction system. J Lab Clin Med. 1994;124(4):507–20.
10. Voskaridou E, Christoulas D, Terpos E. Sickle-cell disease and the heart: review of the current literature. Br J Haematol. 2012;157(6):664–73.
11. Caldas MC, Meira ZA, Barbosa MM. Evaluation of 107 patients with sickle cell anemia through tissue Doppler and myocardial performance index. J Am Soc Echocardiogr. 2008;21(10):1163–7.
12. Alpert BS, Gilman PA, Strong WB, et al. Hemodynamic and ECG responses to exercise in children with sickle cell anemia. Am J Dis Child. 1981;135(4):362–6.
13. Liu P, Olivieri N. Iron overload cardiomyopathies: new insights into an old disease. Cardiovasc Drugs Ther. 1994;8(1):101–10.
14. Buja LM, Roberts WC. Iron in the heart. Etiology and clinical significance. Am J Med. 1971;51(2):209–21.
15. Gladwin MT, Sachdev V, Jison ML, et al. Pulmonary hypertension as a risk factor for death in patients with sickle cell disease. N Engl J Med. 2004;350(9):886–95.
16. Johnson MC, Kirkham FJ, Redline S, et al. Left ventricular hypertrophy and diastolic dysfunction in children with sickle cell disease are related to asleep and waking oxygen desaturation. Blood. 2010;116(1):16–21.
17. Voskaridou E, Tsetsos G, Tsoutsias A, Spyropoulou E, Christoulas D, Terpos E. Pulmonary hypertension in patients with sickle cell/beta thalassemia: incidence and correlation with serum N-terminal pro-brain natriuretic peptide concentrations. Haematologica. 2007;92(6):738–43.
18. Gordeuk VR, Castro OL, Machado RF. Pathophysiology and treatment of pulmonary hypertension in sickle cell disease. Blood. 2016;127(7):820–8.
19. Klings ES, Machado RF, Barst RJ, et al. An official American Thoracic Society clinical practice guideline: diagnosis, risk stratification, and management of pulmonary hypertension of sickle cell disease. Am J Respir Crit Care Med. 2014;189(6):727–40.
20. Barrett O Jr, Saunders DE Jr, McFarland DE, Humphries JO. Myocardial infarction in sickle cell anemia. Am J Hematol. 1984;16(2):139–47.
21. Bode-Thomas F, Hyacinth HI, Ogunkunle O, Omotoso A. Myocardial ischaemia in sickle cell anaemia: evaluation using a new scoring system. Ann Trop Paediatr. 2011;31(1):67–74.
22. Lippman SM, Niemann JT, Thigpen T, Ginzton LE, Laks MM. Abnormal septal Q waves in sickle cell disease. Prevalence and causative factors. Chest. 1985;88(4):543–8.
23. Mansi IA, Rosner F. Myocardial infarction in sickle cell disease. J Natl Med Assoc. 2002;94(6):448–52.
24. Khalique Z, Pavlu J, Lefroy D, Layton M. Erythrocytapheresis in the prevention of recurrent myocardial infarction in sickle cell disease. Am J Hematol. 2010;85(1):91.
25. Banerjee S, Owen C, Chopra S. Sickle cell hepatopathy. Hepatology. 2001;33(5):1021–8.
26. Hurtova M, Bachir D, Lee K, et al. Transplantation for liver failure in patients with sickle cell disease: challenging but feasible. Liver Transpl. 2011;17(4):381–92.

27. Gardner K, Suddle A, Kane P, et al. How we treat sickle hepatopathy and liver transplantation in adults. Blood. 2014;123(15):2302–7.
28. Khalifeh HK, Chamoun CT, Elhoujairy AH, Alkoussa WA, Zeidan Lahoud CI, Masri GA. Acute hepatic crisis in sickle cell anemia: favorable outcome after exchange transfusion. J Hematol. 2016;5(4):138–41.
29. Brunetta DM, Silva-Pinto AC, do Carmo Favarin de Macedo M, et al. Intrahepatic cholestasis in sickle cell disease: a case report. Anemia. 2011;2011:975731.
30. Lacaille F, Lesage F, de Montalembert M. Acute hepatic crisis in children with sickle cell disease. J Pediatr Gastroenterol Nutr. 2004;39(2):200–2.
31. Ahn H, Li CS, Wang W. Sickle cell hepatopathy: clinical presentation, treatment, and outcome in pediatric and adult patients. Pediatr Blood Cancer. 2005;45(2):184–90.
32. Yawn BP, Buchanan GR, Afenyi-Annan AN, et al. Management of sickle cell disease: summary of the 2014 evidence-based report by expert panel members. JAMA. 2014;312(10):1033–48.
33. Lee ES, Chu PC. Reverse sequestration in a case of sickle crisis. Postgrad Med J. 1996;72(850):487–8.
34. Adamkiewicz TV, Abboud MR, Paley C, et al. Serum ferritin level changes in children with sickle cell disease on chronic blood transfusion are nonlinear and are associated with iron load and liver injury. Blood. 2009;114(21):4632–8.
35. Hassan M, Hasan S, Giday S, et al. Hepatitis C virus in sickle cell disease. J Natl Med Assoc. 2003;95(10):939–42.
36. Hasan MF, Marsh F, Posner G, et al. Chronic hepatitis C in patients with sickle cell disease. Am J Gastroenterol. 1996;91(6):1204–6.
37. Kato GJ, Gladwin MT. Sickle cell disease. In: Hall JB, Schmidt GA, Kress JP, editors. Principles of critical care. 4th ed. New York: McGraw-Hill; 2015.
38. Goodwin EF, Partain PI, Lebensburger JD, Fineberg NS, Howard TH. Elective cholecystectomy reduces morbidity of cholelithiasis in pediatric sickle cell disease. Pediatr Blood Cancer. 2017;64(1):113–20.
39. Vichinsky EP, Haberkern CM, Neumayr L, et al. A comparison of conservative and aggressive transfusion regimens in the perioperative management of sickle cell disease. The Preoperative Transfusion in Sickle Cell Disease Study Group. N Engl J Med. 1995;333(4):206–13.
40. Bauer TW, Moore GW, Hutchins GM. The liver in sickle cell disease. A clinicopathologic study of 70 patients. Am J Med. 1980;69(6):833–7.
41. Lama M. Hepatic abscess in sickle cell anaemia: a rare manifestation. Arch Dis Child. 1993;69(2):242–3.
42. Marolf MD, Chaudhary M, Kaplan SL. An hepatic abscess in a patient with sickle cell anemia. Pediatr Infect Dis J. 2016;35(11):1269–70.
43. Jitraruch S, Fitzpatrick E, Deheragoda M, et al. Autoimmune liver disease in children with sickle cell disease. J Pediatr. 2017;189:79–85.e72.
44. Markowitz RI, Harcke HT, Ritchie WG, Huff DS. Focal nodular hyperplasia of the liver in a child with sickle cell anemia. AJR Am J Roentgenol. 1980;134(3):594–7.
45. Ataga KI, Orringer EP. Hypercoagulability in sickle cell disease: a curious paradox. Am J Med. 2003;115(9):721–8.
46. Stein PD, Beemath A, Meyers FA, Skaf E, Olson RE. Deep venous thrombosis and pulmonary embolism in hospitalized patients with sickle cell disease. Am J Med. 2006;119(10):897.e7–e11.
47. Ataga KI, Key NS. Hypercoagulability in sickle cell disease: new approaches to an old problem. Hematology Am Soc Hematol Educ Program. 2007;2007:91–6.
48. Brunson A, Lei A, Rosenberg AS, White RH, Keegan T, Wun T. Increased incidence of VTE in sickle cell disease patients: risk factors, recurrence and impact on mortality. Br J Haematol. 2017;178(2):319–26.
49. Branchford BR, Mourani P, Bajaj L, Manco-Johnson M, Wang M, Goldenberg NA. Risk factors for in-hospital venous thromboembolism in children: a case-control study employing diagnostic validation. Haematologica. 2012;97(4):509–15.

50. Sharathkumar AA, Mahajerin A, Heidt L, et al. Risk-prediction tool for identifying hospitalized children with a predisposition for development of venous thromboembolism: Peds-Clot clinical Decision Rule. J Thromb Haemost. 2012;10(7):1326–34.
51. Meier KA, Clark E, Tarango C, Chima RS, Shaughnessy E. Venous thromboembolism in hospitalized adolescents: an approach to risk assessment and prophylaxis. Hosp Pediatr. 2015;5(1):44–51.
52. Mahajerin A, Branchford BR, Amankwah EK, et al. Hospital-associated venous thromboembolism in pediatrics: a systematic review and meta-analysis of risk factors and risk-assessment models. Haematologica. 2015;100(8):1045–50.
53. Topley JM, Rogers DW, Stevens MC, Serjeant GR. Acute splenic sequestration and hypersplenism in the first five years in homozygous sickle cell disease. Arch Dis Child. 1981;56(10):765–9.
54. Emond AM, Collis R, Darvill D, Higgs DR, Maude GH, Serjeant GR. Acute splenic sequestration in homozygous sickle cell disease: natural history and management. J Pediatr. 1985;107(2):201–6.
55. Smith-Whitley K, Zhao H, Hodinka RL, et al. Epidemiology of human parvovirus B19 in children with sickle cell disease. Blood. 2004;103(2):422–7.
56. Airede AI. Acute splenic sequestration in a five-week-old infant with sickle cell disease. J Pediatr. 1992;120(1):160.
57. Bansil NH, Kim TY, Tieu L, Barcega B. Incidence of serious bacterial infections in febrile children with sickle cell disease. Clin Pediatr (Phila). 2013;52(7):661–6.
58. Asinobi AO, Fatunde OJ, Brown BJ, Osinusi K, Fasina NA. Urinary tract infection in febrile children with sickle cell anaemia in Ibadan, Nigeria. Ann Trop Paediatr. 2003;23(2):129–34.
59. Tsitsikas DA, Gallinella G, Patel S, Seligman H, Greaves P, Amos RJ. Bone marrow necrosis and fat embolism syndrome in sickle cell disease: increased susceptibility of patients with non-SS genotypes and a possible association with human parvovirus B19 infection. Blood Rev. 2014;28(1):23–30.
60. Ohene-Frempong K, Weiner SJ, Sleeper LA, et al. Cerebrovascular accidents in sickle cell disease: rates and risk factors. Blood. 1998;91(1):288–94.
61. Talahma M, Strbian D, Sundararajan S. Sickle cell disease and stroke. Stroke. 2014;45(6):e98–100.
62. Lee LJ, Kidwell CS, Alger J, Starkman S, Saver JL. Impact on stroke subtype diagnosis of early diffusion-weighted magnetic resonance imaging and magnetic resonance angiography. Stroke. 2000;31(5):1081–9.
63. Saposnik G, Barinagarrementeria F, Brown RD Jr, et al. Diagnosis and management of cerebral venous thrombosis: a statement for healthcare professionals from the American Heart Association/American Stroke Association. Stroke. 2011;42(4):1158–92.
64. Kassim AA, Galadanci NA, Pruthi S, DeBaun MR. How I treat and manage strokes in sickle cell disease. Blood. 2015;125(22):3401–10.
65. Hulbert ML, Scothorn DJ, Panepinto JA, et al. Exchange blood transfusion compared with simple transfusion for first overt stroke is associated with a lower risk of subsequent stroke: a retrospective cohort study of 137 children with sickle cell anemia. J Pediatr. 2006;149(5):710–2.
66. Howard J, Malfroy M, Llewelyn C, et al. The Transfusion Alternatives Preoperatively in Sickle Cell Disease (TAPS) study: a randomised, controlled, multicentre clinical trial. Lancet. 2013;381(9870):930–8.
67. Adams RJ, McKie VC, Carl EM, et al. Long-term stroke risk in children with sickle cell disease screened with transcranial Doppler. Ann Neurol. 1997;42(5):699–704.
68. Powars D, Adams RJ, Nichols FT, Milner P, Charache S, Sarnaik S. Delayed intracranial hemorrhage following cerebral infarction in sickle cell anemia. J Assoc Acad Minor Phys. 1990;1(3):79–82.
69. Mammen C, Bissonnette ML, Matsell DG. Acute kidney injury in children with sickle cell disease-compounding a chronic problem. Pediatr Nephrol. 2017;32(8):1287–91.
70. Lebensburger JD, Palabindela P, Howard TH, Feig DI, Aban I, Askenazi DJ. Prevalence of acute kidney injury during pediatric admissions for acute chest syndrome. Pediatr Nephrol. 2016;31(8):1363–8.

71. Baddam S, Aban I, Hilliard L, Howard T, Askenazi D, Lebensburger JD. Acute kidney injury during a pediatric sickle cell vaso-occlusive pain crisis. Pediatr Nephrol. 2017;32(8):1451–6.
72. Yanni E, Grosse SD, Yang Q, Olney RS. Trends in pediatric sickle cell disease-related mortality in the United States, 1983–2002. J Pediatr. 2009;154(4):541–5.
73. Vichinsky EP, Styles LA, Colangelo LH, Wright EC, Castro O, Nickerson B. Acute chest syndrome in sickle cell disease: clinical presentation and course. Cooperative Study of Sickle Cell Disease. Blood. 1997;89(5):1787–92.
74. Mekontso Dessap A, Deux JF, Abidi N, et al. Pulmonary artery thrombosis during acute chest syndrome in sickle cell disease. Am J Respir Crit Care Med. 2011;184(9):1022–9.
75. Cecchini J, Lionnet F, Djibre M, et al. Outcomes of adult patients with sickle cell disease admitted to the ICU: a case series. Crit Care Med. 2014;42(7):1629–39.
76. Boga C, Kozanoglu I, Ozdogu H, Ozyurek E. Plasma exchange in critically ill patients with sickle cell disease. Transfus Apher Sci. 2007;37(1):17–22.
77. Chehal A, Taher A, Shamseddine A. Sicklemia with multi-organ failure syndrome and thrombotic thrombocytopenic purpura. Hemoglobin. 2002;26(4):345–51.
78. Allareddy V, Roy A, Lee MK, et al. Outcomes of acute chest syndrome in adult patients with sickle cell disease: predictors of mortality. PLoS One. 2014;9(4):e94387.
79. Mekontso Dessap A, Leon R, Habibi A, et al. Pulmonary hypertension and cor pulmonale during severe acute chest syndrome in sickle cell disease. Am J Respir Crit Care Med. 2008;177(6):646–53.
80. Boissier F, Katsahian S, Razazi K, et al. Prevalence and prognosis of cor pulmonale during protective ventilation for acute respiratory distress syndrome. Intensive Care Med. 2013;39(10):1725–33.
81. Vieillard-Baron A, Price LC, Matthay MA. Acute cor pulmonale in ARDS. Intensive Care Med. 2013;39(10):1836–8.
82. Mallouh AA, Asha M. Beneficial effect of blood transfusion in children with sickle cell chest syndrome. Am J Dis Child. 1988;142(2):178–82.
83. Lucas SM, Mason DG, Weyman D. A sickle crisis? A report of the national confidential enquiry into patient outcome and death (2008). London: NCEPOD; 2008.
84. Zaki SA, Lad V. Piperacillin-tazobactam-induced hypokalemia and metabolic alkalosis. Indian J Pharmacol. 2011;43(5):609–10.
85. Iannini PB. Cardiotoxicity of macrolides, ketolides and fluoroquinolones that prolong the QTc interval. Expert Opin Drug Saf. 2002;1(2):121–8.
86. McPherson ME, Anderson AR, Castillejo MI, et al. HLA alloimmunization is associated with RBC antibodies in multiply transfused patients with sickle cell disease. Pediatr Blood Cancer. 2010;54(4):552–8.
87. Rosse WF, Gallagher D, Kinney TR, et al. Transfusion and alloimmunization in sickle cell disease. The Cooperative Study of Sickle Cell Disease. Blood. 1990;76(7):1431–7.
88. Fasano RM, Booth GS, Miles M, et al. Red blood cell alloimmunization is influenced by recipient inflammatory state at time of transfusion in patients with sickle cell disease. Br J Haematol. 2015;168(2):291–300.
89. Vidler JB, Gardner K, Amenyah K, Mijovic A, Thein SL. Delayed haemolytic transfusion reaction in adults with sickle cell disease: a 5-year experience. Br J Haematol. 2015;169(5):746–53.
90. Bachmeyer C, Maury J, Parrot A, et al. Rituximab as an effective treatment of hyperhemolysis syndrome in sickle cell anemia. Am J Hematol. 2010;85(1):91–2.
91. Perronne V, Roberts-Harewood M, Bachir D, et al. Patterns of mortality in sickle cell disease in adults in France and England. Hematol J. 2002;3(1):56–60.

Chapter 7
Bone Marrow Failure

Sajad Khazal, Jorge Ricardo Galvez Silva, Monica Thakar, and David Margolis

Acquired Aplastic Anemia

Acquired aplastic anemia in children is a rare disorder (two per million children per year in North America and Europe [1]) associated with variable peripheral blood cytopenias and a hypocellular bone marrow. It can be broadly divided into mild to moderate (non-severe), severe, and very severe depending on the degree or severity of the peripheral blood cytopenias in the presence of a hypocellular marrow. Mild to moderate aplastic anemia is defined as marrow cellularity of <50% and any two of the following: absolute neutrophil count (ANC) <1500/μl, platelet count <100,000/μl, and absolute reticulocyte count (ARC) <40,000/μl [2]. Severe aplastic anemia (SAA) is associated with severe hypoplastic marrow (bone marrow cellularity <25%) and at least two of the following: ANC <500/μl, platelet count <20,000/μl, and absolute reticulocyte count <20,000/μl [3]. Very severe aplastic anemia (vSAA) is defined by fulfilling criteria for SAA plus ANC of <200/μl [4]. Mild to moderate aplastic anemia can be associated with spontaneous resolution or can progress to SAA [5]. Severe and very severe aplastic anemias (SAA) are life-threatening disorders. Major advances in diagnostic and therapeutic (including immunosuppressive therapy or IST) resulted in long-term survival for more than 90% of the cases [6].

S. Khazal (✉)
The University of Texas MD Anderson Cancer Center, Houston, TX, USA
e-mail: sjkhazal@mdanderson.org

J. R. Galvez Silva
Nicklaus Children's Hospital, Miami Children's Health System, Miami, FL, USA
e-mail: jorgericardo.galvezsilva@mch.com

M. Thakar · D. Margolis
Children's Hospital of Wisconsin, Milwaukee, WI, USA
e-mail: mthakar@mcw.edu; dmargoli@mcw.edu

C. N. Duncan et al. (eds.), *Critical Care of the Pediatric Immunocompromised Hematology/Oncology Patient*, https://doi.org/10.1007/978-3-030-01322-6_7

Acquired aplastic anemia can be secondary to irradiation, drugs (e.g., chemotherapy, chloramphenicol, NSAIDs, and benzene), infections (EBV, CMV, HHV6, parvovirus B19, HIV, and hepatitis), pregnancy, nutritional deficiency (e.g., vitamin B12, folate and trace elements), and immune diseases (e.g., SLE) or "idiopathic" when no clear etiology can be identified. There is strong evidence that idiopathic acquired aplastic anemia is an immune destruction-mediated phenomena associated with an abnormal hematopoietic microenvironment [7–9]. The clinical signs and symptoms of aplastic anemia result from the pancytopenias. Spontaneous petechial skin rash, easy bruising, epistaxis, gum bleeding, or heavy menses in postmenarchal females are manifestations of thrombocytopenia. Anemia can present as fatigue, lack of energy, exercise intolerance, respiratory distress, and pallor. Infectious complications (e.g., fever, gingivitis, and skin abscesses) are a consequence of neutropenia. Organomegaly is not a typical clinical finding in aplastic anemia, and its presence should raise the suspicion of other diagnoses (infections and malignancies). Prompt diagnostic evaluation and early therapeutic intervention (IST or hematopoietic stem cell transplantation HSCT) are associated with improved outcomes [10]. Inherited bone marrow failure syndromes (IBMFS) and hypoplastic myelodysplastic syndrome (MDS) can have similar clinical presentation and must be distinguished from idiopathic acquired aplastic anemia. It is important to obtain a detailed history including exposure to medications and chemicals, comprehensive family history, and complete physical examination. Standard laboratory evaluations include complete blood count, reticulocyte count, peripheral smear, chemistries, unilateral bone marrow aspiration, and biopsy for histology and cytogenetics. Chromosomal breakage studies, telomeres' length, and genetic testing may be helpful to rule out IBMFS. Testing for paroxysmal nocturnal hemoglobinuria (PNH) by flow cytometry [11] is also important as PNH can present with marrow failure and pancytopenia and can also be an early clonal evolution in SAA. Once the diagnosis is established, HLA typing of the patient and related family members should be sent. Despite improvement in survival for patients with SAA [12], infection and bleeding remain as major causes of morbidity and mortality [13, 14]. SAA patients are profoundly immunocompromised and at risk of life-threatening infections including fungal infections [15]. Prophylactic antimicrobials (fungal and *Pneumocystis jiroveci* prophylaxis) are recommended [16] especially during periods of prolonged leukopenia and IST. Antibacterial prophylaxis may be considered in patients with vSAA [16]. Fever and neutropenia require immediate medical attention and hospitalization as they can progress rapidly to septic shock. Cultures (blood and urine), imaging (e.g., CT scans or chest X-ray), and prompt initiation of broad-spectrum antimicrobials (including antifungal agents for prolonged fever) are critical and can be lifesaving. Treatment should be initiated without waiting for culture results. There are currently no data to support the routine use of growth factors (GCSF or GMCSF) in patients with SAA. It may shorten the duration of neutropenia but did not improve overall survival, and prolonged use of high doses may be associated with malignant transformation [17, 18]. On the other hand, one large meta-analysis showed no association between the use of growth factors and the progression to MDS, acute leukemia, or PNH [19]. Granulocyte transfusions may be considered in life-threatening infections and neutropenia knowing that there is limited data to support it [20]. Several studies reported a negative impact of the number of blood products transfused prior to HSCT on the outcome after HSCT [21], and a restrictive blood product transfusion policy should be applied in patients with SAA who are candidates for HSCT; that being said, this should not delay a transfusion when indicated. Patients with active bleeding should receive platelet transfusions. Prophylactic platelet transfusion in asymptomatic patients with platelet count of <10,000/μl is recommended [22]. Higher platelet transfusion threshold (<20,000/μl) is recommended in patients at risk of rapid platelet consumption (e.g., fever or patients receiving IST) or those with history of life-threatening bleeding (gastrointestinal or central nervous system bleeding) [16]. There is no data to support the use of non-HLA-matched apheresis platelets over pooled platelets in non-allosensitized patients [23]. HLA-matched single-donor apheresis platelets should be used if the patient is platelet refractory and HLA antibodies are positive [24]. The addition of the thrombopoietin receptor agonist eltrombopag to the standard IST regimen was associated with improved hematologic response after 6 months without increasing the risk of clonal evolution [25]. Red blood cell transfusion is recommended for patients with hemoglobin level <8 g/dl or those with symptomatic anemia, and a higher threshold may be indicated in patients with other comorbidities (cardiac and/or respiratory) [26]. Erythropoietin should be avoided due to the resulting delay in definitive SAA therapy. Transfusions from related family members should be avoided as this may increase the risk of HLA sensitization and graft rejection if a matched related donor (MRD) bone marrow transplant could be an option. Blood products should always be leukoreduced and irradiated [27]. CMV-negative blood products are not routinely recommended if universal leukodepletion is applied [28, 29]. Treatment options for patients with SAA are hematopoietic stem cell transplantation (HSCT) and IST. The backbone of IST is antithymocyte globulin (ATG) in combination with the calcineurin inhibitor cyclosporine. Steroids are used during ATG therapy to prevent serum sickness (fever, rash, bronchospasm, and elevated liver enzymes 2–3 weeks after starting ATG) followed by rapid taper. Prolonged steroid use in SAA is ineffective and can increase the risk of infectious complications and gastrointestinal hemorrhage in the setting of severe thrombocytopenia. Horse ATG was proven to be associated with higher rates of hematologic response (68%) at 6 months and superior overall survival (96% at 3 years) compared to rabbit ATG [13]. ATG can be associated with rare immediate severe allergic (anaphylactic) reaction that can be predicted by skin test followed by desensitization for those who are allergic [30]. Horse ATG should be infused over at least 4 h through a 0.2 to 1 micron inline filter. Strongly consider premedication with antipyretics, antihistamines, and/or corticosteroids to prevent reactions. Cyclosporine blood levels should be closely monitored to avoid toxicities (nephrotoxicity, hypertension, hypertensive encephalopathy, hepatotoxicity, electrolyte abnormalities, and opportunistic infections). The current recommendation of primary therapy is HSCT with a bone marrow graft for patients who have MRD [31, 32]. IST is usually the first line of therapy in patients who lack full HLA-matched related donor and is associated with hematologic recovery in 50–70% of cases with excellent long-term survival [33]. Matched unrelated donor (MUD) or unrelated cord blood HSCT should be offered to all patients who do not respond to IST within 3–6 months [34, 35]. MUD HSCT was reported to be superior to second course of IST [36]. If MUD is unavailable, a second course of IST may be considered. Recent data may suggest that first-line therapy with HSCT forms MUD or even haploidentical donor HSCT is comparable or even superior to IST [37].

Fanconi Anemia

Fanconi anemia (FA) is a genetic disease characterized by marrow failure, predisposition to malignancies, and congenital abnormalities. This disorder was first described by pediatrician Dr. Guido Fanconi in 1927 after describing a family of three brothers with aplastic anemia and developmental defects [38]. FA is the most common of the rare inherited bone marrow failure syndromes, with a heterozygous carrier frequency of 1 in 300, with at least 20 different gene mutations described to date, known as "complementation groups," on which *FANCA* gene mutations are the most common. FA is a widely heterogeneous disease associated with multiple congenital malformations in different organ systems. Examples include the skin (hyper or hypopigmentation), musculoskeletal (thenar hypoplasia, absence or hypoplasia of the radius/thumbs, scoliosis, clubfoot), gastrointestinal (esophageal atresia, tracheoesophageal fistula, duodenal web, anal atresia), cardiopulmonary (ventricular septal defects, patent ductus arteriosus, pulmonary atresia), central nervous system (hydrocephalus, microcephaly), urogenital (undescended testes, micropenis, vaginal hypoplasia, urethral stenosis), renal (horseshoe kidney, hydronephrosis), ears (deafness, low-set ears), and endocrine (failure to thrive, short stature, glucose intolerance, infertility) [39]. FA is not classically associated with mental retardation. Patients with FA are often followed by multiple subspecialists since birth due to these congenital anomalies, which should raise suspicion for the diagnosis. However, up to 25% of patients will not display classic phenotypic features of the disease. A unifying feature is marked chromosomal instability and defects in DNA repair, for which increased breaks and radial formations in chromosomes are seen when cultured with diepoxybutane (DEB) or mitomycin C (MMC). This functional testing should be performed in a CLIA (Clinical Laboratory Improvement Amendments)-approved lab that has established expertise in performing this assay as a reference center. On occasion, patients' blood lymphocytes may not exhibit the degree of hypersensitivity to DEB and MMC crosslinking agents that would be expected for someone with FA, known as revertant somatic mosaicism [40, 41]. This occurs when there is spontaneous functional correction of the gene mutation and can sometimes lead to a milder phenotype of marrow failure. However, this could then create false-negative results on chromosomal fragility testing. If there is strong suspicion for FA, a skin biopsy should be sent to perform DEB/MMC testing on fibroblasts [42]. Greater than 90% of all patients will develop marrow failure before the age of 40 years old, with most presenting within the first decade of life [43]. Patients with FA have increased risk of developing all forms of hematological malignancies, with the most common being acute myeloid leukemia (10–37%) and myelodysplastic syndrome (11–34%), which often presents as refractory cytopenias with multilineage dysplasia. Patients with hematological malignancies frequently present during teenage years or young adulthood [44]. Solid tumor risk is also high, with a 700-fold risk of squamous cell carcinomas compared to the general population. Solid tumors are rare in the FA pediatric population, with exception of those with FANCD1/BRCA2, FANCN/PALB2, and FANCJ/BRIP1 complementation groups. Chemotherapy regimens must be adjusted when treating hematological malignancies and solid tumors for concern of increased toxicity. Most patients will need to undergo bone marrow transplantation for marrow failure. The conditioning regimen must also be limited in doses of agents which cross-link DNA. Fatal sinusoidal obstruction syndrome (SOS) as well as severe mucositis can affect management in the critical care setting. X-rays and CT scans, while necessary, should be thoughtfully used to limit ionizing radiation exposures. Each FA patient's underlying congenital defects must be considered when he or she becomes critically ill. For example, problems with tracheal stenosis could affect airway management; specific heart defects could impact fluid management. Patients who have urogenital concerns could be more prone to urinary tract infections and urosepsis when immunocompromised. Prior transfusion burden could impact iron overload, which can further increase the risk of SOS in FA.

Diamond-Blackfan Anemia

Diamond-Blackfan anemia (DBA) was initially described by Diamond and Blackfan in 1938 [45]. However, it was not until 25 years later that a full case series based on 25 years of experience on congenital hypoplastic anemia was published. This mainly described patients who had normocytic normochromic anemia, lacked erythroid precursors in the bone marrow, and had the absence of clinical leukopenia and/or thrombocytopenia [46]. Since then, despite the advances and efforts in understanding the etiology of the disease, the mainstay therapies remain unchanged. These therapies are packed red blood cells' (PRBCs) transfusion, corticosteroids, and hematopoietic stem cell transplantation (HSCT), the last one reserved for severe non-remission cases. DBA usually presents early in life, even in utero, due to the early severity of anemia (hydrops fetalis). Therefore, the classic phenotype of a patient with DBA is short stature, thumb anomalies, and congenital heart disease. This is in the context of macrocytic normochromic anemia (not described by Blackfan and Diamond) and reticulocytopenia in patients before 1 year of age [47, 48]. Nonetheless, at least 50% of the patients have only one congenital anomaly, and in approximately 25% of the cases, patients may go unnoticed due to the lack of anomalies and present later in life as adolescents or young adults [48–51]. Bone marrow biopsy will confirm normocellular marrow with the lack of erythroid precursors [51]. The diagnosis is further confirmed through an elevated pre-transfusion serum adenosine deaminase (erythrocytes) with a sensitivity and specificity of 84% and 95%, respectively [52]. This can be confirmed with the ongoing increased knowledge of the pathophysiology of DBA, locating the biogenesis in the ribosomes in at least 50% of the cases, with the majority of them inherited in an autosomal dominant pattern with incomplete penetrance [53]. These ribosome gene mutations seem to activate p53 pathways leading to the apoptosis of progenitor cells [54–57]. Among approximately 20 different genes, mutations in the RPS19 gene can be detected in up to 25% of the cases of DBA. In addition, genes such as GATA1 and TSR2 (XLR) have been described [51]. Differential diagnoses are described in this chapter such as Fanconi anemia, Shwachman-Diamond syndrome, dyskeratosis congenita, **or** transient erythroblastopenia of childhood (transient red cell hypoplasia). Once the diagnosis is confirmed, urgent treatment with PRBCs is needed due to severe anemia. Then, corticosteroids should be started at a dose of 2 mg/Kg a day in patients older than 12 months [47]. Corticosteroids may achieve a goal of complete or partial remission in up to 80% of the cases; however eventually a subset of patients will become refractory; only 37% patients will have a sustained response without the need of PRBCs [47, 58]. Response is expected within 4 weeks after initiation of therapy. If patients continue to require transfusion(s), then they are considered to have refractory disease. All data from corticosteroid treatment is based on retrospective studies. Tapering should be slow, and the maintenance dose recommended to avoid toxicities should be less than 0.5 mg/kg/day. In addition, the use of steroids before 1 year of age is avoided due to the significant impact on growth and development. Patients on prolonged steroids warrant close monitoring for steroid-related complications (i.e., bone density, susceptibility to infections). If patients become refractory, then they may require chronic PRBCs transfusions with the goal of keeping the hemoglobin above 8 g/dl to lessen effects on growth and development [49, 59]. The major and most detrimental effect of chronic transfusions is the development of iron overload and the subsequent multiorgan involvement that could increase morbidity and mortality in the transfusion-dependent population. This should be promptly treated with iron chelation, and patient's organs such as the heart and liver should be closely monitored for dysfunction due to iron overload.

In addition, patients with DBA are at increased risk of malignancies such as gastrointestinal carcinomas, myelodysplastic syndromes, and myeloid leukemia, and in rare occasions this could be the initial presentation [47, 60, 61]. HSCT is the only curative option for the hematological manifestations in patients with DBA who are transfusion dependent and steroid refractory or patients with other hematopoietic abnormalities such as MDS/leukemia. Chemotherapy and posttransplant complications require co-management with transplant physicians and a hematologist-oncologist [62].

Dyskeratosis Congenita

Dyskeratosis congenita (DKC) is a rare and highly variable phenotype condition that was initially described in 1906 in a dermatologic conference [63]. The principal triad of abnormal skin pigmentation, nail dystrophy, and mucosal leukoplakia characterizes the most severe phenotype [63–65]. In addition, patients with DKC are at higher risk of bone marrow failure, variable immunodeficiency (severe opportunistic infections), myelodysplastic syndrome/acute myeloid leukemia, solid tumors, and pulmonary fibrosis. Other nonclassical features may develop later in adulthood and include early gray hair, liver cirrhosis, emphysema, esophageal and urethral strictures, and head/neck squamous cell carcinoma, making the diagnosis more difficult and delayed [48]. The sole presence of pulmonary fibrosis and bone marrow failure in a patient has been found to be highly predictive of DKC [66].

The biological finding, however not unique to patients with DKC, is abnormally short telomere length, which encompasses the whole spectrum of telomere biology disorders [67, 68]. Telomeres are essential for maintaining chromosomal (DNA) stability [68]. The measurement can be performed clinically in peripheral lymphocytes via Flow-FISH [69, 70]. Lymphocytes' telomere lengths below the first percentile have a sensitivity and specificity of 97% and 91%, respectively [70]. Genetic mutation identified in 50–60% of the cases can be helpful in confirming the diagnosis. The most common gene mutation is in the DKC1 gene, which is inherited in an X-linked recessive fashion, can be seen in up to 25% of all cases. However, up to 25% of patients with DKC have unknown genetic variants. Other genes include *TERC, TERT* (associated with adult-onset pulmonary fibrosis), RTEL1, *and TINF2* among others (14 pathogenic known genes) that are inherited in autosomal dominant or recessive pattern [71]. The treatment utilized for patients with telomeropathies is based on using derivatives of androgens or synthetic steroids to improve telomere length [62]. Hematologic response is seen in up to 60–80% of the patients. However, common side effects include virilization, dyslipidemias, liver toxicity, splenic peliosis, bone fractures, and muscle cramps [72, 73]. Bone marrow failure in patients with DKC does not respond to immunosuppressive therapy [74]. The aforementioned treatments and complications describe clearly the complexity in managing patients with DKC. Moreover, these patients due to their liver and lung issues and their ongoing supportive therapies should be closely monitored for potential additional toxicities, especially medications that affect the DNA and/or are metabolized in the liver. HSCT is the only potential curative strategy for the patients who do not have a hematological response to medical treatment or for patients with severe bone marrow failure/immunodeficiency [75, 76]. Due to high sensitivity to DNA-disrupting medications, patients are conditioned with reduced intensity preparative regimens for their transplant. As described before, some of the phenotypes may be aggravated by the HSCT, and the complications warrant co-management with the bone marrow transplant physician and the respective specialists [59].

Schwachman-Bodian-Diamond Syndrome

First described by two different groups in 1964 for which the disease has its namesake [77, 78], Schwachman-Bodian-Diamond syndrome (SBDS) is characterized by progressive marrow failure (most commonly with neutropenia), exocrine pancreatic insufficiency, acute myeloid leukemia (AML) or myelodysplastic syndrome (MDS), and skeletal abnormalities. It is inherited in an autosomal recessive fashion with an incidence of 1 in 77,000 and a carrier frequency of 1 in 110 [79]. SBDS is a clinical diagnosis in which a genetic diagnosis can be made in approximately 90% of individuals who have biallelic mutations in the *SBDS* gene, which is located on chromosome 7 [80]. SBDS uniformly has an exocrine pancreatic defect associated with steatorrhea and often failure to thrive, similar to that of a patient with cystic fibrosis. Evaluation includes checking fat-soluble vitamin levels (vitamins A, D, E, K), low serum trypsinogen, elevated fecal fat levels, and MRI imaging of the pancreas demonstrating a small-sized pancreas with fatty replacement [81]. The marrow dysfunction has been characterized as neutropenia, although thrombocytopenia and anemia can also occur. One of the most concerning features of this disease is the risk of transformation to AML or MDS, with an estimated risk of 19% at 20 years and 36% at 30 years [82]. Other concerns for this disease include an association with endocrine abnormalities including insulin-dependent diabetes mellitus, growth hormone deficiency, hypothyroidism, cardiac issues including myocardial necrosis [83], and skeletal abnormalities typically at growth plates, with more than 50% of patients having metaphyseal dysostosis or rib cage abnormalities [84]. Patients are referred to hematopoietic stem cell transplant (HSCT) for progressive cytopenias, development of AML, or MDS with excessive blasts [85]. Congenital defects of the skeletal system and associated endocrine and cardiac dysfunction may create additional concerns in the posttransplant setting when considering fluid management, sepsis, and cardiorespiratory concerns.

Intensive Care Considerations

Patients with bone marrow failure syndromes (congenital and acquired) are at risk of life-threatening complications related to their primary disease or as a result of treatment (Table 7.1). Isolated cytopenias and pancytopenia can result in life-threatening hemorrhage, respiratory and/or cardiac failure, and sepsis. Chronic blood product transfusions is the mainstay of supportive treatment for most marrow failure syndromes which are associated with high risk of iron overload resulting in multiple organs' damage/dysfunction (Table 7.1), risk of transmission of infectious diseases, alloimmunization, and transfusion reactions (including TRALI or transfusion-related acute lung injury). Inherited marrow failure syndromes can be associated with congenital malformations (craniofacial, thoracic cage, cardiac, renal, pulmonary among others) which can impact ICU care in regard to airway management, fluid balance, and risk of infectious complications.

Table 7.1 Common complications of bone marrow failure syndromes and syndrome-specific intensive care considerations

Bone marrow failure syndrome	Intensive care considerations
Common complications associated with all bone marrow failure syndromes are: Pancytopenia-associated complications (bleeding (gastrointestinal hemorrhage, intracranial hemorrhage, menorrhagia), anemia (respiratory distress, ischemic heart disease, and heart failure), and infections (neutropenic fever, sepsis, and septic shock) including fungal, viral, bacterial, and parasitic Progression to myelodysplastic syndrome and acute leukemia Treatment-related (chronic blood transfusion) complications (iron overload resulting in liver fibrosis, cirrhosis and hepatocellular cancer, exocrine and endocrine pancreatic insufficiency, renal insufficiency, adrenal insufficiency, and cardiac failure) and red cell and HLA alloimmunization Risk of difficult airway and intubation (for inherited bone marrow failure syndromes)	
Acquired aplastic anemia	Immunosuppressive therapy-related complications (antithymocyte globulin-associated anaphylactic reaction, calcineurin inhibitor-associated PRES (posterior reversible encephalopathy syndrome), and acute kidney injury)
Fanconi anemia	Skeletal (microcephaly), urogenital (horseshoe, ectopic or absent kidneys, hypospadias, cryptorchidism, uterine malformations), cardiac (septal defects, truncus arteriosus), gastrointestinal (tracheoesophageal fistula, annular pancreas), and central nervous system (absent corpus callosum, hydrocephalus) malformations Hematopoietic stem cell transplantation-related complications (high risk of sinusoidal obstruction syndrome and severe mucositis)
Diamond-Blackfan anemia	Craniofacial (microcephaly, micrognathia, cleft lip/palate), cardiac (septal defects, coarctation of aorta), and urogenital (absent and horseshoe kidney, hypospadias) malformation
Dyskeratosis congenita	Pulmonary fibrosis and respiratory failure (at presentation or post-allogeneic stem cell transplantation), pulmonary arteriovenous malformation Liver fibrosis and cirrhosis Cardiac abnormalities (septal defects, myocardial fibrosis, and dilated cardiomyopathy) Esophageal and upper airway disease and stenosis, risk of esophageal varices and aspiration
Schwachman-Bodian-Diamond syndrome	Severe exocrine and endocrine pancreatic insufficiency (malabsorption, failure to thrive, fat-soluble vitamin deficiency) Cardiac abnormalities (myocardial necrosis and cardiac failure) Skeletal dysplasia (metaphyseal changes in the costochondral junctions and rib cage abnormalities during infancy and early childhood), delayed dentition, dental dysplasia, and craniofacial abnormalities

HLA human leukocyte antigen

References

1. Montane E, Ibanez L, Vidal X, et al. Epidemiology of aplastic anemia: a prospective multicenter study. Haematologica. 2008;93(4):518–23.
2. Howard SC, Naidu PE, Hu XJ, et al. Natural history of moderate aplastic anemia in children. Pediatr Blood Cancer. 2004;43(5):545–51.
3. Camitta BM, Rappeport JM, Parkman R, Nathan DG. Selection of patients for bone marrow transplantation in severe aplastic anemia. Blood. 1975;45(3):355–63.
4. Bacigalupo A, Hows J, Gluckman E, et al. Bone marrow transplantation (BMT) versus immunosuppression for the treatment of severe aplastic anaemia (SAA): a report of the EBMT SAA working party. Br J Haematol. 1988;70(2):177–82.
5. Khatib Z, Wilimas J, Wang W. Outcome of moderate aplastic anemia in children. Am J Pediatr Hematol Oncol. 1994;16(1):80–5.
6. Hartung HD, Olson TS, Bessler M. Acquired aplastic anemia in children. Pediatr Clin N Am. 2013;60(6):1311–36.
7. Young NS, Scheinberg P, Calado RT. Aplastic anemia. Curr Opin Hematol. 2008;15(3):162–8.
8. Young NS, Calado RT, Scheinberg P. Current concepts in the pathophysiology and treatment of aplastic anemia. Blood. 2006;108(8):2509–19.
9. Knospe WH, Crosby WH. Aplastic anaemia: a disorder of the bone-marrow sinusoidal microcirculation rather than stem-cell failure? Lancet. 1971;1(7688):20–2.
10. Locasciulli A, Oneto R, Bacigalupo A, et al. Outcome of patients with acquired aplastic anemia given first line bone marrow transplantation or immunosuppressive treatment in the last decade: a report from the European Group for Blood and Marrow Transplantation (EBMT). Haematologica. 2007;92(1):11–8.
11. Sutherland DR, Kuek N, Davidson J, et al. Diagnosing PNH with FLAER and multiparameter flow cytometry. Cytometry B Clin Cytom. 2007;72(3):167–77.
12. Valdez JM, Scheinberg P, Nunez O, Wu CO, Young NS, Walsh TJ. Decreased infection-related mortality and improved survival in severe aplastic anemia in the past two decades. Clin Infect Dis. 2011;52(6):726–35.
13. Scheinberg P, Nunez O, Weinstein B, et al. Horse versus rabbit antithymocyte globulin in acquired aplastic anemia. N Engl J Med. 2011;365(5):430–8.
14. Tichelli A, Schrezenmeier H, Socie G, et al. A randomized controlled study in patients with newly diagnosed severe aplastic anemia receiving antithymocyte globulin (ATG), cyclosporine, with or without G-CSF: a study of the SAA Working Party of the European Group for Blood and Marrow Transplantation. Blood. 2011;117(17):4434–41.
15. Weinberger M, Elattar I, Marshall D, et al. Patterns of infection in patients with aplastic anemia and the emergence of Aspergillus as a major cause of death. Medicine (Baltimore). 1992;71(1):24–43.
16. Hochsmann B, Moicean A, Risitano A, Ljungman P, Schrezenmeier H. Supportive care in severe and very severe aplastic anemia. Bone Marrow Transplant. 2013;48(2):168–73.
17. Ohara A, Kojima S, Hamajima N, et al. Myelodysplastic syndrome and acute myelogenous leukemia as a late clonal complication in children with acquired aplastic anemia. Blood. 1997;90(3):1009–13.
18. Jeng MR, Naidu PE, Rieman MD, et al. Granulocyte-macrophage colony stimulating factor and immunosuppression in the treatment of pediatric acquired severe aplastic anemia. Pediatr Blood Cancer. 2005;45(2):170–5.
19. Gurion R, Gafter-Gvili A, Paul M, et al. Hematopoietic growth factors in aplastic anemia patients treated with immunosuppressive therapy-systematic review and meta-analysis. Haematologica. 2009;94(5):712–9.
20. Quillen K, Wong E, Scheinberg P, et al. Granulocyte transfusions in severe aplastic anemia: an eleven-year experience. Haematologica. 2009;94(12):1661–8.
21. Champlin RE, Horowitz MM, van Bekkum DW, et al. Graft failure following bone marrow transplantation for severe aplastic anemia: risk factors and treatment results. Blood. 1989;73(2):606–13.

22. Marsh JC, Ball SE, Cavenagh J, et al. Guidelines for the diagnosis and management of aplastic anaemia. Br J Haematol. 2009;147(1):43–70.
23. Schrezenmeier H, Seifried E. Buffy-coat-derived pooled platelet concentrates and apheresis platelet concentrates: which product type should be preferred? Vox Sang. 2010;99(1):1–15.
24. Laundy GJ, Bradley BA, Rees BM, Younie M, Hows JM. Incidence and specificity of HLA antibodies in multitransfused patients with acquired aplastic anemia. Transfusion. 2004;44(6):814–25.
25. Townsley DM, Scheinberg P, Winkler T, et al. Eltrombopag added to standard immunosuppression for aplastic anemia. N Engl J Med. 2017;376(16):1540–50.
26. Welte M. Erythrocyte transfusion: update of the guidelines "therapy with blood components and plasma derivatives". Anaesthesist. 2009;58(11):1150–8.
27. Marsh J, Socie G, Tichelli A, et al. Should irradiated blood products be given routinely to all patients with aplastic anaemia undergoing immunosuppressive therapy with antithymocyte globulin (ATG)? A survey from the European Group for Blood and Marrow Transplantation Severe Aplastic Anaemia Working Party. Br J Haematol. 2010;150(3):377–9.
28. Nichols WG, Price TH, Gooley T, Corey L, Boeckh M. Transfusion-transmitted cytomegalovirus infection after receipt of leukoreduced blood products. Blood. 2003;101(10):4195–200.
29. Vamvakas EC. Is white blood cell reduction equivalent to antibody screening in preventing transmission of cytomegalovirus by transfusion? A review of the literature and meta-analysis. Transfus Med Rev. 2005;19(3):181–99.
30. Bielory L, Wright R, Nienhuis AW, Young NS, Kaliner MA. Antithymocyte globulin hypersensitivity in bone marrow failure patients. JAMA. 1988;260(21):3164–7.
31. Yoshida N, Kobayashi R, Yabe H, et al. First-line treatment for severe aplastic anemia in children: bone marrow transplantation from a matched family donor versus immunosuppressive therapy. Haematologica. 2014;99(12):1784–91.
32. Bacigalupo A, Brand R, Oneto R, et al. Treatment of acquired severe aplastic anemia: bone marrow transplantation compared with immunosuppressive therapy--The European Group for Blood and Marrow Transplantation experience. Semin Hematol. 2000;37(1):69–80.
33. Bacigalupo A. How I treat acquired aplastic anemia. Blood. 2017;129(11):1428–36.
34. Samarasinghe S, Steward C, Hiwarkar P, et al. Excellent outcome of matched unrelated donor transplantation in paediatric aplastic anaemia following failure with immunosuppressive therapy: a United Kingdom multicentre retrospective experience. Br J Haematol. 2012;157(3):339–46.
35. Pagliuca S, Peffault de Latour R, Volt F, et al. Long-term outcomes of cord blood transplantation from an HLA-identical sibling for patients with bone marrow failure syndromes: a report from eurocord, cord blood committee and severe aplastic anemia Working Party of the European Society for Blood and Marrow Transplantation. Biol Blood Marrow Transplant. 2017;23(11):1939–48.
36. Kosaka Y, Yagasaki H, Sano K, et al. Prospective multicenter trial comparing repeated immunosuppressive therapy with stem-cell transplantation from an alternative donor as second-line treatment for children with severe and very severe aplastic anemia. Blood. 2008;111(3):1054–9.
37. Cheng Y, Xu Z, Zhang Y, et al. First-line choice for severe aplastic anemia in children: transplantation from a haploidentical donor vs immunosuppressive therapy. Clin Transpl. 2017 PMID: 29297952
38. Fanconi G. Familiaere infantile pernizisaartige anaemie. Jahrbuch Kinderheild. 1927;117: 257–80.
39. Triemstra J, Rhodes L, Waggoner DJ, Onel K. A review of Fanconi anemia for the practicing pediatrician. Pediatr Ann. 2015;44(10):444–5, 448, 450, 452
40. Soulier J, Leblanc T, Larghero J, et al. Detection of somatic mosaicism and classification of Fanconi anemia patients by analysis of the FA/BRCA pathway. Blood. 2005;105(3):1329–36.
41. Gregory JJ Jr, Wagner JE, Verlander PC, et al. Somatic mosaicism in Fanconi anemia: evidence of genotypic reversion in lymphohematopoietic stem cells. Proc Natl Acad Sci U S A. 2001;98(5):2532–7.

42. Fargo JH, Rochowski A, Giri N, Savage SA, Olson SB, Alter BP. Comparison of chromosome breakage in non-mosaic and mosaic patients with Fanconi anemia, relatives, and patients with other inherited bone marrow failure syndromes. Cytogenet Genome Res. 2014;144(1):15–27.
43. Kutler DI, Singh B, Satagopan J, et al. A 20-year perspective on the International Fanconi Anemia Registry (IFAR). Blood. 2003;101(4):1249–56.
44. Peffault de Latour R, Soulier J. How I treat MDS and AML in Fanconi anemia. Blood. 2016;127(24):2971–9.
45. Diamond LK, Blackfan KD. Hypoplastic anemia. Am J Dis Child. 1938;56:464.
46. Diamond LK, Allen DM, Magill FB. Congenital (erythroid) hypoplastic anemia. A 25-year study. Am J Dis Child. 1961;102:403–15.
47. Vlachos A, Muir E. How I treat Diamond-Blackfan anemia. Blood. 2010;116(19):3715–23.
48. West AH, Churpek JE. Old and new tools in the clinical diagnosis of inherited bone marrow failure syndromes. Hematology Am Soc Hematol Educ Program. 2017;2017(1):79–87.
49. Vlachos A, Ball S, Dahl N, et al. Diagnosing and treating Diamond Blackfan anaemia: results of an international clinical consensus conference. Br J Haematol. 2008;142(6):859–76.
50. Wilson DB, Link DC, Mason PJ, Bessler M. Inherited bone marrow failure syndromes in adolescents and young adults. Ann Med. 2014;46(6):353–63.
51. Clinton C, Gazda HT. Diamond-Blackfan Anemia. In: Adam MP, Ardinger HH, Pagon RA, et al., editors. GeneReviews((R)). Seattle: University of Washington; 1993.
52. Fargo JH, Kratz CP, Giri N, et al. Erythrocyte adenosine deaminase: diagnostic value for Diamond-Blackfan anaemia. Br J Haematol. 2013;160(4):547–54.
53. Narla A, Ebert BL. Ribosomopathies: human disorders of ribosome dysfunction. Blood. 2010;115(16):3196–205.
54. McGowan KA, Li JZ, Park CY, et al. Ribosomal mutations cause p53-mediated dark skin and pleiotropic effects. Nat Genet. 2008;40(8):963–70.
55. Fumagalli S, Di Cara A, Neb-Gulati A, et al. Absence of nucleolar disruption after impairment of 40S ribosome biogenesis reveals an rpL11-translation-dependent mechanism of p53 induction. Nat Cell Biol. 2009;11(4):501–8.
56. Dutt S, Narla A, Lin K, et al. Haploinsufficiency for ribosomal protein genes causes selective activation of p53 in human erythroid progenitor cells. Blood. 2011;117(9):2567–76.
57. Keel SB, Doty RT, Yang Z, et al. A heme export protein is required for red blood cell differentiation and iron homeostasis. Science. 2008;319(5864):825–8.
58. Lipton JM, Atsidaftos E, Zyskind I, Vlachos A. Improving clinical care and elucidating the pathophysiology of Diamond Blackfan anemia: an update from the Diamond Blackfan Anemia Registry. Pediatr Blood Cancer. 2006;46(5):558–64.
59. Calado RT, Cle DV. Treatment of inherited bone marrow failure syndromes beyond transplantation. Hematology Am Soc Hematol Educ Program. 2017;2017(1):96–101.
60. Vlachos A, Rosenberg PS, Kang J, Atsidaftos E, Alter BP, Lipton JM. Myelodysplastic syndrome and gastrointestinal carcinomas characterize the cancer risk in Diamond Blackfan anemia: a report from the Diamond Blackfan anemia registry. Blood. 2016;128(122):333.
61. Vlachos A, Rosenberg PS, Atsidaftos E, Alter BP, Lipton JM. Incidence of neoplasia in Diamond Blackfan anemia: a report from the Diamond Blackfan Anemia Registry. Blood. 2012;119(16):3815–9.
62. Alter BP. Inherited bone marrow failure syndromes: considerations pre- and posttransplant. Hematology Am Soc Hematol Educ Program. 2017;2017(1):88–95.
63. Savage SA, Bertuch AA. The genetics and clinical manifestations of telomere biology disorders. Genet Med. 2010;12(12):753–64.
64. Dokal I. Dyskeratosis congenita in all its forms. Br J Haematol. 2000;110(4):768–79.
65. Dokal I. Dyskeratosis congenita. Hematology Am Soc Hematol Educ Program. 2011;2011:480–6.
66. Parry EM, Alder JK, Qi X, Chen JJ, Armanios M. Syndrome complex of bone marrow failure and pulmonary fibrosis predicts germline defects in telomerase. Blood. 2011;117(21):5607–11.
67. Vulliamy TJ, Marrone A, Knight SW, Walne A, Mason PJ, Dokal I. Mutations in dyskeratosis congenita: their impact on telomere length and the diversity of clinical presentation. Blood. 2006;107(7):2680–5.

68. Savage SA, Alter BP. The role of telomere biology in bone marrow failure and other disorders. Mech Ageing Dev. 2008;129(1–2):35–47.
69. Baerlocher GM, Lansdorp PM. Telomere length measurements in leukocyte subsets by automated multicolor flow-FISH. Cytometry A. 2003;55(1):1–6.
70. Alter BP, Baerlocher GM, Savage SA, et al. Very short telomere length by flow fluorescence in situ hybridization identifies patients with dyskeratosis congenita. Blood. 2007;110(5):1439–47.
71. Alter BP, Rosenberg PS, Giri N, Baerlocher GM, Lansdorp PM, Savage SA. Telomere length is associated with disease severity and declines with age in dyskeratosis congenita. Haematologica. 2012;97(3):353–9.
72. Khincha PP, Wentzensen IM, Giri N, Alter BP, Savage SA. Response to androgen therapy in patients with dyskeratosis congenita. Br J Haematol. 2014;165(3):349–57.
73. Townsley DM, Dumitriu B, Young NS. Danazol treatment for telomere diseases. N Engl J Med. 2016;375(11):1095–6.
74. Al-Rahawan MM, Giri N, Alter BP. Intensive immunosuppression therapy for aplastic anemia associated with dyskeratosis congenita. Int J Hematol. 2006;83(3):275–6.
75. Dietz AC, Orchard PJ, Baker KS, et al. Disease-specific hematopoietic cell transplantation: nonmyeloablative conditioning regimen for dyskeratosis congenita. Bone Marrow Transplant. 2011;46(1):98–104.
76. Gadalla SM, Sales-Bonfim C, Carreras J, et al. Outcomes of allogeneic hematopoietic cell transplantation in patients with dyskeratosis congenita. Biol Blood Marrow Transplant. 2013;19(8):1238–43.
77. Bodian M, Sheldon W, Lightwood R. Congenital hypoplasia of the exocrine pancreas. Acta Paediatr. 1964;53:282–93.
78. Shwachman H, Diamond LK, Oski FA, Khaw KT. The syndrome of pancreatic insufficiency and bone marrow dysfunction. J Pediatr. 1964;65:645–63.
79. Goobie S, Popovic M, Morrison J, et al. Shwachman-Diamond syndrome with exocrine pancreatic dysfunction and bone marrow failure maps to the centromeric region of chromosome 7. Am J Hum Genet. 2001;68(4):1048–54.
80. Boocock GR, Morrison JA, Popovic M, et al. Mutations in SBDS are associated with Shwachman-Diamond syndrome. Nat Genet. 2003;33(1):97–101.
81. Toiviainen-Salo S, Raade M, Durie PR, et al. Magnetic resonance imaging findings of the pancreas in patients with Shwachman-Diamond syndrome and mutations in the SBDS gene. J Pediatr. 2008;152(3):434–6.
82. Donadieu J, Leblanc T, Bader Meunier B, et al. Analysis of risk factors for myelodysplasias, leukemias and death from infection among patients with congenital neutropenia. Experience of the French Severe Chronic Neutropenia Study Group. Haematologica. 2005;90(1):45–53.
83. Savilahti E, Rapola J. Frequent myocardial lesions in Shwachman's syndrome. Eight fatal cases among 16 Finnish patients. Acta Paediatr Scand. 1984;73(5):642–51.
84. Burroughs L, Woolfrey A, Shimamura A. Shwachman-Diamond syndrome: a review of the clinical presentation, molecular pathogenesis, diagnosis, and treatment. Hematol Oncol Clin North Am. 2009;23(2):233–48.
85. Dror Y, Donadieu J, Koglmeier J, et al. Draft consensus guidelines for diagnosis and treatment of Shwachman-Diamond syndrome. Ann N Y Acad Sci. 2011;1242:40–55.

Chapter 8
Hematopoietic Stem Cell Transplant and Cellular Therapy

Priti Tewari, Rajinder Bajwa, Agne Taraseviciute, Jerelyn Moffet, David McCall, and Kris M. Mahadeo

Overview of HCT + CT

Hematopoietic cell transplantation (HCT) and cellular therapy (CT) offer potentially curative treatment for patients with a wide array of high-risk malignancies and nonmalignant diseases (Table 8.1) [1–3]. Autologous HCT refers to infusion of the patient's own hematopoietic stem cells (HSCs) which were previously collected and cryopreserved, usually following myeloablative chemotherapy and/or radiation; this facilitates the patient's hematopoietic recovery following high-dose consolidation therapy [4–7]. Allogeneic HCT refers to infusion of HSCs from a donor, who (i) may be related (MRD) or unrelated (MUD), and (ii) full histocompatible match (10/10 or 8/8) or mismatched (including haplo-identical) donors. Allogeneic graft source may be from bone marrow or peripheral blood stem cells (PBSC). Related and unrelated umbilical cord blood HSCs are also used for allogeneic HCT with permissive mismatch (4/6–6/6) given the relatively naïve T cells in these units (provided there is an adequate cell dose per unit); double cord units may be used to overcome limited cell dose of a single unit [8]. Cell therapies such as chimeric

P. Tewari · D. McCall · K. M. Mahadeo (✉)
University of Texas MD Anderson Cancer Center, Houston, TX, USA
e-mail: KMMahadeo@mdanderson.org

R. Bajwa
Nationwide Children's Hospital, Columbus, OH, USA

A. Taraseviciute
Children's Hospital Los Angeles, University of Southern California, Los Angeles, CA, USA

J. Moffet
Duke Children's Hospital, Durham, NC, USA

C. N. Duncan et al. (eds.), *Critical Care of the Pediatric Immunocompromised Hematology/Oncology Patient*, https://doi.org/10.1007/978-3-030-01322-6_8

Table 8.1 Evidence-based indications for allogeneic and autologous stem cell transplantation [1–3]

Allogeneic		Autologous
High-risk/relapsed/refractory malignant disease	Nonmalignant disease	High-risk/relapsed/ refractory
Acute myeloid leukemia	Severe aplastic anemia	Neuroblastoma
Acute lymphoblastic leukemia	Hemoglobinopathy Sickle cell disease Thalassemia	Germ cell tumor
Acute promyelocytic leukemia	Bone marrow failure syndromes Severe aplastic anemia Dyskeratosis congenita Diamond-Blackfan anemia Congenital amegakaryocytic thrombocytopenia Severe congenital neutropenia Fanconi anemia	Medulloblastoma
Chronic myeloid leukemia	Immunodeficiencies Severe combined immunodeficiency IPEX syndrome Chronic granulomatous disease Wiskott-Aldrich syndrome	Hodgkin's lymphoma
Lymphoma T-cell non-Hodgkin lymphoma Lymphoblastic B-cell non-Hodgkin lymphoma Burkitt's lymphoma Hodgkin lymphoma Anaplastic large cell lymphoma	Inherited metabolic disorders Hurler syndrome Hunter syndrome Krabbe disease Metachromatic leukodystrophy	Non-Hodgkin lymphoma
Treatment related AML/MDS	Adrenoleukodystrophy	Burkitt's lymphoma
Myelodysplastic syndromes	Osteopetrosis	Anaplastic large cell lymphoma
	Hemophagocytic disorders	Diffuse large B-cell lymphoma

antigen receptor T-cell therapy (CAR-T) have been used to successfully treat children and young adults with relapsed and/or refractory pre-B cell CD-19+ acute lymphoblastic leukemia (ALL) or young adults with CD-19+ lymphoma [9]. Clinical trials exploring the role of gene therapy and editing for the cure of nonmalignant diseases are ongoing [10].

While up to 35% of the more than 2500 children who undergo HCT in the United States each year require intensive care support for life-threatening complications [11], the number of pediatric HCT patients who survive following PICU admission is increasing. Unfortunately, these patients may have up to eight times greater odds for pediatric intensive care unit (PICU) mortality than do other critically ill children

[12]. Importantly, for pediatric HCT patients who survive intensive care admission, their 1-year survival and organ function are similar to those pediatric HCT patients who never require intensive care [12, 13]. While almost half of pediatric and young adult patients who received tisagenlecleucel CAR therapy on the pivotal clinical trial required intensive care support, the outcomes among this high-risk disease cohort are quite promising [14].

HCT Timeline

In some cases, even when initial disease presentation warrants care in the intensive care setting, an HCT evaluation may be necessary around the time of diagnosis. Early referral to HCT, prior to development of organ toxicity and comorbidity may significantly improve outcomes. The National Marrow Donor Program® (NMDP)/ Be The Match® and the American Society for Blood and Marrow Transplantation (ASBMT) have developed guidelines for the prompt referral to HCT [15]. This allows for appropriate planning and early donor identification (or optimal time to autologous collection) and avoids delays in progression to HCT (Fig. 8.1).

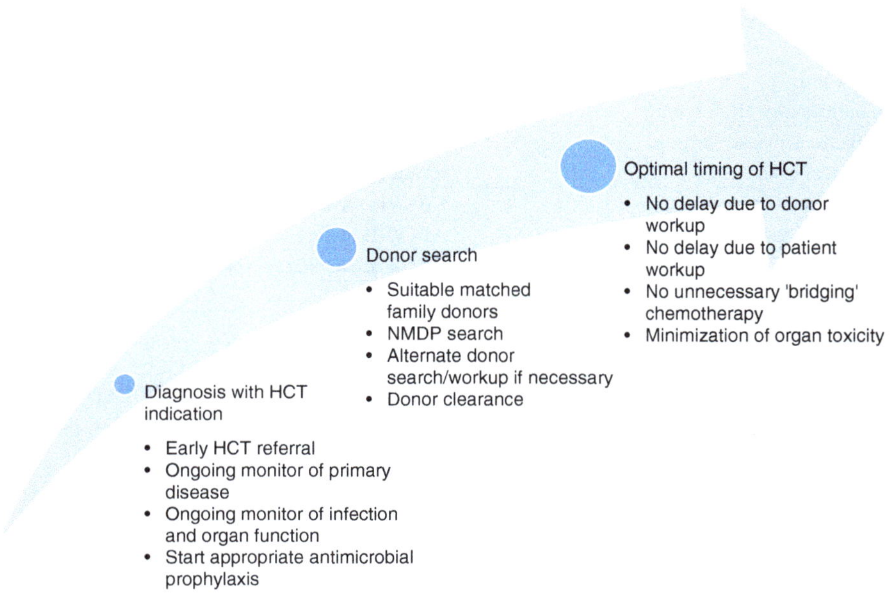

Fig. 8.1 Optimal timing of consultation of hematopoietic stem cell transplant service. Early referral to Hematopoietic Stem Cell Transplant (HCT) Service for a patient with HCT indication is important to organize timing of patient/donor workup; this should prevent unnecessary delays and faciliate timely and safe HCT

Autologous Apheresis and Mobilization

Stem cell mobilization refers to the process of stimulating stem cells out of the bone marrow space into peripheral circulation for apheresis. Mobilization regimens may include growth factor alone or in combination with chemotherapy or immunostimulants [16, 17]. Typically, autologous HSC apheresis should occur as early in the treatment course as possible to ensure sufficient marrow mobilization for collection. Some have suggested that the more immunocompetent the host at the time of apheresis (pre-mobilization T-cell status), the better the survival after HCT [18–20]. Prior to stem cell mobilization, the patient will undergo pre-collection testing (Table 8.2) [21] to ensure that he/she is medically appropriate to proceed. The patient should be hemodynamically stable and able to tolerate fluid shifts and be free of active infection. If a patient requires intensive care support at the time of apheresis, consider obtaining an echocardiogram to assess for evidence of systolic or diastolic dysfunction and pulmonary hypertension. Institutional guidelines will generally outline specific hematologic criteria to proceed with collection. Due to the relatively low circulatory volume and narrow vessels of pediatric patients, hypotension, hypocalcemia, and catheter-related pain are not infrequent side effects during

Table 8.2 Standard components of HCT donor/recipient medical clearance

Pre-HCT workup	
Donor	Patient
HLA testing	HLA testing
Confirmatory HLA typing	Confirmatory HLA typing
Infectious disease testing	Infectious disease testing
Physical exam	Physical exam
CBC/chemistries	CBC/chemistries
ABO/RH testing	ABO/RH testing
Pregnancy testing (if applicable)	Pregnancy testing (if applicable)
EKG	EKG
CXR	CXR
Sickledex/hemoglobinopathy assessment	Echo
High-risk behavior assessment	Performance status (Lansky/Karnofsky)
Health history questionnaire	Pulmonary function testing
Clearance by an independent provider[a]	Renal function testing
	Chest/sinus CT scan (optional)
	Dental evaluation
	Primary disease assessment/management[b]
	Final selection of appropriate preparative regimen

HLA human leukocyte antigen, *CBC* complete blood count, *CT* computed tomography
[a]HCT donors should have a medical evaluation also performed by an independent physician not involved in the recipient's care
[b]Evaluation may be tailored based upon individual scenarios prior to HCT [21]

pediatric apheresis [22–26]. Monitoring of ionized calcium (iCa) in blood with anticipatory calcium supplementation may avoid hypocalcemic tetany, especially among infants and younger children who may be unable to articulate symptoms. The use of albumin in addition to irradiated packed red blood cells to prime the collection pathway in patients weighing less than 30 kg may avoid hypovolemia. Once sufficient autologous HSC cells are obtained, they are cryopreserved for later use. Prior to high-dose consolidation chemotherapy with autologous HCT, patients must be again evaluated to determine eligibility to safely proceed. A preparative regimen will be finalized, with dose adjustments made for current renal function and other regimen changes as necessary based on organ function assessment.

Allogeneic Donor Search

Human leukocyte antigen (HLA) typing is used to match patients and donors for allogeneic HCT. If a patient is considered an allogeneic HCT candidate, high-resolution HLA typing of the patient and potential family donors should be completed early after diagnosis. If no histocompatible matches are found, a preliminary search of the unrelated donor and cord blood registries may be performed to identify a matched unrelated donor (MUD). At some institutions and depending upon the disease indication for HCT, a related haplo-identical donor may be prioritized over a MUD donor. Once an optimal donor has been selected, this donor will undergo HLA confirmatory typing and a medical examination to confirm donor eligibility. If the selected donor is found to be ineligible, the process is repeated with the next best available donor, until a donor is confirmed. This process can take several weeks to be completed, so early initiation of a donor search is important.

Pre-HCT and CT Evaluation

A comprehensive evaluation is performed to confirm that the HCT-CT recipient/patient is medically suitable to proceed (Table 8.2) [21]. This typically includes assessment of cardiac, lung, and renal function and screening for the presence of occult infection. Disease-specific screening may also be performed to ensure the patient has not advanced beyond the potential benefit of HCT-CT.

Chimeric Antigen Receptor (CAR) Therapy

Chimeric antigen receptors (CAR) consist of an extracellular antigen-recognition domain, linked to at least one intracellular signaling. The extracellular portion of the CAR allows recognition of a specific antigen, and the signaling domain(s) stimulate T-cell proliferation, cytolysis, and cytokine secretion to eliminate the target cell. The patients' cells are isolated, activated, and genetically modified to generate CAR cells [9, 27–41].

The first step in generating autologous (CAR) T cells is to collect CD3+ lymphocytes by apheresis of the patient. However, patients requiring intensive care support may have leukopenia and/or other disease-related complications, which make adequate collection more challenging. Early leukapheresis that is timed to avoid administration of chemotherapy and other agents that may diminish circulating T cells may optimize chances of successful collection. Eligibility for leukapheresis collection is performed as described above. Once an adequate collection is achieved, production of CAR-T cells may take 2–4 weeks. A major limitation of autologous CAR therapy is the time required for manufacture. Bridging chemotherapy may be required during this period. Patients should be monitored for tumor lysis syndrome and receive anti-microbial prophylaxis if indicated. Allogeneic CAR cells may allow for an off-the-shelf third-party approach to therapy [42]. Once CAR cells are available, the patient typically receives lympho-depleting chemotherapy followed by infusion of the cells.

Preparative or Lympho-depletion Regimen

On the day of initiation of the preparative or lympho-depletion regimen, an interim assessment should be performed to ensure that the patient still meets eligibility criteria. This usually includes screening for signs/symptoms of active infection and/or new organ toxicity and confirming no significant interval height/weight changes. Good communication between intensive care and HCT-CT teams ensures that adjustments are made if indicated. Review of side effects related to specific drugs/treatment modalities used in the preparative regimen may be useful to the patient/caregivers as well as to the treatment team. Prophylactic medication orders should be confirmed (such as anticonvulsants used with busulfan, proton-pump inhibitor, nausea, and antimicrobial prophylaxis). Myelosuppressive medications should be discontinued prior to infusion of the cell therapy product when appropriate.

Infusion of Hematopoietic Stem Cells or CAR-T Cells

Oxygen, suction, and emergency medications (epinephrine, diphenhydramine, and corticosteroids) should be readily available prior to infusion. The patient/caregiver should be counselled to report symptoms such as shortness of breath, rash, chills, chest pain, and back pain. Infusion should occur through the largest patent lumen. Whether an in-line filter is indicated or contraindicated will depend upon the product being infused and should be confirmed prior to infusion. Premedications with drugs such as acetaminophen and diphenhydramine should be administered.

Corticosteroids should not be routinely used for premedication and may be contraindicated for CAR infusions. Vital signs and urine output should be monitored closely and diuresis considered when larger volume infusions occur.

Infusion of cellular therapy products is generally safe, but serious adverse reactions may occur in approximately 11% of cell therapy infusions [43]. In a retrospective study of pediatric HCT recipients, independent risk factors for developing a serious adverse reaction included stem cell source (PBSC vs marrow (odds ratio (OR) 1.8; 95% confidence interval (CI), 0.4–9); cord vs marrow (OR 7.3; 95% CI, 1.3–40), overall $P = 0.0001$). White blood cell count and granulocyte content were not found to be risk factors in this pediatric population [43]. Dimethyl sulfoxide (DMSO) is a cryoprotectant used in cell products as a preservative when a given product needs to be cryopreserved while a patient awaits HCT or CT. It preserves cell viability, durability, and ability for stem cells to successfully repopulate marrow and is a critical component of autologous, cord blood transplant products, and CT products [44]. Characteristic adverse reactions associated with *DMSO* have been reported. These include nausea, vomiting, abdominal pain, chills, fever, and rarely severe respiratory depression, neurotoxicity, and cardiac arrhythmias [43, 45–52]. Hydration, allopurinol administration, slowing the rate of infusion, and reduction of cryopreservation volume (and DMSO content) are all strategies used to reduce DMSO toxicity [26].

During HCT acute hemolytic infusion reactions may occur when there is donor-recipient ABO or other red cell antigen incompatibility. Symptoms include fever, tachycardia, chills, dyspnea, back and chest pain, bleeding, shock, disseminated intravascular coagulation (DIC), and hypotension. Abnormal laboratory parameters may include hemoglobinemia, hemoglobinuria, hyperbilirubinemia, and a positive direct antiglobulin test. Measures to restore blood pressure, urine output, and correct coagulopathy are important management strategies. Delayed hemolytic transfusion reactions may occur as up to 2 weeks following cell therapy infusion. Unexplained anemia, jaundice, low-grade fevers, and hemoglobinuria may be present. Febrile nonhemolytic infusion reactions occur when the patient has an increase in baseline body temperature by at least 1° centigrade with/without chills. Allergic infusion reactions may be due to atopic substances which interact with antibodies present in the donor or recipient plasma. Urticaria, facial/glottal edema, wheezing, pulmonary edema, and anaphylaxis may occur. Anaphylactoid infusion reactions may be characterized by dyspnea, laryngeal spasm, bronchospasm, pulmonary and/or laryngeal edema. Transfusion-related acute lung injury (TRALI) caused by white blood cells and/or their components usually from the donor (and rarely the recipient) presents most often as transient non-cardiogenic pulmonary edema with/without leukopenia. These reactions usually respond to antihistamines, corticosteroids, and/or epinephrine. Transfusion-associated circulatory overload (TACO) results from volume overload with cardiogenic pulmonary edema.

Bacterial infusion reactions occur from infusion of contaminated products, typically with gram-negative organisms. Prompt treatment with appropriate antibiotics and supportive care are important to preclude death [53].

General management principles for cell therapy infusion reactions include (i) consideration of slowing/halting the infusion, (ii) activation of emergency supportive care measures, and (iii) confirmation of product details for accuracy. If symptoms resolve uneventfully without intervention, an infusion-related event is unlikely. If an infusion-related event is considered likely, a transfusion reaction laboratory evaluation should be initiated [53].

Overview of PICU Outcomes

The leading cause of admission to the PICU among pediatric HCT patients is respiratory failure followed by severe septic shock [54]. Pediatric HCT patients who require PICU care for severe sepsis have a 30–40% mortality rate compared to 12% for pediatric cancer (non-HCT) patients [55–57]. While HCT patients like non-HCT cancer patients may have neutropenia when septic, HCT patients are more profoundly immunocompromised with various arms of the immune system simultaneously affected. Other variables associated with a negative impact on the event-free survival of HCT patients admitted to the PICU include (1) the type of transplantation, (2) the need for inotropic support, (3) an elevated C-reactive protein level (>10 mg/dL), and (4) a high oncological-PRISM (O-PRISM) score [56, 58, 59]. On multivariate analysis, only the O-PRISM score influenced event-free survival (≤10 points, 54.6 +/− 15.3%; >10 points, 8.6 +/− 5.8%; $P = 0.007$) [58].

Despite the fact that HCT patients are usually no longer severely neutropenic following initial hospital discharge, they remain significantly immunocompromised and at risk for infectious complications. Thus, it is not surprising that in studies evaluating hospital readmission risk factors in post-HCT patients, the most common identified cause was infection. Other causes of readmission include graft failure, extramedullary relapse, GVHD, and bleeding disorders [60]. Recipients of allogeneic HCT are twice as likely to be readmitted compared to recipients of autologous HCT [61]. Patients who are readmitted to the hospital in the first 6 months following HCT may have a decreased 1-year OS compared to patients who were not readmitted [61, 62].

Toxicities Following HCT and CT

Preparative regimens preceding HCT typically consist of a combination of chemotherapeutic agents and/or irradiation with nonoverlapping toxicities. The choice of higher intensity myeloablative versus reduced intensity and/or non-ablative regimens may depend upon the primary disease, graft, and clinical characteristics of the recipient (such as disease burden and/or clinical comorbidities). Reduced intensity and non-ablative regimens may result in reversible myelosuppression (if given without HCT) and may be associated with a lower rate of non-hematologic toxicity [63]. Unique toxicities associated with individual agents should be reviewed from trusted sources prior to administration.

In general, HCT preparative regimens may be associated with cytopenias (that may require transfusion support with irradiated blood products as well as growth factors), profound immunocompromised state that may require antimicrobial prophylaxis and precautions, mucositis, nausea/vomiting and malnutrition, veno-occlusive disease (VOD) (also known as sinusoidal obstruction syndrome (SOS)), acute fluid overload, multi-organ failure, graft-versus-host disease, and death. Patients who receive a preparative regimen followed by HCT or a lympho-depletion regimen followed by CAR therapy will require time to achieve hematologic recovery and immune reconstitution. The length of time for this to occur will depend upon the preparative regimen, the primary disease, clinical status of the host, and cell source used [64, 65]. Unique post-infusion toxicities associated with CAR therapy include cytokine release syndrome (CRS) and CAR-T related encephalopathy syndrome (CRES) [65].

Toxicity Related to Hematologic Recovery and Immune Reconstitution

The duration of cytopenia following HCT and CT may vary based upon intensity of the preparative regimen, pre-existing clinical variable of the recipient, and donor source. Patients may require transfusion support with irradiated packed red blood cells and platelets until they achieve hematologic recovery. Patients with graft failure and/or acute graft rejection may undergo prolonged cytopenia until autologous recovery occurs and/or they undergo a second HCT. Common transfusion thresholds for HCT patients are 7–8 gm/dL for blood and 20×10^9/l for platelets or for symptomatic anemia and thrombocytopenia. Appropriately matched, irradiated blood products should be used for HCT patients. A higher platelet transfusion threshold of 30×10^9/l is used for patients with veno-occlusive disease (VOD) on treatment with defibrotide or other thrombolytic therapy. HCT patients with VOD, multi-organ dysfunction, respiratory failure, or other comorbidities like severe mucositis, liver dysfunction, and refractory hypertension as well as those requiring dialysis and/or who experience or at high risk for CRES, may be at a higher risk of bleeding and require a higher platelet threshold. Low-dose platelet transfusions given more frequently are preferred to high-dose platelets [66], and these should be infused over 30 min, unless there are concerns due to small patient size. Platelets can be infused once, twice daily, or more frequently to achieve the desired threshold, and a continuous infusion may be helpful in refractory cases. Volume-reduced platelets can be used in small patients with fluid overload issues.

Acute life-threatening bleeding is a rare complication during HCT and more commonly seen in patients with VOD and multi-organ failure and/or on thrombolytic therapy and those requiring ventilator or renal replacement therapy (RRT). Patients with life-threatening bleeding have a poor 3-year survival (17%) as compared to those without bleeding (67%). Management of such bleeding involves treatment of shock, platelet and blood transfusions, discontinuation of thrombolytic therapy, and control of coagulopathy by infusion of FFP and cryoprecipitate or rarely use of recombinant activated factor VII [67–69]. Diffuse alveolar hemorrhage (DAH) is a life-threatening bleeding complication associated with rapid decompensation along with very high mortality. This clinicopathologic diagnosis is characterized by acute dyspnea, decrease in hemoglobin, hypoxemia, and new infiltrate on chest radiograph (CXR) with/without hemoptysis. Bronchiolar lavage (BAL) may show progressively more bloody sequential fluid aliquots. Treatment is challenging. Management strategies may include (i) platelet transfusion support, (ii) use of intravenous, instilled, or inhaled recombinant factor VIIa, (iii)aminocaproic acid, or tranexamic acid (iv) increased mean airway pressure through the use of mechanical ventilation to help tamponade bleeding and/or (v) use of highdose steroids [70]. Extracorporeal membrane oxygenation (ECMO) has been explored as a supportive care management option for patients with DAH [71]. To date, there is no proven therapy for DAH and further research is needed.

Growth factor support may be used to promote hematologic recovery following HCT. Eltrombopag is an oral thrombopoietin receptor agonist which has been used for persistent thrombocytopenia after allogeneic HCT [72, 73]. Granulocyte colony-stimulating factor (G-CSF) may decrease the period of neutropenia and/or hasten recovery if the patient develops an infection following HCT [74, 75]. Infection prevention practices and prophylaxis are important, even following resolution of neutropenia, since patients may not recover normal lymphocyte counts for several months after HCT-CT [75]. Immunosuppressive medications to prevent graft-versus-host disease (GVHD) impair immune function even in the presence of adequate cell counts. Impaired cellular and humoral immunity may persist for months and sometimes years following HCT rendering patients at risk for life-threatening infections from encapsulated bacteria, fungal and viral pathogens [75]. Active GVHD may prolong this period and exacerbate risk. Serum immunoglobulin levels may reflect survival of long-lived plasma cells that have survived preparative regimens and may not reflect immunity to specific pathogens [75]. Environmental exposure and revaccination stimulate the memory B lymphocyte pool to restore humoral immune responses [75]. For patient receiving CD19+ directed CAR therapy, transient or permanent B cell aplasia and hypogammaglobinemia/agammaglobulinemia may be seen. Adjunctive administration of intravenous immune globulin may be indicated for these patients to maintain adequate trough levels (> 400 μg/L) and/or provide specific immunity during active infection.

Typically infectious risk stratification should include consideration of the clinical scenario along with timing post HCT or CAR infusion (Table 8.3) [76–84]. The risk of bacterial sepsis is highest among patients who have not yet achieved neutrophil recovery (absolute neutrophil count >500/mm^3 for 3 consecutive days) follow-

Table 8.3 Common infections by timeline following HCT [76–84]

	Prior to engraftment (day 0–30)	Post-engraftment to day 100	>100 days post BMT	Risk factors	Monitoring/detection
Bacterial	Staphylococcus Alpha hemolytic streptococcus Gram-negative Bacilli	Gram-negative bacilli	Encapsulated organisms	Neutropenia Indwelling catheters Mucositis/mucosal barrier injury GVHD	Blood/tissue culture
Fungal	Candida Aspergillus	Candida Aspergillus	Aspergillus Pneumocystis	Primary immunodeficiency Relapsed/refractory disease History of invasive fungal infection GVHD Endemic area	Galactomannan Beta-D-glucan assays Radiographic imaging Biopsy
Virus	Herpes simplex virus Community respiratory viruses (CRV) Gastrointestinal virus	Cytomegalovirus (CMV) Community respiratory virus (CRV) BK virus Human herpes virus-6 (HHV-6)	Varicella Zoster Virus (VZV) CMV	Pre-existing immunodeficiency GVHD Poor immune reconstitution (may be related to graft failure, graft source)	Blood viral PCR Nasal wash/BAL viral PCR Stool PCR Culture

ing HCT. Pediatric patients undergoing HCT require high vigilance for sepsis as they may not manifest more common signs/symptoms such as fevers while they are leukopenic and/or receiving immunosuppressive therapies.

Patients undergoing HCT who develop severe sepsis have shown a fourfold higher mortality rate, compared to those without HCT, and are more likely to develop end-organ dysfunction. While patients with immune dysfunction represent a known group predisposed to severe sepsis, even higher mortality is observed among patients undergoing HCT compared to immunocompromised who have not received HCT, despite similar ventilator-free days and vasoactive infusion-free days [57]. HCT patients may have an increased risk of bacterial sepsis due to prolonged central venous catheter line days, mucosal barrier injuries from mucositis, and skin breakdown secondary to preparative regimens. Close clinical monitoring and prompt empiric treatment of a suspected infection with or without fevers with broad-spectrum antibiotics are imperative after sending appropriate cultures. Empiric antimicrobial therapy may be tailored based upon risk factors such as mucositis, multidrug resistance risk profile, and prior infectious history [85]. A de-escalation empiric sepsis treatment strategy that employs an upfront regimen covering the most dangerous resistant pathogens may be appropriate among HCT patients [86]. Patients with refractory fevers and/or symptoms may require a change in therapy. For patients with severe sepsis and ongoing neutropenia, donor granulocyte infusions may be considered [87, 88].

Viral infections are another significant cause of infectious morbidity and mortality following HCT. Tables 8.3 and 8.4 summarize potential viral pathogens seen among patients following HCT as well as diagnostic and therapeutic considerations [76, 77, 81, 83, 84]. Patients are typically screened for signs and symptoms of community respiratory viral infections prior to HCT. Patients with community viral infections prior to HCT may be delayed. Strict adherence to infection prevention practices on units (including PICUs) with immune-compromised HCT patients is imperative to prevent nosocomial infection-related mortality. Other opportunistic viral infections may be associated with hemorrhagic cystitis, pneumonitis, colitis, encephalitis, and/or graft failure/rejection (Tables 8.3 and 8.4) [76, 77, 81, 83, 84].

The overall incidence of invasive fungal infections (IFI) among pediatric HCT recipients was 14.5% in one retrospective single center study [80]. Predominant organisms included *Candida* species (51%) and *Aspergillus* species (26%); *Candida albicans* accounted for 18.8% of all fungal species identified; there was a strong trend toward an increase in rare molds in more recent years [80]. The respiratory tract was the main site of infection (52.6%), with urine and blood also noted as significant sites [80]. Antifungal prophylaxis strategies, infection prevention practices, and the use of serum biomarkers (galactomannan and beta-D-glucan assays) may assist in prevention and early detection of invasive fungal infections [80]. While culture and histopathology are needed to prove fungal infection, radiographic and serum biomarkers may allow for noninvasive methods of detection of probable IFIs. Therapeutic drug monitoring when available should be used to ensure optimal therapeutic effect while minimizing toxicity [81].

Table 8.4 Viral pathogens/therapy options [76, 77, 81, 83, 84]

Virus	Disease manifestations	Detection methods	Evidence-based therapeutic options/agent	References
CMV	Pneumonia Colitis Retinitis Meningitis Ventriculitis	Antigenemia Blood Tissue Stool PCR Blood Tissue Nasal wash BAL	Foscarnet Ganciclovir Brincidofovir[a] Viral cytotoxic lymphocytes[a] Valacyclovir Letermovir	[75, 89–92]
RSV	Upper respiratory disease Lower respiratory disease	PCR Nasal wash BAL	Ribavirin	[93–95]
Parainfluenza	Upper respiratory disease Lower respiratory disease	PCR Nasal wash BAL	DAS181[a]	[96]
Influenza	Upper respiratory disease Lower respiratory disease	PCR Nasal wash BAL	Oseltamivir	[94]
Adenovirus	Upper respiratory disease Lower respiratory disease Disseminated disease Hepatitis Colitis	PCR Nasal wash BAL Stool	Cidovifor Brincidofovir[a] Viral cytotoxic lymphocytes[a]	[97–99]
HHV6	Encephalitis	PCR Blood CSF	Foscarnet	[100]
BK	Cystitis Nephritis	PCR Blood Urine	Cidofovir Viral cytotoxic lymphocytes[a]	[101, 102]
VZV	Zoster Encephalitis	PCR Swab of vesicle fluid Blood	Acyclovir Foscarnet	[75]
EBV	Post-transplant lymphoproliferative disorder	PCR Blood	Rituximab Viral cytotoxic lymphocytes Decrease immunosuppression when possible	[105], [104]

(continued)

Table 8.4 (continued)

Virus	Disease manifestations	Detection methods	Evidence-based therapeutic options/agent	References
JC	Encephalitis Cystitis	PCR CSF Blood	Decrease immune suppression when possible Viral cytotoxic lymphocytes[a]	[105, 106]
HSV 1, HSV 2	Mucocutaneous disease	PCR Vesicle Fluid Blood	Acyclovir	[75]
			Foscarnet	

Summary of common viral infections, their disease manifestation, most common detection methods along with therapeutic options
[a]Currently under investigation

Mucositis

Oral mucositis (OM) is a potentially debilitating early adverse effect associated with the intensity of the preparative regimen during HCT and has been more commonly associated with myeloablative conditioning regimens as well as GVHD prophylaxis regimens with methotrexate. Intensive oral hygiene may reduce the incidence and severity of mucositis [107, 108]. Herpes simplex infections of the oropharynx may mimic severe oral mucositis. HCT patients who experience mucositis may have a higher incidence of fever, serious infection, use of narcotics, parenteral nutrition, increased length of hospitalization, and mortality [109–111]. Please refer to Table 8.5 for classification and management of OM [107–110, 113–121].

Acute Fluid Overload

Acute fluid overload (AFO) may result from an excess of fluid intake and/or may be related to acute kidney injury (AKI) as a result of various factors affecting renal blood flow and tubular function. Excess fluid intake may occur during HCT due to hyperhydration for cyclophosphamide, increased need for intravenous medications, and blood product support. Early AKI is generally related to acute tubular necrosis (ATN), veno-occlusive disease, septic shock, and nephrotoxicity induced by medications (chemotherapeutics, antibiotics, and immunosuppressants) [123]. Aggressive fluid resuscitation for hypotension following bleeding, sepsis, or dehydration may result in AFO, especially in the setting of compromised renal function [124]. In these instances, earlier initiation of vasopressor support in lieu of repeat fluid bolus administration may be beneficial. Strict monitoring of intake and output, daily or more frequent weight, and clinical assessments can result in earlier detection of

Table 8.5 Mucositis [107–120]

Grade	0	1	2	3	4
NCI CTCAE	No symptoms	Asymptomatic or mild symptoms	Moderate pain, not interfering with oral intake; modified diet	Severe pain, interfering with oral intake	Life-threatening Mucositis
Clinical description (upper)	No findings	Painless ulcers, erythema	Patchy ulceration, pseudomembranes	Confluent ulcerations, bleeding	Tissue necrosis, spontaneous bleeding
Clinical description (lower)	No findings	Asymptomatic	Mild symptoms, abdominal discomfort, diarrhea	Stool incontinence	
Management		Topical anesthetics Intermittent narcotics	Soft foods, liquid diet Topical anesthetics	Assessment for total parenteral nutrition Adjust oral medications to intravenous when possible	Total parenteral nutrition Adjust oral medications to intravenous when possible Continuous intravenous narcotic infusion Intubation for airway protection
Additional risk factors			Risk of bacteriemia (bacterial translocation) with mucosal barrier injury	Risk of bacteriemia (bacterial translocation) with mucosal barrier injury	Risk of bacteriemia (bacterial translocation) with mucosal barrier injury Risk of Respiratory failure, may require intubation for airway protection
Supportive care/ prevention strategies	Keratinocyte growth factor Oral rinses Cryotherapy Low-level light therapy				

AFO. HCT patients who experience prolonged hospitalizations and require intensive care unit (ICU) support may require reassessment for “dry weight” as the fluid and nutritional status may have changed from admission. Euvolemic assessments should consider intake and output, hospital admission weight, nutritional status, weight trends, insensible losses, and clinical judgment [124].

Fluid restriction may be utilized to achieve fluid balance. However, this may be challenging among HCT patients who often require multiple intravenous medications and blood product support. Careful attention must be made to maintain nutrition and an appropriate hydration status during administration of nephrotoxic medications. HCT patients with 5% fluid overload (FO) should be started on diuretics such as furosemide (if no contraindication) and titrated to achieve euvolemia without affecting hemodynamic stability. In HCT patients with hypoproteinemia (as in patients with VOD), combining furosemide with albumin administration may improve hemodynamics, oxygenation, and fluid balance [125, 126].

Patients with 10% FO with or without renal impairment should be initiated on CRRT if there are no contraindications [123, 124, 127]. Early initiation of CRRT to allow for sufficient blood product and nutrition administration while preventing FO has been associated with improved outcomes [123, 128, 129].

SIADH

Syndrome of inappropriate antidiuretic hormone (SIADH) is the continuous release of ADH by the pituitary leading to the retention of free water by the kidneys with a decrease in plasma osmolality. Objective findings include oliguria, hyponatremia, hypoosmolality, continued urinary excretion of sodium, increased urine specific gravity, and normal renal and adrenal function [130–133]. Common causes in a transplant setting include high-dose cyclophosphamide, melphalan, cisplatin, and vincristine and underlying central nervous system tumors [130, 131]. Frequent serum sodium, serum osmolality, and urine-specific gravity monitoring is helpful to monitor for SIADH [132]. Treatment consists of fluid restriction and 3% hypertonic saline (up to 2 ml/kg) for patients with symptomatic hyponatremia. Overall correction of hyponatremia should occur slowly to prevent osmotic demyelination (avoid more than 8–10 mEq/L over the first 24 h) [134].

Hepatic Veno-occlusive Disease

VOD or sinusoidal obstruction syndrome (SOS) is a potentially fatal complication, occurring in up to 30% of children undergoing HCT. The spectrum of clinical features is varied, and most patients with mild to moderate VOD are usually managed on the HCT units, while patients with severe VOD can develop life-threatening multi-organ dysfunction and require pediatric intensive care unit (PICU) support.

Chemotherapy and radiation given as part of preparative regimens for HCT lead to toxic injury to the endothelial cells lining the hepatic sinusoids and hepatocytes. This leads to occlusive thrombotic clots in the sinusoids, obstructing blood flow to the central vein [135]. There are no specific or sensitive biomarkers for diagnosis of VOD. Endothelial injury, cytokine-mediated inflammation, and complement may have a role in the pathogenesis of VOD. Severe VOD (S-VOD) is associated with development of multi-organ failure (MOF) including renal failure (54%), pulmonary failure (23%), cardiac failure (63%), and changes in mental status (78%). Mortality for patients who develop S-VOD has ranged between 75 and 98% with the most common causes of death being MOF or sepsis [136]. In S-VOD, extravasation of fluid leads to weight gain, edema, ascites, pleural and pericardial effusions, and depletion of the intravascular volume. Increased intra-abdominal pressure from worsening ascites can cause decreased renal perfusion by direct pressure on the renal vasculature and pulmonary dysfunction due to decreased excursion of the diaphragms [137]. Hypoxia, renal dysfunction, and sudden onset multi-organ failure (MOF) are the common reasons for patients with VOD to be transferred to the PICU.

Fluid overload, hepatomegaly, and hyperbilirubinemia were the main clinical features of the modified Seattle and the Baltimore Criteria proposed for diagnosis of VOD in adults in the 1980s. For lack of better alternatives, this was applied to children until 2017 [138–140]. It is now well known that up to 30% of pediatric patients never develop hyperbilirubinemia throughout the course of VOD [141, 142]. In 2017 the European group for Blood and Marrow Transplantation (EBMT) published criteria for the diagnosis and grading of severity of VOD in children (Table 8.6) [122].

Early initiation of specific therapy with defibrotide and supportive care are critical to improved outcomes in VOD. Defibrotide was approved in the United States for the treatment of S-VOD in 2016. While the majority of cases of VOD fall into the mild or moderate category, approximately 25% of cases are severe [136, 138, 139, 143–146]. Treatment with defibrotide is recommended for 21 days or until resolution of MOF and signs of VOD. The ideal time to commence defibrotide therapy is not certain. Cryoprecipitate transfusion is suggested to maintain fibrinogen >150 mg/dl in a VOD patient with bleeding, but correction of abnormal clotting tests results by infusion of fresh frozen plasma or cryoprecipitate is not recommended [137].

Table 8.6 EBMT diagnostic criteria for hepatic SOS/VOD in children. (With permission from …. [122])

No limitation for time of onset of SOS/VOD
The presence of two or more of the following[a]
Unexplained consumptive and transfusion-refractory thrombocytopenia[b]
Otherwise unexplained weight gain on 3 consecutive days despite the use of diuretics or a weight gain >5% above baseline value
[c]Hepatomegaly (best if confirmed by imaging) above baseline value
[c]Ascites (best if confirmed by imaging) above baseline value
Rising bilirubin from a baseline value on 3 consecutive days or bilirubin ≥2 mg/dL within 72 h

Abbreviations: *CT* computed tomography, *HCT* hematopoietic cell transplantation, *MRI* magnetic resonance imaging, *SOS/VOD* sinusoidal obstruction syndrome/veno-occlusive disease, *US* ultrasonography. [a]With the exclusion of other potential differential diagnoses. [b]≥1 weight-adjusted platelet substitution/day to maintain institutional transfusion guidelines. [c]Suggested: imaging (US, CT, or MRI) immediately before HCT to determine baseline value for both hepatomegaly and ascites

Given the high fatality rate of S-VOD and the limited options for treatment, several groups have generated consensus statements regarding the treatment of S-VOD [147–149]. Fluid restriction (50–75% of normal maintenance fluids) may be critical for patients with acute fluid overload. Blood products and medications alone may be equal to the daily fluid requirements for small children. Controlled diuresis may be necessary to achieve euvolemia in patients with VOD [137]. Worsening renal function with electrolyte imbalance and fluid overload refractory to diuresis suggest the need to start renal replacement therapy (RRT). Paracentesis should be considered in the management of ascites if conservative management fails or in the setting of intra-abdominal hypertension/abdominal compartment syndrome or among patients developing pulmonary dysfunction due to tense ascites [137]. Volume controlled drainage at a rate of 5 ml/kg/h may be adequate in most circumstances with close monitoring for hypotension and hypothermia. Continuous pump controlled drainage or manual setup for a continuous drainage is preferred, and open drainage to gravity is discouraged to prevent hypovolemic shock due to rapid fluid shifts from intravascular to extravascular spaces (peritoneum). Infusion of 5% or 25% albumin is helpful to correct hypoalbuminemia after paracentesis. A consensus report on the supportive care management of children with VOD covered many aspects related to care of children with VOD and peritoneal and pleural drains [137], including time of insertion and removal. According to these guidelines, VOD patients with pleural effusions causing pulmonary dysfunction may benefit from thoracocentesis to maintain adequate oxygenation. In VOD for patients with both pleural effusions and ascites who become hypoxic, a peritoneal drain may improve the pulmonary dysfunction and avoid insertion of a pleural drain [150]. The pleural drains can be clamped once the drainage is <3 ml/kg/day for 24 h, and if no further accumulation occurs, the drain can be removed.

Transplant-Associated Thrombotic Microangiopathy (TA-TMA)

Transplant-associated thrombotic microangiopathy (TA-TMA) is considered in the differential diagnosis in a patient undergoing HCT with hypertension, anemia, thrombocytopenia, elevated LDH, and proteinuria. Risk factors which have been associated with the development of TA-TMA include exposure to irradiation, busulfan, cisplatin, fludarabine and rapamycin, and calcineurin inhibitors (CNI) as well as viral infections and possibly acute graft-versus-host disease (aGVHD) [151, 152]. A series of six patients who developed TA-TMA and had a high prevalence of deletion in the complement Factor H (CFH)-related genes and CFH autoantibodies were reported in 2013 [153]. The authors postulated that dysregulation of the alternative complement pathway may have a role in the pathogenesis of TA-TMA. Encouraging response to treatment with eculizumab, a monoclonal antibody which prevents the formation of C5b-9, has further supported the role of complement in the pathogenesis of TA-TMA and aHUS [154, 155].

Diagnostic criteria for TA-TMA are listed in Table 8.7 [156]. TA-TMA should be suspected among patients undergoing HCT, who develop proteinuria ≥30 mg/dL, severe hypertension, and acute elevation of lactate dehydrogenase (LDH) [156]. The management of TA-TMA includes supportive care with withdrawal of the offending agents like CNI, treatment of hypertension and underlying infection(s) if any, and treatment of aGVHD. If CNI are weaned off, alternative GVHD prophylaxis may be indicated. Patients with polyserositis may require drainage of the pericardial, pleural, or ascitic fluids. In rare cases a pericardial-pleural window may be indicated. Specific treatment of TA-TMA is targeted therapy with eculizumab to achieve complete blockade of the upregulated complement activation pathway [155–158]. Weight-based dosing (600 mg for patient wt. 10–40 kg, 900 mg for wt. >40 kg and 300 mg for wt. between 5 and 10 kg) of eculizumab for induction may be used with dose titration recommended until the desired level (CH50 < 10%) is achieved [154]. Eculizumab should be continued until the signs and symptoms of TA-TMA have resolved, after which maintenance therapy is initiated [154]. During maintenance, eculizumab is given every 2 weeks for approximately four doses, after which further treatment may be discontinued. Among patients receiving simultaneous renal replacement therapy, dosing titration may be indicated.

Table 8.7 Diagnostic criteria for TA-TMA. (With permission to reprint from… [156])

A. Microangiopathy diagnosed on tissue biopsy	
or	
B. Laboratory and clinical markers indicating TMA	
Laboratory or clinical marker	Description
Lactate dehydrogenase (LDH)[a]	Elevated above the upper limit of normal for age
Proteinuria[a, b]	A random urinalysis protein concentration of ≥30 mg/dL
Hypertension[a, b]	<18 years of age: blood pressure at the 95th percentile value for age, sex, and height
	≥18 years of age: blood pressure ≥ 140/90 mm Hg
De novo thrombocytopenia[b]	Thrombocytopenia with a platelet count $<50 \times 10^9$/L or a ≥50% decrease in the platelet count
De novo anemia[b]	A hemoglobin below the lower limit of normal for age or anemia requiring transfusion support
Evidence of microangiopathy[b]	The presence of schistocytes in the peripheral blood or histologic evidence of microangiopathy on a tissue specimen
Terminal complement activation[b]	Elevated plasma concentration of sC5b-9 above upper normal laboratory limit

[a]Present: consider diagnosis of TA-TMA. Monitor very closely

[b]At TA-TMA diagnosis indicate high features associated with poor outcome: consider therapeutic intervention

GVHD

Graft-versus-host disease (GVHD) is a potentially devastating complication associated with allogeneic HCT; alloreactive donor lymphocytes trigger a dysregulated immune response in healthy host tissue resulting in inflammation and damage to those tissues. Acute GVHD occurs following neutrophil recovery (engraftment) and typically affects the skin, gastrointestinal (GI) tract, and liver. Acute GVHD was traditionally thought to occur prior to day +100 following HCT, but the diagnosis is now based on clinical symptoms [159]. The skin is the most commonly affected organ in acute GVHD and can present with a spectrum from self-limited areas of skin erythema to macular pruritic rashes to even full thickness skin bullae and blisters resulting in life-threatening desquamation.

Upper GI acute GVHD is characterized by unexplained abdominal pain, nausea, anorexia, and/or vomiting; lower GI GVHD is characterized by abdominal pain with diarrhea and, in severe cases, ileus [159, 160]. Using severity stratification, quantification of stool output based on the weight of the child may upstage the grade of GI GVHD and guide treatment strategies. Although several biomarkers are under investigation, GVHD remains a clinical diagnosis. Acute hepatic GVHD most commonly is associated with cholestatic jaundice and transaminitis. Isolated hepatic GVHD is rare. When present, hepatic GVHD is typically associated with progression of uncontrolled GI GVHD or shortly following wean of immunosuppressive medications.

With rare exceptions, allogeneic HCT recipients receive primary GVHD prophylaxis. Common GVHD prophylaxis medications include calcineurin inhibitors (cyclosporine/tacrolimus) with other immune modulators such as methotrexate, mycophenolate mofetil, and corticosteroids. Stringent therapeutic drug monitoring (TDM) of calcineurin inhibitors (cyclosporine, tacrolimus, sirolimus) is important to maintain therapeutic and avoid toxic levels. Post-HCT cyclophosphamide is another prophylaxis strategy used to promote tolerance in alloreactive host and donor T cells, leading to suppression of both graft rejection and GVHD after allogeneic HCT [161, 162].

Patients with acute GVHD will typically resume or continue their calcineurin inhibitors and initiate first-line treatment with administration of corticosteroids. While this is effective in up to 60% of cases [163, 164], it confers an added risk of immunosuppression, along with significant side effects of hypertension, hyperglycemia, pancreatitis, osteopenia, avascular necrosis, emotional lability, and psychosis. Patients with steroid-refractory or steroid-unresponsive GVHD require a second-line treatment option. Potential second-line agents include infliximab, basiliximab, and ruxolitinib. Extracorporeal photopheresis (ECP) is a promising second-line therapy for refractory GVHD which is immunomodulatory rather than immunosuppressive. During this procedure T lymphocytes are functionally inactivated following treatment with psoralen plus ultraviolet A therapy. While the mechanism of photopheresis is not clearly understood, photoinactivation of the exposed T lymphocytes occurs [165, 166]. Patients typically undergo leukapheresis procedure several times a week; the procedure requires technical expertise with appropriately trained staff and an indwelling pheresis catheter. During the procedure patients undergo fluid shifts; smaller patients with lower body weights require diligent hemodynamic monitoring, and frequently the ECP circuit may require priming with either irradiated PRBC or albumin to maintain hemodynamic status [166, 167]. Prior to each ECP procedure, patients should have stable fluid status, along with adequate baseline hematocrit. Ex vivo cultured adult human mesenchymal stromal cells have been studied for the treatment of steroid-refractory acute GVHD in pediatric patients (as an immunomodulatory agent) and show promising results [168].

Chronic GVHD may occur in 20–50% of children undergoing allogeneic HCT [169–172]. Its pathogenesis remains poorly understood, but T and B lymphocytes are thought to play a role in disease development [173–176]. Chronic GVHD has features resembling autoimmune and other immunologic disorders such as scleroderma, bronchiolitis obliterans (BO), immune cytopenias, and chronic immunodeficiency [177]. The management of chronic GVHD has historically mirrored the management of acute GVHD [177, 178]. Recent reports support the hypothesis that the reestablishment of normal numbers of functional rTregs is required for the clinical resolution of chronic GVHD, which provide insight toward future directions in the management of this potentially debilitating morbidity [179, 180].

Neurologic Complications of HCT

Neurologic complications may be frequently encountered among pediatric patients following HCT [181–184]. The most common clinical symptoms, as listed in Table 8.8, include seizures, encephalopathy, and motor dysfunction [183, 184]. In a large study of 405 pediatric HCT patients, 25 (6.2%) developed encephalopathy in the first 100 days post-HCT [185]. In a single institution study of 383 pediatric patients (<19 years of age) who underwent allogeneic HCT between 2000 and 2012, neurologic complications were present in 70 (18%) of these patients, with 63% of neurologic episodes, occurring in the first 100 days following HCT [182].

Table 8.8 Neurological complications

	Associations	Clinical manifestations	Treatment
Posterior reversible encephalopathy syndrome (PRES)	Calcineurin inhibitors	Increased blood pressure, headaches, neurological changes, seizure	Blood pressure control, hold calcineurin inhibitor if possible, adjust drug dosage if level high
Encephalopathy	TBI, busulfan	Mental status change	Supportive care
Encephalitis	HHV6, HSV, VZV, JC, West Nile Virus	Mental status change Seizure Neurological deficits	Antiviral agents (Foscarnet) Supportive care, decrease immunosuppression (if feasible)
Seizure	Busulfan	Seizure	Antiepileptic prophylaxis (and treatment when indicated)

Chemotherapy used as part of preparative regimens for HCT such as (i) high-dose carmustine (BCNU) frequently used as part of the BEAM preparative regimen for Hodgkin and non-Hodgkin lymphoma and (ii) busulfan have been associated with seizures [183, 186]. It is standard practice to administer anticonvulsant medications such as levetiracetam prior to busulfan conditioning [183, 186]. Among HCT patients who receive cranial radiation or intrathecal chemotherapy as part of their preparative regimens, leukoencephalopathy may occur days to months after HCT and is characterized by dysarthria, ataxia, confusion, and dysphagia [184, 185].

Among patients with neurologic complications, the following risk factors for mortality have been reported: days to neutrophil engraftment, extensive chronic GVHD, and presence of neurologic sequelae [182]. In the early neutropenic and lymphopenic post-HCT period as well as during times of increased immunosuppression for the treatment of GVHD, infection-related neurologic complications are more common [181, 184]. CNS infections include bacterial meningitis, aspergillus infection of the brain, cerebral toxoplasmosis, or viral encephalitis (caused by HSV, VZV, HHV-6, EBV, and polyomavirus JC) [183, 184, 187]. Central nervous system (CNS) complications may be observed more commonly in pediatric patients undergoing unrelated allogeneic transplantation, compared to related allogeneic or autologous HCT [184, 188, 189]. Patients with GVHD require extended courses of immunosuppression and may have a higher risk of neurologic complications due to an increased incidence of CNS infections, intracranial hemorrhage, metabolic derangements, medication-related toxicities, and CNS involvement of the primary disease [183–185]. Use of calcineurin inhibitors (CNIs) such as tacrolimus or cyclosporine for GVHD prophylaxis and treatment has been associated with neurotoxicity. CNI-related neurologic toxicity is characterized by headache, tremor, seizures, cortical blindness, coma, akinetic mutism, or mental status changes [182, 183, 190] and is more likely to occur if CNI serum drug levels exceed the therapeutic range; this should be reversible once CNI is held [186]. Patients with sickle cell anemia undergoing HCT have a higher risk of CNI-associated neurotoxicity and typically receive simultaneous anti-seizure prophylaxis; medications, preferably valproic acid or levetiracetam, which do not affect cytochrome p450 activity and thereby alter CSA and Tacrolimus levels, are used for CNI-associated seizure prophylaxis and management [183]. Furthermore, CNIs cause magnesium wasting which can further decrease the seizure threshold.

Posterior reversible encephalopathy syndrome (PRES) is another CNI-related complication, which may occur among pediatric HCT patients [183, 191]. PRES presents with refractory hypertension, headache, vomiting, visual disturbances, mental status changes, and seizures. Magnetic resonance imaging (MRI) may show vasogenic edema predominantly in subcortical gray and white matter in the posterior regions of the brain [191]. The pathophysiology of PRES remains unknown with a commonly accepted theory of a hyperperfusion injury model. A failure of cerebral autoregulation in relation to the sudden increase in mean arterial pressure (MAP) can lead to arteriolar dilation, hyperperfusion, endothelial vascular damage, and disruption of the blood-brain barrier [192]. The management of PRES includes control of hypertension and seizures as well as changing the CNI in favor of a different immunosuppressive agent [183, 191]. PRES is usually reversible; however, severe life-threatening complications and irreversible neurologic damage can occur, such as cerebral hemorrhage, cerebellar herniation, and refractory status epilepticus [191].

Neurovascular complications such as intracerebral hemorrhage in a patient with refractory thrombocytopenia, thromboembolic episodes, subdural hemorrhages, and thrombotic thrombocytopenic purpura (TTP) have been reported among pediatric HCT patients [183, 185].

Cardiac Complications of HCT

The overall incidence of fatal cardiac complications in pediatric patients post-HCT was previously reported to be quite low (<1%); however, patients who developed heart failure had a very high incidence of mortality [193]. More recent data from Cincinnati Children's Hospital suggests that cardiac complications may be more common than previously reported when routine screening echocardiograms are performed on day +7 after transplant and on admission to the ICU for any reason [194, 195]. Abnormal echocardiography in the early post-HCT period was present in 30% of patients and revealed pericardial effusions, elevated right ventricular pressure, and decreased LV function [194]. Cardiac complications post-HCT may manifest as heart failure, pulmonary hypertension, pericardial tamponade, and dysrhythmias [193, 196, 197]. Among pediatric patients, cardiac complications may present either in the acute setting, (i.e., in the first 100 days post-HCT), or later, often after years following HCT [198].

Exposure to medications such as anthracyclines (prior to HCT) and cyclophosphamide, alemtuzumab, and total body irradiation (TBI) (during HCT preparative regimens) as well as iron overload from frequent red blood cell transfusions increase the risk of cardiotoxicity [196, 199–202]. Anthracycline-related cardiac toxicity is cumulative and dose-dependent. Risk factors include younger age at exposure, female sex, and prior chest radiation [202]. Furthermore, the exposure to high-dose cyclophosphamide during conditioning (>150 mg/kg), and prior cumulative anthracycline exposure (>100 mg/m2), may increase the risk of cardiac events [197]. High-dose cyclophosphamide can lead to myocardial necrosis and result in clinical symptoms of dyspnea, tachycardia, hypotension, and pericardial effusion within 10 days of administration (reported in post-HCT adult series with total cyclophosphamide doses >120–180 mg/kg), culminating in heart failure in 28% of cases [198]. Dose reduction of cyclophosphamide has been associated with a lower incidence of heart failure (2%) [203]. A recent study also found that cumulative anthracycline doses >250 mg/m2 were associated with a tenfold increased risk of cardiac complications in HCT survivors, especially in those who were very young at the time of exposure or female [202]. Additionally, recent studies also point to genetic susceptibility factors that modulate the risk of developing cardiac complications. These include polymorphisms in the NAD(P)H oxidase subunit RAC2 and the carbonyl reductase CBR1 [203].

During stem cell infusion, cardiac events, including bradyarrhythmias and cardiac death, attributed to DMSO, have been reported [196]. Following HCT, cardiac function can be further compromised by hyperhydration, blood product administration, impaired renal function, and sepsis [193, 203]. Patients may develop pericardial effusions with or without cardiac tamponade. Pericardial effusions may be a manifestation of acute cardiac GVHD or transplant associated-thrombotic microangiopathy (TA-TMA) and/or infection [196]. In critically ill pediatric HCT patients, echocardiographic abnormalities that require intervention or further screening were found in 50% of patients and included elevated RV pressure, LVSD, and moderate to large pericardial effusions [195]. In addition to pericardial effusions, pulmonary artery hypertension is commonly observed in patients with TA-TMA and among patients with sickle cell anemia [193]. Interestingly, when routine echocardiography was performed in pediatric patients post-HCT, if elevated RV pressure was observed on day +7 post-HCT, this finding was significantly associated with TA-TMA [194].

Attention to repletion of electrolytes, avoidance of acute fluid overload, and careful selection of medications which affect cardiac contractility may reduce serious cardiac complications during HCT. Patients with metabolic diseases such as Hurler's syndrome undergoing HCT with pre-existing cardiomyopathy may benefit from early cardiology evaluation for judicious management of hypertension, fluid status, and heart rate control.

Late cardiovascular complications include the development of life-threatening cardiovascular disease (CVD), constrictive pericarditis, valvular heart disease, and conduction abnormalities [202, 203]. Long-term survivors are at risk for cardiovascular disease at a rate four times higher than the general population [198].

Pulmonary Complications Among Pediatric HCT-CT Patients

Lung injury following HCT remains a challenging problem, with increased mortality, both in the acute peri-HCT period as well as during long-term follow-up [54, 204–206]. As many as 75% of pediatric patients undergoing HCT experience pulmonary complications. The presence of respiratory signs or symptoms may pose a diagnostic dilemma. Differentiating infectious from noninfectious lung injury is important (Tables 8.9 and 8.10), especially among patients with GVHD, where management is typically divergent.

Infectious causes of pulmonary compromise in children undergoing HCT may vary based upon the immune status of the child (see Tables 8.9). This in turn may depend upon such variables as primary disease, preparative regimen, type of donor, and time since HCT. Isolation precautions and good hospital ventilation may reduce the rate of hospital acquired infection [75, 207]. Frequent serum galactomannan surveillance is usually performed among children undergoing HCT during phases of immune compromise; a positive result (optical density index ≥ 0.5) may suggest

Table 8.9 Infectious pulmonary complications following HCT

Infection	Risk Factors	Diagnosis	Treatment
Invasive fungal infections (IFI) Molds Yeast [a]Pneumocystis jirovecii (PJP)	All HCT recipients, especially if h/o multiple relapsed leukemia; primary immune deficiency; graft-versus-host disease; resides in areas with endemic fungal pathogens	Culture and histopathology proves IFI, radiographic and serum biomarkers may allow diagnosis of probable and possible IFIs Early BAL and/or transbronchial biopsy may be helpful	Triazoles Amphotericin B Echinocandins Therapeutic drug monitoring may improve efficacy/ toxicity in children (difference in clearance) In severe cases, combination treatments may provide synergy PJP[a] Pentamidine (IH/IV) Bactrim (myelosuppressive, may negatively impact hematologic recovery, donor engraftment status)
Bacterial infections *Gram-negative* *Pseudomonas aeruginosa*, *Klebsiella pneumoniae*, and *Enterobacter cloacae* *Gram-positive* *Staphylococcus aureus* and α-hemolytic streptococci	Prolonged neutropenia Asplenia	Consolidation on imaging Positive cultures (blood/BAL)	Empiric therapy should include agents with good lung penetration with gram-positive and gram-negative coverage and consider prior infectious history. A de-escalation antimicrobial strategy to cover multidrug-resistant organisms should be used
Viral infections Respiratory syncytial virus Parainfluenza Influenza Human metapneumovirus Adenovirus Cytomegalovirus Human herpes virus-6 (HHV-6) Rhinovirus	Recent viral infection and/ or exposure Recipient (virus+ history)/ donor (virus - history) Impaired T-lymphocyte immunity, immunosuppressive therapy, GVHD	Patchy diffuse infiltrates on imaging, Positive viral PCR from nasopharyngeal specimens and/or BAL	Oseltamivir Ribavirin Ganciclovir Foscarnet Cidofovir Supportive care: Consideration of intravenous immune globulin (IVIG) and/or CMV-immune globulin (cytogam)

Infectious pulmonary complications: These are more common in the early HCT period but may occur in the late post-HCT period among patients with poor immune reconstitution and/or graft-versus-host disease

[a]PJP treatment is different to mold and yeast

Table 8.10 Noninfectious pulmonary complication following HCT

Complication	Onset	Diagnosis	Treatment
Idiopathic pneumonia syndrome(IPS)	Usually within 120 days of HCT	Widespread alveolar injury Absence of active lower respiratory tract infection Absence of cardiac dysfunction, acute renal failure, or acute fluid overload	*General management guidelines:* Ensure antimicrobial prophylaxis and high vigilance for superimposing infection, with prompt empiric therapy Administer intravenous immunoglobulin (IVIG) for levels <500 mg/dL or when specific immunity is needed in response to pathogen Minimize gastroesophageal reflux (GERD), optimize GERD prophylaxis Optimize nutrition Some patients may benefit from higher hemoglobin (10 g/dL) *See below for specific treatment considerations*
Engraftment syndrome	Within 5–7 days of neutrophil engraftment	Fever, dyspnea, and hypoxemia	Corticosteroids
Diffuse alveolar hemorrhage (DAH)	Usually within 100 days of HCT	Progressive cough, dyspnea, hemoptysis Progressively bloody lavage Diffuse infiltrates on imaging	Treat shock Transfuse platelet and packed red blood cells as needed Discontinue thrombolytic therapy Correct coagulopathy by infusion of fresh frozen plasma (FFP) or cryoprecipitate or use of recombinant activated factor VII Consider maintaining INR >1.5 (FFP), fibrinogen >100 (cryoprecipitate), and platelets >50 k/uL
Bronchiolitis obliterans organizing pneumonia (BOOP)/ cryptogenic organizing pneumonia (COP)	Within 2–12 months	Fever, dry cough, dyspnea Patchy infiltrates, ground-glass opacities on imaging Peribronchiolar infiltration/fibrosis, intraluminal granulation tissue	*Early cases*: Inhaled fluticasone, azithromycin, and montelukast (FAM) with brief steroid burst (1 mg/kg per day prednisone) and rapid taper (0.25 mg/kg per week) *Advanced cases:* Corticosteroids (2 mg/kg/day) Immunomodulation Tumor necrosis factor Inhibitors Continuous veno-venous Hemofiltration (CVVH)

Table 8.10 (continued)

Complication	Onset	Diagnosis	Treatment
Bronchiolitis obliterans syndrome (BOS)	Within 3–24 months	Cough, dyspnea, wheezing, afebrile Obstructive lung disease Usually normal chest x-ray CT: bronchiectasis, ground glass Lymphocytic bronchitis; bronchiolar inflammation with luminal obliteration	*Early cases:* Inhaled fluticasone, azithromycin, and montelukast (FAM) with brief steroid burst (1 mg/kg per day prednisone) and rapid taper (0.25 mg/kg per week) *Advanced cases:* Corticosteroids (2 mg/kg/day) Immunomodulation Tumor necrosis factor Inhibitors Continuous veno-venous Hemofiltration (CVVH)

risk of an invasive fungal infection (IFI) [82]. The diagnostic evaluation for children undergoing HCT with fever and/or pulmonary infiltrates may include blood cultures (including fungal cultures), serum galactomannan and β-D-glucan, respiratory viral panel, serum viral polymerase chain reaction (PCR) testing, computed tomography (CT) scan, bronchoscopy, and/or transbronchial biopsy. Rising β-D-glucan (BDG) levels suggest pneumocystis jirovecii pneumonia (PJP) among immunocompromised patients who are hypoxic with a high sensitivity; a negative result makes the diagnosis unlikely [208]. If a bronchoscopy is performed, a galactomannan optical density index of ≥1 from the lavage is suggestive of IFI. Positive fungal cultures would confirm the diagnosis. The diagnostic yield of bronchoscopy is variable (31–80%) but may be improved if performed early and prior to prolonged empiric use of antimicrobials and potential clinical decline in the patient's status [209–211]. In a retrospective single center study of over 2000 non-intubated adult HCT recipients, earlier bronchoscopy was more than twice as likely to yield a diagnosis of infection compared to late examination (73 vs 31%, $P < 0.0001$) [211]. The role of transbronchial biopsy was examined in another retrospective single center cohort among 130 adult HCT recipients; non-specific interstitial pneumonitis was seen among 18% of cases. However, pathogens were rarely identified (<5%), suggesting that transbronchial biopsy may contribute to the diagnostic management of noninfectious lung injury post-HCT but is less useful in the management of infectious pulmonary complications of HCT [212].

Highly immunocompromised children with invasive fungal infections may not have characteristic radiographic findings such as pulmonary nodules with halo, air crescent sign, or cavitation, seen more typically among adults with mold-associated pneumonia. Imaging findings may often be non-specific, especially among younger children [82]. Ground-glass opacities, especially if concurrent with positive serologic markers such as galactomannan, may indicate an IFI, particularly aspergillus. Candida and mucor are other important fungal pathogens [82]. A high index of suspicion and prompt empiric therapy may optimize outcomes [82, 213].

Lobar infiltrates on imaging may be more suggestive of bacterial pathogens, while patchy, diffuse infiltrates may be more suggestive of viral infections. Gram-negative bacilli causing bacterial pneumonia include *Pseudomonas aeruginosa*, *Klebsiella pneumoniae*, and *Enterobacter cloacae.* Important gram-positive organisms causing bacterial pneumonia are *Staphylococcus aureus* and α-hemolytic streptococci (e.g., *Streptococcus mitis*) [83]. Community respiratory viral infections such as respiratory syncytial virus (RSV), parainfluenza, influenza, human metapneumovirus, and adenovirus are important viral causes of respiratory compromise in the immunocompromised child. Cytomegalovirus (CMV) pneumonitis is less frequently seen among children undergoing HCT but remains a significant cause of morbidity and mortality [83].

For immunocompromised children with fever, pulmonary infiltrates, and/or respiratory compromise, empiric broad-spectrum antibiotics should be initiated after cultures have been obtained. Choice of broad-spectrum coverage may be influenced by the patient's prior infectious history (multidrug resistance risk profile), renal and liver function, drug mechanism of action (bacteriostatic versus bactericidal), and potential lung tissue penetration [214, 215]. Rapid initiation of appropriate antimicrobial therapy may be a critical factor to achieving optimal outcomes [214]. Trimethoprim-sulfamethoxazole is a first-line agent for patients with PJP pneumonia, but its use among HCT patients may be associated with delayed hematologic recovery and even graft failure [75, 84, 216, 217]. The myelosuppressive risks of antimicrobial agents should be weighed against potential benefits. HCT recipients usually receive antifungal prophylaxis during phases of immune compromise [75, 82]. For pediatric HCT recipients with >3 days of fever of unclear etiology that is unresponsive to broad-spectrum antibacterial agents and those with suspected IFI, empiric antifungal treatment with an echinocandin or liposomal amphotericin is recommended [82]. For patients already receiving mold-active antifungal prophylaxis who require empiric antifungal treatment, it is reasonable to consider switching to a different mold-active class or optimizing to treatment doses [82]. For profoundly immunocompromised children and those with concerns of rapid clinical deterioration due to IFI, adjunctive administration of granulocyte-macrophage colony-stimulating factor (GM-CSF), donor granulocyte infusions, aerosolized amphotericin B lipid complex, or combination antifungal therapies have been used [213, 218–225].

Patients with community respiratory viral (CRV) infections may benefit from antiviral agents such as oseltamivir and ribavirin (oral, inhaled, or intravenous) [75, 95, 226–230]. Intravenous immune globulin (IVIG) infusion may provide specific immunity and provide adjunctive therapy [229]. Ganciclovir is a typical first-line agent for CMV pneumonitis, but among HCT recipients, foscarnet may serve as a first-line agent, if there is concern regarding myelosuppression associated with ganciclovir. Cytomegalovirus intravenous immune globulin may provide adjunctive therapy for children with CMV pneumonitis [231, 232].

The management of children with infectious respiratory complications should consider general management principles for those undergoing HCT. Therapeutic drug monitoring (TDM) should be performed frequently given the multiple medication interactions that are possible for HCT recipients. TDM for drugs such as azoles and antibiotics such as vancomycin are important to avoid toxicity and may require more frequent testing than customary for non-HCT recipients. For patients on dialysis or with renal impairment, appropriate medication dose adjustments may be indicated to account for renal clearance [233].

Noninfectious lung injury, as depicted in Table 8.10, following HCT can occur in the acute and chronic settings. Idiopathic pneumonia syndrome (IPS) occurs acutely following HCT when there is (i) diffuse alveolar injury, (ii) absence of lower respiratory tract infection, and (iii) absence of cardiac, renal, or iatrogenic causes of pulmonary symptoms [234]. The spectrum of IPS encompasses an array of disorders including pediatric acute respiratory distress syndrome (PARDS), diffuse alveolar hemorrhage (DAH), interstitial pneumonitis, peri-engraftment syndrome, capillary leak syndrome, bronchiolitis obliterans organizing pneumonia (BOOP), and bronchiolitis obliterans syndrome (BOS), though BOOP and BOS are typically seen as later complications. IPS likely results from direct toxicity of the preparative regimen, undiagnosed pulmonary infections, and/or inflammatory cytokines. T-lymphocyte activation may occur in response to injury, and lipopolysaccharide (LPS) entry into circulation via the intestinal mucosa may trigger the gut-liver-lung axis of inflammation [235]. Patients with IPS may require critical care support with oxygen supplementation and mechanical ventilation. A single-arm multicenter phase II study of inhaled fluticasone, azithromycin, and montelukast (FAM) with brief steroid burst (1 mg/kg per day prednisone) and rapid taper (0.25 mg/kg per week) has been associated with a halt in pulmonary decline among newly diagnosed IPS [236]. First-line treatment for more advanced disease typically involves corticosteroids 2 mg/kg/day and inhibitors of tumor necrosis factor α (TNF-α) [235, 237]. In a multicenter phase II trial investigating a soluble TNF-binding protein, etanercept (Enbrel, Amgen, Thousand Oaks, CA), 28 pediatric patients with IPS received systemic corticosteroids (2.0 mg/kg/day) plus etanercept (0.4 mg/kg twice weekly × 8 doses). This regimen was associated with a high response rate, with 89% overall survival at 28 days, 71% with no oxygen requirement and alive at 28 days, and 63% alive at 1 year. The median time to response was 10 days (range 1–24 days) [237].

Chronic noninfectious lung injury following HCT may be characterized as restrictive or obstructive based on pulmonary function testing. Restrictive lung disease may present within the first 3 months following HCT, with obstructive disease typically occurring later. Symptoms may be similar, and they are typically differentiated based on differences in (i) the ratio of forced expiratory volume in 1 sec (FEV1) to forced vital capacity (FVC) which is normal in restrictive lung disease and decreased in obstructive lung disease and (ii) total lung capacity which is normal in obstructive but decreased in restrictive lung disease. The diffusing capacity of the lung for carbon dioxide (DLCO) is typically decreased in both forms of chronic lung injury. The pathophysiology of chronic lung injury following HCT remains poorly understood but is likely related to ongoing inflammatory injury after initial insult(s). The treatment of chronic lung injury following

HCT is largely supportive with oxygen supplementation, broad-spectrum antimicrobial coverage, and, more recently, etanercept [238].

Noninfectious pulmonary injury may be detected early with prospective pulmonary function testing. Early signs and symptoms of pulmonary compromise should prompt a thorough diagnostic evaluation. Empiric antimicrobial treatment may be initiated, while cultures are pending. Antimicrobial prophylaxis is indicated with initiation of immunosuppressive medications. Etanercept and pulse steroids are considered in more advanced cases [236, 238, 239].

Endocrine Complications

Patients undergoing HCT may be at risk for adrenal insufficiency based on prior corticosteroid exposure for management of their primary disease (such as acute lymphoblastic leukemia) or for supportive care management (such as treatment of GVHD) [240]. Patients with adrenoleukodystrophy may have adrenal insufficiency as a manifestation of their primary disease [241, 242]. These patients usually require stress-dose steroid administration prior to anesthesia or invasive procedures and during periods of stress such as sepsis [241]. The recommended stress dose for suspected adrenal crisis is an immediate parenteral injection of 50 mg/m^2 hydrocortisone, followed by appropriate fluid resuscitation and 50–100 mg/m^2 of hydrocortisone/24 h (via continuous iv therapy or divided every 6 h) [243]. If patients are already receiving high-dose steroids as part of their other management, additional steroids may not be required. Prophylaxis against gastrointestinal bleeding with antiacid therapy is recommended during periods of stress and steroid administration.

In a retrospective single center review, the prevalence of endocrine complications among pediatric HCT patients was as follows: 1.2% primary hypothyroidism, 7% compensated hypothyroidism, 2.4% hyperthyroidism, 22.4% hypergonadotropic hypogonadism, 2.4% abnormal bone density, and 1.2% secondary diabetes mellitus [244]. Thyrotoxicosis, though rare, has been reported among pediatric HCT patients [245]. The prevalence of endocrine complications of adult patients who are survivors of HCT is higher, suggesting that long-term monitoring of endocrine complications following HCT is important [246]. Patients with GVHD may be at a disproportionately higher risk of hypothyroidism [244]. Patients undergoing HCT who receive parenteral nutrition and steroids and/or who have sepsis are at risk for hyperglycemia which may require insulin administration. Insulin management during HCT admissions require careful monitoring for labile blood sugars, which may fluctuate with steroid and nutrition adjustments. For patients with pre-existing diabetes who are undergoing HCT or admitted for critical care management, consideration of an insulin drip over home regimens should be considered during the acute admission phase.

Cytokine Release Syndrome (CRS), CAR-T-Related Encephalopathy Syndrome (CRES), and CAR-T-Related Hemophagocytic Lymphohistiocytosis (HLH)

Immune effector cell-based therapies, including monoclonal antibodies (mAbs) and chimeric antigen receptor (CAR-T) cells, have been associated with unique toxicities such as cytokine release syndrome (CRS), CAR-T-related encephalopathy syndrome (CRES), and CAR-T-related hemophagocytic lymphohistiocytosis (HLH) [41, 247, 248]. CRS is a well-described albeit non-specific systemic inflammatory response typically characterized by tachycardia, fever, hypoxia, hypotension, and multi-organ dysfunction [248]. The development of CRS is associated with CAR-T engagement and proliferation and subsequent cytokine elevation [249]. Cytokine elevations of interleukin-6 (IL-6), interferon gamma (IFN-γ), and interleukin-10 (IL-10) have been noted among patients with CRS. Yet, this is not a universal finding among all patients who develop CRS and levels of elevation when present do not always correlate with severity [249, 250]. In a phase 2, single-cohort, 25-center, global study of tisagenlecleucel among pediatric and young adult patients with CD19+ relapsed or refractory B-cell acute lymphoblastic leukemia (ALL), CRS occurred in 77% of patients. Among these patients, transient increases in serum IL-6, IFN-γ, and ferritin levels were seen with CRS and tended to be more pronounced among patients with more severe CRS [14]. Anti-IL-6 therapy with tocilizumab was used among 48% of patients, and almost half of the patients required critical care support (median stay 7 days) with high-dose vasopressors (25%), oxygen supplementation (44%), mechanical ventilation (13%), or dialysis (9%) [14]. Guidelines for the diagnosis, grading, and management of CRS among children are summarized in Table 8.11. Early signs and symptoms of CRS may be mild with sinus tachycardia and fever at presentation. CRS should be suspected if at least one of the following four symptoms or signs is present during the CRS risk period following CAR-T infusion: (i) fever ≥ 38 °C, (ii) hypotension (age 1–10 years: systolic blood pressure < [70 + (2 × age in years)] mmHg; age > 10 years: SBP < 90 mmHg; change from baseline and/or reduced requirements for chronic anti-hypertensive medications), (iii) hypoxia with an arterial oxygen saturation of <90% on room air, and/or (iv) evidence of organ toxicity [251–253]. Attention to pediatric guidelines for age-appropriate norms and considerations is important. For example, the Pediatric Acute Lung Injury Consensus Conference (PALICC) guidelines for diagnosis and management of pediatric acute respiratory distress syndrome (PARDS) and Pediatric RIFLE (Risk, Injury, Failure, Loss, End Stage Renal Disease) and KDIGO (Kidney Disease: Improving Global Outcomes) definitions of oliguria should be considered [252–255]. Vigilance for prompt recognition of hemodynamic shock in the child is crucial. The baseline blood pressure range of the child should be reviewed pre CAR-T infusion so that relative hypotension from an elevated baseline is not missed. Reduced requirements for chronic antihypertensive medications may also indicate relative hypotension. It is also important that providers use their clinical judgment to determine CRS attribution [251].

Table 8.11 CRS/CRES [251]

Cytokine release syndrome (CRS) grading and management		
Step 1 **Age, signs and symptoms**	**Step 2** **CRS grading**	**Step 3** **Management**
Temperature greater than or equal to 38 °C No hypotension No hypoxia Grade 1 CTCAE v5.0 Organ Toxicity *Pediatric consideration:* Asymptomatic sinus tachycardia (above age specific normal range or baseline) Hypotension: (1–10 years: SBP < [70 + (2 × age in years)] mmHg; > 10 years: SBP < 90 mmHg)	*Grade 1*	Acetaminophen as needed for fever Evaluate for infectious etiologies (blood, urine cultures, and chest X-ray) Consider broad spectrum antibiotics and filgrastim (if neutropenic) Assess for adequate hydration Consider IL-6 antagonist for persistent or refractory fever[a] Symptomatic management of constitutional symptoms and organ toxicities
Any temperature and any of the following: Hypotension that responds to IV fluids or low-dose vasopressor FiO2 requirement <40% (SpO2 < 90% on room air) to keep SpO2 > 88% Grade 2 CTCAE v5.0 organ toxicity *Pediatric consideration:* Hypotension: (1–10 years: SBP < [70 + (2 × age in years)] mmHg; > 10 years: SBP < 90 mmHg)	*Grade 2*	Perform grade 1 management (if applicable) IV fluid bolus of 10–20 ml/kg normal saline; repeat as necessary to maintain SBP above baseline or age normal range Consider IL-6 antagonist (tocilizumab 12 mg/kg/dose for <30 kg, 8 mg/kg/dose for ≥30 kg maximum 800 mg/dose IV every 8 h (titrate frequency based on response up to 3 doses/24 h) for hypotension refractory to fluid boluses or hypoxia If hypotension persists after two fluid boluses and IL-6 antagonist, start vasopressors, transfer patient to PICU, and obtain ECHO Use supplemental oxygen as needed If high risk for severe CRS, hypotension persists after IL-6 antagonist and/or there are signs of hypoperfusion or rapid deterioration, use stress-dose hydrocortisone (50–100 mg/m^2/day divided every 6 h) or dexamethasone (0.5 mg/kg/dose; maximum 10 mg/dose) IV every 6 h or methylprednisolone (1–2 mg/kg/day divided q6–q12 h)

Table 8.11 (continued)

Any temperature and any of the following: Hypotension (1–10 years: SBP < [70 + (2 × age in years)] mmHg; >10 years: SBP < 90) that needs high-dose or multiple vasopressors FiO2 requirement ≥40% and/or requiring BiPAP to keep SpO2 > 88% Grade 3 CTCAE v5.0 organ toxicity Grade 4 transaminitis (> 20.0 × ULN) *Pediatric consideration:* Oliguria (< 0.5 ml/kg/h for 8 h)	*Grade 3*	Perform grade 1 and 2 management Transfer patient to PICU, and obtain ECHO if not performed already Dexamethasone 0.5 mg/kg/dose (maximum 10 mg/dose) IV every 6 h may increase to 20 mg IV every 6 h if refractory (alternatively methylprednisolone 1–2 mg/kg/day divided q6–q12 h)[b] Use supplemental oxygen including high-flow oxygen delivery and noninvasive positive-pressure ventilation
Any temperature and any of the following: Persistent hypotension despite fluid resuscitation and multiple vasopressors Mechanical ventilation Grade 4 CTCAE v5.0 organ toxicity (except grade 4 transaminitis) *Pediatric consideration:* Anuria (<0.3 ml/kg/h for 24 h or anuric for 12 h)	*Grade 4*	IV fluids, IL-6 antagonist, corticosteroids, vasopressors, and hemodynamic monitoring as in Grade 1, 2, 3 If lower doses of corticosteroids do not lead to clinical improvement, consider high-dose methylprednisolone (1 g daily for 3 days followed by rapid taper based on clinical response)

Early recognition and intervention is essential to avoid life-threatening complications
CRS should be suspected if any of the above-listed signs and symptoms are present within the first 3 weeks of CAR cell therapy, or for CRES, within the first 4 weeks of CAR T-cell therapy
Patients at higher risk of severe CRS: early onset (<3 days) of CRS signs and symptoms, bulky disease, and comorbidities
CRS grading should be performed at least twice a day and when there is change in the patient clinical status
Persistent fever >3 days or fever > = 39 for >10 h unresponsive to acetaminophen
[b]It is not unreasonable for simultaneous administration of both corticosteroids and IL-6 antagonists or to wait for a response to IL-6 antagonists only (may vary based on products/risk factors)
CTCAE v5.0 common terminology criteria for adverse events version 5.0, *SBP* systolic blood pressure, *mmHg* millimeter mercury, *ULN* upper limit normal, *IV* intravenous, *FiO2* fraction of inspired oxygen, *BiPAP* bi-level positive airway pressure, *ml* milliliter, *kg* kilograms, *h* hour, *IL-6* interleukin 6, *mg* milligrams, *PICU* pediatric intensive care unit, *ECHO* echocardiography

(continued)

Table 8.11 (continued)

CAR-T-cell-related encephalopathy syndrome (CRES) grading and management		
Step 1 **Age, signs, and symptoms**	**Step 2** **CRES grading**	**Step 3** **Management**
>12 years (and age-appropriate cognitive performance) [a]Grade 1 (per CTCAE v5.0) somnolence, confusion, encephalopathy, dysphasia, seizure (brief partial seizure, no LOC), tremor Neurologic assessment score 7–9 *≤12 years* Grade 1 CNS toxicities as above and CAPD score <9	*Grade 1*	Vigilant supportive care; aspiration precautions; IV hydration Withhold oral intake of food/ medicines/fluids and assess swallowing Convert all oral medications and/or nutrition to IV if swallowing is impaired Avoid medications that cause CNS depression Low doses of lorazepam (0.05 mg/kg (max 1 mg) IV every 8 h) or haloperidol (0.05 mg/kg (max 1 mg) IV every 6 h) may be used for agitated patients with careful monitoring Neurology consultation MRI brain with and without contrast; diagnostic lumbar puncture with OP; MRI spine if focal peripheral neurological deficits; CT scan of brain may be performed if MRI brain is not feasible Perform EEG; if no seizures on EEG, continue levetiracetam If EEG shows nonconvulsive status epilepticus, treat per algorithm A Consider IL-6 antagonist if associated with concurrent CRS
>12 years (and age-appropriate cognitive performance) [a]Grade 2 (per CTCAE v5.0) somnolence, confusion, encephalopathy, dysphasia, seizure (brief generalized seizure), tremor Neurologic assessment score 3–6 *≤12 years* Grade 2 CNS toxicities as above and CAPD score <9	*Grade 2*	Supportive care and neurological workup as per grade 1 IL-6 antagonist if associated with concurrent CRS Dexamethasone 0.5 mg/kg/dose (maximum 10 mg/dose) IV every 6 h or methylprednisolone 1–2 mg/kg/day divided q6–q12 h for CRES not associated with concurrent CRS, or if refractory to IL-6 antagonist therapy when it is administered Consider PICU transfer if associated with grade 2 or greater CRS

Table 8.11 (continued)

>12 years (and age-appropriate cognitive performance) [a]Grade 3 (per CTCAE v5.0) somnolence, confusion, encephalopathy, dysphasia, seizure (multiple seizures despite medical interventions), tremor and incontinence or motor weakness, raised ICP (stage 1 or 2 papilledema with CSF OP <20 mmHg) Neurologic assessment score 0–2 *≤12 years* CAPD score >9	*Grade 3*	Supportive care and neurological work-up as per grade 1 PICU transfer is recommended IL-6 antagonist, if associated with concurrent CRS if not administered previously Dexamethasone 0.5 mg/kg/dose (maximum 10 mg/dose) IV every 6 h; increase to 20 mg IV every 6 h if refractory or methylprednisolone 1–2 mg/kg/day divided q6–q12 h around the clock, if symptoms worsen despite IL-6 antagonist therapy or for CRES without concurrent CRS Continue corticosteroids until improvement to grade 1 and then taper or stop Stage 1 or 2 papilledema with CSF OP <20 mmHg, treat per algorithm C Consider repeat neuroimaging (CT or MRI) q 2–3 days if persistent CRES greater than or equal to grade 3
Critical/obtunded/unable to perform CAPD High grade (Stage 3, 4, or 5) papilledema, CSF OP ≥ 20 mm Hg, or cerebral edema Life-threatening prolonged repetitive seizure Requirement of mechanical ventilation	*Grade 4*	Supportive care and neurological workup as per grade 1 PICU monitoring; consider mechanical ventilation for airway protection Neurosurgical evaluation Consider repeating CT scans Chemistry panels frequently medication adjustment and osmotherapy to prevent rebound cerebral edema, renal failure, hypovolemia/hypotension, and electrolyte abnormalities IL-6 antagonist and repeat neuroimaging as per grade 3 Consider high-dose corticosteroids (e.g. methylprednisolone IV 1 g/day × 3 days followed by rapid taper) Continue corticosteroids until improvement to grade 1 and then taper For convulsive status epilepticus, treat per algorithm B Stage 3,4 or 5 papilledema, CSF OP ≥20 mmHg, or cerebral edema treat per algorithm D

(continued)

Table 8.11 (continued)

CRES grading with history, physical examination, neurologic assessment score, or Cornell assessment of pediatric delirium tool (CAPD) should be performed at least twice a day and when there is change in the patient clinical status
The trend in CAPD scores within an individual subject is important; increasing scores can be used as a marker for CRES severity
Papilledema scoring according to modified Frisen graded scale of papilledema
[a]CTCAE neurologic toxicities should be assessed for etiology, in a similar manner to fevers. If toxicities are thought to be attributable to CRES, then symptoms should be treated per the algorithm
LOC loss of consciousness, *CNS* central nervous system, *CTCAE* common terminology criteria for adverse events, *CSF* cerebrospinal fluid, *OP* opening pressure, *IV* intravenous, *mg* milligrams, *max* maximum, *EEG* electroencephalography, *CT* computed tomography, *MRI* magnetic resonance imaging, *PICU* pediatric intensive care unit, *IL-6* interleukin 6

CAR-T-related encephalopathy syndrome (CRES) may present concurrently with CRS, after its resolution or without antecedent CRS [41, 247, 248]. CRES can also present with a wide range of symptoms including handwriting difficulty, delirium, seizures, and cerebral edema [65, 251]. CRES occurred in 40% of children with ALL who received tisagenlecleucel during the phase 2 global study [14]. The Cornell Assessment of Pediatric Delirium (CAPD) provides a validated screening tool for recognition of delirium among children and adolescents (ages birth to 21 years old) [256]. CAPD screening with use of developmental anchor points may be used to perform developmentally appropriate delirium screening for children during their CRES risk period [251]. A CAPD score greater than 8 is indicative of delirium, with a trend of increasing scores worrisome for CRES severity [251]. Alternatively, a neurological assessment score may be performed for older patients as previously described [41]. While delirium and handwriting difficulty may represent the earliest signs of CRES, seizures, papilledema, and cerebral edema are some of the most worrisome signs. Patients who receive products associated with a reasonable likelihood of CRES may receive anti-seizure prophylaxis with non-cardiotoxic medications such as levetiracetam. Grading and management of CRES are outlined in Table 8.11 [251]. Children who show signs and symptoms of CRES may require early assessment by neurology and critical care teams. Seizure precautions, airway management considerations, serial funduscopic examinations, and appropriate planning for possible status epilepticus and cerebral edema may mitigate negative outcomes.

Diagnostic criteria and considerations for CAR-T-related hemophagocytic lymphohistiocytosis (HLH) have been previously described [9, 41, 247, 251]. Children may be diagnosed with CAR-T-related HLH/MAS if they have a peak ferritin >10,000 ng/ml during their CRS phase and develop two of the following: grade ≥ 3 organ toxicities involving the liver, kidney, or lung, or hemophagocytosis in the bone marrow or other organs [9, 41, 247, 251].

Early recognition and close monitoring for worsening status and prompt treatment with anti-IL-6 therapy such as tocilizumab (competitively inhibits the binding of IL-6 to its receptor IL-6R) and siltuximab (monoclonal antibody (MAb) against IL-6) may mitigate severe manifestations of CRS/CRES and CAR-T-related HLH [14, 257, 258]. Routine administration of corticosteroids to patients receiving CAR-T therapy is usually avoided in the absence of CRS as its impact on CAR-T expansion remains to be determined. However, prompt steroid administration in the setting of significant sequelae, particularly if refractory to tocilizumab, may be appropriate [251]. Safety mechanisms to eliminate transduced cells have also been added to some CAR cells, such as (i) CD19 CAR with a truncated EGFR (EGFRt) that can be inactivated with administration of cetuximab [259], (ii) functional co-expression of RQR8 ligand sensitive to the monoclonal antibody rituximab, and (iii) inducible caspase-9 (iC9) that can be pharmacologically activated to eliminate transduced cells [251, 260–262]. Anticipatory preparation and precautions for severe sequelae such as management of hemodynamic shock, status epilepticus, and cerebral edema are important. It is important to consider the differential diagnoses in the management of these sequelae. For example, broad-spectrum antibiotics may be appropriate with fever, and fluid resuscitation may be indicated for hypotension (without triggering acute fluid overload and cardiorespiratory compromise).

References

1. Majhail NS, et al. Indications for autologous and allogeneic hematopoietic cell transplantation: guidelines from the American Society for Blood and Marrow Transplantation. Biol Blood Marrow Transplant. 2015;21:1863–9.
2. Peffault de Latour R, et al. Recommendations on hematopoietic stem cell transplantation for inherited bone marrow failure syndromes. Bone Marrow Transplant. 2015;50:1168–72.
3. Sureda A, et al. Indications for Allo- and auto-Sct for haematological diseases, solid tumours and immune disorders: current practice in Europe, 2015. Bone Marrow Transplant. 2015;50:1037–56.
4. Fish JD, Grupp SA. Stem cell transplantation for neuroblastoma. Bone Marrow Transplant. 2008;41:159–65.
5. Kasenda B, et al. High-dose chemotherapy with autologous haematopoietic stem cell support for relapsed or refractory primary Cns lymphoma: a prospective multicentre trial by the German cooperative primary central nervous system lymphoma study broup. Leukemia. 2017;31:2623–9.
6. DeFilipp Z, et al. High-dose chemotherapy with Thiotepa, Busulfan, and cyclophosphamide and autologous stem cell transplantation for patients with primary central nervous system lymphoma in first complete remission. Cancer. 2017;123:3073–9.
7. Baird K, et al. Reduced intensity allogeneic stem cell transplantation in children and young adults with ultra-high risk pediatric sarcomas. Biol Blood Marrow Transplant. 2012;18:698–707.
8. Eapen M, et al. Umbilical cord blood transplantation in children with acute leukemia: impact of conditioning on transplantation outcomes. Biol Blood Marrow Transplant. 2017;23:1714–21.
9. Grupp SA, et al. Chimeric antigen receptor – modified T cells for acute lymphoid leukemia. N Engl J Med. 2013;368:1509–18.
10. Kumar SRP, Markusic DM, Biswas M, High KA, Herzog RW. Clinical development of gene therapy: results and lessons from recent successes. Mol Ther Methods Clin Dev. 2016;3:16034.

11. Zinter MS, et al. Pediatric hematopoietic cell transplant patients who survive critical illness frequently have significant but recoverable decline in functional status. Biol Blood Marrow Transplant. 2018;24:330–6.
12. Zinter MS, Dvorak CC, Spicer A, Cowan MJ, Sapru A. New insights into multicenter Picu mortality among pediatric hematopoietic stem cell transplant patients. Crit Care Med. 2015;43:1986–94.
13. Duncan CN, et al. Clinical outcomes of children receiving intensive cardiopulmonary support during hematopoietic stem cell transplant. Pediatr Crit Care Med. 2013;14:261–7.
14. Maude SL, et al. Tisagenlecleucel in children and young adults with B-cell lymphoblastic leukemia. N Engl J Med. 2018;378:439–48.
15. https://bethematchclinical.org/workarea/downloadasset.aspx?id=3545
16. Samaras P, et al. Mobilization of hematopoietic progenitor cells with standard or reduced dose Filgrastim after Vinorelbine in multiple myeloma patients. A randomized prospective single center phase ii study. Biol Blood Marrow Transplant. 2018;24(4):694–9. https://doi.org/10.1016/j.bbmt.2017.12.775. Epub 2017 Dec 12.
17. Clark RE, et al. Plerixafor is superior to conventional chemotherapy for first-line stem cell mobilisation, and is effective even in heavily pretreated patients. Blood Cancer J. 2014;4:e255.
18. Holtan SG, et al. Timing of autologous stem cell transplantation from last chemotherapy affects lymphocyte collection and survival in non-Hodgkin lymphoma. Br J Haematol. 2006;133:628–33.
19. Porrata LF, et al. Infused peripheral blood autograft absolute lymphocyte count correlates with day 15 absolute lymphocyte count and clinical outcome after autologous peripheral hematopoietic stem cell transplantation in non-Hodgkin's lymphoma. Bone Marrow Transplant. 2004;33:291–8.
20. Rosinski SL, et al. Prognostic analysis of pre-transplant peripheral T-cell levels in patients receiving an autologous hematopoietic progenitor-cell transplant. Bone Marrow Transplant. 2005;36:425–30.
21. Bitan M, et al. Determination of eligibility in related pediatric hematopoietic cell donors: ethical and clinical considerations. Recommendations from a Working Group of the Worldwide Network for Blood and Marrow Transplantation Association. Biol Blood Marrow Transplant. 2016;22:96–103.
22. Michon B, et al. Complications of apheresis in children. Transfusion. 2007;47:1837–42.
23. Gorlin JB, et al. Pediatric large volume peripheral blood progenitor cell collections from patients under 25kg: a primer. J Clin Apher. 1996;11:195–203.
24. Carausu L, Clapisson G, Philip I, Sebban H, Marec-Beard P. Use of totally implantable catheters for peripheral blood stem cell apheresis. Bone Marrow Transplant. 2007;40:417–22.
25. Koristek Z, Sterba J, Havranova D, Mayer J. Technique for Pbsc harvesting in children of weight under 10 kg. Bone Marrow Transplant. 2002;29:57–61.
26. Ohara Y, et al. Comprehensive technical and patient-care optimization in the Management of Pediatric Apheresis for peripheral blood stem cell harvesting. Transfus Apher Sci. 2016;55:338–43.
27. Abate-Daga D, Davila ML. Car models: next-generation Car modifications for enhanced T-cell function. Mol Ther Oncolytics. 2016;3:16014.
28. Brentjens RJ, et al. Cd19-targeted T cells rapidly induce molecular remissions in adults with chemotherapy-refractory acute lymphoblastic leukemia. Sci Transl Med. 2013;5:177.
29. Cruz CR, et al. Infusion of donor-derived Cd19-redirected virus-specific T cells for B-cell malignancies relapsed after allogeneic stem cell transplant: a phase 1 study. Blood. 2013;122:2965–73.
30. Davila ML, et al. Efficacy and toxicity management of 19–28z Car T cell therapy in B cell acute lymphoblastic leukemia. Sci Transl Med. 2014;6:224ra225.
31. Kochenderfer JN, et al. Donor-derived Cd19-targeted T cells cause regression of malignancy persisting after allogeneic hematopoietic stem cell transplantation. Blood. 2013;122:4129–39.

32. Kochenderfer JN, et al. Chemotherapy-refractory diffuse large B-cell lymphoma and indolent B-cell malignancies can be effectively treated with autologous T cells expressing an anti-Cd19 chimeric antigen receptor. J Clin Oncol. 2015;33:540–9.
33. Kochenderfer JN, et al. Eradication of B-lineage cells and regression of lymphoma in a patient treated with autologous T cells genetically engineered to recognize Cd19. Blood. 2010;116:4099–102.
34. Maus MV, Levine BL. Chimeric antigen receptor T-cell therapy for the community oncologist. Oncologist. 2016;21:608–17.
35. Porter DL, Levine BL, Kalos M, Bagg A, June CH. Chimeric antigen receptor-modified T cells in chronic lymphoid leukemia. N Engl J Med. 2011;365:725–33.
36. Lee DW, et al. T cells expressing Cd19 chimeric antigen receptors for acute lymphoblastic Leukaemia in children and young adults: a phase 1 dose-escalation trial. Lancet. 2015;385:517–28.
37. Garfall AL, et al. Chimeric antigen receptor T cells against Cd19 for multiple myeloma. New Engl J Med. 2015;373:1040–7.
38. Brudno JN, et al. Allogeneic T cells that express an anti-Cd19 chimeric antigen receptor induce remissions of B-cell malignancies that Progress after allogeneic hematopoietic stem-cell transplantation without causing graft-versus-host disease. J Clin Oncol. 2016;34:1112.
39. Turtle CJ, et al. Durable molecular remissions in chronic lymphocytic leukemia treated with Cd19-specific chimeric antigen receptor-modified T cells after failure of Ibrutinib. J Clin Oncol. 2017;35:3010–20.
40. Locke FL, et al. Product characteristics associated with in vivo expansion of anti-Cd19 Car T cells in patients treated with Axicabtagene Ciloleucel (Axi-Cel). J Clin Oncol. 2017;35:3023.
41. Neelapu SS, et al. Axicabtagene Ciloleucel Car T-cell therapy in refractory large B-cell lymphoma. New Engl J Med. 2017;377:2531–44.
42. Rezvani K, Rouce R, Liu E, Shpall E. Engineering natural killer cells for Cancer immunotherapy. Mol Ther. 2017;25:1769–81.
43. Truong TH, et al. Adverse reactions during stem cell infusion in children treated with autologous and allogeneic stem cell transplantation. Bone Marrow Transplant. 2016;51:680–6.
44. Berz D, McCormack EM, Winer ES, Colvin GA, Quesenberry PJ. Cryopreservation of hematopoietic stem cells. Am J Hematol. 2007;82:463–72.
45. Davis JM, Rowley SD, Braine HG, Piantadosi S, Santos GW. Clinical toxicity of cryopreserved bone marrow graft infusion. Blood. 1990;75:781–6.
46. Stroncek DF, et al. Adverse reactions in patients transfused with cryopreserved marrow. Transfusion. 1991;31:521–6.
47. Zambelli A, et al. Clinical toxicity of cryopreserved circulating progenitor cells infusion. Anticancer Res. 1998;18:4705–8.
48. Zenhausern R, Tobler A, Leoncini L, Hess OM, Ferrari P. Fatal cardiac arrhythmia after infusion of dimethyl sulfoxide-cryopreserved hematopoietic stem cells in a patient with severe primary cardiac amyloidosis and end-stage renal failure. Ann Hematol. 2000;79:523–6.
49. Hoyt R, Szer J, Grigg A. Neurological events associated with the infusion of cryopreserved bone marrow and/or peripheral blood progenitor cells. Bone Marrow Transplant. 2000;25:1285–7.
50. Otrock ZK, et al. Transient global amnesia associated with the infusion of Dmso-cryopreserved autologous peripheral blood stem cells. Haematologica. 2008;93:e36–7.
51. Miniero R, Vai S, Giacchino M, Giubellino C, Madon E. Severe respiratory depression after autologous bone marrow infusion. Haematologica. 1992;77:98–9.
52. Cruz CR, et al. Adverse events following infusion of T cells for adoptive immunotherapy: a 10-year experience. Cytotherapy. 2010;12:743–9.
53. AABB. Standards for blood banks and transfusion Medicine. 30th ed. Bethesda: AABB; 2016.
54. Rowan CM, et al. Invasive mechanical ventilation and mortality in pediatric hematopoietic stem cell transplantation: a multicenter study. Pediatr Crit Care Med. 2016;17:294–302.

55. Demaret P, Pettersen G, Hubert P, Teira P, Emeriaud G. The critically-ill pediatric Hemato-oncology patient: epidemiology, management, and strategy of transfer to the pediatric intensive care unit. Ann Intensive Care. 2012;2:14.
56. Weiss SL, et al. Global epidemiology of pediatric severe Sepsis: the Sepsis prevalence, outcomes, and therapies study. Am J Respir Crit Care Med. 2015;191:1147–57.
57. Lindell RB, et al. High levels of morbidity and mortality among pediatric hematopoietic cell transplant recipients with severe Sepsis: insights from the Sepsis prevalence, outcomes, and therapies international point prevalence study. Pediatr Crit Care Med. 2017;18:1114–25.
58. González-Vicent M, Marín C, Madero L, Sevilla J, Díaz MA. Risk score for pediatric intensive care unit admission in children undergoing hematopoietic stem cell transplantation and analysis of predictive factors for survival. J Pediatr Hematol Oncol. 2005;27:526–31.
59. Schneider DT, et al. Introduction of the oncological pediatric risk of mortality score (O-Prism) for Icu support following stem cell transplantation in children. Bone Marrow Transplant. 2000;25:1079.
60. Jaing TH, et al. Evaluation of readmission in children receiving allogeneic hematopoietic stem cell transplantation: an institutional experience. Transplant Proc. 2008;40:3643–5.
61. Shulman DS, London WB, Guo D, Duncan CN, Lehmann LE. Incidence and causes of hospital readmission in pediatric patients after hematopoietic cell transplantation. Biol Blood Marrow Transplant. 2015;21:913–9.
62. Maher OM, et al. Etiologies and impact of readmission rates in the first 180 days after hematopoietic stem cell transplantation in children, adolescents, and young adults. J Pediatr Hematol Oncol. 2017;39:609–13.
63. Giralt S, et al. Reduced-intensity conditioning regimen workshop: defining the dose spectrum. Report of a workshop convened by the center for international blood and marrow transplant research. Biol Blood Marrow Transplant. 2009;15:367–9.
64. Tomblyn MB, et al. Myeloablative hematopoietic cell transplantation for acute lymphoblastic leukemia: analysis of graft sources and long-term outcome. J Clin Oncol. 2009;27:3634–41.
65. Neelapu SS, et al. Chimeric antigen receptor T-cell therapy – assessment and management of toxicities. Nat Rev Clin Oncol. 2018;15:47–62.
66. Nahirniak S, et al. Guidance on platelet transfusion for patients with hypoproliferative thrombocytopenia. Transfus Med Rev. 2015;29:3–13.
67. Pihusch M, et al. Recombinant activated factor Vii in treatment of bleeding complications following hematopoietic stem cell transplantation. J Thromb Haemost. 2005;3:1935–44.
68. Franchini M, Veneri D, Lippi G. The potential role of recombinant activated Fvii in the management of critical hemato-oncological bleeding: a systematic review. Bone Marrow Transplant. 2007;39:729–35.
69. Tang Y, et al. Use of recombinant factor Viia in uncontrolled gastrointestinal bleeding after hematopoietic stem cell transplantation among patients with thrombocytopenia. Pak J Med Sci. 2015;31:1389–93.
70. Park JA. Diffuse alveolar hemorrhage and recombinant factor Viia treatment in pediatric patients. Korean J Pediatr. 2016;59:105–13.
71. Abrams D, et al. Extracorporeal membrane oxygenation in the management of diffuse alveolar hemorrhage. ASAIO J. 2015;61:216–8.
72. Garnock-Jones KP, Keam SJ. Eltrombopag. Drugs. 2009;69:567–76.
73. Tanaka T, et al. Eltrombopag for treatment of thrombocytopenia after allogeneic hematopoietic cell transplantation. Biol Blood Marrow Transplant. 2016;22:919–24.
74. Vose JM, Armitage JO. Clinical applications of hematopoietic growth factors. J Clin Oncol. 1995;13:1023–35.
75. Tomblyn M, et al. Guidelines for preventing infectious complications among hematopoietic cell transplantation recipients: a global perspective. Biol Blood Marrow Transplant. 2009;15:1143–238.

76. Balian C, Garcia M, Ward J. A retrospective analysis of bloodstream infections in pediatric allogeneic stem cell transplant recipients: the role of central venous catheters and mucosal barrier injury. J Pediatr Oncol Nurs. 2018;35:210–7.
77. Mehta RS, Rezvani K. Immune reconstitution post allogeneic transplant and the impact of immune recovery on the risk of infection. Virulence. 2016;7:901–16.
78. Dandoy CE, et al. Healthcare burden, risk factors, and outcomes of mucosal barrier injury laboratory-confirmed bloodstream infections after stem cell transplantation. Biol Blood Marrow Transplant. 2016;22:1671–7.
79. Cesaro S, et al. Incidence, risk factors and long-term outcome of acute leukemia patients with early Candidemia after allogeneic stem cell transplantation. A study by the acute leukemia and infectious diseases working parties of Ebmt. Clin Infect Dis. 2018;67(4):564–72.
80. Simms-Waldrip T, et al. Invasive fungal infections in pediatric hematopoietic stem cell transplant patients. Infect Dis (Lond). 2015;47:218–24.
81. Abdel-Azim H, et al. A survey of infectious disease clinical practices among pediatric blood and marrow transplant programs in the United States. Pediatr Blood Cancer. 2015;62(4):731–5. https://doi.org/10.1002/pbc.25355. Epub 2015 Jan 3.
82. Groll AH, et al. Fourth European conference on infections in Leukaemia (Ecil-4): guidelines for diagnosis, prevention, and treatment of invasive fungal diseases in Paediatric patients with Cancer or allogeneic Haemopoietic stem-cell transplantation. Lancet Oncol. 2014;15:327–40.
83. Veys P, Owens C. Respiratory infections following Haemopoietic stem cell transplantation in children. Br Med Bull. 2002;61:151–74.
84. Winston DJ. Prophylaxis and treatment of infection in the bone marrow transplant recipient. Curr Clin Top Infect Dis. 1993;13:293–321.
85. Collin BA, Leather HL, Wingard JR, Ramphal R. Evolution, incidence, and susceptibility of bacterial bloodstream isolates from 519 bone marrow transplant patients. Clin Infect Dis. 2001;33:947–53.
86. Averbuch D, et al. European guidelines for empirical antibacterial therapy for febrile Neutropenic patients in the era of growing resistance: summary of the 2011 4th European conference on infections in leukemia. Haematologica. 2013;98:1826–35.
87. Lee JJ, et al. Clinical efficacy and prediction of response to granulocyte transfusion therapy for patients with neutropenia-related infections. Haematologica. 2004;89:632–3.
88. Lee JJ, et al. Clinical efficacy of granulocyte transfusion therapy in patients with neutropenia-related infections. Leukemia. 2001;15:203–7.
89. Busca A, et al. Oral valganciclovir as preemptive therapy for cytomegalovirus infection post allogeneic stem cell transplantation. Transpl Infect Dis. 2007;9:102–7.
90. Tzannou I, et al. Off-the-shelf virus-specific T cells to treat Bk virus, human herpesvirus 6, cytomegalovirus, epstein-barr virus, and adenovirus infections after allogeneic hematopoietic stem-cell transplantation. J Clin Oncol. 2017;35:3547–57.
91. Marty FM, et al. Cmx001 to prevent cytomegalovirus disease in hematopoietic-cell transplantation. N Engl J Med. 2013;369:1227–36.
92. El-Haddad D, et al. Brincidofovir (Cmx-001) for refractory and resistant cmv and Hsv infections in immunocompromised Cancer patients: a single-center experience. Antivir Res. 2016;134:58–62.
93. Shah DP, et al. Impact of aerosolized ribavirin on mortality in 280 allogeneic haematopoietic stem cell transplant recipients with respiratory syncytial virus infections. J Antimicrob Chemother. 2013;68:1872–80.
94. Dignan FL, et al. Bcsh/Bsbmt/Uk clinical virology network guideline: diagnosis and management of common respiratory viral infections in patients undergoing treatment for haematological malignancies or stem cell transplantation. Br J Haematol. 2016;173:380–93.
95. Boeckh M, et al. Randomized controlled multicenter trial of aerosolized ribavirin for respiratory syncytial virus upper respiratory tract infection in hematopoietic cell transplant recipients. Clin Infect Dis. 2007;44:245–9.

96. MEdicine, N.U.S.N.L.o. An open label study to examine the effects of Das181 administered by dry powder inhaler or nebulized formulation in immunocompromised subjects with parainfluenza infection. 2018. [cited 2018 April 16, 2018]. Available from: https://clinicaltrials.gov/ct2/show/NCT01924793?cond=Parainfluenza&rank=1.
97. Hiwarkar P, et al. Brincidofovir is highly efficacious in controlling adenoviremia in pediatric recipients of hematopoietic cell transplant. Blood. 2017;129:2033–7.
98. O'Reilly RJ, Prockop S, Hasan AN, Koehne G, Doubrovina E. Virus-specific T-cell banks for 'Off the Shelf' adoptive therapy of refractory infections. Bone Marrow Transplant. 2016;51:1163–72.
99. Ramsay ID, et al. Disseminated adenovirus infection after allogeneic stem cell transplant and the potential role of Brincidofovir – case series and 10 year experience of management in an adult transplant cohort. J Clin Virol. 2017;96:73–9.
100. Greco R, et al. Human herpesvirus 6 infection following haploidentical transplantation: immune recovery and outcome. Biol Blood Marrow Transplant. 2016;22:2250–5.
101. Mayer K, et al. Intravesical cidofovir application in Bk virus cystitis after allogeneic hematopoetic stem cell transplantation (Hsct) is safe and highly effective. Bone Marrow Transplant. 2018;53(4):495–8.
102. Harkensee C, Vasdev N, Gennery AR, Willetts IE, Taylor C. Prevention and Management of Bk-Virus Associated Haemorrhagic Cystitis in children following Haematopoietic stem cell transplantation—a systematic review and evidence-based guidance for clinical management. Br J Haematol. 2008;142:717–31.
103. Coppoletta S, et al. Rituximab treatment for epstein-barr virus dnaemia after alternative-donor hematopoietic stem cell transplantation. Biol Blood Marrow Transplant. 2011;17:901–7.
104. Barker JN, et al. Successful treatment of Ebv-associated posttransplantation lymphoma after cord blood transplantation using third-party Ebv-specific cytotoxic T lymphocytes. Blood. 2010;116:5045–9.
105. Du Pasquier RA, Kuroda MJ, Zheng Y, Jean-Jacques J, Letvin NL, Koralnik IJ. A prospective study demonstrates an association between JC virus-specific cyto toxic T lymphocytes and the early control of progressive multifocal leukoencepha lopathy. Brain. 2004;127(Pt 9):1970–8. Epub 2004 Jun 23.
106. Tummala S, Rezvani K. Treating progressive multifocal leukoen cephalopathy with expanded third party BK virus specific cytoxic T cells in acute myeloid leukemia patient following cord blood transplantation (S41.004). Neurology. 2018;90(15 Supplement):S41.004.
107. Elad S, et al. Basic Oral Care for Hematology-Oncology Patients and Hematopoietic Stem Cell Transplantation Recipients: a position paper from the joint task force of the multinational Association of Supportive Care in Cancer/International Society of Oral Oncology (Mascc/Isoo) and the European Society for Blood and Marrow Transplantation (Ebmt). Support Care Cancer. 2015;23:223–36.
108. Miller MM, Donald DV, Hagemann TM. Prevention and treatment of oral mucositis in children with cancer. J Pediatr Pharmacol Ther. 2012;17:340–50.
109. Herbers AH, de Haan AF, van der Velden WJ, Donnelly JP, Blijlevens NM. Mucositis not neutropenia determines bacteremia among hematopoietic stem cell transplant recipients. Transpl Infect Dis. 2014;16:279–85.
110. Van Der Velden WJ, Herbers AH, Netea MG, Blijlevens NM. Mucosal barrier injury, fever and infection in neutropenic patients with cancer: introducing the paradigm febrile mucositis. Br J Haematol. 2014;167:441–52.
111. Sonis ST. Pathobiology of mucositis. Semin Oncol Nurs. 2004;20:11–5.
112. Al-Dasooqi N, et al. Emerging evidence on the pathobiology of mucositis. Support Care Cancer. 2013;21:2075–83.
113. Chaudhry HM, et al. The incidence and severity of oral mucositis among allogeneic hematopoietic stem cell transplantation patients: a systematic review. Biol Blood Marrow Transplant. 2016;22:605–16.

114. Schmidt V, et al. Efficacy and safety of keratinocyte growth factor (Palifermin) for prevention of oral mucositis in Tbi-based allogeneic hematopoietic stem cell transplantation. Bone Marrow Transplant. 2018;53(9):1188–92.
115. Sonis ST, et al. Perspectives on cancer therapy-induced mucosal injury: pathogenesis, measurement, epidemiology, and consequences for patients. Cancer. 2004;100:1995–2025.
116. Sung L, et al. Guideline for the prevention of oral and oropharyngeal mucositis in children receiving treatment for cancer or undergoing haematopoietic stem cell transplantation. BMJ Support Palliat Care. 2017;7:7–16.
117. Morris J, et al. Safety, pharmacokinetics, and efficacy of palifermin in children and adolescents with acute leukemias undergoing myeloablative therapy and allogeneic hematopoietic stem cell transplantation: a pediatric blood and marrow transplant consortium trial. Biol Blood Marrow Transplant. 2016;22:1247–56.
118. Dunbar PJ, Buckley P, Gavrin JR, Sanders JE, Chapman CR. Use of patient-controlled analgesia for pain control for children receiving bone marrow transplant. J Pain Symptom Manag. 1995;10:604–11.
119. Pillitteri LC, Clark RE. Comparison of a patient-controlled analgesia system with continuous infusion for administration of diamorphine for mucositis. Bone Marrow Transplant. 1998;22:495–8.
120. U.S. Department of Health and Human Services, N.I.o.H., National Cancer Institute. Common Terminology Criteria for Adverse Events (Ctcae) Version 5.0. 2017 November 27, 2017 [cited 2018 April 16, 2018]; 5.0:[available from: https://ctep.cancer.gov/protocoldevelopment/electronic_applications/docs/CTCAE_v5_Quick_Reference_5x7.pdf.
121. Al-Dasooqi N, et al. Emerging evidence on the pathobiology of mucositis. Support Care Cancer. 2013;21:3233–41.
122. Corbacioglu S, et al. Diagnosis and severity criteria for sinusoidal obstruction syndrome/Veno-occlusive disease in pediatric patients: a new classification from the European society for blood and marrow transplantation. Bone Marrow Transplant. 2018;53(2):138–45. https://doi.org/10.1038/bmt.2017.161. Epub 2017 Jul 31.
123. Michael M, Kuehnle I, Goldstein SL. Fluid overload and acute renal failure in pediatric stem cell transplant patients. Pediatr Nephrol. 2004;19:91–5.
124. Lombel RM, et al. Implications of different fluid overload definitions in pediatric stem cell transplant patients requiring continuous renal replacement therapy. Intensive Care Med. 2012;38:663–9.
125. Ingelse SA, et al. Pediatric acute respiratory distress syndrome: fluid management in the PICU. Front Pediatr. 2016;4:21. https://doi.org/10.3389/fped.2016.00021. eCollection 2016.
126. Arikan AA, et al. Fluid overload is associated with impaired oxygenation and morbidity in critically ill children. Pediatr Crit Care Med. 2012;13:253–8.
127. Elbahlawan L, Morrison RR. Continuous renal replacement therapy in children post-hematopoietic stem cell transplantation: the present and the future. Curr Stem Cell Res Ther. 2012;7:381–7.
128. Elbahlawan L, et al. Impact of continuous renal replacement therapy on oxygenation in children with acute lung injury after allogeneic hematopoietic stem cell transplantation. Pediatr Blood Cancer. 2010;55:540–5.
129. Raina R, Abusin GA, Vijayaraghavan P, Auletta JJ, Cabral L, Hashem H, Vogt BA, Cooke KR, Abu-Arja RF. The role of continuous renal replacement therapy in the management of acute kidney injury associated with sinusoidal obstruction syndrome following hematopoietic cell transplantation. Pediatr Transplant. 2018;22(2) https://doi.org/10.1111/petr.13139. Epub 2018 Feb 1. PMID:29388370.
130. Sorensen JB, Andersen MK, Hansen HH. Syndrome of inappropriate secretion of antidiuretic hormone (Siadh) in malignant disease. J Intern Med. 1995;238:97–110.
131. Lim YJ, Park EK, Koh HC, Lee YH. Syndrome of inappropriate secretion of antidiuretic hormone as a leading cause of hyponatremia in children who underwent chemotherapy or stem cell transplantation. Pediatr Blood Cancer. 2010;54:734–7.

132. Abe T, et al. Syndrome of inappropriate antidiuretic hormone secretion (Siadh) in children undergoing high-dose chemotherapy and autologous peripheral blood stem cell transplantation. Pediatr Hematol Oncol. 1995;12:363–9.
133. Shiminski-Maher T. Diabetes insipidus and syndrome of inappropriate secretion of antidiuretic hormone in children with midline suprasellar brain tumors. J Pediatr Oncol Nurs. 1991;8:106–11.
134. Moritz ML, Ayus JC. New aspects in the pathogenesis, prevention, and treatment of hyponatremic encephalopathy in children. Pediatr Nephrol. 2010;25:1225–38.
135. Vion AC, Rautou PE, Durand F, Boulanger CM, Valla DC. Interplay of inflammation and endothelial dysfunction in bone marrow transplantation: focus on hepatic Veno-occlusive disease. Semin Thromb Hemost. 2015;41:629–43.
136. McDonald GB, Hinds MS, Fisher LD, Schoch HG, Wolford JL, Banaji M, et al. Veno-occlusive disease of the liver and multiorgan failure after bone marrow transplantation: a cohort study of 355 patients. Ann Intern Med. 1993;118:255–67.
137. Mahadeo KM, et al. Consensus report by the pediatric acute lung injury and Sepsis investigators and pediatric blood and marrow transplant consortium joint working committees on supportive care guidelines for Management of Veno-Occlusive Disease in children and adolescents: part 2-focus on ascites, fluid and electrolytes, renal, and transfusion issues. Biol Blood Marrow Transplant. 2017;23(12):2023–33.
138. Jones RJ, et al. Venoocclusive disease of the liver following bone marrow transplantation. Transplantation. 1987;44:778–83.
139. McDonald GB, Sharma P, Matthews DE, Shulman HM, Thomas ED. Venocclusive disease of the liver after bone marrow transplantation: diagnosis, incidence, and predisposing factors. Hepatology. 1984;4:116–22.
140. Shulman HM, Hinterberger W. Hepatic veno-occlusive disease – liver toxicity syndrome after bone marrow transplantation. Bone Marrow Transplant. 1992;10:197–214.
141. Naples JC, et al. Anicteric veno-occlusive disease after hematopoietic stem cell transplantation in children. Bone Marrow Transplant. 2015;51(1):135.
142. Myers KC, Dandoy C, El-Bietar J, Davies SM, Jodele S. Veno-occlusive disease of the liver in the absence of elevation in bilirubin in pediatric patients after hematopoietic stem cell transplantation. Biol Blood Marrow Transplant. 2015;21:379–81.
143. Carreras E, et al. The incidence of Veno-occlusive disease following allogeneic hematopoietic stem cell transplantation has diminished and the outcome improved over the last decade. Biol Blood Marrow Transplant. 2011;17:1713–20.
144. Coppell JA, et al. Hepatic veno-occlusive disease following stem cell transplantation: incidence, clinical course, and outcome. Biol Blood Marrow Transplant. 2010;16:157–68.
145. Sakai M, et al. Severe hepatocellular injury after hematopoietic cell transplant: incidence, etiology and outcome. Bone Marrow Transplant. 2009;44:441–7.
146. Woods WG, et al. Fatal veno-occlusive disease of the liver following high dose chemotherapy, irradiation and bone marrow transplantation. Am J Med. 1980;68:285–90.
147. Dignan FL, Wynn RF, Hadzic N, Karani J, Quaglia A, Pagliuca A, Veys P, Potter MN. Bchs guideline: diagnosis and management of veno-occlusive disease (sinusoidal obstruction syndrome) following haematopoietic stem cell transplantation. Br J Haematol. 2013;163:444–57.
148. Bajwa RPS, et al. Consensus report by pediatric acute lung injury and Sepsis investigators and pediatric blood and marrow transplantation consortium joint working committees: supportive care guidelines for management of veno-occlusive disease in children and adolescents, part 1: focus on investigations, prophylaxis, and specific treatment. Biol Blood Marrow Transplant. 2017;23(11):1817–25.
149. Ovchinsky N, Frazier W, Auletta JJ, Dvorak CC, Ardura M, Song E, McArthur J, Jeyapalan A, Tamburro R, Mahadeo KM, Traube C, Duncan CN, Bajwa RPS. Consensus report by the pediatric acute lung injury and sepsis investigators and pediatric blood and marrow transplantation consortium joint working committees on supportive care guidelines for management of veno-occlusive disease in children and adolescents, part 3: focus on cardiorespiratory

dysfunction, infections, liver dysfunction, and delirium. Biol Blood Marrow Transplant. 2018;24(2):207–18. https://doi.org/10.1016/j.bbmt.2017.08.035. Epub 2017 Sep 1. PMID: 28870776.
150. Havelock T, Teoh R, Laws D, Gleeson F, BTS Pleural Disease Guideline Group. Pleural procedures and thoracic ultrasound: British Thoracic Society pleural disease guideline 2010. Thorax. 2010;65(Suppl 2):ii61–76.
151. Willems E, et al. Comparison of thrombotic microangiopathy after allogeneic hematopoietic cell transplantation with high-dose or nonmyeloablative conditioning. Bone Marrow Transplant. 2010;45:689–93.
152. Rosenthal J, et al. Transplant-associated thrombotic microangiopathy in pediatric patients treated with sirolimus and tacrolimus. Pediatr Blood Cancer. 2011;57:142–6.
153. Jodele S, et al. Abnormalities in the alternative pathway of complement in children with hematopoietic stem cell transplant-associated thrombotic microangiopathy. Blood. 2013;122:2003–7.
154. Jodele S, et al. Eculizumab therapy in children with severe hematopoietic stem cell transplantation-associated thrombotic microangiopathy. Biol Blood Marrow Transplant. 2014;20:518–25.
155. Legendre CM, et al. Terminal complement inhibitor eculizumab in atypical hemolytic-uremic syndrome. N Engl J Med. 2013;368:2169–81.
156. Jodele S, et al. A new paradigm: diagnosis and management of Hsct-associated thrombotic microangiopathy as multi-system endothelial injury. Blood Rev. 2015;29:191–204.
157. Hillmen P, et al. Long-term safety and efficacy of sustained eculizumab treatment in patients with paroxysmal nocturnal haemoglobinuria. Br J Haematol. 2013;162:62–73.
158. Peffault de Latour R, et al. Successful use of eculizumab in a patient with post-transplant thrombotic microangiopathy. Br J Haematol. 2013;161:279–80.
159. Przepiorka D, et al. Consensus conference on acute Gvhd grading. Bone Marrow Transplant. 1994;15(1995):825–8.
160. Rowlings PA, et al. Ibmtr severity index for grading acute graft-versus-host disease: retrospective comparison with Glucksberg grade. Br J Haematol. 1997;97:855–64.
161. Kanakry CG, et al. Multi-institutional study of post-transplantation cyclophosphamide as single-agent graft-versus-host disease prophylaxis after allogeneic bone marrow transplantation using myeloablative busulfan and fludarabine conditioning. J Clin Oncol. 2014;32:3497–505.
162. Luznik L, Fuchs EJ. High-dose, post-transplantation cyclophosphamide to promote graft-host tolerance after allogeneic hematopoietic stem cell transplantation. Immunol Res. 2010;47:65–77.
163. Weisdorf D, et al. Treatment of moderate/severe acute graft-versus-host disease after allogeneic bone marrow transplantation: an analysis of clinical risk features and outcome. Blood. 1990;75:1024–30.
164. MacMillan ML, et al. Response of 443 patients to steroids as primary therapy for acute graft-versus-host disease: comparison of grading systems. Biol Blood Marrow Transplant. 2002;8:387–94.
165. Messina C, et al. Extracorporeal photochemotherapy for paediatric patients with graft-versus-host disease after haematopoietic stem cell transplantation. Br J Haematol. 2003;122:118–27.
166. Komanduri KV, Couriel D, Champlin RE. Graft-versus-host disease after allogeneic stem cell transplantation: evolving concepts and novel therapies including Photopheresis. Biol Blood Marrow Transplant. 2006;12:1–6.
167. DeSimone RA, Schwartz J, Schneiderman J. Extracorporeal photopheresis in pediatric patients: practical and technical considerations. J Clin Apher. 2017;32:543–52.
168. Chaudhury S, et al. A phase 3 single-arm, prospective study of remestemcel-L, ex-vivo cultured adult human mesenchymal stromal cells, for the treatment of steroid refractory acute Gvhd in pediatric patients. Biol Blood Marrow Transplant. 2018;24:S171–2.
169. Storb R, et al. Predictive factors in chronic graft-versus-host disease in patients with aplastic-Anemia treated by marrow transplantation from Hla-identical siblings. Ann Intern Med. 1983;98:461–6.

170. Atkinson K, et al. Risk-factors for chronic graft-versus-host disease after Hla-identical sibling bone-marrow transplantation. Blood. 1990;75:2459–64.
171. Sullivan KM, et al. Chronic graft versus host-disease in 52 patients – adverse natural course and successful treatment with combination immunosuppression. Blood. 1981; 57:267–76.
172. Ochs LA, et al. Predictive factors for chronic graft-versus-host disease after Histocompatible sibling donor bone-marrow transplantation. Bone Marrow Transplant. 1994;13:455–60.
173. Rouquettegally AM, Boyeldieu D, Prost AC, Gluckman E. Autoimmunity after allogeneic bone-marrow transplantation – a study of 53 long-term-surviving patients. Transplantation. 1988;46:238–40.
174. Quaranta S, et al. Autoantibodies in human chronic graft-versus-host disease after hematopoietic cell transplantation. Clin Immunol. 1999;91:106–16.
175. Allan SE, et al. Activation-induced Foxp3 in human T effector cells does not suppress proliferation or cytokine production. Int Immunol. 2007;19:345–54.
176. Schultz KR, Paquet J, Bader S, Hayglass KT. Requirement for B-cells in T-cell priming to minor histocompatibility antigens and development of graft-versus-host disease. Bone Marrow Transplant. 1995;16:289–95.
177. Filipovich AH, et al. National Institutes of Health consensus development project on criteria for clinical trials in chronic graft-versus-host disease: I. diagnosis and staging working group report. Biol Blood Marrow Transplant. 2005;11:945–56.
178. Lee SJ, Vogelsang G, Flowers ME. Chronic graft-versus-host disease. Biol Blood Marrow Transplant. 2003;9:215–33.
179. Mahadeo KM, et al. Immunologic resolution of human chronic graft-versus-host disease. Biol Blood Marrow Transplant. 2014;20:1508–15.
180. Koreth J, et al. Interleukin-2 and regulatory T cells in graft-versus-host disease. New Engl J Med. 2011;365:2055–66.
181. Barba P, et al. Early and late neurological complications after reduced-intensity conditioning allogeneic stem cell transplantation. Biol Blood Marrow Transplant. 2009;15:1439–46.
182. Kang J-M, et al. Neurologic complications after allogeneic hematopoietic stem cell transplantation in children: analysis of prognostic factors. Biol Blood Marrow Transplant. 2015;21:1091–8.
183. Schmidt K, Schulz AS, Debatin K-M, Friedrich W, Classen CF. Cns complications in children receiving chemotherapy or hematopoietic stem cell transplantation: retrospective analysis and clinical study of survivors. Pediatr Blood Cancer. 2008;50:331–6.
184. Weber C, et al. Diagnostic and therapeutic implications of neurological complications following paediatric haematopoietic stem cell transplantation. Bone Marrow Transplant. 2008;41:253–9.
185. Woodard P, et al. Encephalopathy in pediatric patients after allogeneic hematopoietic stem cell transplantation is associated with a poor prognosis. Bone Marrow Transplant. 2004;33:1151–7.
186. Azik F, et al. Neurological complications after allogeneic hematopoietic stem cell transplantation in children, a single center experience. Pediatr Transplant. 2014;18:405–11.
187. Openshaw H, Chen BT. Neurologic complications of hematopoietic cell transplantation. Wiley; 2015. https://onlinelibrary.wiley.com/doi/10.1002/9781118416426.ch105.
188. Uckan D, et al. Life-threatening neurological complications after bone marrow transplantation in children. Bone Marrow Transplant. 2005;35:71–6.
189. Zaucha-Prazmo A, et al. Neurologic complications in children after hemaopoietic stem cell transplantation: a single-center experience. Transplant Proc. 2007;39:2905–7.
190. Najera JE, Alousi A, Lima MD, Ciurea SO. Akinetic mutism – a serious complication to tacrolimus-based Gvhd prophylaxis. Bone Marrow Transplant. 2013;48:157.
191. Masetti R, et al. Pres in children undergoing hematopoietic stem cell or solid organ transplantation. Pediatrics. 2015;135:890–901.
192. Hedna VS, et al. Posterior reversible encephalopathy syndrome (Pres) and Ct perfusion changes. Int J Emerg Med. 2012;5:12.

193. McArthur J, Duncan C, Rajapreyar P, Talano J-A, Tamburro RT. Critical illness involving children undergoing hematopoietic cell transplantation: cardiac complications. In: *Pediatric clinical care*. 5th ed. Philadelphia: Elsevier; 2017.
194. Dandoy CE, et al. Abnormal echocardiography 7 days after stem cell transplantation may be an early Indicator of thrombotic microangiopathy. Biol Blood Marrow Transplant. 2015;21:113–8.
195. Dandoy CE, et al. Team-based approach to identify cardiac toxicity in critically ill hematopoietic stem cell transplant recipients. Pediatr Blood Cancer. 2017;64:e26513.
196. Tichelli A, Bhatia S, Socié G. Cardiac and cardiovascular consequences after haematopoietic stem cell transplantation. Br J Haematol. 2008;142:11–26.
197. Peres E, et al. Cardiac complications in patients undergoing a reduced-intensity conditioning hematopoietic stem cell transplantation. Bone Marrow Transplant. 2010;45:149–52.
198. Blaes A, Konety S, Hurley P. Cardiovascular complications of hematopoietic stem cell transplantation. Curr Treat Options Cardiovasc Med. 2016;18:25.
199. Majhail NS, Lazarus HM, Burns LJ. Iron overload in hematopoietic cell transplantation. Bone Marrow Transplant. 2008;41:997.
200. Yeh ETH, et al. Cardiovascular complications of cancer therapy: diagnosis, pathogenesis, and management. Circulation. 2004;109:3122–31.
201. Yoon J-H, et al. Early left ventricular dysfunction in children after hematopoietic stem cell transplantation for acute leukemia: a case control study using speckle tracking echocardiography. Korean Circ J. 2015;45:51–8.
202. Armenian SH, Chow EJ. Cardiovascular disease in survivors of hematopoietic cell transplantation. Cancer. 2014;120:469–79.
203. Armenian SH, Ryan TD, Khouri MG. Cardiac dysfunction and heart failure in hematopoietic cell transplantation survivors: emerging paradigms in pathophysiology, screening, and prevention. Heart Fail Clin. 2017;13:337–45.
204. Cerveri I, et al. Late pulmonary sequelae after childhood bone marrow transplantation. Thorax. 1999;54:131–5.
205. Griese M, et al. Pulmonary complications after bone marrow transplantation in children: twenty-four years of experience in a single pediatric center. Pediatr Pulmonol. 2000;30:393–401.
206. Leneveu H, et al. Respiratory function in children undergoing bone marrow transplantation. Pediatr Pulmonol. 1999;28:31–8.
207. Sokol KA, et al. Masks for prevention of respiratory viruses on the Bmt unit: results of a quality initiative. Transpl Infect Dis. 2016;18:965–7.
208. Karageorgopoulos DE, et al. Accuracy of beta-D-glucan for the diagnosis of pneumocystis jirovecii pneumonia: a meta-analysis. Clin Microbiol Infect. 2013;19:39–49.
209. Jain P, et al. Role of flexible bronchoscopy in immunocompromised patients with lung infiltrates. Chest. 2004;125:712–22.
210. Murray PV, et al. Use of first line bronchoalveolar lavage in the immunosuppressed oncology patient. Bone Marrow Transplant. 2001;27:967–71.
211. Shannon VR, Andersson BS, Lei X, Champlin RE, Kontoyiannis DP. Utility of early versus late Fiberoptic bronchoscopy in the evaluation of new pulmonary infiltrates following hematopoietic stem cell transplantation. Bone Marrow Transplant. 2010;45:647–55.
212. O'Dwyer DN, et al. Transbronchial biopsy in the management of pulmonary complications of hematopoietic stem cell transplantation. Bone Marrow Transplant. 2018;53(2):193–8. https://doi.org/10.1038/bmt.2017.238. Epub 2017 Oct 23.
213. Tissot F, et al. Ecil-6 guidelines for the treatment of invasive candidiasis, aspergillosis and mucormycosis in leukemia and hematopoietic stem cell transplant patients. Haematologica. 2017;102:433–44.
214. Deresinski S. Principles of antibiotic therapy in severe infections: optimizing the therapeutic approach by use of laboratory and clinical data. Clin Infect Dis. 2007;45:S177–83.
215. Gustinetti G, Mikulska M. Bloodstream infections in neutropenic cancer patients: a practical update. Virulence. 2016;7:280–97.

216. Woods WG, Daigle AE, Hutchinson RJ, Robison LL. Myelosuppression associated with co-trimoxazole as a prophylactic antibiotic in the maintenance phase of childhood acute lymphocytic leukemia. J Pediatr. 1984;105:639–44.
217. Winston D. Infections in bone marrow transplant recipients. In: *Principles and practice of infectious disease*; 1995. p. 2717–22.
218. Wan L, et al. Effect of granulocyte-macrophage colony-stimulating factor on prevention and treatment of invasive fungal disease in recipients of allogeneic stem-cell transplantation: a prospective multicenter randomized phase Iv trial. J Clin Oncol. 2015;33:3999–4006.
219. Bodey GP, Anaissie E, Gutterman J, Vadhan-Raj S. Role of granulocyte-macrophage colony-stimulating factor as adjuvant treatment in neutropenic patients with bacterial and fungal infection. Eur J Clin Microbiol Infect Dis. 1994;13(Suppl 2):S18–22.
220. Tewari P, Allison J, Waters-Pick B, Cash JV, Kurtzberg J, Prasad VK. Collection of G-Csf-mobilized granulocytes from related donors to support hematopoietic stem cell transplant recipients at high risk of infection is safe and feasible. ASBMT. 2011;17, A1–A10:S149–386.
221. Safdar A, Rodriguez GH. Aerosolized amphotericin B lipid complex as adjunctive treatment for fungal lung infection in patients with cancer-related immunosuppression and recipients of hematopoietic stem cell transplantation. Pharmacotherapy. 2013;33:1035–43.
222. Cugno C, Deola S, Filippini P, Stroncek DF, Rutella S. Granulocyte transfusions in children and adults with hematological malignancies: benefits and controversies. J Transl Med. 2015;13:362.
223. Le J, Schiller DS. Aerosolized delivery of antifungal agents. Curr Fungal Infect Rep. 2010;4:96–102.
224. Hertenstein B, et al. Low incidence of invasive fungal infections after bone marrow transplantation in patients receiving amphotericin B inhalations during neutropenia. Ann Hematol. 1994;68:21–6.
225. Busca A, Pagano L. Antifungal therapy in hematopoietic stem cell transplant recipients. Mediterr J Hematol Infect Dis. 2016;8:e2016039.
226. Machado CM, et al. Use of oseltamivir to control influenza complications after bone marrow transplantation. Bone Marrow Transplant. 2004;34:111–4.
227. Sparrelid E, et al. Ribavirin therapy in bone marrow transplant recipients with viral respiratory tract infections. Bone Marrow Transplant. 1997;19:905–8.
228. Whimbey E, et al. Combination therapy with aerosolized ribavirin and intravenous immunoglobulin for respiratory syncytial virus disease in adult bone marrow transplant recipients. Bone Marrow Transplant. 1995;16:393–9.
229. Shachor-Meyouhas Y, Ben-Barak A, Kassis I. Treatment with oral ribavirin and Ivig of severe human metapneumovirus pneumonia (Hmpv) in immune compromised child. Pediatr Blood Cancer. 2011;57:350–1.
230. Adams RJ, Christenson JC, Petersen FB, Beatty PG. Pre-emptive use of aerosolized ribavirin in the treatment of asymptomatic pediatric marrow transplant patients testing positive for Rsv. Bone Marrow Transplant. 1999;24:661–4.
231. Jacobsen N, Schafer U, Ostendorf P, Kubaneck B, Wolf H. Intravenous Hyperimmune globulin prophylaxis against cytomegalovirus interstitial pneumonitis after allogenic bone marrow transplantation. Tokai J Exp Clin Med. 1985;10:193–5.
232. Alexander BT, et al. Use of cytomegalovirus intravenous immune globulin for the adjunctive treatment of cytomegalovirus in hematopoietic stem cell transplant recipients. Pharmacotherapy. 2010;30:554–61.
233. Kempke AP, Leino AS, Daneshvar F, Lee JA, Mueller BA. Antimicrobial doses in continuous renal replacement therapy: a comparison of dosing strategies. Crit Care Res Prac. 2016;2016:3235765.
234. Clark JG, Hansen JA, Hertz MI, et al. Idiopathic pneumonia syndrome after bone marrow transplantation. Am Rev Respir Dis. 1993;147(6 Pt I):1601–6.
235. Cooke KR, et al. Hyporesponsiveness of donor cells to lipopolysaccharide stimulation reduces the severity of experimental idiopathic pneumonia syndrome: potential role for a gut-lung axis of inflammation. J Immunol. 2000;165:6612–9.

236. Williams KM, et al. Fluticasone, azithromycin, and montelukast treatment for new-onset bronchiolitis obliterans syndrome after hematopoietic cell transplantation. Biol Blood Marrow Transplant. 2016;22:710–6.
237. Yanik GA, et al. Tnf-receptor inhibitor therapy for the treatment of children with idiopathic pneumonia syndrome. A joint pediatric blood and marrow transplant consortium and Children's oncology group study (Asct0521). Biol Blood Marrow Transplant. 2015;21:67–73.
238. Yanik GA, et al. Etanercept for sub-acute lung injury following allogeneic stein cell transplantation. Blood. 2003;102:471a–471a.
239. Williams KM. How I treat bronchiolitis obliterans syndrome after hematopoietic stem cell transplantation. Blood. 2017;129:448–55.
240. Zeiser R, Blazar BR. Acute graft-versus-host disease – biologic process, prevention, and therapy. N Engl J Med. 2017;377:2167–79.
241. Petryk A, Polgreen LE, Chahla S, Miller W, Orchard PJ. No evidence for the reversal of adrenal failure after hematopoietic cell transplantation in X-linked adrenoleukodystrophy. Bone Marrow Transplant. 2012;47:1377–8.
242. Mitchell R, et al. Outcomes of Haematopoietic stem cell transplantation for inherited metabolic disorders: a report from the Australian and New Zealand Children's Haematology oncology group and the Australasian bone marrow transplant recipient registry. Pediatr Transplant. 2013;17:582–8.
243. Bornstein SR, et al. Diagnosis and treatment of primary adrenal insufficiency: an endocrine society clinical practice guideline. J Clin Endocrinol Metab. 2016;101:364–89.
244. Ho J, Lewis V, Guilcher GMT, Stephure DK, Pacaud D. Endocrine complications following pediatric bone marrow transplantation. J Pediatr Endocrinol Metab. 2011;24:327–32.
245. Sag E, et al. Hyperthyroidism after allogeneic hematopoietic stem cell transplantation: a report of four cases. J Clin Res Pediatr Endocrinol. 2015;7:349–54.
246. Savani BN, et al. Prolonged chronic graft-versus-host disease is a risk factor for thyroid failure in long-term survivors after matched sibling donor stem cell transplantation for hematologic malignancies. Biol Blood Marrow Transplant. 2009;15:377–81.
247. Minoia F, et al. Development and initial validation of the macrophage activation syndrome/primary hemophagocytic lymphohistiocytosis score, a diagnostic tool that differentiates primary hemophagocytic lymphohistiocytosis from macrophage activation syndrome. J Pediatr. 2017;189:72–8 e73.
248. Lee DW, et al. Current concepts in the diagnosis and management of cytokine release syndrome. Blood. 2014;124:188–95.
249. Maude SL, Barrett D, Teachey DT, Grupp SA. Managing cytokine release syndrome associated with novel T cell-engaging therapies. Cancer J. 2014;20:119–22.
250. Klinger M, et al. Immunopharmacologic response of patients with B-lineage acute lymphoblastic leukemia to continuous infusion of T cell-engaging Cd19/Cd3-Bispecific bite antibody blinatumomab. Blood. 2012;119:6226–33.
251. Mahadeo KM, Khazal SJ, Abdel-Azim H, Fitzgerald JC, Taraseviciute A, Bollard CM, Tewari P, Duncan C, Traube C, McCall D, Steiner ME, Cheifetz IM, Lehmann LE, Mejia R, Slopis JM, Bajwa R, Kebriaei P, Martin PL, Moffet J, McArthur J, Petropoulos D, O'Hanlon Curry J, Featherston S, Foglesong J, Shoberu B, Gulbis A, Mireles ME, Hafemeister L, Nguyen C, Kapoor N, Rezvani K, Neelapu SS, Shpall EJ. Pediatric Acute Lung Injury and Sepsis Investigators (PALISI) network. Management guidelines for paediatric patients receiving chimeric antigen receptor T cell therapy. Nat Rev Clin Oncol. 2018. https://doi.org/10.1038/s41571-018-0075-2. [Epub ahead of print] Review. PMID: 30082906.
252. Chong SL, et al. A retrospective review of vital signs and clinical outcomes of febrile infants younger than 3 months old presenting to the emergency department. PLoS One. 2018;13:e0190649.
253. Pediatric Acute Lung Injury Consensus Conference, G. Pediatric acute respiratory distress syndrome: consensus recommendations from the pediatric acute lung injury consensus conference. Pediatr Crit Care Med. 2015;16:428–39.

254. Akcan-Arikan A, et al. Modified rifle criteria in critically ill children with acute kidney injury. Kidney Int. 2007;71:1028–35.
255. Kidney Disease: Improving Global Outcomes (KDIGO) Acute Kidney Injury Work Group. KDIGO Clinical Practice Guideline for Acute Kidney Injury. Kidney Int. 2012;2:124–38.
256. Traube C, et al. Cornell assessment of pediatric delirium: a valid, rapid, observational tool for screening delirium in the Picu. Crit Care Med. 2014;42:656–63.
257. Chen F, et al. Measuring Il-6 and Sil-6r in serum from patients treated with tocilizumab and/ or siltuximab following Car T cell therapy. J Immunol Methods. 2016;434:1–8.
258. FDA. Actemra® (Tocilizumab) injection, for intravenous or subcutaneous use: highlights of prescribing information. 2010. https://www.accessdata.fda.gov/drugsatfda_docs/label/2017/125276s114lbl.pdf, FDA.
259. Gardner, R.S.C.s.H. A pediatric and young adult trial of genetically modified T cells directed against Cd19 for relapsed/refractory Cd19+ Leukemia. 2018, April 10. Available from: https://clinicaltrials.gov/ct2/show/NCT02028455.
260. Liu E, et al. Cord blood Nk cells engineered to express Il-15 and a Cd19-targeted Car show long-term persistence and potent antitumor activity. Leukemia. 2018;32:520–31.
261. Philip B, Kokalaki E, Mekkaoui L, Thomas S, Straathof K, Flutter B, Marin V, Marafioti T, Chakraverty R, Linch D, Quezada SA, Peggs KS, Pule M. A highly compact epitope-based marker/suicide gene for easier and safer T-cell therapy. Blood. 2014;124(8):1277–87. https://doi.org/10.1182/blood-2014-01-545020. Epub 2014 Jun 26.
262. Trials C. A pediatric and young adult trial of genetically modified T cells directed against Cd19 for relapsed/refractory Cd19+ leukemia. ClinicalTrials.gov. Study Record Detail 2014 [cited]. Available from: https://clinicaltrials.gov/ct2/show/NCT02028455.

Chapter 9
Diagnosis, Treatment, and Management of Hemophagocytic Lymphohistiocytosis in the Critical Care Unit

Melissa Hines, Neel Bhatt, and Julie-An M. Talano

Introduction

Definitions, HLH Nomenclature, and Clinical Presentation

Hemophagocytic lymphohistiocytosis (HLH) is a hyperinflammatory syndrome characterized by significant CD8 T-cell and macrophage activation and severe hypercytokinemia. This hypercytokinemia can lead to severe multi-organ dysfunction which often requires aggressive supportive care within the intensive care unit. Given the syndromic nature of the disease, HLH is defined by the constellation of certain physical exam findings and laboratory criteria that were initially defined by the Histiocyte Society in the HLH-94 protocol [1, 2] and then updated in the HLH-2004 protocol [3]. While these diagnostic criteria were initially intended as inclusion criteria for these protocols, they remain the most widespread and accepted clinical diagnostic criteria. In the initial HLH-94 definition, patients had to meet five of five diagnostic criteria to be included within the study, including fever, splenomegaly, hemophagocytosis, hypertriglyceridemia and/or hypofibrinogenemia, and cytopenias [1, 2]. With the HLH-2004 protocol, the diagnostic criteria were updated to include elevated soluble IL-2 receptor, reduced or absent NK-cell cytotoxic function, and hyperferritinemia [3]. Patients were required to meet at least 5 of 8 criteria or harbor genetic defects known to cause HLH for inclusion in the study protocol (Table 9.1) [3].

M. Hines (✉)
Department of Pediatric Medicine, Division of Critical Care, St. Jude Children's Research Hospital, Memphis, TN, USA
e-mail: Melissa.Hines@STJUDE.ORG

N. Bhatt · J.-A. M. Talano
Department of Pediatrics, Division of Pediatric Hematology/Oncology, Medical College of Wisconsin, Children's Hospital of Wisconsin, Milwaukee, WI, USA

C. N. Duncan et al. (eds.), *Critical Care of the Pediatric Immunocompromised Hematology/Oncology Patient*, https://doi.org/10.1007/978-3-030-01322-6_9

Table 9.1 HLH diagnostic criteria from HLH-2004 protocol

Five of criteria below
Fever
Splenomegaly
Cytopenias (affecting ≥2 of 3 lineages in the peripheral blood)
Hemoglobin < 9 g/dl (10 g/dl in infants less than 4 weeks)
Platelets < 100 × 10^9/L
Neutrophils < 1 × 10^9/L
Hypertriglyceridemia and/or hypofibrinogenemia
Fasting triglycerides ≥265 mg/dl
Fibrinogen ≤150 g/dl
Presence of hemophagocytosis in bone marrow or other tissue
Low or absent NK-cell activity
Ferritin ≥500 microgram/L
Soluble IL-2 receptor (CD25) ≥2400 U/ml

HLH is often differentiated into primary or familial HLH (fHLH) or secondary HLH (sHLH) based on whether a genetic defect associated with HLH can be identified. Those with a genetic defect are classified as having fHLH, whereas those with secondary HLH are thought to have overwhelming immune system activation due to infection, malignancy, or another cause rather than disease caused by an underlying genetic defect. The pathophysiology and the current understanding about the differentiation of fHLH and sHLH is evolving as many secondary HLH patients are found to have other genetic changes that can predispose them to the development of HLH. This will be discussed in more detail in the HLH pathophysiology section. Regardless, experts typically use the HLH-2004 diagnostic criteria as a guide for diagnosis of both fHLH and sHLH. Macrophage activation syndrome (MAS) refers to the cytokine storm and inflammation that can be associated with rheumatologic disease. While MAS is often categorized as a form of secondary HLH, new diagnostic criteria have been formed in recent years to specifically define MAS associated with systemic juvenile idiopathic arthritis (sJIA; Table 9.2), but there are no currently diagnostic criteria for MAS associated with other rheumatologic diseases.

Fever (91%) and splenomegaly (84%) are two of the most common clinical features described in HLH [4]. Fever in HLH patients is particularly notable as it tends to be high and persistent despite antimicrobial therapy [5]. Primary HLH patients in particular have very prominent organomegaly (hepatomegaly and splenomegaly) that often progresses with time [5]. Cytopenias, especially thrombocytopenia (97%) and anemia (88%), are common laboratory findings [2]. Neutropenia is less common (69%) at the time of diagnosis [2]. These patients can also have DIC with significant hypofibrinogenemia, but this finding is more variable (primary HLH 60–65%; secondary HLH 40%) [6]. When hypofibrinogenemia is present, it is highly suggestive of HLH and can be helpful in differentiating patients with HLH from patients with sepsis who tend to have DIC with hyperfibrinogenemia [5]. Elevated ferritin is a marker of inflammatory response and macrophage activation

Table 9.2 Diagnostic criteria for macrophage activation syndrome in sJIA

Suspected or confirmed diagnosis of sJIA
Fever
Ferritin >684 ng/ml
AND any two of the following:
Platelet count $\leq$*181* $\times$ *10*^{9}*/L*
Aspartate aminotransferase >48 u/L
Triglycerides >156 mg/dl
Fibrinogen $\leq$*360 mg/dl*

and is seen in up to 93% of HLH cases. Hyperferritinemia, particularly >10,000 μg/L, is a highly sensitive (90%) and specific (96%) test for HLH and can differentiate hyperferritinemia seen in other conditions such as liver disease, chronic transfusions, and infections [7]. Hypertriglyceridemia is common (80%), but is not specific for HLH and thought to be secondary to elevated TNF-alpha levels [5, 8]. In addition to ferritin, elevated serum-soluble IL-2 receptor (α chain; sCD25), a marker of T-cell activation, is helpful for diagnosis and disease monitoring [9]. Other HLH testing included in the HLH-2004 diagnostic criteria includes tissue or bone marrow biopsy with the presence of hemophagocytosis and NK-cell function. Decreased or absent NK-cell function is suggestive of HLH but can be normal in both primary and secondary HLH [10]. Similarly, the presence of hemophagocytosis can be suggestive of HLH if other clinical and laboratory criteria are met, but is not specific or necessary for the diagnosis of HLH [11].

There are several other important clinical and laboratory findings that are not part of the HLH-2004 diagnostic criteria which are often found in HLH patients. For example, liver dysfunction evident by elevated transaminases and bilirubin (typically direct hyperbilirubinemia) is a common associated finding [2, 5, 9]. Cases of fulminant liver failure and hydrops fetalis have been reported in patients who have ultimately been diagnosed with HLH [12]. Elevated AST, ALT, and bilirubin have been reported in 76%, 76%, and 51% of the patients, respectively. Other common abnormal laboratory findings include elevated LDH, hyponatremia, and hypoalbuminemia [1–3, 8]. More variable clinical findings include edema, ascites, respiratory failure, lymphadenopathy, rash (30–65%), and CNS involvement [2, 5, 13]. Symptoms concerning for CNS involvement include seizures, mental status changes, or focal neurologic findings and can be seen in up to 75% of the pediatric HLH cases [2, 4, 13, 14]. In the HLH-94 study, patients with CNS HLH (n = 122) presented with either abnormal CSF studies (CSF pleocytosis, elevated protein; 41%) or neurological symptoms (17%) or both (42%) [14]. MRI findings are just as broad as the neurologic symptoms in HLH and include leptomeningeal enhancement, hemorrhage, and T2 and FLAIR hyperattenuation [15, 16]. Both MRI changes and CSF findings can be seen in patients that have no CNS symptomatology. Rare cases of isolated CNS HLH (i.e., no or few systemic HLH manifestations) have also been reported in the literature which makes the diagnosis challenging [17–19]. Skin manifestations such as rashes are present in up to 65% of the cases [9]. Types of rashes range from generalized maculopapular to petechiae and purpura [20]. These signs and symptoms can be seen in patients with or without an identifiable trigger, such as infection. In short, while the presentation of HLH is extremely variable, patients that raise suspicion for HLH include those who are persistently febrile with cytopenia and hepatosplenomegaly and are often critically ill with some evidence of liver dysfunction and/or DIC with hypofibrinogenemia.

Incidence and Mortality

The incidence of familial HLH has been estimated to be 1 in 50,000 live births with average survival of 2 months and a mortality of greater than 90% without therapy [4, 21]. The estimated incidence of both primary and secondary HLH is not known but has been reported to be 1 in 3000 inpatient admissions in a retrospective review at a single center [7]. While mortality has significantly improved over the last 20 years, it remains high for both adult and pediatric HLH patients. Mortality in the adult population has been reported to be 22–59% [22–24]. With the introduction of etoposide-based immunochemotherapy, pediatric HLH survival has improved from less than 10% to a 5-year survival of 55% to 61% [1, 2, 25]. Familial HLH patients that receive a bone marrow transplant have a reported survival of 64% at 3 years and 58–66% at 5 years [1, 2, 25, 26].

HLH Pathophysiology

Primary HLH

The understanding of the pathophysiology of HLH has grown dramatically over the last 15 years with the discovery of loss-of-function germline mutations in the *PRF1* gene, which encodes the protein perforin, in familial HLH patients [27–29]. Prior to this discovery, it was recognized that HLH patients often exhibited NK cytotoxic dysfunction, but the cause of the dysfunction was unknown [30, 31]. Since this initial discovery, several other genes have been identified to cause the HLH phenotype, many of these involving the sorting, trafficking, docking, and fusion of cytotoxic granules containing granzymes A and B and perforin to the cell membrane (including the proteins LYST, AP-3 complex, Rab27a, Munc 13–4, Munc 18–2, Syntaxin 11) [9, 32, 33]. In these cases, the cytotoxic granules do not contain perforin, or they are unable to stably dock and/or fuse with the cell membrane, preventing optimal perforin pore formation and granzymes A and B delivery to the target cell (Fig. 9.1). Typically, once the cytotoxic granule saddles up to the cell membrane and fuses, perforin proteins come together to form a pore-like structure allowing the release of granzymes A and B from the granule of the NK or cytotoxic T cell into the target cell. Once in the target cell, granzymes A and B stimulate the apoptosis cascade

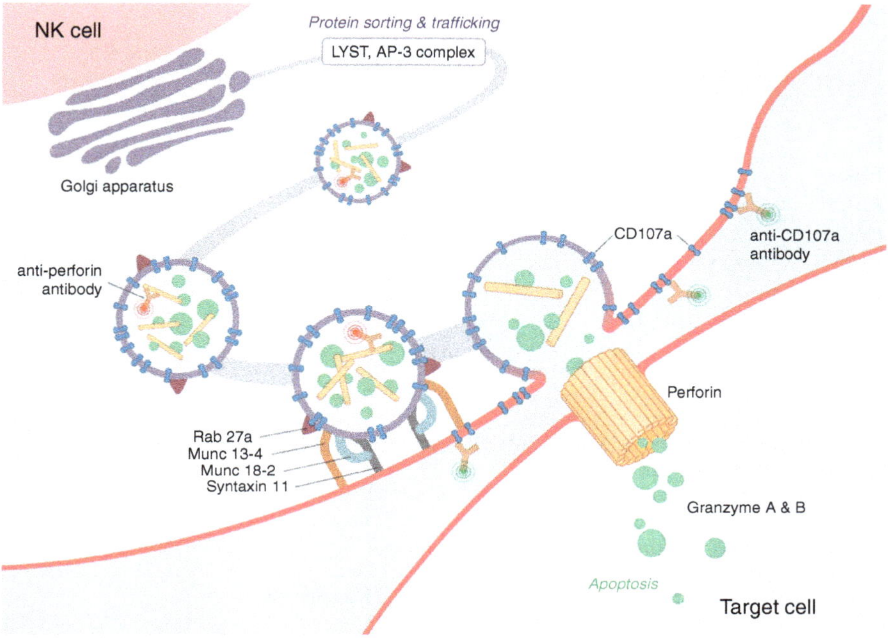

Fig. 9.1 *Function of HLH-related proteins and cytotoxic cell function and the use of CD107a and perforin expression assays for diagnosis.* LYST (function not fully understood) and AP-3 function in protein trafficking and sorting from the Golgi apparatus to the formation of the cytotoxic granules. As seen in the figure, granzymes A and B, as well as perforin, are packaged in the cytotoxic granules. Rab27a function is in cytotoxic vesicle trafficking and cytotoxic vesicle membrane fusion to the effector cell membrane. Munc 13–4, Munc 14–2, and Syntaxin 11 assist in the docking, priming, and fusion of the cytotoxic granule to the effector cell membrane for degranulation. Once the cytotoxic vesicle fuses with the effector cell membrane, individual perforin proteins come together to form a pore-like structure that allows granzymes packaged in the cytotoxic granules to pass from the effector cell to the target cell causing target cell death. CD107a is found within the membrane of the cytotoxic granule and is expressed in the cell membrane once the cytotoxic membrane fuses with the cell membrane during cytotoxic granule degranulation. Perforin and CD107a expression testing uses fluorescently conjugated anti-perforin and anti-CD107a antibodies and detects and quantifies the amount of florescence by flow cytometry. Perforin expression assay determines the amount of perforin within the cytotoxic vesicles within the cell. In CD107a expression testing, NK and cytotoxic T cells are stimulated to degranulate. After degranulation, anit-CD107a antibodies attach to CD107a expressed on the cell membrane (This figure was originally published in *Blood*. Hines and Nichols [34])

leading to cell death [35]. In the case of *PFR1* mutations (codes the perforin protein), the cytotoxic granule is appropriately trafficked and can fuse with the cell membrane, but there is a decreased or an absent perforin. Therefore, no perforin pore is made, and granzyme A or granzyme B is not delivered to the target cell to induce apoptosis [32, 33, 36]. These known gene mutations account for FHL 2–5 (*PFR1*, *UNC13D*, *STX11*, *STXBP2*) and three other immunodeficiency disorders, Griscelli syndrome type 2, Chediak-Higashi syndrome, and Hermansky-Pudlak

Table 9.3 Genetic causes of HLH and associated tests

Disease	Gene name	Encoded protein	Perforin expression	CD107a upregulation	NK cell cytotoxicity
FHL2	*PRF1*	Perforin	↓↓	Normal	↓ or 0
FHL3	*UNC13D*	Munc13–4	Normal	↓↓	↓ or 0
FHL4	*STX11*	Syntaxin 11	Normal	↓↓	↓ or 0
FHL5	*STXBP2*	Munc18–2	Normal	↓↓	↓ or 0
Griscelli	*RAB27A*	Rab27a	Normal	↓↓	↓ or 0
Chediak-Higashi	*LYST*	LYST	Normal	↓↓	↓ or 0
XLP1[a]	*SH2D1A*	SAP[b]	Normal[d]	Normal[d]	↓ or normal
XLP2	*BIRC4*	XIAP[c]	Normal[e]	Normal[e]	↓ or normal
HPS2[f]	*AP3B1*	AP3[g]	Normal	↓↓	↓

[a]X-linked lymphoproliferative syndrome
[b]signaling lymphocytic activation molecule (SLAM)-associated protein
[c]X-linked inhibitor of apoptosis
[d]SAP expression decreased
[e]XIAP expression decreased
[f]Hermansky-Pudlak syndrome type 2
[g]adaptor protein 3 complex
This figure was originally published in *Blood*. Hines and Nichols [34]

syndrome type 2 (*RAB27A*, *LYST*, *AP3B1*; Table 9.3), which are all inherited in an autosomal recessive fashion [9, 32]. In addition to these disorders, there are two X-linked disorders that can lead to an HLH phenotype [3, 9, 32]. X-linked lymphoproliferative disease types 1 and 2 are caused by a defect in the genes *SH2D1A* and *BIRC4*, which code for the SAP and XIAP proteins, respectively. SAP protein is thought to play a role in effector function of multiple immune cells including NK, NKT, and T cells by relaying proper signaling for the polarization of granules [32]. Due to the defect in effector function, there can be impaired NK and CD8 T-cell cytotoxic dysfunction that is thought to lead to the HLH phenotype, particularly after EBV infection [32, 37, 38]. XIAP is an anti-apoptotic protein that inhibits caspase activity, but how a defect in this protein leads to HLH pathophysiology is not as well understood [32].

How do these defects in cytotoxic function lead to a cytokine storm? Familial or primary HLH is an immunodeficiency as well as a hyperinflammatory syndrome. The effector function of NK and CD8 T cells kills cells with intracellular infection as well as cells that are dysfunctional, such as cancer cells. In addition to the surveillance function that these cells serve, they also play a crucial role in controlling the immune response by eliminating immune cells that are no longer needed, including antigen-presenting cells. Based on what we know from murine models, both CD8 T cells and interferon-gamma are imperative to the formation of the cytokine storm and clinical findings of primary HLH [39]. In an HLH flare, the initial immune response including immune activation is appropriate but is later complicated by persistent antigenemia, persistent antigen presentation, uncontrolled monoclonal expansion of CD8 T cells, and hypercytokinemia (predominately INF-gamma) [33, 39–41]. Once there is a triggering event, such as a viral infection, CD8 T cells are activated by antigen-presenting cells (APCs) and monoclonally expand both in the blood and in the tissue and secrete interferon-gamma. Interferon-gamma activates and then recruits macrophages to the area [32, 33]. Macrophages in turn secrete multiple cytokines, including IL-18, IL-10, IL-6, IL-1beta, and TNF-alpha, which provide a feedback loop for further CD8 T-cell activation and proliferation [32, 39, 42]. This process of CD8 T-cell activation continues, since virally infected cells cannot be eliminated due to defective degranulation of CD8 T cells and NK cells, leading to persistent antigenemia and cytokine production [33, 40, 43]. APCs are typically removed by NK and CD8 T cells but remain in this case due to the ineffective cytotoxic function of these cells [33, 40, 41]. Continued activation and expansion of the CD8 T cells lead to massive amounts of interferon-gamma [39]. NK and CD8 T cells with degranulation defects have prolonged contact with the target cells, which can cause a fivefold increased release of interferon-gamma and promote hypercytokinemia [44]. All aspects of this immune dysfunction lead to signs and symptoms of HLH, including hyperferritinemia, increased soluble IL-2 receptor (sIL2R), cytopenias, splenomegaly, hemophagocytosis, hypertriglyceridemia, fever, and hypofibrinogenemia [5].

Secondary HLH

sHLH patients have the same HLH phenotype as those with fHLH, but they lack the known HLH-associated genetic mutations. Secondary HLH can be induced by infection, rheumatologic disease, or malignancy. Infection-associated HLH can be due to viral, bacterial, fungal, or parasitic infection [45]. The most common viral culprits are the DNA viruses, including EBV, HHV6, parvovirus, HSV, CMV, and adenovirus [45]. HLH secondary to influenza and HIV (typically with superinfection) has also been described. Bacterial-associated HLH has been described particularly with *Mycobacterium*, as well as *Staphylococcus aureus*, *Ehrlichia*, *Rickettsia*, and *Mycoplasma* [45]. Parasitic infections are a common cause of HLH in countries outside of the United States, and causative agents include *Leishmania* (particularly visceral leishmaniasis), *Plasmodium*, and *Toxoplasma*. *Histoplasmosis* (particularly disseminated), *Candida*, and *Cryptococcus* are fungal agents that have been associated with HLH in the literature [33, 45].

HLH-like presentation associated with rheumatologic disease is typically referred to as MAS or MAS-HLH. The rheumatologic disease most commonly associated with MAS is sJIA [46]. Up to 10% of sJIA patients develop overt MAS, but there is evidence that up to 30% of patients may have subclinical MAS [47]. In addition, MAS has been described in SLE, adult-onset Still's disease, dermatomyositis, Kawasaki's disease, rheumatoid arthritis, and inflammatory bowel disease [46]. Malignancy-associated HLH is more commonly seen in adult patients but can also be seen in pediatric patients. It is most often associated with lymphomas, particularly T cell or NK cell, or leukemias [48]. It is thought that HLH may manifest due to immune dysregulation from dysfunctional leukemic or lymphoma cells with ensuing hypercytokinemia. Often there is a concomitant viral infection, particularly EBV [33, 48]. In addition to HLH resulting directly from the malignancy, there are reports of HLH resulting after bone marrow transplant [49, 50], as well as malignancy-related therapies including chemotherapy and immunomodulation [33, 48]. The majority (88%) of patients that develop HLH related to cancer-directed therapy often have a concomitant infection, so infectious disease work-up is important in these patients [48].

The pathophysiology for secondary HLH is not as well understood as fHLH. Unlike the pathophysiology of primary HLH, secondary HLH pathophysiology cannot be completely explained by a defect in cytotoxic function, as many secondary HLH patients have normal NK-cell cytotoxic function when tested [10, 51]. Cytotoxic dysfunction and the sizable innate immune activation appear to work in concert leading to the subsequent cytokine storm and phenotype of HLH. It also appears that depending on the etiology of the secondary HLH, the predominance of innate immune system activation versus cytotoxic cell dysfunction may vary. The cytotoxic dysfunction that may occur in secondary HLH can be due to a direct, but reversible, defect in cytotoxic function or a relative cytotoxic dysfunction due to decreased numbers of NK or CD8 T cells [33, 52]. The acquired cytotoxic dysfunction is particularly important in certain viral infections, such as EBV, influenza, and HSV, where the cytotoxic dysfunction is virally induced [44, 53, 54]. Prolonged increased IL-6, which can be seen in infection but is particularly common in rheumatologic disorders, can also play a role in acquired cytotoxic dysfunction by decreasing perforin and granzyme B expression [55]. In addition to acquired defects in cytotoxicity, overactivation of the innate immune system also plays an important role in the development of HLH, particularly MAS and sepsis or bacterial-induced HLH. Both sepsis and MAS are characterized largely by innate immune system activation by Toll-like receptors (TLRs) as well as high levels of IL-6, which have been shown to amplify TLR signaling [56]. In a recent murine model, it was demonstrated that blatant HLH phenotype with hypercytokinemia could be produced by repeated stimulation of TLR9 [57]. Contrary to primary HLH murine models, this process does not appear to be dependent on CD8 T-cell activation or interferon-gamma secretion [57, 58]. Based on multiple murine cytokine neutralization studies, there is no single cytokine that is responsible for driving HLH/MAS pathophysiology [33, 43]. IL-1 family, IL-6, IL-10, IL-18, and INF-gamma all appear to play a role in the pathophysiology and the MAS/HLH phenotype [33, 43, 57, 58]. While the differences between primary and secondary HLH or MAS may seem esoteric, the differences in pathophysiology will be crucial in predicting the best novel therapies, such as cytokine neutralization, that will be the most effective.

Evolving Understanding of Secondary HLH

Traditionally, secondary HLH has referred to patients that have the phenotype of HLH, but do not have bi-allelic mutations in HLH-associated genes. The distinction between primary and secondary HLH has become more complex as we have learned that some secondary HLH patients also carry polymorphisms (of unknown significance) or mono-allelic mutations in HLH-associated genes, although it is controversial if the reported polymorphism cause disease [36, 59–63]. In addition to mutations or polymorphisms in HLH-associated genes, there have been mutations and other variants found in secondary HLH patients with whole-genome sequencing, including mutations in genes involved with microtubule organization, vesicle transport, NK-cell receptors, cytokine production and signaling, inflammasome activation, and TLR signaling [33, 64]. This is an interesting concept as it suggests that these variants or mono-allelic mutations could lead to a small decrease in cytotoxic function or other immunopathology that may predispose an individual to develop HLH with an infectious or rheumatologic trigger. This may be an explanation why some individuals are predisposed to the development of HLH with infection while others may not.

HLH Versus Sepsis Pathophysiology

Are sepsis and HLH really that different? There are many similarities, but there are some very important differences between the immune response in HLH compared to sepsis. The best understanding that we have about immune function during the initial phases of sepsis and an HLH flare is from genomic expression profiling within the pediatric population and serum cytokines from both adult and pediatric studies. According to genomic expression profiling in sepsis, there is initially a large activation of the innate immune system, likely due to DAMPs (damage-associated molecular patterns) and/or PAMPs (pathogen-associated molecular patterns), and then the cytokine storm [65]. In sepsis, there is an immediate downregulation of adaptive immunity, increased apoptosis particularly of T cells, as well as decreased antigen presentation over the ensuing days (due to IL-4 and IL-10) [65]. However, in a primary HLH flare, there is a similar downregulation in genes related to adaptive immunity but also a downregulation in innate immunity and proteins related to promoting apoptosis [66]. Contrary to serum cytokine profiles, in genomic expression profiling, both HLH and sepsis patients demonstrated upregulation of genes related to the same cytokines, including IL-6, IL-10, and IL-1 family [65, 66]. Serum cytokine levels in HLH patients usually show an overwhelming predominance of INF-gamma (consistent with overwhelming CD8 T-cell activation) and IL-10 (released in an attempt to control the immune response) [42, 67–69]. TNF-alpha and IL-6 are elevated within the HLH group, but not predominant [36, 42, 67–69]. In sepsis, IL-6 and IL-10 levels tend to predominate with some elevation of TNF-alpha [36, 68, 70, 71]. Interestingly in sepsis, a low INF-gamma is associated with a poorer prognosis [72], most likely a herald for overwhelming immune suppression and lack of T cells. In summary, both syndromes have a similar initial release of cytokines with subsequent cytokine storm with a paradoxical but needed early attempt to control the immune response with the downregulation of multiple genes related to adaptive immunity.

In primary HLH, this attempted downregulation of the immune system is ineffective due to the lack of cytotoxic function of NK and CD8 T cells to appropriately dampen activated immune cells resulting in continued, unrestricted immune system activation and cytokine release. In sepsis, the term for this reactive downregulation of the immune system has been coined compensatory downregulation syndrome (CDS) [73, 74]. In sepsis, downregulation of the immune system can be adequate, over-exaggerated, or inadequate. If the CDS is adequate, then the infection is cleared and the immune system returns to homeostasis and the patient will slowly improve. If CDS is overexaggerated, then immunoparalysis (defined as TNF-alpha release <200 pg/ml with ex vivo lipopolysaccharide stimulation or monocyte HLA-DR) can occur with inadequate clearance of initial infectious agent or new nosocomial infection with multi-organ dysfunction syndrome (MODS) and increased risk of mortality [74, 75]. Interestingly, there is another newly described phenotype of MODS/sepsis in the literature, MAS-like MODS or macrophage activation-like syndrome [76–81]. This entity is thought to be caused by inadequate downregulation of the immune system with continued inflammation. Unfortunately, there is no consistent definition of these patients. Some fulfill five of eight HLH diagnostic criteria or the H-score [80, 82], while other studies describe sepsis characterized by hyperferritinemia, hepatobiliary dysfunction, and DIC with or without cytopenias [36, 76, 78, 81, 83]. The leading hypothesis for the pathophysiology for this subgroup of sepsis is thought to be partly due to CDS. Due to sepsis-related CDS, there is thought to be a decreased overall number of NK cells and/or function leading to impaired pruning of activated immune cells, including antigen-presenting cells and macrophages, as well as overactivation of the innate immune system via TLRs. While the literature is still young, those with hyperferritinemic (>1980 ng/ml or >4420 ng/ml) sepsis represent an at-risk group with high mortality (44–46%) [78, 81]. These MAS-like MODS/sepsis patients may not fit all HLH criteria, but they may represent patients in the HLH spectrum of inflammation that may benefit from some amount of immunosuppression [78, 80, 82, 83]. Despite this growing evidence for MAS-like MODS/sepsis, much work still needs to be done including more clearly defining this phenotype of sepsis within the literature and determining best therapy.

In conclusion based on emerging data, there are many potential reasons why sepsis and HLH appear phenotypically the same, particularly at initial presentation. There is a growing body of evidence to suggest that the amount of inflammation seen in sepsis, HLH, and MAS is not dissimilar, but rather each entity is represented on a spectrum of inflammation.

HLH Evaluation and Testing

There are several tests (Table 9.4) that can be sent immediately with a quick turnaround that can assist in the diagnosis of HLH. This includes complete blood cell count, coagulation studies with fibrinogen, ferritin level, lactate dehydrogenase

Table 9.4 Initial testing for diagnosis and suggested testing are listed in the table. Those indicated with an astericks (*) represent tests that often require specialized testing at a send-out lab with varying expected return times. NK cell function, CD25 level, CD107a mobilization, perforin expression, XIAP, and SAP expression usual takes 2 to 5 days for results to return. Time for HLH genetic testing often requires 4 to 6 weeks

Recommended laboratory and diagnostic studies for HLH	
Initial testing	
Complete blood count	
Basic metabolic panel	
LDH	
Coagulation studies including fibrinogen	
Albumin	
Liver function panel	
Ferritin	
Soluble IL-2 receptor or CD25 level*	
NK-cell function*	
Bone marrow biopsy	
Hemophagocytosis	
Optional:	
Abdominal ultrasound to determine hepatosplenomegaly if not palpable	
Tests to consider in primary HLH	
Lumbar puncture	
CSF cell count	
CSF protein level	
MRI head with and without contrast	
CD107a mobilization*	
Perforin/granzyme B expression*	
HLH genetic panel*	
In males:	
XIAP and SAP expression*	
Tests for HLH monitoring	
Ferritin	Once to twice weekly
Soluble IL-2 receptor or CD25 level	Once weekly

(LDH), albumin, bilirubin (total and direct), and liver function studies. Other tests that are helpful for HLH diagnosis include soluble IL-2 receptor level (also known as CD25) and NK-cell function; however, in most institutions these are send-out labs and do not have a quick turnaround time. Soluble IL-2 receptor level acts as a barometer for the amount of T-cell activation and can be helpful in the diagnosis of HLH and following disease activity. The use of NK-cell function for HLH diagnosis is more nuanced as many secondary HLH patients will have normal NK-cell function [10, 51]. In addition steroids can cause NK-cell dysfunction making the study invalid once patients have received steroids. NK-cell function can also be normal in primary HLH patients, so a normal NK-cell function result does not rule out primary HLH [10]. Soluble CD163 is a marker of scavenger macrophage activation and may aid in making the diagnosis along with other tests. Patients with sepsis or infectious mononucleosis could also show elevated sCD163 levels; however there is minimal overlap compared to the levels seen in patients with HLH [84]. Bone marrow biopsy for the evaluation of hemophagocytosis can be helpful for the diagnosis of HLH, particularly in patients where the cause of persistent cytopenias is unclear, specifically in the context of a possible HLH at malignancy diagnosis, chemotherapy-related HLH, or HLH in the setting of bone marrow transplant. The result of the bone marrow biopsy must be considered in the whole of the clinical picture and alone cannot prove or disprove the diagnosis of HLH. Primary HLH patients can have a normal bone marrow biopsy particularly early in their illness [5, 11]. In addition, hemophagocytosis can be found in critically ill patients without HLH, and hemophagocytosis is not always seen in HLH patients [36, 85–87]. Because of these reasons, hemophagocytosis is considered neither a sensitive nor a specific finding to diagnose HLH, and HLH diagnosis should not solely depend on the finding of hemophagocytosis but rather the complete clinical picture [86]. DIC or coagulopathy does not necessarily preclude performing bone marrow biopsy as the risk of bleeding is low. In addition, there are two functional flow cytometry tests that determine perforin/granzyme B expression and CD107a mobilization that typically have a turnaround time of 2–5 days (Fig. 9.1) [10, 51]. These tests have been found to be both sensitive and specific for predicting the presence of an HLH-associated gene mutation [10, 51]. There are two other flow cytometry tests, SAP and XIAP expression, which should be sent in male patients for work-up for possible X-linked lymphoproliferative disease. Please see Table 9.3 for expected results for NK-cell function, CD107a mobilization, and perforin expression for different HLH-associated mutations.

While primary or familial HLH is most commonly thought of in neonates or those under 1 year of age, many familial HLH patients may not present until later in life depending on the severity of their mutation (i.e., and thus the degree of cytotoxic dysfunction). Due to this reason, genetic testing should be considered in all pediatric patients to determine if they have germline mutations associated with fHLH, especially in patients less than 1 year of age, or if perforin/granzyme B, SAP, XIAP expression, or CD107a mobilization testing is abnormal. For HLH genetic testing, next-generation sequencing (NGS)-based assays are commercially available to test for the genetic syndromes responsible for abnormal T-cell and NK-cell cytotoxicity leading to HLH development [88]. These tests take several weeks to result and should be sent early in the work-up in cases of high clinical suspicion.

In addition to testing required for HLH diagnosis, there are some additional tests that are helpful in determining additional type of HLH-specific therapy required, as well as response to therapy. Most patients with high suspicion of HLH should have a baseline MRI head and lumbar puncture with CSF studies (CSF cell count and differential and CSF protein level) [2, 15, 16]. These studies should be performed even if patients have no neurologic findings, as CSF pleocytosis and MRI findings can be seen in patients that are asymptomatic [14, 16]. Due to higher mortality and significant morbidity in patients with abnormal CSF at diagnosis, patients with neurologic symptoms, CSF pleocytosis, and/or MRI findings may require additional intrathecal therapy [2, 14, 16, 36]. In addition to CSF studies, all patients need a full infectious work-up including blood cultures, common viral etiologies (EBV, CMV, hepatitis viruses, adenovirus, influenza), and possible fungal etiologies even if there is suspicion of primary HLH. Rheumatology may need to be consulted to assist in further investigation of a possible underlying rheumatologic disorder. Both ferritin and soluble IL-2 receptor can be followed weekly to twice weekly to monitor patients' progress on therapy [2, 30].

Intensive Care Presentation and Management

In addition to the early diagnosis of HLH, most of the ICU (intensive care unit) management for HLH patients hinges on anticipation of HLH-related multi-system organ failure and providing adequate supportive care while getting immunosuppressive therapies initiated in a timely fashion. Another key point of management is the understanding that the severity of disease can change drastically in a matter of hours (sometimes as little as 6–12 h). Given this factor, another important aspect for care of HLH/MAS patients is frequent reevaluation and communication with the oncology, immunology, and/or rheumatology teams, especially if there is worsening in the patient's status, to determine if another agent or additional doses of agents, such as steroids, etoposide, anakinra, alemtuzumab, or a novel therapy, need to be given.

ICU care is centered around the management of quickly evolving multi-system organ failure, including cardiovascular, renal, hepatobiliary, neurological, respiratory, and hematological systems, including cytopenias and coagulopathy [89]. Reported reasons for ICU admission in the limited literature for HLH ICU patients (total of 80 patients described) include respiratory failure or ARDS (30–50%), neurologic decompensation (encephalopathy, seizure; 20–21%), shock or hypotension (18–22%), acute renal failure (16%), fulminant liver failure (7–30%), and bleeding (5%; Table 9.5) [90–92]. HLH patients had failure of two or greater organs at ICU admission [90, 92]. There were 44% of patients that were not diagnosed with HLH prior to ICU admission [90], which highlights the need for intensivists to have a low threshold for ruling out this diagnosis in the ICU particularly in patients with quickly decompensating MODS. These patients typically require multiple forms of interventional support including mechanical ventilation (57–100%), vasopressors (43–80%), and renal replacement therapy (17–75%; Table 9.5) [90–93]. ARDS was described in as many as 90% of the patients in one study [92]. In addition to respiratory failure secondary to parenchymal disease, respiratory failure can occur due to significant organomegaly with decreased thoracic compliance and respiratory impingement. As many as 90% have been reported to have hepatomegaly and 76% with splenomegaly [2, 90–92]. In the pediatric cohort, many patients required aggressive respiratory and cardiac support. The use of the high-frequency oscillatory ventilation and/or inhaled nitric oxide was described in three patients (20%) that required mechanical ventilation, and 22% of the cohort required three or more vasopressors [91]. While up to one third of the ICU patients described required renal replacement therapy, clinical indication for renal replacement therapy (i.e., fluid overload vs. acute renal failure vs. oliguria) was not described; however, these

Table 9.5 This table describes the described causes of ICU admission as well as the extensive supportive measures that are often required

Reasons for ICU admission	
Respiratory failure	30–50%
Encephalopathy or seizure	20–21%
Hypotension/shock	18–22%
Acute renal failure	16%
Fulminant liver failure	7–30%
Bleeding or coagulopathy	5%
ICU supportive care requirements	
Vasopressors	43–88%
Mechanical ventilation	57–100%
iNO and/or oscillator (pediatric)	20%
Renal replacement therapy	17–75%
Frequent blood product transfusions	~8.5 units of product (adult)
Packed red blood cells	1–7 transfusions (average pediatric)
Fresh frozen plasma	0–4.5 transfusions (average pediatric)
Platelets	0–12.5 transfusions (average pediatric)

patients can have extremely low albumin levels (1.6–3.2), capillary leak, and edema secondary to the severity of cytokine storm [2, 92]. Anecdotally, these patients often have severe fluid overload and may benefit from continuous renal replacement therapy. In addition, many critically ill HLH patients require support with multiple transfusions, particularly platelet (mean platelet count 48–61 × 10^9/L) and FFP or cryoprecipitate transfusions (mean INR 1.4, mean PTT 57.3, mean fibrinogen 130–157 mg/dl) [90–92]. Anemia (mean hemoglobin 8.3–10 g/dl) can be present, but is not as severe or as prominent as thrombocytopenia [90–92]. In one study, patients required an average of 8.5 units of product per person [92]. In a pediatric study, non-survivors required more blood products than survivors with a mean of 7 packed red cell transfusions, 4.5 transfusions of FFP, and 12.5 transfusions of platelets [91]. Many of these patients will have some amount of liver dysfunction ranging from transaminitis (41%) and hyperbilirubinemia (mean bilirubin 6.45 mg/dl) to fulminant liver failure (7–30%) [90, 92]. Exploration of possible infectious etiologies needs to be performed and infections aggressively treated. HLH ICU non-survivors had higher organ dysfunction and mortality indexes at ICU admission compared to survivors and more often required supportive therapies including mechanical ventilation, renal replacement therapy, inotropes, and transfusion [90, 91]. Average length of ICU stay is 5.7–8.5 days [90–92]. Despite aggressive supportive therapy, ICU mortality is high in this subset of patients ranging from 35% to 70% [90–92].

If these supportive measures are ineffective, extracorporeal life support (ECLS) can be considered within this patient cohort. Initiation of ECLS may allow time for immunosuppressive therapies to be effective. A recent study evaluating the survival of pediatric HLH patients on ECLS showed a survival rate of only 30% [94]. This is significantly lower than the general pediatric ECLS survival of 59% but is comparable to other immunocompromised pediatric cohort survival (31%) and neonatal cardiac and E-CPR (extracorporeal cardiopulmonary resuscitation) patients (38%) [94]. Indication for ECLS included respiratory failure, cardiac failure, and E-CPR with 63% being placed on venoarterial ECLS [94]. Unfortunately, no clear risk factors could be identified for increased mortality (including age, sex, time of ventilation prior to cannulation, vasopressors, or nitric oxide use), but all of the patients that were placed on ECLS for cardiac failure or E-CPR died [94]. There was also no indication whether these patients were primary or secondary HLH [94]. Care should be taken when managing anticoagulation on the circuit as many of these patients have underlying coagulopathy (DIC; 17%) and the most common complication reported was bleeding with >50% of patients reported to have bleeding at the cannula site and 17% with pulmonary or intracranial hemorrhage [94]. Infection status should also be considered when evaluating for ECLS candidacy, particularly in primary HLH patients since viremia or fungal diseases are more likely to persist due to their underlying cytotoxic defect which can complicate their ECLS course. Other patients with secondary HLH with infection (influenza, tick-borne diseases) have successfully cleared infection on ECLS [95–98].

A unique consideration within this group of patients is the various neurologic symptoms that can manifest including seizure, encephalopathy, focal deficits, ataxia, generalized hypotonia or hypertonia, or meningismus [15, 16]. With new onset symptoms, CT scan can be helpful to rule out intracerebral hemorrhage or significant cerebral edema. An attempt to manage cerebral edema with hypertonic therapy can be considered, but this has not been studied within the HLH population. Neurosurgical consult should be considered with both hemorrhage and cerebral edema for possible surgical intervention since both are potentially reversible phenomena once immunosuppressive therapy is started. Early initiation of HLH therapy is imperative to prevent or decrease the severity of long-term neurological sequelae [15, 16]. MRI and lumbar puncture should be obtained once the patient is stable.

HLH-Directed Therapy

Because of the diagnostic challenges and significant mortality associated with HLH, when there is a high degree of suspicion, treatment often needs to be started before all HLH-specific testing has resulted. Patients often develop disease characteristics over time, and the delay in diagnosis could make it too late to initiate therapy. Organ failure (high sequential organ failure score) has been associated with significantly increased mortality in adult patients admitted to the ICU [99]; therefore an early consultation of an HLH expert is of utmost importance.

In broad terms, the management of familial or primary HLH includes a short-term approach in a critically ill child controlling over-inflammation, targeting activated immune cells, and treating infections and a long-term approach replacing the defective immune system through a hematopoietic cell transplant (HCT) in familial HLH or refractory secondary HLH. Etoposide, an epipodophyllotoxin, was first used in the 1980s for HLH therapy and has become a mainstay in familial HLH therapy [100]. The mechanism for use in HLH is thought to be due to its ability to reverse defective apoptosis and to target activated T cells which are a known important driving force for the development of primary HLH [101, 102]. Similarly, corticosteroids have been the mainstay of HLH therapy and have been successfully used in combination with vinblastine/etoposide/teniposide/antithymocyte globulin [33, 35–37] [21, 103–105]. In 1994, the Histiocyte Society implemented the first international protocol (HLH-94) to treat previously untreated children and adolescents (<16 years of age) with primary and secondary HLH. [1, 106] Patients were treated with an 8-week regimen using the combination of dexamethasone (10 mg/m^2 for the initial 2 weeks followed by a taper over 2 months), and etoposide (150 mg/m^2 twice weekly for 2 weeks, followed by 150 mg/m^2 once a week for 6 weeks), and cyclosporine (CSA) in a continuation phase, starting at week 9 (Fig. 9.2). Patients with CNS HLH received intrathecal methotrexate, and patients with familial HLH were bridged to HCT. A total of 249 patients received the therapy with a 5-year overall survival of 54% (95% CI: 48–60%) [2]. Pre-HCT mortality was 29% [2]. The HLH-2004 protocol aimed to improve the pre-HCT morbidity and mortality seen in HLH-94 trial by using CSA up front [25]. Additionally, prednisolone was given intrathecally to reduce the late neurological sequelae (19%) seen in HLH-94 protocol. Between 2004 and 2011, a total of 369 children were enrolled. Overall survival was 61% (56–67%) in the entire cohort, but the pre-HCT mortality was non-different compared to HLH-94 (27% vs. 19%, p = 0.064) [25]. Therefore, upfront CSA approach was deemed not necessary. It is important to note that both trials used dexamethasone as the corticosteroid of choice due to its higher concentration in CSF compared to prednisolone [107] and the poor prognosis associated with CNS HLH. Children with abnormal CSF studies were at higher risk of mortality and late neurological sequelae in HLH-94 study [14].

When patients are initially treated, they typically will show improvement/stabilization within the first 48 h after they receive their initial dose of dexamethasone and etoposide. However, if no improvement or worsening is noted after the first week on therapy, we would consider them refractory to frontline therapy.

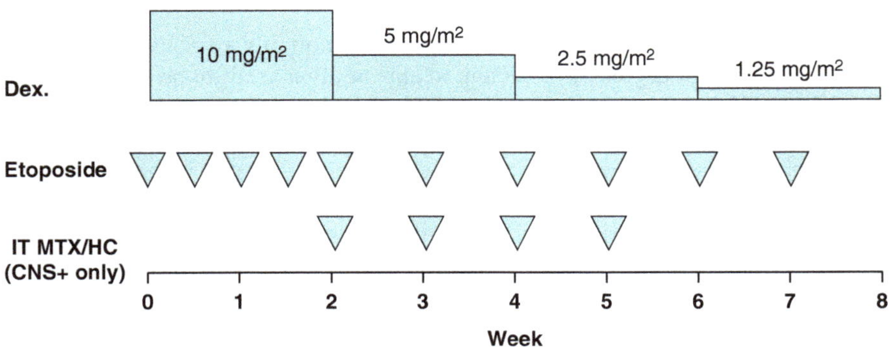

Fig. 9.2 Standard-of-care induction treatment for HLH (*Dex.* dexamethasone, etoposide dosing 150 mg/m^2, IT MTX/HC, intrathecal methotrexate and hydrocortisone for patients with active CNS disease at week 2)

Approximately 25–50% of patients will fail to achieve a complete response to the standard-of-care therapy or relapse and may require additional treatment with the same drugs or alternative "salvage" agents. Alemtuzumab, anakinra, and antithymocyte globulin have been reported in small studies as options for salvage therapy; however this has not been extensively studied [108, 109]. Future clinical trials are desperately needed in this patient population.

Secondary/Acquired HLH

Patients with secondary HLH in the ICU need prompt initiation of HLH-specific therapy regardless of the type of HLH (familial vs. acquired) [9, 110]. Often at diagnosis, it is impossible to distinguish between the primary and secondary HLH unless the patient has a known trigger, such as a malignancy or rheumatologic disorder. Efforts should be made to identify underlying trigger in patients with acquired or secondary HLH, especially infection and malignancy, which could be treated with appropriate antimicrobials or cancer-directed therapy, respectively. Decision for type and length of immunosuppression in this patient population must be made in consideration of patient's trajectory and severity of illness. There is a subset of patients with secondary HLH who will respond to steroids alone or in conjunction with IVIG that will have a good outcome without etoposide-based therapy. Decision to add etoposide is based on the severity of illness and clinical evolution and should be made early in the course, usually with a reassessment within 24–48 h after starting dexamethasone. Any worsening during a patient's clinical course should also trigger a reassessment for the addition of etoposide therapy. Additionally, in patients with EBV-associated HLH, the addition of rituximab (a CD20-specific antibody which targets B cells) to steroid or etoposide should be considered [111]. Those with chemotherapy-related HLH are a specialized group that require much careful consideration as further immunosuppression/myelosuppression in an neutropenic patient with concurrent infection may not be therapeutic. In these patients, it is often prudent to hold chemotherapy and agressively treat the infection. It is often helpful for determining need for immunosup
presion in this group to obtain a bone marrow biopsy to determine if continued cytopenias are related to HLH or continued effect of previous chemotherapy [48].

Treatment of MAS is unique within the secondary HLH group. The mainstay of MAS therapy is high-dose pulse intravenous steroids with or without the addition of CSA or IVIG [112]. New cytokine inhibitors have shown promise in MAS and some secondary HLH patients. Anakinra, an interleukin-1 inhibitor, concurrently with steroids has been found to be helpful in the treatment of both MAS and MAS-like sepsis and is the most common biologic used for sJIA MAS therapy [82, 83, 112–114]. Similarly, tocilizumab (IL-6 inhibitor) has also shown durable responses in patients with adult-onset Still's disease [115]. While etoposide is not a mainstay of MAS therapy, if there is clinical deterioration or laboratory findings of worsening inflammation despite steroids, cyclosporine, or other disease-specific therapy, it is sometimes necessary to escalate treatment to include etoposide or other HLH salvage therapy (such as ATG or Campath), or HCT.

Novel Therapeutics

Currently several novel agents are being studied for the management of HLH. Blockade of interferon-gamma (IFNγ) has shown therapeutic benefit in two models of perforin- and Rab27a-deficient mice infected with lymphocytic choriomeningitis virus. Increased survival was noted in perforin-deficient mice, and resolution of cytopenias, reduction of cytokines, and hemophagocytosis were noted in both models [39, 116]. Subsequently, NI-0501, a human anti-interferon-gamma monoclonal antibody (anti-IFNγ mAb), was used in a phase-2 trial setting including pediatric patients with primary HLH ($n = 13$) and showed a satisfactory response (69%) [117]. Twelve patients received NI-0501 as a second-line agent, and 7 proceeded to allogeneic hematopoietic cell transplant. Resolution of CNS signs and symptoms was noticed in two evaluable patients. At 8-week follow-up, 11 patients were alive. Based on the promise shown in this trial, a multi-institutional clinical trial is currently studying the role of NI-0501 in pediatric patients with primary HLH (NCT01818492). Another ongoing clinical trial aims to study the safety and efficacy of anti-IFNγ mAb in pediatric patients with systemic juvenile idiopathic arthritis developing MAS/secondary HLH (NCT03311854).

Ruxolitinib, a Janus kinase (JAK) 1/Janus kinase (JAK) 2 inhibitor, has been used as a therapeutic strategy in murine models of HLH. Ruxolitinib significantly improved cytopenias, organomegaly, and cytokinemia in murine models of HLH [118]. A trial is ongoing to study the effects of ruxolitinib in adults with secondary HLH (NCT02400463). It has also been used on an individual basis as a salvage therapy in pediatric and adult patients with HLH. Broglie et al. used it in an 11-year-old boy with HLH refractory to HLH-directed therapy and anakinra [119]. The patient was noted to have improvement in liver dysfunction, inflammatory markers, and resolution of fevers within 24 h of the medication administration. A critically ill adult patient with rheumatoid arthritis with secondary HLH responded within 48 h and survived [120]. Sin and colleagues published a case report describing the use of ruxolitinib in an adult patient with EBV-associated HLH [121]. The patient was also noted to have improvement in ferritin, LDH, and liver function within 3 days, but bone marrow did not recover and patient had continued pancytopenia [121]. In the future, we anticipate potential use of newer less toxic pharmacologic options as first-line therapy options in critically ill patients who may not otherwise tolerate conventional chemotherapy.

Conclusion and Future Directions

The best care of HLH patients hinges on early recognition and initiation of immunosuppressive therapy as well as the aggressive supportive intensive care physicians are able to provide. Our understanding of HLH has evolved quickly over the last 30 years, but continued investigation of novel therapies will be imperative for further improvement in HLH patient outcomes.

References

1. Henter JI, Samuelsson-Horne A, Arico M, et al. Treatment of hemophagocytic lymphohistiocytosis with HLH-94 immunochemotherapy and bone marrow transplantation. Blood. 2002;100(7):2367–73.
2. Trottestam H, Horne A, Arico M, et al. Chemoimmunotherapy for hemophagocytic lymphohistiocytosis: long-term results of the HLH-94 treatment protocol. Blood. 2011;118(17):4577–84.
3. Henter JI, Horne A, Arico M, et al. HLH-2004: diagnostic and therapeutic guidelines for hemophagocytic lymphohistiocytosis. Pediatr Blood Cancer. 2007;48(2):124–31.
4. Henter JI, Elinder G, Soder O, Ost A. Incidence in Sweden and clinical features of familial hemophagocytic lymphohistiocytosis. Acta Paediatr Scand. 1991;80(4):428–35.
5. Janka GE. Familial and acquired hemophagocytic lymphohistiocytosis. Eur J Pediatr. 2007;166(2):95–109.
6. George MR. Hemophagocytic lymphohistiocytosis: review of etiologies and management. J Blood Med. 2014;5:69–86.
7. Allen CE, Yu X, Kozinetz CA, McClain KL. Highly elevated ferritin levels and the diagnosis of hemophagocytic lymphohistiocytosis. Pediatr Blood Cancer. 2008;50(6):1227–35.
8. Arico M, Janka G, Fischer A, et al. Hemophagocytic lymphohistiocytosis. Report of 122 children from the International Registry. FHL Study Group of the Histiocyte Society. Leukemia. 1996;10(2):197–203.
9. Jordan MB, Allen CE, Weitzman S, Filipovich AH, McClain KL. How I treat hemophagocytic lymphohistiocytosis. Blood. 2011;118(15):4041–52.
10. Rubin TS, Zhang K, Gifford C, Lane A, Bleesing JJ, Marsh RA. Perforin and CD107a testing are superior to NK cell function testing for screening patients for genetic HLH. Blood. 2017;129(22):2993–9.
11. Gupta A, Tyrrell P, Valani R, Benseler S, Weitzman S, Abdelhaleem M. The role of the initial bone marrow aspirate in the diagnosis of hemophagocytic lymphohistiocytosis. Pediatr Blood Cancer. 2008;51(3):402–4.
12. Stapp J, Wilkerson S, Stewart D, Coventry S, Mo JQ, Bove KE. Fulminant neonatal liver failure in siblings: probable congenital hemophagocytic lymphohistiocytosis. Pediatr Dev Pathol. 2006;9(3):239–44.
13. Henter JI, Nennesmo I. Neuropathologic findings and neurologic symptoms in twenty-three children with hemophagocytic lymphohistiocytosis. J Pediatr. 1997;130(3):358–65.
14. Horne A, Trottestam H, Aricò M, et al. Frequency and spectrum of central nervous system involvement in 193 children with haemophagocytic lymphohistiocytosis. Br J Haematol. 2008;140(3):327–35.
15. Horne A, Trottestam H, Arico M, et al. Frequency and spectrum of central nervous system involvement in 193 children with haemophagocytic lymphohistiocytosis. Br J Haematol. 2008;140(3):327–35.
16. Horne A, Wickstrom R, Jordan MB, et al. How to treat involvement of the central nervous system in hemophagocytic lymphohistiocytosis? Curr Treat Options Neurol. 2017;19(1):3.
17. Chong KW, Lee JH, Choong CT, et al. Hemophagocytic lymphohistiocytosis with isolated central nervous system reactivation and optic nerve involvement. J Child Neurol. 2012;27(10):1336–9.
18. Henter JI, Elinder G. Cerebromeningeal haemophagocytic lymphohistiocytosis. Lancet. 1992;339(8785):104–7.
19. Shinoda J, Murase S, Takenaka K, Sakai N. Isolated central nervous system hemophagocytic lymphohistiocytosis: case report. Neurosurgery. 2005;56(1):E187–90.

20. Morrell DS, Pepping MA, Scott JP, Esterly NB, Drolet BA. Cutaneous manifestations of hemophagocytic lymphohistiocytosis. Arch Dermatol. 2002;138(9):1208–12.
21. Janka GE. Familial hemophagocytic lymphohistiocytosis. Eur J Pediatr. 1983;140(3):221–30.
22. Dhote R, Simon J, Papo T, et al. Reactive hemophagocytic syndrome in adult systemic disease: report of twenty-six cases and literature review. Arthritis Rheum. 2003;49(5):633–9.
23. Kaito K, Kobayashi M, Katayama T, et al. Prognostic factors of hemophagocytic syndrome in adults: analysis of 34 cases. Eur J Haematol. 1997;59(4):247–53.
24. Risdall RJ, Brunning RD, Hernandez JI, Gordon DH. Bacteria-associated hemophagocytic syndrome. Cancer. 1984;54(12):2968–72.
25. Bergsten E, Horne A, Arico M, et al. Confirmed efficacy of etoposide and dexamethasone in HLH treatment: long term results of the cooperative HLH-2004 study. Blood. 2017;130(25):2728–38.
26. Ouachee-Chardin M, Elie C, de Saint BG, et al. Hematopoietic stem cell transplantation in hemophagocytic lymphohistiocytosis: a single-center report of 48 patients. Pediatrics. 2006;117(4):e743–50.
27. Goransdotter Ericson K, Fadeel B, Nilsson-Ardnor S, et al. Spectrum of perforin gene mutations in familial hemophagocytic lymphohistiocytosis. Am J Hum Genet. 2001;68(3):590–7.
28. Molleran Lee S, Villanueva J, Sumegi J, et al. Characterisation of diverse PRF1 mutations leading to decreased natural killer cell activity in North American families with haemophagocytic lymphohistiocytosis. J Med Genet. 2004;41(2):137–44.
29. Stepp SE, Dufourcq-Lagelouse R, Le Deist F, et al. Perforin gene defects in familial hemophagocytic lymphohistiocytosis. Science. 1999;286(5446):1957–9.
30. Egeler RM, Shapiro R, Loechelt B, Filipovich A. Characteristic immune abnormalities in hemophagocytic lymphohistiocytosis. J Pediatr Hematol Oncol. 1996;18(4):340–5.
31. Schneider EM, Lorenz I, Muller-Rosenberger M, Steinbach G, Kron M, Janka-Schaub GE. Hemophagocytic lymphohistiocytosis is associated with deficiencies of cellular cytolysis but normal expression of transcripts relevant to killer-cell-induced apoptosis. Blood. 2002;100(8):2891–8.
32. Brisse E, Wouters CH, Matthys P. Hemophagocytic lymphohistiocytosis (HLH): a heterogeneous spectrum of cytokine-driven immune disorders. Cytokine Growth Factor Rev. 2015;26(3):263–80.
33. Brisse E, Wouters CH, Matthys P. Advances in the pathogenesis of primary and secondary haemophagocytic lymphohistiocytosis: differences and similarities. Br J Haematol. 2016;174(2):203–17.
34. Hines M, Nichols KE. Going with the flow: perforin and CD107a in HLH. Blood. 2017;129(22):2954–5.
35. de Saint BG, Sepulveda FE, Maschalidi S, Fischer A. Cytotoxic granule secretion by lymphocytes and its link to immune homeostasis. *F1000Res*. 2015;4(F1000 Faculty Rev):930.
36. Abdalgani M, Filipovich AH, Choo S, et al. Accuracy of flow cytometric perforin screening for detecting patients with FHL due to PRF1 mutations. Blood. 2015;126(15):1858–60.
37. Pachlopnik Schmid J, Canioni D, Moshous D, et al. Clinical similarities and differences of patients with X-linked lymphoproliferative syndrome type 1 (XLP-1/SAP deficiency) versus type 2 (XLP-2/XIAP deficiency). Blood. 2011;117(5):1522–9.
38. Sumegi J, Seemayer TA, Huang D, et al. A spectrum of mutations in SH2D1A that causes X-linked lymphoproliferative disease and other Epstein-Barr virus-associated illnesses. Leuk Lymphoma. 2002;43(6):1189–201.
39. Jordan MB, Hildeman D, Kappler J, Marrack P. An animal model of hemophagocytic lymphohistiocytosis (HLH): CD8+ T cells and interferon gamma are essential for the disorder. Blood. 2004;104(3):735–43.
40. Terrell CE, Jordan MB. Perforin deficiency impairs a critical immunoregulatory loop involving murine CD8(+) T cells and dendritic cells. Blood. 2013;121(26):5184–91.
41. Lykens JE, Terrell CE, Zoller EE, Risma K, Jordan MB. Perforin is a critical physiologic regulator of T-cell activation. Blood. 2011;118(3):618–26.

42. Henter JI, Elinder G, Soder O, Hansson M, Andersson B, Andersson U. Hypercytokinemia in familial hemophagocytic lymphohistiocytosis. Blood. 1991;78(11):2918–22.
43. Behrens EM, Koretzky GA. Review: cytokine storm syndrome: looking toward the precision medicine era. Arthritis Rheumatol. 2017;69(6):1135–43.
44. Jenkins MR, Rudd-Schmidt JA, Lopez JA, et al. Failed CTL/NK cell killing and cytokine hypersecretion are directly linked through prolonged synapse time. J Exp Med. 2015;212(3):307–17.
45. Rouphael NG, Talati NJ, Vaughan C, Cunningham K, Moreira R, Gould C. Infections associated with haemophagocytic syndrome. Lancet Infect Dis. 2007;7(12):814–22.
46. Atteritano M, David A, Bagnato G, et al. Haemophagocytic syndrome in rheumatic patients. A systematic review. Eur Rev Med Pharmacol Sci. 2012;16(10):1414–24.
47. Behrens EM, Beukelman T, Paessler M, Cron RQ. Occult macrophage activation syndrome in patients with systemic juvenile idiopathic arthritis. J Rheumatol. 2007;34(5):1133–8.
48. Lehmberg K, Sprekels B, Nichols KE, et al. Malignancy-associated haemophagocytic lymphohistiocytosis in children and adolescents. Br J Haematol. 2015;170(4):539–49.
49. Abdelkefi A, Ben Jamil W, Torjman L, et al. Hemophagocytic syndrome after hematopoietic stem cell transplantation: a prospective observational study. Int J Hematol. 2009;89(3):368–73.
50. Takagi S, Masuoka K, Uchida N, et al. High incidence of haemophagocytic syndrome following umbilical cord blood transplantation for adults. Br J Haematol. 2009;147(4):543–53.
51. Bryceson YT, Pende D, Maul-Pavicic A, et al. A prospective evaluation of degranulation assays in the rapid diagnosis of familial hemophagocytic syndromes. Blood. 2012;119(12):2754–63.
52. Grom AA, Villanueva J, Lee S, Goldmuntz EA, Passo MH, Filipovich A. Natural killer cell dysfunction in patients with systemic-onset juvenile rheumatoid arthritis and macrophage activation syndrome. J Pediatr. 2003;142(3):292–6.
53. Chuang HC, Lay JD, Hsieh WC, et al. Epstein-Barr virus LMP1 inhibits the expression of SAP gene and upregulates Th1 cytokines in the pathogenesis of hemophagocytic syndrome. Blood. 2005;106(9):3090–6.
54. Mao H, Tu W, Qin G, et al. Influenza virus directly infects human natural killer cells and induces cell apoptosis. J Virol. 2009;83(18):9215–22.
55. Cifaldi L, Prencipe G, Caiello I, et al. Inhibition of natural killer cell cytotoxicity by interleukin-6: implications for the pathogenesis of macrophage activation syndrome. Arthritis Rheumatol. 2015;67(11):3037–46.
56. Strippoli R, Carvello F, Scianaro R, et al. Amplification of the response to toll-like receptor ligands by prolonged exposure to interleukin-6 in mice: implication for the pathogenesis of macrophage activation syndrome. Arthritis Rheum. 2012;64(5):1680–8.
57. Behrens EM, Canna SW, Slade K, et al. Repeated TLR9 stimulation results in macrophage activation syndrome-like disease in mice. J Clin Invest. 2011;121(6):2264–77.
58. Canna SW, Wrobel J, Chu N, Kreiger PA, Paessler M, Behrens EM. Interferon-gamma mediates anemia but is dispensable for fulminant toll-like receptor 9-induced macrophage activation syndrome and hemophagocytosis in mice. Arthritis Rheum. 2013;65(7):1764–75.
59. Wang Y, Wang Z, Zhang J, et al. Genetic features of late onset primary hemophagocytic lymphohistiocytosis in adolescence or adulthood. PLoS One. 2014;9(9):e107386.
60. Zhang K, Biroschak J, Glass DN, et al. Macrophage activation syndrome in patients with systemic juvenile idiopathic arthritis is associated with MUNC13-4 polymorphisms. Arthritis Rheum. 2008;58(9):2892–6.
61. Zhang K, Jordan MB, Marsh RA, et al. Hypomorphic mutations in PRF1, MUNC13-4, and STXBP2 are associated with adult-onset familial HLH. Blood. 2011;118(22):5794–8.
62. Zhang M, Behrens EM, Atkinson TP, Shakoory B, Grom AA, Cron RQ. Genetic defects in cytolysis in macrophage activation syndrome. Curr Rheumatol Rep. 2014;16(9):439.

63. Zhang M, Bracaglia C, Prencipe G, et al. A heterozygous RAB27A mutation associated with delayed cytolytic granule polarization and hemophagocytic lymphohistiocytosis. J Immunol. 2016;196(6):2492–503.
64. Kaufman KM, Linghu B, Szustakowski JD, et al. Whole-exome sequencing reveals overlap between macrophage activation syndrome in systemic juvenile idiopathic arthritis and familial hemophagocytic lymphohistiocytosis. Arthritis Rheumatol. 2014;66(12):3486–95.
65. Wong HR, Cvijanovich N, Allen GL, et al. Genomic expression profiling across the pediatric systemic inflammatory response syndrome, sepsis, and septic shock spectrum. Crit Care Med. 2009;37(5):1558–66.
66. Sumegi J, Barnes MG, Nestheide SV, et al. Gene expression profiling of peripheral blood mononuclear cells from children with active hemophagocytic lymphohistiocytosis. Blood. 2011;117(15):e151–60.
67. Tang Y, Xu X, Song H, et al. Early diagnostic and prognostic significance of a specific Th1/Th2 cytokine pattern in children with haemophagocytic syndrome. Br J Haematol. 2008;143(1):84–91.
68. Xu XJ, Tang YM, Song H, et al. Diagnostic accuracy of a specific cytokine pattern in hemophagocytic lymphohistiocytosis in children. J Pediatr. 2012;160(6):984–90. e981
69. Osugi Y, Hara J, Tagawa S, et al. Cytokine production regulating Th1 and Th2 cytokines in hemophagocytic lymphohistiocytosis. Blood. 1997;89(11):4100–3.
70. Damas P, Canivet JL, de Groote D, et al. Sepsis and serum cytokine concentrations. Crit Care Med. 1997;25(3):405–12.
71. Rau M, Schiller M, Krienke S, Heyder P, Lorenz H, Blank N. Clinical manifestations but not cytokine profiles differentiate adult-onset Still's disease and sepsis. J Rheumatol. 2010;37(11):2369–76.
72. Jekarl DW, Kim JY, Lee S, et al. Diagnosis and evaluation of severity of sepsis via the use of biomarkers and profiles of 13 cytokines: a multiplex analysis. Clin Chem Lab Med. 2015;53(4):575–81.
73. Bone RC. Sir Isaac Newton, sepsis, SIRS, and CARS. Crit Care Med. 1996;24(7):1125–8.
74. Hall MW, Knatz NL, Vetterly C, et al. Immunoparalysis and nosocomial infection in children with multiple organ dysfunction syndrome. Intensive Care Med. 2011;37(3):525–32.
75. Muszynski JA, Nofziger R, Greathouse K, et al. Early adaptive immune suppression in children with septic shock: a prospective observational study. Crit Care. 2014;18(4):R145.
76. Carcillo JA, Podd B, Aneja R, et al. Pathophysiology of pediatric multiple organ dysfunction syndrome. *Pediatr Crit Care Med.* 2017;18(3_suppl Suppl 1):S32–45.
77. Carcillo JA, Podd B, Simon DW. From febrile pancytopenia to hemophagocytic lymphohistiocytosis-associated organ dysfunction. Intensive Care Med. 2017;43(12):1853–5.
78. Carcillo JA, Sward K, Halstead ES, et al. A systemic inflammation mortality risk assessment contingency table for severe sepsis. Pediatr Crit Care Med. 2017;18(2):143–50.
79. Castillo L, Carcillo J. Secondary hemophagocytic lymphohistiocytosis and severe sepsis/systemic inflammatory response syndrome/multiorgan dysfunction syndrome/macrophage activation syndrome share common intermediate phenotypes on a spectrum of inflammation. Pediatr Crit Care Med. 2009;10(3):387–92.
80. Demirkol D, Yildizdas D, Bayrakci B, et al. Hyperferritinemia in the critically ill child with secondary hemophagocytic lymphohistiocytosis/sepsis/multiple organ dysfunction syndrome/macrophage activation syndrome: what is the treatment? Crit Care. 2012;16(2):R52.
81. Kyriazopoulou E, Leventogiannis K, Norrby-Teglund A, et al. Macrophage activation-like syndrome: an immunological entity associated with rapid progression to death in sepsis. BMC Med. 2017;15(1):172.
82. Rajasekaran S, Kruse K, Kovey K, et al. Therapeutic role of anakinra, an interleukin-1 receptor antagonist, in the management of secondary hemophagocytic lymphohistiocytosis/sepsis/multiple organ dysfunction/macrophage activating syndrome in critically ill children*. Pediatr Crit Care Med. 2014;15(5):401–8.
83. Shakoory B, Carcillo JA, Chatham WW, et al. Interleukin-1 receptor blockade is associated with reduced mortality in sepsis patients with features of macrophage activation syndrome: reanalysis of a prior phase III trial. Crit Care Med. 2016;44(2):275–81.

84. Schaer DJ, Schleiffenbaum B, Kurrer M, et al. Soluble hemoglobin–haptoglobin scavenger receptor CD163 as a lineage-specific marker in the reactive hemophagocytic syndrome. Eur J Haematol. 2005;74(1):6–10.
85. Francois B, Trimoreau F, Vignon P, Fixe P, Praloran V, Gastinne H. Thrombocytopenia in the sepsis syndrome: role of hemophagocytosis and macrophage colony-stimulating factor. Am J Med. 1997;103(2):114–20.
86. Gupta A, Weitzman S, Abdelhaleem M. The role of hemophagocytosis in bone marrow aspirates in the diagnosis of hemophagocytic lymphohistiocytosis. Pediatr Blood Cancer. 2008;50(2):192–4.
87. Strauss R, Neureiter D, Westenburger B, Wehler M, Kirchner T, Hahn EG. Multifactorial risk analysis of bone marrow histiocytic hyperplasia with hemophagocytosis in critically ill medical patients--a postmortem clinicopathologic analysis. Crit Care Med. 2004;32(6):1316–21.
88. Filipovich AH, Chandrakasan S. Pathogenesis of hemophagocytic lymphohistiocytosis. Hematol/Oncol Clin. 2015;29(5):895–902.
89. Creput C, Galicier L, Buyse S, Azoulay E. Understanding organ dysfunction in hemophagocytic lymphohistiocytosis. Intensive Care Med. 2008;34(7):1177–87.
90. Buyse S, Teixeira L, Galicier L, et al. Critical care management of patients with hemophagocytic lymphohistiocytosis. Intensive Care Med. 2010;36(10):1695–702.
91. Leow EH, Soh SY, Tan AM, Mok YH, Chan MY, Lee JH. Critically Ill children with hemophagocytic lymphohistiocytosis: a case series of 14 patients. J Pediatr Hematol Oncol. 2017;39(6):e303–6.
92. Rajagopala S, Singh N, Agarwal R, Gupta D, Das R. Severe hemophagocytic lymphohistiocytosis in adults-experience from an intensive care unit from North India. Indian J Crit Care Med. 2012;16(4):198–203.
93. Wohlfarth P, Agis H, Gualdoni GA, et al. Interleukin 1 receptor antagonist anakinra, intravenous immunoglobulin, and corticosteroids in the management of critically Ill adult patients with hemophagocytic lymphohistiocytosis. J Intensive Care Med. 2017; https://doi.org/10.1177/0885066617711386.
94. Cashen K, Chu RL, Klein J, Rycus PT, Costello JM. Extracorporeal membrane oxygenation outcomes in children with hemophagocytic lymphohistiocytosis. Perfusion. 2017;32(2):151–6.
95. Cheng A, Williams F, Fortenberry J, Preissig C, Salinas S, Kamat P. Use of extracorporeal support in hemophagocytic lymphohistiocytosis secondary to ehrlichiosis. Pediatrics. 2016;138(4):e20154176.
96. Henter JI, Palmkvist-Kaijser K, Holzgraefe B, Bryceson YT, Palmer K. Cytotoxic therapy for severe swine flu A/H1N1. Lancet. 2010;376(9758):2116.
97. Saites VA, Hadler R, Gutsche JT, Laudanski K. Extracorporeal membrane oxygenation for hemophagocytic lymphohistiocytosis. Am J Case Rep. 2016;17:686–9.
98. Wu ET, Huang SC, Sun LC, Ko WJ. Reactive hemophagocytic syndrome treated with extracorporeal membrane oxygenation. Pediatr Int. 2008;50(5):706–8.
99. Barba T, Maucort-Boulch D, Iwaz J, et al. Hemophagocytic lymphohistiocytosis in intensive care unit: a 71-case strobe-compliant retrospective study. Medicine. 2015;94(51):e2318.
100. Ambruso DR, Hays T, Zwartjes WJ, Tubergen DG, Favara BE. Successful treatment of lymphohistiocytic reticulosis with phagocytosis with epipodophyllotoxin VP 16–213. Cancer. 1980;45(10):2516–20.
101. Fadeel B, Orrenius S, Henter JI. Induction of apoptosis and caspase activation in cells obtained from familial haemophagocytic lymphohistiocytosis patients. Br J Haematol. 1999;106(2):406–15.
102. Johnson TS, Terrell CE, Millen SH, Katz JD, Hildeman DA, Jordan MB. Etoposide selectively ablates activated T cells to control the immunoregulatory disorder hemophagocytic lymphohistiocytosis. J Immunol. 2014;192(1):84–91.
103. Fischer A, Virelizier JL, Arenzana-Seisdedos F, Perez N, Nezelof C, Griscelli C. Treatment of four patients with erythrophagocytic lymphohistiocytosis by a combination of epipodophyllotoxin, steroids, intrathecal methotrexate, and cranial irradiation. Pediatrics. 1985;76(2):263–8.

104. Henter J-I, Elinder G, Finkel Y, Söder O. Successful induction with chemotherapy including teniposide in familial erythrophagocytic lymphohistiocytosis. Lancet. 1986;328(8520):1402.
105. Mahlaoui N, Ouachee-Chardin M, de Saint BG, et al. Immunotherapy of familial hemophagocytic lymphohistiocytosis with antithymocyte globulins: a single-center retrospective report of 38 patients. Pediatrics. 2007;120(3):e622–8.
106. Henter JI, Aricò M, Egeler RM, et al. HLH-94: a treatment protocol for hemophagocytic lymphohistiocytosis. Pediatr Blood Cancer. 1997;28(5):342–7.
107. Balis FM, Lester CM, Chrousos GP, Heideman RL, Poplack DG. Differences in cerebrospinal fluid penetration of corticosteroids: possible relationship to the prevention of meningeal leukemia. J Clin Oncol. 1987;5(2):202–7.
108. Marsh RA, Jordan MB, Talano JA, et al. Salvage therapy for refractory hemophagocytic lymphohistiocytosis: a review of the published experience. Pediatr Blood Cancer. 2017;64(4). https://doi.org/10.1002/pbc26308.
109. Marsh RA, Allen CE, McClain KL, et al. Salvage therapy of refractory hemophagocytic lymphohistiocytosis with alemtuzumab. Pediatr Blood Cancer. 2013;60(1):101–9.
110. Haytoglu Z, Yazici N, Erbay A. Secondary hemophagocytic lymphohistiocytosis: do we really need chemotherapeutics for all patients? J Pediatr Hematol Oncol. 2017;39(2):e106–9.
111. Chellapandian D, Das R, Zelley K, et al. Treatment of Epstein Barr virus-induced haemophagocytic lymphohistiocytosis with rituximab-containing chemo-immunotherapeutic regimens. Br J Haematol. 2013;162(3):376–82.
112. Minoia F, Davi S, Horne A, et al. Clinical features, treatment, and outcome of macrophage activation syndrome complicating systemic juvenile idiopathic arthritis: a multinational, multicenter study of 362 patients. Arthritis Rheumatol. 2014;66(11):3160–9.
113. Behrens EM, Kreiger PA, Cherian S, Cron RQ. Interleukin 1 receptor antagonist to treat cytophagic histiocytic panniculitis with secondary hemophagocytic lymphohistiocytosis. J Rheumatol. 2006;33(10):2081–4.
114. Miettunen PM, Narendran A, Jayanthan A, Behrens EM, Cron RQ. Successful treatment of severe paediatric rheumatic disease-associated macrophage activation syndrome with interleukin-1 inhibition following conventional immunosuppressive therapy: case series with 12 patients. Rheumatology (Oxford). 2011;50(2):417–9.
115. Sakai R, Nagasawa H, Nishi E, et al. Successful treatment of adult-onset Still's disease with tocilizumab monotherapy: two case reports and literature review. Clin Rheumatol. 2012;31(3):569–74.
116. Pachlopnik Schmid J, Ho CH, Chretien F, et al. Neutralization of IFNgamma defeats haemophagocytosis in LCMV-infected perforin- and Rab27a-deficient mice. EMBO Mol Med. 2009;1(2):112–24.
117. Allen C, De Benedetti F, Grom AA, et al. A novel targeted approach to the treatment of hemophagocytic lymphohistiocytosis (HLH) with an anti-interferon gamma (IFNγ) monoclonal antibody (mAb), NI-0501: first results from a pilot phase 2 study in children with primary HLH. 2015.
118. Das R, Guan P, Sprague L, et al. Janus kinase inhibition lessens inflammation and ameliorates disease in murine models of hemophagocytic lymphohistiocytosis. Blood. 2016;127(13):1666–75.
119. Broglie L, Pommert L, Rao S, et al. Ruxolitinib for treatment of refractory hemophagocytic lymphohistiocytosis. Blood Adv. 2017;1(19):1533–6.
120. Slostad JPJ, Tefferi A. Ruxolitinib as first-line treatment in secondary hemophagocytic lymphohistiocytosis: a single patient experience. Am J Hematol. 2017;93(2):E47–9.
121. Sin JH, Zangardi ML. Ruxolitinib for secondary hemophagocytic lymphohistiocytosis: first case report. Hematol Oncol Stem Cell Ther. 2017. https://doi.org/10.1016/jhemonc.2017.07.002.

Part II
Critical Care Management

Chapter 10
Early Recognition of Critical Illness

Asya Agulnik

Introduction

Inpatient cardiopulmonary arrests in hospitalized pediatric patients are infrequent, occurring in approximately 1.4% of pediatric intensive care unit (PICU) admissions [1] and 0.08% of hospital admissions (1 in every 1300 pediatric hospitalizations) [2]. Survival to hospital discharge following cardiopulmonary resuscitation, however, remains low, ranging from 27% to 48% in recent studies [1–5]. Hospitalized pediatric patients with cancer and those who have received hematopoietic stem cell transplant (HSCT) are more likely to experience a cardiopulmonary arrest [2] and have lower survival compared with other pediatric patients [2, 3]. Beyond cardiopulmonary arrest, hospitalized pediatric hemato-oncology patients have frequent clinical deterioration requiring critical care—one in every three to four patients will require at least one PICU admission during the course of their treatment [6]. These patients are at higher risk of, and have higher mortality following, episodes of severe sepsis [7, 8]. Early identification of critical illness and prevention of cardiopulmonary arrests in hospitalized pediatric oncology and post-HSCT patients are an integral part of improving overall hospital outcomes and survival.

Defining Clinical Deterioration

Because inpatient cardiopulmonary arrests are infrequent, other measures of critical illness must be used to evaluate strategies to improve hospital outcomes. Unplanned transfers to the PICU, defined as hospitalized floor patients requiring an emergency

A. Agulnik (✉)
Department of Global Pediatric Medicine, Division of Critical Care, St. Jude Children's Research Hospital, Memphis, TN, USA
e-mail: asya.agulnik@stjude.org

C. N. Duncan et al. (eds.), *Critical Care of the Pediatric Immunocompromised Hematology/Oncology Patient*, https://doi.org/10.1007/978-3-030-01322-6_10

PICU transfer (not following scheduled surgery), represent a group of hospitalized patients with clinical deterioration. Compared with other PICU admissions, unplanned PICU transfers have higher mortality and longer PICU length-of-stay (LOS) [9, 10]. As a high-risk population, oncology patients make up a large percentage of unplanned PICU transfers [9], highlighting the importance of appropriate identification of critical illness in this group.

Another approach to describe critical illness in hospitalized pediatric patients is the concept of "critical deterioration," unplanned PICU transfers requiring noninvasive ventilation, intubation, or vasoactive infusions within 12 h of PICU admission [11]. Critical deterioration was found to be eightfold more common than cardiac and respiratory arrests in hospitalized patients and is associated with a greater than 13-fold increased risk of in-hospital death [11].

Delays in Identification of Clinical Deterioration and Outcomes

There is an extensive literature regarding the relationship between delayed transfer to the intensive care unit and mortality in hospitalized patients. Adult studies demonstrate that delays in intensive care unit (ICU) transfer for critically ill floor patients are frequent and result in increasing organ dysfunction, longer ICU LOS, and higher hospital mortality [12–14]. A large multicenter study demonstrated that every hour of delay in ICU transfer after the start physiologic deterioration was associated with a 3% increase in odds of mortality [15]. Preliminary analysis suggests that ICU transfer delays are related to failure to recognize physiologic changes in hospitalized patients, delays in notification of treating physicians of these changes, or lack of prompt bedside patient evaluation [13].

As in adults, pediatric data suggest that changes in vital signs occur 12–24 h prior to unplanned PICU transfer in hospitalized patients [9]; however, these changes are frequently not recognized or acted upon by clinical staff. Recently, data from a global epidemiologic study of pediatric severe sepsis demonstrate that nearly a third of episodes of severe sepsis requiring PICU care originate from the hospital wards, where patients have more comorbidities (including cancer) [7]. Similar to adult data, there is evidence that delay in PICU admission for hospitalized pediatric oncology patients requiring unplanned PICU transfer is associated with higher mortality [16]. Among critically ill post-HSCT patients with severe sepsis, two-thirds originated from inpatient wards and had higher PICU mortality compared to severe sepsis admissions from other locations (operating room, emergency room), providing a potential opportunity for earlier sepsis recognition and intervention [8]. These findings suggest systems that aid in early identification, evaluation, and management for hospitalized patients with deterioration may improve hospital outcomes and overall survival. This is particularly true for patients with a higher underlying risk of deterioration such as children with cancer or post-HSCT.

Rapid Response Teams (RRTs)

Hospitals use a number of strategies to improve early identification and ICU transfer for patients with clinical deterioration. In 2004, the Institute for Healthcare Improvement's 100,000 Lives Campaign recommended that hospitals implement rapid response teams (RRTs) charged with identifying non-intensive care unit patients at risk for rapid deterioration [17]. RRTs are components of emergency response systems (Fig. 10.1) designed to identify patients with deterioration using a set trigger (physiologic change, staff or family concern→afferent limb) and activate a responding team of trained providers, usually composed of a physician, nurse, and respiratory therapist, to assess the patient and aid in management or facilitate ICU transfer (efferent limb). A recent meta-analysis of adult hospital outcomes after implementing RRTs and/or medical emergency teams (MET) demonstrated a significant decrease in hospital mortality and number of non-ICU cardiac arrests [18]. Pediatric data similarly demonstrates that RRT/MET implementation is associated with a reduction in risk of respiratory and cardiopulmonary arrest in hospitalized children outside of the PICU and reduces the frequency of critical deterioration [19, 20].

Because the success of RRTs is largely dependent on the appropriate identification of patients with deterioration (afferent limb), it is important to identify the best trigger system to activate an RRT, MET, or clinician evaluation. Adult evidence demonstrates that aggregate weighted scoring system (multicomponent scoring systems based on a number of physiologic and patient factors) performs better at identifying patients with deterioration than single parameter systems (i.e., staff concern only) [21]. As a result, recent work has focused on the development of adult and pediatric early warning scores to serve as the afferent limb of emergency systems to improve the hospital care of patients with deterioration.

Little data exists regarding the impact of RRT implementation specifically on hospitalized oncology and post-HSCT patients. Adult data suggests that, due to a higher underlying risk of deterioration, RRT activations are more common in hospitalized oncology patients compared to general medical admissions [22], and RRT implementation decreases severity of illness and organ dysfunction at time of ICU transfer in hospitalized post-HSCT patients [23]. As a high-risk population, hospi-

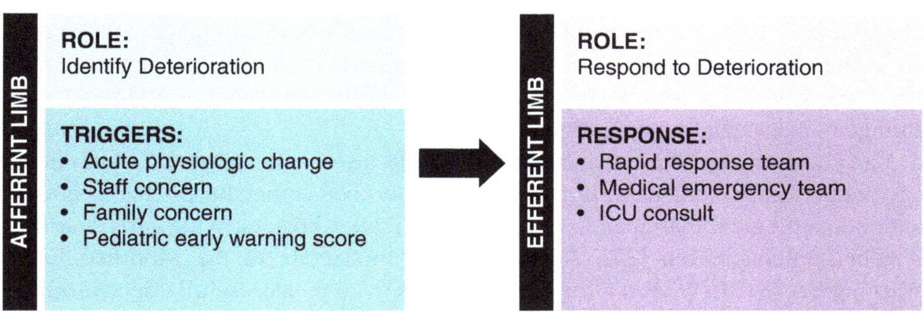

Fig. 10.1 Emergency response systems

talized pediatric oncology and post-HSCT patients are likely to disproportionally benefit from emergency response systems designed to identify and proactively manage clinical deterioration outside the ICU.

Pediatric Early Warning Systems (PEWS)

Pediatric early warning systems (PEWS) are multicomponent scoring tools (afferent limb) associated with an action algorithm (efferent limb) designed to aid in identification and management of hospitalized children with clinical deterioration. The PEWS score is typically calculated by the bedside nurse or an electronic system with every set of vital signs in hospitalized patients. While a variety of PEWS scoring tools have been described in the literature [24], the majority are based on a combination of vital signs, physical exam findings, and treatment necessities. The PEWS score is interpreted by the bedside team using an action algorithm, typically with specific triggers for physician evaluation, RRT activation [20], or PICU consultation [25].

Implementation of PEWS scoring tools paired with an escalation algorithm as part of an emergency response system has been shown to reduce hospital mortality and rates of cardiac and respiratory arrests outside of the PICU [20, 24, 26], as well as severity of illness on PICU transfer [27]. A recent cluster-randomized study of PEWS implementation in 21 inpatient pediatric units failed to show an improvement in all-cause hospital mortality but did demonstrate a reduction in frequency of significant clinical deterioration events [28]. Qualitative work has shown that PEWS implementation facilitates patient safety by alerting clinicians of concerning clinical changes in hospitalized patients, provides less-experience nurses with easily accessible vital sign references, and empowers nurses to overcome barriers to escalating care [29]. There is also evidence that PEWS are cost-effective, resulting in cost savings as a result of averted critical deterioration events [30, 31].

Although a number of PEWS scoring tools are used by different hospitals, different tools have ranging validity in identifying patients with clinical deterioration [24, 32, 33]. Because pediatric in-patient cardiopulmonary arrests are rare, PEWS validation studies typically use other outcomes, such as unplanned transfer to the PICU, to evaluate a given's score's utility in predicting deterioration. Despite variability in performance, a number of PEWS tools have been shown to be accurate in identifying hospitalized patients with deterioration through multicenter studies [34] and across a range of subspecialty populations [25, 35].

Early warning systems have been successfully used in hospitalized adult oncology patients [36]. Adult data suggest improved survival among hospitalized patients with hematological malignancies or post-HSCT after hospital-wide early warning system implementation [37]. Addition of serum lactate to the Modified Early Warning Score (MEWS) as a trigger for RRT activation successfully decreased the number of codes in hospitalized adult oncology patients, without increasing the frequency of unplanned ICU transfers [38].

PEWS are widely used in hospitals caring for pediatric oncology patients [39], and two scoring tools have been specifically validated to identify need for unplanned PICU transfer in hospitalized pediatric oncology and post-HSCT patients [35, 40] (Fig. 10.2 shows one example). One study demonstrated that PEWS scores increase 12–24 h prior to unplanned PICU transfer (and an average of 8 h prior to notification of the PICU team of patient deterioration) and patients arriving to the PICU with higher scores have longer PICU length of stay and higher mortality [40].

It is important to note that while each hospital adapts the PEWS scoring tool to reflect the medical language and escalation pathways of their center, validation of PEWS for pediatric oncology and HCT patients has not required adaptation of the score specifically for this population. Despite differences in this patient population, PEWS tools used for general pediatrics and other subspecialties function well to identify critical illness in these patients. In fact, due to the increased frequency of clinical deterioration in these patients, the "number needed to evaluate" (number of patients screened to identify one patient with deterioration) among pediatric oncology patients is approximately half that of general medical and surgical patients [35]. Adaptation of the escalation algorithm, however, is integral to ensure the system reflects established mechanisms for the management of hospitalized patients with deterioration, such as RRTs, ICU consults, and code blue teams.

Our team recently implemented a modified version of a PEWS validated in pediatric oncology and HCT patients (Fig. 10.2) at St. Jude Children's Research Hospital (SJCRH), a dedicated hematology-oncology/HSCT hospital. Implementation of PEWS resulted in increased frequency of RRT activations with a higher proportion of clinical deterioration events arriving to the PICU via an organized escalation pathway, without an increase in overall unplanned PICU transfers [41]. As has been described at other centers, we feel these changes represent an improvement in the culture of safety at the bedside in our hospital.

Resource-Limited Settings

Although this chapter and textbook primarily focus on the management of the critically ill immunocompromised pediatric hematology-oncology patients in high-resource settings, pediatric cancer is a global challenge; low- and middle-income countries (LMICs) account for 80% of pediatric cancer cases and over 90% of global childhood cancer deaths [42]. Hospitals in LMICs face a number of resource challenges affecting their ability to identify and respond to clinical deterioration in hospitalized patients, resulting in more frequent cardiopulmonary arrests [43] with higher mortality [43–45]. As access to cancer-directed therapy increases worldwide, hospitals in LMIC are increasingly presented with the dual challenge of caring for a high-risk patient population with limited staff and infrastructure, resulting in poor hospital outcomes and high rates of toxic deaths.

Although research is limited, there is evidence that PEWS implementation is feasible in resource-limited settings. A group in Malawi demonstrated a modified

Component	0	1	2	3	Score
Behavior/ neurologic	• Playing or sleeping appropriately • Alert at patient's baseline	• Sleepy, somnolent when not disturbed	• Irritable, difficult to console • Increase in patient's baseline seizure activity	• Lethargic, confused, and floppy • Reduced response to pain • Prolonged or frequent seizures • Pupils asymmetric or sluggish	
Cardiovascular	• Skin tone appropriate for patient • Capillary refill ≤2 s	• Pale • Capillary refill 3–4 s • Mild tachycardia • Intermittent ectopy or irregular heart rhythm (not new)	• Grey • Capillary refill 4–5 s • Moderate tachycardia	• Grey and mottled • Capillary refill >5 s • Severe tachycardia • New onset bradycardia • New onset/increase in ectopy, irregular heart rhythm, or heart block	
	• Within normal • parameters • No retractions	• Mild tachypnea • Mild increased WOB (flaring and retracting) • Up to 40% supplemental • O_2 via mask	• Moderate increased • WOB (flaring, retracting, grunting, and use of accessory muscles) • 40–60% O_2 via mask	• Severe tachypnea • Respiratoty rate below normal for age • Severe increased WOB (i.e ., head bobbing, paradoxical, breathing) • > 60% O_2 via mask	

Fig. 10.2 Example pediatric early warning system scoring tool [40]

Respiratory		• Up to 1 LNC>patient's baseline need • Mild desaturation • Intermittent apnea self-resolving	• 1–2 LNC > patient's baseline need • Nebulizations every • 1–2 hr • Moderate desaturation • Apnea requiring repositioning or stimulation	• > 2 LNC > patient's baseline need • Nebulizations every 30 min to 1 hr • Severe desaturation • Apnea requiring interventions other than repositioning or stimulation	
Staff concern	Not concerned	Concerned			
Family concern	Not concerned	Concerned or absent			
				Total score	

Vital Sign	Age	Mild	Moderate	Severe
Respiratory rate and heart rate	Infant	≥ 10% ↑ for age	≥ 15% ↑ for age	≥ 25% ↑ for age
	Toddler and older ≥ 10% ↑ for age	≥ 10% ↑ for age	≥ 25% ↑ for age	≥ 50% ↑ for age
Desaturation from patient's baseline O_2 saturation	All ages	5 % below	10 % below	15 % below

WOB = work of breathing. NC = nasal cannula.

Fig. 10.2 (continued)

PEWS is accurate in identifying general pediatric patients at risk of death in the hospital [46], and implementation of PEWS increased the frequency of patient assessment and reduced hospital mortality [26].

Our team recently described the successful implementation of PEWS in a resource-limited pediatric oncology hospital in Guatemala [47]. Implementation resulted in decreased frequency of unplanned PICU transfers and improved PICU utilization in the hospital [47]. The PEWS was accurate in identifying hospitalized patients requiring unplanned PICU transfer in this setting, with abnormal scores beginning as early as 24 h prior to PICU admission and higher scores on PICU transfer predicting organ dysfunction, septic shock, and need for early intensive interventions [48]. Implementation of PEWS was highly cost-effective, resulting in over $350,000 in annual cost savings as a result of reduction in unplanned PICU transfers [31]. These findings suggest that tools that aid in early identification and management of pediatric oncology and post-HSCT patients with clinical deterioration, such as PEWS, can improve hospital outcomes and survival for these patients in hospitals of all resource levels.

References

1. Berg RA, Nadkarni VM, Clark AE, et al. Incidence and outcomes of cardiopulmonary resuscitation in PICUs. Crit Care Med. 2016;44(4):798–808.
2. Knudson JD, Neish SR, Cabrera AG, et al. Prevalence and outcomes of pediatric in-hospital cardiopulmonary resuscitation in the United States: an analysis of the Kids' inpatient database*. Crit Care Med. 2012;40(11):2940–4.
3. Del Castillo J, Lopez-Herce J, Canadas S, et al. Cardiac arrest and resuscitation in the pediatric intensive care unit: a prospective multicenter multinational study. Resuscitation. 2014;85(10):1380–6.
4. Girotra S, Spertus JA, Li Y, et al. Survival trends in pediatric in-hospital cardiac arrests: an analysis from get with the guidelines-resuscitation. Circ Cardiovasc Qual Outcomes. 2013;6(1):42–9.
5. Nadkarni VM, Larkin GL, Peberdy MA, et al. First documented rhythm and clinical outcome from in-hospital cardiac arrest among children and adults. JAMA. 2006;295(1):50–7.
6. Demaret P, Pettersen G, Hubert P, Teira P, Emeriaud G. The critically-ill pediatric hemato-oncology patient: epidemiology, management, and strategy of transfer to the pediatric intensive care unit. Ann Intensive Care. 2012;2(1):14.
7. Weiss SL, Fitzgerald JC, Pappachan J, et al. Global epidemiology of pediatric severe sepsis: the sepsis prevalence, outcomes, and therapies study. Am J Respir Crit Care Med. 2015;191(10):1147–57.
8. Lindell RB, Gertz SJ, Rowan CM, et al. High levels of morbidity and mortality among pediatric hematopoietic cell transplant recipients with severe Sepsis: insights from the Sepsis PRevalence, OUtcomes, and therapies international point prevalence study. Pediatr Crit Care Med. 2017;18(12):1114–25.
9. Tume L. The deterioration of children in ward areas in a specialist children's hospital. Nurs Crit Care. 2007;12(1):12–9.
10. Humphreys S, Totapally BR. Rapid response team calls and unplanned transfers to the pediatric intensive care unit in a pediatric hospital. Am J Crit Care. 2016;25(1):e9–13.
11. Bonafide CP, Roberts KE, Priestley MA, et al. Development of a pragmatic measure for evaluating and optimizing rapid response systems. Pediatrics. 2012;129(4):e874–81.

12. Cardoso LT, Grion CM, Matsuo T, et al. Impact of delayed admission to intensive care units on mortality of critically ill patients: a cohort study. Crit Care. 2011;15(1):R28.
13. Young MP, Gooder VJ, McBride K, James B, Fisher ES. Inpatient transfers to the intensive care unit: delays are associated with increased mortality and morbidity. J Gen Intern Med. 2003;18(2):77–83.
14. Sankey CB, McAvay G, Siner JM, Barsky CL, Chaudhry SI. "Deterioration to door time": an exploratory analysis of delays in escalation of care for hospitalized patients. J Gen Intern Med. 2016;31(8):895–900.
15. Churpek MM, Wendlandt B, Zadravecz FJ, Adhikari R, Winslow C, Edelson DP. Association between intensive care unit transfer delay and hospital mortality: a multicenter investigation. J Hosp Med. 2016;11(11):757–62.
16. Fausser JL, Tavenard A, Rialland F, et al. Should we pay attention to the delay before admission to a pediatric intensive care unit for children with Cancer? Impact on 1-month mortality. A report from the French children's oncology study group, GOCE. J Pediatr Hematol Oncol. 2017;39(5):e244–8.
17. 100K Lives campaign—getting started kit: rapid response teams. http://www.ihi.org/IHI/Programs/Campaign/Campaign.htm. Accessed 7 Feb 2018.
18. Solomon RS, Corwin GS, Barclay DC, Quddusi SF, Dannenberg MD. Effectiveness of rapid response teams on rates of in-hospital cardiopulmonary arrest and mortality: a systematic review and meta-analysis. J Hosp Med. 2016;11(6):438–45.
19. Brilli RJ, Gibson R, Luria JW, et al. Implementation of a medical emergency team in a large pediatric teaching hospital prevents respiratory and cardiopulmonary arrests outside the intensive care unit. Pediatr Crit Care Med. 2007;8(3):236–46. quiz 247
20. Bonafide CP, Localio AR, Roberts KE, Nadkarni VM, Weirich CM, Keren R. Impact of rapid response system implementation on critical deterioration events in children. JAMA Pediatr. 2013;168(1):25–33.
21. McNeill G, Bryden D. Do either early warning systems or emergency response teams improve hospital patient survival? A systematic review. Resuscitation. 2013;84(12):1652–67.
22. Austin CA, Hanzaker C, Stafford R, et al. Utilization of rapid response resources and outcomes in a comprehensive cancer center*. Crit Care Med. 2014;42(4):905–9.
23. Hayani O, Al-Beihany A, Zarychanski R, et al. Impact of critical care outreach on hematopoietic stem cell transplant recipients: a cohort study. Bone Marrow Transplant. 2011;46(8):1138–44.
24. Chapman SM, Wray J, Oulton K, Peters MJ. Systematic review of paediatric track and trigger systems for hospitalised children. Resuscitation. 2016;109:87–109.
25. McLellan MC, Gauvreau K, Connor JA. Validation of the children's hospital early warning system for critical deterioration recognition. J Pediatr Nurs. 2017;32:52–8.
26. Olson D, Preidis GA, Milazi R, et al. Task shifting an inpatient triage, assessment and treatment programme improves the quality of care for hospitalised Malawian children. Tropical Med Int Health. 2013;18(7):879–86.
27. Sefton G, McGrath C, Tume L, Lane S, Lisboa PJ, Carrol ED. What impact did a paediatric early warning system have on emergency admissions to the paediatric intensive care unit? An observational cohort study. Intensive Crit Care Nurs. 2015;31(2):91–9.
28. Parshuram CS, Dryden-Palmer K, Farrell C, et al. Effect of a pediatric early warning system on all-cause mortality in hospitalized pediatric patients: the EPOCH randomized clinical trial. JAMA. 2018;319(10):1002–12.
29. Bonafide CP, Roberts KE, Weirich CM, et al. Beyond statistical prediction: qualitative evaluation of the mechanisms by which pediatric early warning scores impact patient safety. J Hosp Med. 2013;8(5):248–53.
30. Bonafide CP, Localio AR, Song L, et al. Cost-benefit analysis of a medical emergency team in a children's hospital. Pediatrics. 2014;134(2):235–41.
31. Agulnik A, Antillon-Klussmann F, Soberanis Vasquez DJ, et al. Cost effectiveness of implementing a pediatric early warning system (PEWS) at a pediatric oncology hospital in a low-middle income country. Pediatr Blood Cancer. 2017;64(Suppl 3):S39.

32. Chapman SM, Wray J, Oulton K, Pagel C, Ray S, Peters MJ. 'The score matters': wide variations in predictive performance of 18 paediatric track and trigger systems. Arch Dis Child. 2017;102(6):487–95.
33. Lambert V, Matthews A, MacDonell R, Fitzsimons J. Paediatric early warning systems for detecting and responding to clinical deterioration in children: a systematic review. BMJ Open. 2017;7(3):e014497.
34. Parshuram CS, Duncan HP, Joffe AR, et al. Multicentre validation of the bedside paediatric early warning system score: a severity of illness score to detect evolving critical illness in hospitalised children. Crit Care. 2011;15(4):R184.
35. Dean NP, Fenix JB, Spaeder M, Levin A. Evaluation of a pediatric early warning score across different subspecialty patients. Pediatr Crit Care Med. 2017;18(7):655–60.
36. Olsen M, Mooney K, Evans E. Implementation of an early warning scoring system to identify patients with cancer at risk for deterioration. Clin J Oncol Nurs. 2016;20(4):374–6.
37. Bokhari SW, Munir T, Memon S, Byrne JL, Russell NH, Beed M. Impact of critical care reconfiguration and track-and-trigger outreach team intervention on outcomes of haematology patients requiring intensive care admission. Ann Hematol. 2010;89(5):505–12.
38. Young RS, Gobel BH, Schumacher M, Lee J, Weaver C, Weitzman S. Use of the modified early warning score and serum lactate to prevent cardiopulmonary arrest in hematology-oncology patients: a quality improvement study. Am J Med Qual. 2014;29(6):530–7.
39. Demmel KM, Williams L, Flesch L. Implementation of the pediatric early warning scoring system on a pediatric hematology/oncology unit. J Pediatr Oncol Nurs. 2010;27(4):229–40.
40. Agulnik A, Forbes PW, Stenquist N, Rodriguez-Galindo C, Kleinman M. Validation of a pediatric early warning score in hospitalized pediatric oncology and hematopoietic stem cell transplant patients. Pediatr Crit Care Med. 2016;17(4):e146–53.
41. Agulnik A, Johnson S, Wilkes R, Faughnan L, Carrillo A, Morrison R. Impact of implementing a pediatric early warning system (PEWS) in a pediatric oncology hospital. Crit Care Med. 2018;46(1:Supplement):631.
42. Rodriguez-Galindo C, Friedrich P, Alcasabas P, et al. Toward the cure of all children with cancer through collaborative efforts: pediatric oncology as a global challenge. J Clin Oncol. 2015;33:3065–73.
43. Ocen D, Kalungi S, Ejoku J, et al. Prevalence, outcomes and factors associated with adult in hospital cardiac arrests in a low-income country tertiary hospital: a prospective observational study. BMC Emerg Med. 2015;15:23.
44. Lopez-Herce J, Del Castillo J, Matamoros M, et al. Factors associated with mortality in pediatric in-hospital cardiac arrest: a prospective multicenter multinational observational study. Intensive Care Med. 2013;39(2):309–18.
45. Olotu A, Ndiritu M, Ismael M, et al. Characteristics and outcome of cardiopulmonary resuscitation in hospitalised African children. Resuscitation. 2009;80(1):69–72.
46. Olson D, Davis NL, Milazi R, et al. Development of a severity of illness scoring system (inpatient triage, assessment and treatment) for resource-constrained hospitals in developing countries. Tropical Med Int Health. 2013;18(7):871–8.
47. Agulnik A, Mora Robles LN, Forbes PW, et al. Improved outcomes after successful implementation of a pediatric early warning system (PEWS) in a resource-limited pediatric oncology hospital. Cancer. 2017;123(15):2965–74.
48. Agulnik A, Mendez Aceituno A, Mora Robles LN, et al. Validation of a pediatric early warning system for hospitalized pediatric oncology patients in a resource-limited setting. Cancer. 2017;123(24):4903–13.

Chapter 11
Acute Respiratory Failure and Management

Prakadeshwari Rajapreyar, Whitney Kopp, and Adrienne Randolph

Acute Respiratory Failure

Acute respiratory failure is a common reason for admission to the pediatric intensive care unit in oncology patients [1]. Acute respiratory complications are also common after pediatric hematopoietic stem cell transplant (HSCT), accounting for a high proportion of HSCT-related morbidity and mortality [2–4]. When pulmonary disease in HSCT patients progresses to acute respiratory failure, they often require emergent intubation and support with invasive mechanical ventilation (IMV) [3, 5]; many children develop refractory hypoxemia and multi-organ failure. Tamburro et al. reported outcomes in a cohort of mechanically ventilated pediatric oncology and HSCT patients. The non-HSCT patients had better outcomes than the HSCT patients with 6-month survival at 60% [6]. While the outcomes are better in the oncology patients, they are nevertheless worse than immunocompetent patients. Their immunocompromised status and chemotherapy-related multi-organ failure are likely complicating factors affecting outcomes in this cohort.

Focusing on the more complicated HSCT patients, intubation for HSCT-related acute lung injury (ALI) often led to early redirection of care due to high fatality two decades ago; recent reports show that outcomes have improved with improved

P. Rajapreyar (✉) · W. Kopp
Division of Pediatric Critical Care Medicine,
Medical College of Wisconsin/Children's Hospital of Wisconsin,
Milwaukee, WI, USA
e-mail: prajaprey@mcw.edu

A. Randolph
Division of Critical Care Medicine, Department of Anesthesia, Critical Care and Pain Medicine, Boston Children's Hospital, Boston, MA, USA

Departments of Anesthesia and Pediatrics, Harvard Medical School,
Boston, MA, USA

C. N. Duncan et al. (eds.), *Critical Care of the Pediatric Immunocompromised Hematology/Oncology Patient*, https://doi.org/10.1007/978-3-030-01322-6_11

survival [6–8]. Tamburro et al. demonstrated 6-month survival of 25% in the HSCT cohort, while van Gestel et al. showed a 6-month survival of 35% [6–9]. Improved outcomes are likely multifactorial, influenced by increased willingness to deliver intensive care therapies with earlier rescue and support and innovations in transplant management leading to less lung toxicity.

Acute respiratory failure with hypoxemia due to inflammation following a known clinical insult is defined as acute respiratory distress syndrome (ARDS). Oncology and HSCT patients should be closely monitored for development of pediatric ARDS (PARDS), with stratification of severity of illness to allow early and appropriate escalation of respiratory support. In 2015, the Pediatric Acute Lung Injury Consensus Conference (PALICC) guidelines defined PARDS and stratified severity [10] using the following definition:

1. Evidence of acute pulmonary parenchymal disease with unilateral of bilateral infiltrates on chest imaging
2. Hypoxemia as documented and stratified by measures of oxygenation (oxygenation index {OI}, oxygen saturation index {OSI}, arterial oxygen saturation/FiO2 ratio {P/F ratio}, oxygen saturation/Fio2 ratio {S/F ratio})
3. Symptoms of hypoxemia and chest imaging changes within 7 days of a known clinical insult
4. Above criteria not explained by left ventricular dysfunction

Lung injury in the pediatric oncology patients is related to their immunocompromised status and direct pulmonary toxicity from chemotherapy and/or radiation. Chemotherapeutic agents most commonly implicated in lung injury include bleomycin, cyclophosphamide, nitrosureas, cyclophosphamide, chlorambucil, methotrexate, procarbazine, mitomycin, cytarabine, vinca alkaloids, and alkylating agents such as busulfan [11]. Of these, bleomycin, busulfan, cyclophosphamide, and the nitrosureas are most commonly implicated in pediatric patients [11, 12]. Toxicity from radiation therapy is dose dependent with patients receiving fractionated doses having less risk for toxicity than patients receiving the same total dose given at one time. Patients typically develop symptoms within 1–3 months of receiving radiation therapy and present with cough, dyspnea, and pink-tinged sputum during the inflammatory phase. This can progress to the fibrotic stage which progresses over 1–2 years. Patients in this phase develop increasing dyspnea, oxygen requirement, and declining pulmonary function tests.

Toxicity from chemotherapeutic agents may occur early in the form of a hypersensitivity reaction which presents with rales, fever, and dyspnea while receiving the medication. Patients typically respond well to stopping the medication and administration of steroids. Endothelial injury and vascular leak causing non-cardiogenic pulmonary edema is another early pulmonary toxicity seen from drugs such as methotrexate, cytarabine, ifosfamide, cyclophosphamide, IL-2, ATRA (all trans-retinoic acid), and bleomycin. Both types of early toxicity respond well to supportive care and have a relatively good prognosis. Later pulmonary toxicity occurring several months to years after receiving the chemotherapeutic agent leads to fibrotic lung injury and has a much worse prognosis [11]. If patients respond to steroids, weaning of steroids should occur slowly and cautiously as it can reactivate the underlying disease process.

The lung injury that occurs in post-HSCT patients can be grossly classified as infectious or noninfectious [3, 13], although it could be multifactorial in some patients. Alternatively, pulmonary complications can be classified as early and late [13]. The classification into early and late (within and beyond 100 days respectively) is not absolute but may help the clinician to develop a differential diagnosis [13]. Early complications tend to be related to immune suppression, endothelial/alveolar injury, and/or neutrophil recovery. For this review, we will first focus on early or acute complications of infectious and noninfectious etiologies and later address late complications.

HSCT Patients

Initial Workup of the HSCT Patient with Acute Pulmonary Complications

Noninfectious complications after HSCT are often treated with immune suppression. Therefore, the first step in management of a HSCT patient with acute hypoxia and/or hypercarbia is to perform a thorough workup to confirm or rule out infectious etiologies (Table 11.1). These children are at high risk of death if their infection is not identified early and treated and their immune dysregulation appropriately addressed. Bacterial, viral, and fungal infections are all considerations in

Table 11.1 Workup of a child presenting with acute lung injury after HSCT

A. Respiratory testing for respiratory pathogens: (a) Viral testing extended panel of organisms with NP swab in non-intubated patients and endotracheal or bronchoalveolar lavage (BAL) when possible (b) Sensitive polymerase chain reaction (PCR) testing for respiratory syncytial virus, HSV, VZV, influenza virus, parainfluenza virus, adenovirus, human metapneumovirus, rhinovirus, coronavirus, and HHV6 at a minimum (c) Consider testing for acid fast bacilli, *Nocardia*, *Legionella* (d) Polymerase chain reaction for *Chlamydia*, *Mycoplasma*, and *Aspergillus* species (e) Consider PCP risk factors and send sensitive PCR test if present
B. Other testing to identify pathogens: (a) Routine cultures of indwelling lines for bacteria and fungi (b) Urine for legionella (c) Shell vial culture for CMV (d) Serum galactomannan ELISA for *Aspergillus* species
C. Rule out non-pulmonary causes or contributors of pulmonary dysfunction: (a) Echocardiogram to rule out cardiac dysfunction (b) Evaluation of renal function (c) Evaluate fluid status and rule out and manage iatrogenic fluid overload

Modified from https://www.atsjournals.org/doi/pdf/10.1164/rccm.2007-413ST [14]

posttransplant patients given their immunosuppression and presence of indwelling catheters and invasive lines. Identification of specific organism can help clinicians target antimicrobial therapy. Unfortunately, broad-spectrum empiric treatment is often prolonged due to delays in turnaround times and insensitivity of microbiological testing.

It is thought that a BAL should be strongly considered in patients with diffuse lung injury posttransplant [3]. However, it is prudent to consider the risk-benefit ratio and optimal timing of the BAL due to the potential for worsening lung mechanics. Triebwasser et al. in 2018 in a retrospective chart review of 593 patients of different age groups that underwent a BAL reported identification of pathogens in 30% of cases [15]. They reported that the BAL led to changes in patient management in 55% of cases, including alteration in antibiotics (37%) and immunosuppression (25%). BAL complications included hypoxemia (1%), hemorrhage (2%), and respiratory failure (1%) in patients not requiring mechanical ventilation prior to the BAL. This would suggest that an early BAL would be safe and may alter the treatment plan in more than half of cases. Prophylaxis and preemptive screening for invasive fungal and CMV infections have resulted in a decrease in their incidence posttransplant [3]. Improved molecular diagnostic techniques will likely result in improved testing yield and decreased need for prolonged empiric therapy.

Noninfectious Complications in HSCT Patients

Once infection is ruled out, children with lung injury are then categorized as either acute idiopathic pneumonia syndrome (IPS), engraftment syndrome, diffuse alveolar hemorrhage, or other lung injury syndromes. In 1993 a National Institutes of Health workshop defined IPS as widespread alveolar injury in the absence of active lower respiratory infection, cardiogenic causes, renal failure, or iatrogenic fluid overload after HSCT [3, 16]. This definition was further classified based on anatomy as interstitial, vascular, airway tissue, or unclassifiable [3, 14]. T-cell-mediated injury is supported as the primary pathophysiology by murine models. TNF-α levels have been shown to be increased in the BAL fluid of mice with IPS. This is supported by the clinical observation that patients who receive T-cell-depleted grafts have a lower incidence of pulmonary complications [13]. However other TNF- α-independent pathways may also contribute to the pathophysiology of IPS [3]. Given the TNF-α pathway-mediated injury, the soluble TNF-α-binding protein, etanercept, has been tested in a trial for treatment of IPS [17]. Early recognition of the disorder, ruling out other infectious etiologies, and initiation of corticosteroids along with other anti-inflammatory targeted therapies may improve outcomes after IPS [3].

Engraftment syndrome (ES) is characterized by fever, rash, and non-cardiogenic pulmonary edema occurring at the time of neutrophil recovery after HSCT [3, 18]. ES may be related to a graft-versus-host response or in some cases a host-versus-graft response [13]. Chang et al. reported a higher risk for developing GVHD and non-relapse-related mortality in patients with ES [19]. Corticosteroids are often effective in patients with ES [3].

Diffuse alveolar hemorrhage (DAH) originates from the pulmonary microvasculature in response to alveolar injury which may be noninfectious etiology, secondary to chemotherapy, radiation, immune-mediated events, or other systemic/pulmonary infections [3, 20]. In some cases, it is a type of IPS. Progressive bloody return is noted on BAL when performed. High-dose corticosteroids were reported to not alter the outcomes in these patients in a prospective cohort study of 103 adult HSCT patients [3, 20]. However, Rathi et al. reported that patients who received low-dose steroids had lower mortality in comparison to medium- and high-dose steroids in a cohort study of 119 adult HSCT patients [3, 21]. Wanko et al. reported a decrease in 100-day mortality (44% versus 83%) in a small group of eight adult patients with DAH, treated with concomitant aminocaproic acid and steroids [22]. Recombinant factor VIIa has been used in some patients for refractory bleeding but has not shown to improve duration of mechanical ventilation or survival [3, 13, 23].

The other lung injury syndromes to consider include radiation pneumonitis, pulmonary veno-occlusive disease, pulmonary cytolytic thrombi, transfusion-related acute lung injury, pulmonary arterial hypertension, and pulmonary thromboembolism [3, 24, 25].

Specific Infectious Complications in HSCT Patients

The type of infection identified influences patient prognosis and treatment in HSCT patients. Preemptive antiviral therapy has reduced the incidence of cytomegalovirus (CMV) infection after HSCT. Ganciclovir is typically used for treatment of CMV infection. Foscarnet can be used when cytopenias are present. Newer drugs under evaluation are maribavir, letermovir, and brincidofovir [26].

Adenovirus can cause a disseminated infection with significant mortality in HSCT patients [27]. Adenovirus titers in the serum are often used to monitor viral load and response to treatment. Cidofovir and brincidofovir have been used to treat adenoviral infection with the latter not demonstrating significant nephrotoxicity [27].

Respiratory syncytial virus (RSV) infection in immunocompromised children can rapidly progress to lower respiratory tract infection. Lower respiratory tract infection in these children has been associated with mortality attributed to RSV [28]. A recent multicenter investigation reported a low incidence of RSV infections in posttransplant patients with low utilization of critical care services and mortality [29]. It should however be noted that all patients who required critical care received treatment with ribavirin, although its benefit has not been rigorously proven in this population.

Invasive fungal infections in HSCT patients are associated with poor outcomes. Abassi et al. reported an 85% mortality within the first year after diagnosis of aspergillus infection in immunosuppressed pediatric patients [3, 30]. However, invasive fungal infections of the lung have decreased with better antifungal prophylaxis [3,

30–33]. Fungal infections also often require aggressive surgical intervention due to the patients underlying immunosuppression.

Pneumocystis jiroveci pneumonia (PJP) develops in 5–15% of pediatric HSCT patients, without prophylaxis, with a mortality rate higher than 50%. However this is rare with the advent of routine prophylaxis [34].

Late Pulmonary Complications in HSCT Patients

Bronchiolitis obliterans syndrome (BOS) and cryptogenic organizing pneumonia (COP) are late-onset noninfectious pulmonary complications of HSCT [13] often requiring chest computed tomography (CT) or lung biopsy to make the diagnosis. BOS is a progressive obstructive disease with onset 3–24 months posttransplant. Patients typically present with wheezing and dyspnea. Chest CT may demonstrate air trapping, centrilobular nodules, or bronchiectasis. Histology demonstrates bronchiolar inflammation with luminal obstruction [3]. COP is a restrictive lung disease with onset 2–12 months posttransplant with acute onset fever, cough, and dyspnea. Chest CT may demonstrate patchy airspace disease or nodular opacities. Histology reveals intraluminal organizing fibrosis in distal airspaces with mild interstitial inflammation [3]. Both BOS and COP are related to T-cell-mediated injury to lung epithelial cells, and Initial therapy is usually high-dose corticosteroids burst with a prolonged taper over months [3, 13]. Other therapies such as azithromycin, cyclosporine, and etanercept have been described and need further evaluation [3, 13]. A recent trial of inhaled fluticasone, azithromycin, and montelukast in patients with new-onset bronchiolitis obliterans showed that the combination therapy had improvement in ability to stabilize disease progression when compared to historical controls [35].

Respiratory Support

The transition from negative pressure ventilation to positive pressure ventilation results in significant changes in cardiopulmonary interactions. This is well known in patients with mediastinal masses impinging on great vessels or large pericardial effusions. Maintaining spontaneous ventilation, using specialized equipment (fiber-optic bronchoscope), avoiding the use of paralytics, and having extracorporeal membrane oxygenation (ECMO) equipment on standby are important considerations [13]. This transition can also result in cardiopulmonary collapse in patients with right heart failure and in patients who are intravascularly depleted such as patients in septic shock or hypovolemic shock. The former may be seen due to cardiac toxicity from chemotherapy and/or radiation or from pulmonary hypertension. Optimization of intravascular volume, use of inotropes to augment ventricular function, and availability of inhaled nitric oxide to avert a pulmonary hypertensive crisis might help prevent the need for cardiopulmonary resuscitation during this transition.

Noninvasive Ventilation (NIV)

Endotracheal intubation is associated with many complications, with highest concern being that of ventilator associated pneumonia [36]. Noninvasive positive pressure ventilation consists of continuous positive airway pressure (CPAP) and bi-level positive airway pressure (BiPAP). These modalities can assist in oxygenation and ventilation in patients with respiratory distress and acute respiratory failure while potentially avoiding the complications of invasive mechanical ventilation (IMV) [37]. Continuous positive airway pressure (CPAP) maintains positive pressure and prevents airway and alveolar collapse in patients who are spontaneously breathing [38]. BiPAP is triggered by the patient's breath and an inspiratory positive airway pressure (IPAP) is provided while preventing airway and alveolar collapse with expiratory positive airway pressure (EPAP) [36–38]. A respiratory rate is also set on BiPAP, which can sometimes lead to dysynchrony between the mandatory breaths and the patient's innate respiratory efforts.

While NIV can potentially allow the avoidance of intubation and IMV, there are certain clinical scenarios that are considered contraindications to the use of NIV [36, 39]. The contraindications relate to the patient's inability to protect their airway with risk of aspiration, worsening gastric distension, and/or inability to provide consistent intrathoracic positive pressure with associated risks. The contraindications for NIV use can be listed as follows:

1. High risk of respiratory or cardiac arrest
2. Hemodynamic instability (dysrhythmias or shock)
3. Absent or weak cough or gag with inability to protect airway
4. Glasgow coma score < 8
5. Rapidly progressive neuromuscular weakness
6. Inability for good mask fit (facial surgery, trauma, burns, etc.)
7. Untreated pneumothorax
8. Vomiting and risk of aspiration
9. Poor skin integrity leading to skin breakdown

Much of NIV data available is in the immunocompromised patients with a dearth of data in the more specific hematopoietic stem cell transplant (HSCT) patients. NIV has been shown in some adult studies to reduce intubation rates, shorten ICU length of stay, and reduce the cost of hospitalization [40–44]. A meta-analysis by Wang et al. [45] looked at NIV versus IMV in all immunocompromised patients; the ICU length of stay was significantly shorter in the NIV group. This was however in patients with lower severity of illness scores [45]. Additionally, this group found a significant decrease in hospital mortality in NIV groups compared to IMV groups though there was high degree of heterogeneity. Within the hematologic and solid tumors subgroups, the 30-day mortality was significantly reduced with OR 0.34 (95% CI 0.22–0.54) when NIV was compared to IMV [45, 46]. Similarly, in a retrospective review of immunocompromised pediatric patients receiving NIV, Pancera et al. found that in the NIV group, there was a higher probability of 30-day survival (46.8%) when compared to the IMV (23.3%) [37]. However, more patients in the IMV group had markers of higher illness severity as evidenced by more than two organ failure, cardiovascular dysfunction, and therapeutic interventions scoring system score of ≥40.

NIV is not uniformly successful, and a growing body of evidence is aimed at determining factors that lead to failure of this modality in this at-risk population [37, 39, 47]. Literature reports a NIV success rate in immunocompromised pediatric patients of 54.5% with diagnosis of acute respiratory distress syndrome and up to 74.2% with diagnosis of respiratory failure [37, 47]. Among all patients with acute respiratory failure who received NIV, $FiO_2 > 80\%$ 1 h after initiation predicted failure of NIV [48]. Within pediatric immunocompromised patients, those who failed NIV were more likely to have severe sepsis and septic shock than those in the success group [47]. Patients in the NIV success group had early and sustained improvement compared to those who failed; therefore, lack of early improvement is discussed with the threshold of improvement being between 1 h and 2–4 h [47–50]. Munoz-Bonet et al. determined that an improvement in respiratory rate and pCO_2 2–4 h after NIV was associated with NIV success. Patients who had improvement of their PaO_2/FiO_2 ratio within the first hour of NIV initiation also were more likely to be in the NIV success group [49]. Therefore, a lack of improvement in physiologic parameters, such as weaning FiO2 or decreasing respiratory rate, within 2–4 h of NIV initiation should be considered an indication for endotracheal intubation (Fig. 11.1) [36]. Additionally, it appears prudent to consider patients with escalating hemodynamic support to have failed NIV trial.

NIV is associated with pressure-related pain/skin breakdown due to face masks and straps which at extremes may necessitate intubation if not addressed early [49]. NIV requires synchrony between the patient and ventilator, without which a patient may also fail NIV; however, there is little to no mention of this in the literature [36]. NIV can also be used in palliative care situations to alleviate air hunger [36] and in adult studies has been shown to decrease dyspnea and reduce the amount of morphine used [51].

NIV is a viable method of oxygenation and ventilation in immunocompromised patients with respiratory failure. However, controversy exists on the use of NIV in patients with acute respiratory failure due to potential for prolonging time to intubation, ultimately leading to worse outcomes [52].

It is therefore important to understand that while NIV potentially avoids complications of IMV, its utilization requires constant monitoring of the patient to ensure improvement. Lack of physiologic improvement should be considered an indication for endotracheal intubation, provided that would be reasonable for the patient's underlying disease and consistent with goals of care outlined by the family.

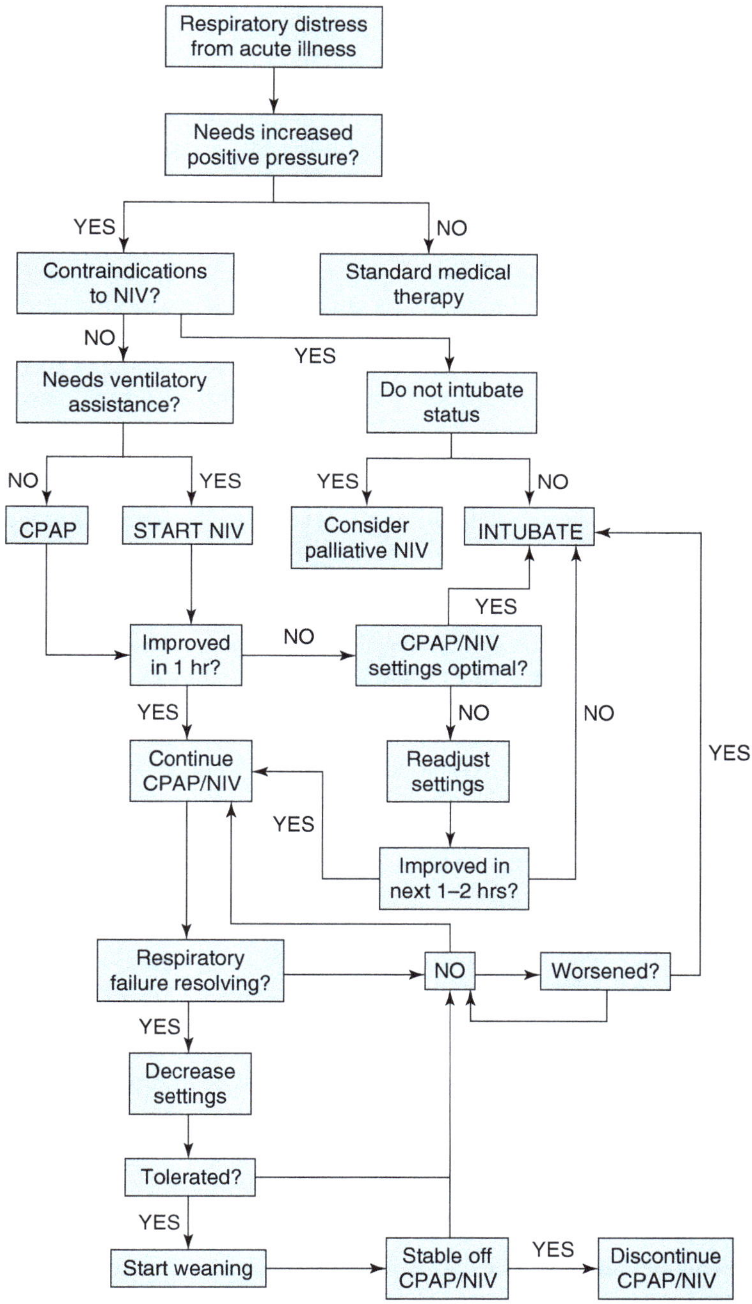

Fig. 11.1 Algorithm for initiation and weaning of NIV [36]. (Used with permission)

Invasive Mechanical Ventilation

Mortality with respiratory failure in pediatric oncology and HSCT patients varies depending on the underlying clinical diagnosis and etiology. Tamburro et al. reported an overall survival of 59% to extubation and discharge, in mechanically ventilated pediatric oncology patients and HSCT patients [6]. Aspesberro et al. cited 25% survival at 6 months in pediatric HSCT patients who were mechanically ventilated [53]. The reason for intubation such as elective for a procedure or emergent due to lung failure and the degree of lung injury is important to consider. Given the high mortality, it is important to urgently rediscuss goals of care and code status for patients with irreversible underlying disease and a few months or less to live, where it may prolong suffering. In a multicenter retrospective cohort study between 2009 and 2014 of 242 HSCT patients, the PICU mortality was noted to be 60.4%. Patients ventilated longer than 15 days had 2.4 times higher odds of death, and 40% of patients were placed on high-frequency oscillatory ventilation (HFOV) with a higher mortality of 76.5%. Transition to HFOV within 2 days of start of invasive mechanical ventilation resulted in a 76% decrease in the odds of death compared to those who were transitioned later [52]. The study suggests that early and aggressive lung protective ventilation strategies may result in improved outcomes in these patients.

In hypoxemic respiratory failure, the more common reason for hypoxemia is likely alveolar derecruitment. Optimizing alveolar recruitment using adequate positive end expiratory pressure (PEEP) while limiting peak inspiratory pressures (PIP) thereby avoiding further ventilator-induced lung injury (VILI) should be the goal with invasive mechanical ventilation. Permissive hypercapnia and hypoxia while ensuring adequate end-organ oxygen delivery would help achieve these goals in these patients. Severity of lung injury in intubated patients with hypoxemic respiratory failure can be estimated using OI and OSI [10]. OI has shown to also be a predictor of mortality [54–56]. An OI $\geq$ 20 at any point during ventilation in post-transplant patients has been shown to be associated with 94% mortality, while an OI $\geq$ 25 was associated with 100% mortality [55].

Consistent with optimizing lung recruitment and preventing further ventilator-induced lung injury, the Pediatric Acute Lung Injury Consensus Conference (PALICC) guidelines recommend utilization of moderately elevated levels of PEEP titrated to observed oxygenation and hemodynamic response and recommend tidal volumes of 3–6 and 5–8 ml/kg ideal body weight based on respiratory system compliance. High PEEP levels may be required in children with large abdominal masses or ascites causing significant mechanical constraints on the diaphragm, interfering with lung mechanics and causing significant lung derecruitment.

PALICC guidelines recommend consideration of HFOV when plateau pressures exceed 28 cm H_2O. Thereby, if one is not able to achieve lung recruitment without utilization of high ventilation strategies, one should consider escalation to other non-conventional modalities that are considered lung protective [10]. Airway pressure release ventilation (APRV) is another modality that has been used by some centers. Rowan et al. in a retrospective multicenter database study reported on 85 pediatric

HSCT patients with severe PARDS managed with HFOV. The study suggested that in that cohort, early use of HFOV was associated with improved survival compared to late implementation of HFOV, and the subjects had outcomes similar to those treated only with conventional mechanical ventilation [57]. There continues to be a need for more outcome data with HFOV and APRV use in pediatric patients with respiratory failure. Yehya et al. in a cohort of pediatric patients, refractory to conventional mechanical ventilation requiring transition to HFOV or APRV, demonstrated that HFOV was associated with more frequent neuromuscular blockade with no difference in mortality [56]. Perhaps more important is to observe the improvement in OI at 6–24 h after transition to HFOV and APRV which has been associated with survival, likely reflecting severity of lung disease and/or the ability to re-recruit the lungs [54, 56, 58]. In conclusion, lung protective ventilation should be implemented early in this cohort of children given the high risk of mortality and morbidity.

Extracorporeal Membrane Oxygenation (ECMO) as Rescue Therapy

Pediatric oncology and HSCT patients with severe PARDS should be evaluated for possible ECMO support when lung protective strategies result in inadequate gas exchange [10]. Immunocompromised status was demonstrated to be an independent risk factor for hospital mortality in adult patients with respiratory failure on ECMO [59]. Establishing set criteria for ECMO cannulation in this population is challenging given their immunocompromised status, thrombocytopenia, unique/varying range of pathologies, and multi-organ dysfunction. Gow et al. in 2006 reported a 21% survival rate to decannulation in a small cohort of 19 pediatric HSCT patients [60]. Renal complications and multi-organ dysfunction were reported to be risk factors for death. It thereby appears prudent to make the decision regarding cannulation by utilizing a multidisciplinary approach early in the disease process, to determine candidacy and timing of cannulation and allow serial evaluation. The patient's family should be appropriately counseled and informed consent obtained prior to ECMO cannulation given the high risk of complications in this patient population.

Ancillary Therapies (Fluid Management, Inhaled Nitric Oxide, and Surfactant)

Fluid overload is common in HSCT patients who develop PARDS. Initiation of empiric broad-spectrum antimicrobial treatment often exacerbates this situation. Tight fluid management is imperative along with initiation of diuretics in many patients. Clinical orders to limit total fluids at maintenance, to concentrate all medications and infusions, and to evaluate the need for medications that have a high volume of fluid should be done early to avoid worsening fluid overload. Acute renal failure is not an uncommon complication in posttransplant patients, and it makes fluid management extremely challenging. Fluid overload associated with acute renal failure leads to worsening respiratory function, prolonged ventilation, increased ICU stay, and mortality [61–66]. Early consultation of renal specialists and intervention with diuretics and advanced therapies for fluid removal is imperative. In a retrospective chart review of 113 critically ill pediatric patients receiving continuous veno-venous hemofiltration, median fluid overload percentage was significantly lower in survivors versus non-survivors (7.8% vs. 15.1%) [65]. Michael et al. reviewed 26 HSCT patients with acute renal failure and noted a fluid overload of <10% was associated with improved survival [66]. Ellbahlawan et al. demonstrated a significant improvement in the PaO2/FiO2 ratio in HSCT patients after initiation of continuous renal replacement therapy, which significantly correlated, with reduction of fluid balance [67]. Initiation of CRRT for treatment of fluid overload may improve oxygenation and survival [3].

The use of inhaled nitric oxide can be considered in patients with documented pulmonary hypertension or severe right ventricular dysfunction [10]. PALICC guidelines also recommend consideration of use as a rescue or bridge to ECMO [10].

Surfactant use in immunocompromised children with acute lung injury was associated with improved oxygenation in a post hoc analysis of data from a previous randomized control trial [68]. A subsequent FDA-funded multicenter trial that attempted to investigate utility of surfactant in this cohort was unfortunately stopped due to low enrollment. Therefore, there remains a lack of evidence supporting the efficacy of surfactant use in this patient population.

Conclusion

Immunocompromised oncology patients, including HSCT patients are a unique patient population with unique pathologies and other organ dysfunction leading to respiratory failure. Evaluation of a HSCT patient with acute hypoxia and/or hypercarbia requires a workup to confirm or rule out infectious etiologies prior to treatment for potential noninfectious causes. Utilization of NIV requires constant monitoring of the patient to ensure improvement. The lack of physiological improvement on NIV should be considered an indication for endotracheal intubation. Early and aggressive lung protective ventilation strategies upon intubation with close monitoring for fluid overload may result in improved outcomes in these patients. Further research is required to look at other modifiable clinical factors/management techniques and to assess outcomes after the use of NIV, IMV, and ECMO in this unique population.

References

1. Sivan Y, Schwrtz PH, Schonfeld T, et al. Outcome of oncology patients in the pediatric intensive care unit. Intensive Care Med. 1991;17:11–5.
2. Eikenberry M, Bartakova H, Defor T, et al. Natural history of pulmonary complications in children after bone marrow transplantation. Biol Blood Marrow Transplant. 2005;11:56–64.
3. Elbahlawan L, Srinivasan A, Morrison RR. A critical care and transplant-based approach to acute respiratory failure after hematopoietic stem cell transplantation in children. Biol Bood Marrow Transplant. 2016;22(4):617–26.
4. Crawford SW, Hackman RC. Clinical course of idiopathic pneumonia after bone marrow transplantation. Am Rev Resp Dis. 1993;147:1393–400.
5. Clark JG, Madtes DK, Martin TR, et al. Idiopathic pneumonia after bone marrow transplantation: cytokine activation and lipopolysaccharide amplification in the bronchoalveolar compartment. Crit Care Med. 1999;27:1800–6.
6. Tamburro RF, Barfield RC, Shaffer ML, et al. Changes in out- comes (1996–2004) for pediatric oncology and hematopoietic stem cell transplant patients requiring invasive mechanical ventilation. Pediatr Crit Care Med. 2008;9(3):270–7.
7. van Gestel JPJ, Bollen CW, Bierings MB, et al. Survival in a recent cohort of mechanically ven- tilated allogeneic hematopoietic stem cell transplantation recipients. Biol Blood Marrow Transplant. 2008;14(12):1385–93.
8. Aspesberro F, Guthrie KA, Woolfrey AE, et al. Outcome of pediatric stem cell transplant recipients requiring mechanical ventilation. J Intensive Care Med. 2014;29(1):31–7.
9. Rowan CM, Smith LS, Loomis A, et al. Pediatric acute respiratory distress syndrome in pediatric allogeneic hematopoietic stem cell transplants: a multicenter study. Pediatr Crit Care Med. 2017;18:304–9.
10. The Pediatric Acute Lung Injury Consensus Conference Group. Pediatric acute respiratory distress syndrome: consensus recommendations from the pediatric acute lung injury consensus conference. Pediatr Crit Care Med. 2015;16(5):428–39.
11. Schwartz C, Hobbie WL, Constine LS, Ruccione K. Chapter 11: Pulmonary effects of antineoplastic therapy. In: Survivors of childhood and adolescent cancer: a multidisciplinary approach. 3rd ed. New York: Springer International Publishing; 2015. p. 201–27.
12. Huang TT, Hudson MM, Stokes DC, Krasin MJ, Spunt SL, Ness KK. Pulmonary outcomes in survivors of childhood cancer a systematic review. Chest. 2011;140(4):881–901.
13. Fuhrmann BP, Zimmerman J. Chapter 38: Critical illness involving children undergoing hematopoietic progenitor cell transplantation. In: Pediatric critical care. 5th ed. Philadelphia: Elsevier Inc; 2016. p.1325–42.
14. Panoskaltsis-Mortari A, Griese M, Madtes DK, et al. An official American Thoracic Society research statement: noninfectious lung injury after hematopoietic stem cell transplantation: idiopathic pneumonia syndrome. Am J Respir Crit Care Med. 2011;183:1262–79.
15. Triebwasser M, Duvall A, Hoffman T, et al. Impact of broncho-alveolar lavage on the diagnosis and management of pulmonary complications following hematopoietic cell transplantation. Biol Blood Marrow Transplant. 2018;24(3):s98.
16. Clark JG, Hertz MI, Parkman R, et al. Idiopathic pneumonia syndrome after bone marrow transplantation. Am Rev Respir Dis. 1993;147:1601–6.
17. Yanik GA, Grupp SA, Pulsipher MA, et al. TNF-receptor inhibitor therapy for the treatment of children with idiopathic pneumonia syndrome. A joint pediatric blood and marrow transplant consortium and children's oncology group study (ASCT0521). Biol Blood Marrow Transplant. 2015;21:67–73.
18. Spitzer TR. Engraftment syndrome following hematopoietic stem cell transplantation. Bone Marrow Transplant. 2001;27:893–8.
19. Chang L, Frame D, Braun T, et al. Engraftment syndrome following allogeneic hematopoietic cell transplantation predicts poor outcomes. Biol Blood Marrow Transplant. 2014;20:1407–17.

20. Majhail NS, Parks K, Defor TE, et al. Diffuse alveolar hemorrhage and infection- associated alveolar hemorrhage following hematopoietic stem cell transplantation: related and high-risk clinical syndromes. Biol Blood Marrow Transplant. 2006;12:1038–46.
21. Rathi NK, Tanner AR, Dinh A, et al. Low-, medium-and high dose steroids with or without aminocaproic acid in adult hematopoietic SCT patients with diffuse alveolar hemorrhage. Bone Marrow Transplant. 2015;50:420–6.
22. Wanko SO, Broadwater G, Folz RJ, et al. Diffuse alveolar hemorrhage: retrospective review of clinical outcome in allogeneic transplant recipients treated with aminocaproic acid. Biol Blood Marrow Transplant. 2006;12:949–53.
23. Elinoff JM, Bagci U, Moriyama B, et al. Recombinant human factor VIIa for aleveolar hemorrhage following allogeneic stem cell transplantation. Biol Blood Marrow Transplant. 2014;20:969–78.
24. Troussard X, Bernaudin JF, Cordonnier C, et al. Pulmonary veno-occlusive disease after bone marrow transplantation. Thorax. 1984;39:956–7.
25. Woodard JP, Gulbahce E, Shreve M, et al. Pulmonary cytolytic thrombi: a newly recognized complication of stem cell transplantation. Bone Marrow Transplant. 2000;25:293–300.
26. Boeckh M, Murphy WJ, Peggs KS. Recent advances in cytomegalovirus: an update on pharmacologic and cellular therapies. Biol Blood Marrow Transplant. 2015;21:24–9.
27. Hiwarkar P, Amrolia P, Sivaprakasam P, et al. Brincidofovir is highly efficacious in controlling adenoviremia in pediatric recipients of hematopoietic cell transplant. Blood. 2017;129:2033–7.
28. Khanna N, Widmer AF, Decker M, et al. Respiratory syncytial virus infection in patients with hematological diseases: single center study and review of literature. Clin Infect Dis. 1999;29:1210–9.
29. Rowan CM, Gertz SJ, Zinter MS, et al. A multicenter investigation of respiratory syncytial viral infection in children with hematopietic cell transplantation. Transpl Infect Dis. 2018; doi:https://doi.org/10.1111/tid.12882 (epub ahead of print).
30. Abbasi S, Shenep JL, Hughes WT, et al. Aspergillosis in children with cancer: a 34-year experience. Clin Infect Dis. 1999;29:1210–9.
31. Alsharif M, Cameron SEH, Young JAH, et al. Time trends in fungal infections as a cause of death in hematopoietic stem cell transplant recipients. Am J Clin Pathol. 2009;132:746–55.
32. van Burik JH, Leisenring W, Myerson D, et al. The effect of prophylactic fluconazole on the clinical spectrum of fungal disease in bone marrow transplant recipients with special attention to hepatic candidiasis. An autopsy study of 355 patients. Medicine. 1998;77:246–54.
33. Maron GM, Hayden RT, Rodriguez A, et al. Voriconazole prophylaxis in children with cancer: changing outcomes and epidemiology of fungal infections. Pediatr Infect Dis J. 2013;32:e451–5.
34. Levy ER, Musick L, Zinter MS, et al. Safe and effective prophylaxis with bimonthly pentamidine in the pediatric hematopoietic stem cell transplant population. Pediatr Infect Dis J. 2016;35:135–41.
35. Williams KM, Cheng GS, Pusic I, Jagasia M, Burns L, Ho VT, Pidala J, Palmer J, Johnston L, Mayer S, Chien JW, Jacobsohn DA, Pavletic SZ, Martin PJ, Storer BE, Inamoto Y, Chai X, Flowers MED, Lee SJ. FAM treatment for new onset bronchiolitis obliterans syndrome after hematopoietic cell transplantation. Biol Blood Marrow Transplant. 2016;22(4):710–6.
36. Venkataraman S. Noninvasive ventilation: concepts and practice. In: Pediatric critical care. Elsevier, Inc: Philadelphia; 2017. p. 770–84.
37. Pancera CF, Hayashi M, Fregnani JH, et al. Noninvasive ventilation in immunocompromised pediatric patients: eight years of experience in a pediatric oncology intensive care unit. J Pediatr Hematol Oncol. 2008;30(7):533–8.
38. Fuhrmann BP, Zimmerman J. Airway management. In: Pediatric critical care. 5th. Elsevier Inc: Philadelphia; 2016.
39. Bello G, De Pascale G, Antonelli M. Noninvasive ventilation for the immunocompromised patient: always appropriate? Curr Opin Crit Care. 2012;18(1):54–60.
40. Popat B, Jones AT. Invasive and non-invasive mechanical ventilation. Medicine. 2012;40(6):298–304.

41. Yanez LJ, Yunge M, Emilfork M, et al. A prospective, randomized, controlled trial of noninvasive ventilation in pediatric acute respiratory failure. Pediatr Crit Care Med. 2008;9(5):484–9.
42. Mayordomo-Colunga J, Pons M, Lopez Y, et al. Predicting non-invasive ventilation failure in children from the SpO2/FiO2 (SF) ratio. Intensive Care Med. 2013;39(6):1095–103.
43. Mehta S, Hill NS. Noninvasive ventilation. Am J Respir Crit Care Med. 2001;163(2):540–77.
44. Carron M. A new horizon for the use of non-invasive ventilation in patients with acute respiratory distress syndrome. Ann Transl Med. 2016;4(18):348.
45. Wang T, Zhang L, Luo K, et al. Noninvasive versus invasive mechanical ventilation for immunocompromised patients with acute respiratory failure: a systematic review and meta-analysis. BMC Pulm Med. 2016;16(1):129.
46. Azoulay E, Alberti C, Bronstain C, et al. Improved survival in cancer patients requiring mechanical ventilatory support: impact of noninvasive mechanical ventilatory support. Crit Care Med. 2001;29(3):519–25.
47. Piastra M, De Luca D, Pietrini D, et al. Noninvasive pressure-support ventilation in immunocompromised children with ARDS: a feasibility study. Intensive Care Med. 2009;35(8):1420–7.
48. Bernet V, Hug MI, Frey B. Predictive factors for the success of noninvasive mask ventilation in infants and children with acute respiratory failure. Pediatr Crit Care Med. 2005;6(6):660–4.
49. Munoz-Bonet JI, Flor-Macian EM, Brines J, et al. Predictive factors for the outcome of noninvasive ventilation in pediatric acute respiratory failure. Pediatr Crit Care Med. 2010;11(6):675–80.
50. Piastra M, De Luca D, Marzano L, et al. The number of failing organs predicts non-invasive ventilation failure in children with ALI/ARDS. Intensive Care Med. 2011;37(9):1510–6.
51. Nava S, Ferrer M, Esquinas A, et al. Palliative use of non-invasive ventilation in end-of-life patients with solid tumours: a randomised feasibility trial. Lancet Oncol. 2013;14(3):219–27.
52. Rowan CM, Gertz SJ, McArthur J, et al. Invasive mechanical ventilation and mortality in pediatric hematopoietic stem cell transplantation: a muticenter study. Pediatr Crit Care Med. 2016;17(4):294–302.
53. Aspesberro F, Guthrie KA, Woolfrey AE, et al. Outcome of pediatric hematopoietic stem cell transplant recipients requiring mechanical ventilation. J Intensive Care Med. 2014;29(1):31–7.
54. Sarnaik AP, Meert KL, Pappas MD, et al. Predicting outcome in children with severe acute respiratory failure treated with high-frequency ventilation. Crit Care Med. 1996;24(8):1396–402.
55. Rowan CM, Hege KM, Speicher RH, et al. Oxygenation index predicts mortality in pediatric stem cell transplant recipients requiring mechanical ventilation. Pediatr Transplant. 2012;16(6):645–50.
56. Yehya N, Topjian AA, Lin R, et al. High frequency oscillation and airway pressure release ventilation in pediatric respiratory failure. Pediatr Pulmonol. 2014;49(7):707–15.
57. Rowan CM, Loomis A, McArthur J, et al. High-frequency oscillatory ventilation use and severe PARDS in the pediatric hematopoietic stem cell transplant recipient. Respir Care. 2018;63(4):404–11.
58. Yehya N, Topijan AA, Thomas NJ, et al. Improved oxygenation 24 hours after transition to airway pressure release ventilation or high-frequency oscillatory ventilation accurately discriminated survival in immunocompromised pediatric patients with acute respiratory distress syndrome. Pediatr Crit Care Med. 2014;15:e147–56.
59. Schmidt M, Bailey M, Sheldrake J, et al. Predicting survival after extracorporeal membrane oxygenation for severe acute respiratory failure: the Respiratory Extracorporeal Membrane Oxygenation Survival Prediction (RESP) score. Am J Respir Crit Care Med. 2014;189:1374–82.
60. Gow KW, Wulkan ML, Heiss KF, et al. Extracorporeal membrane oxygenation for support of children after hematopoietic stem cell transplantation: the extracorporeal life support Oragnization experience. J Pediatr Surg. 2006;41:662–7.
61. Mehta RL, Pasual MT, Soroko S, et al. PICARD study group: diuretics, mortality, and nonrecovery of renal function in acute renal failure. JAMA. 2002;288:2547–53.

62. Flynn JT. Choice of dialysis modality for management of pediatric acute renal failure. Pediatr Nephrol. 2002;17:61–9.
63. Smoyer WE, McAdams C, Kaplan BS, et al. Determinants of survival in pediatric continuous hemofiltration. J Am Soc Nephrol. 1995;6:1401–9.
64. Klee KM, Greenleaf K, Fouser L, et al. Continuous venovenous hemofiltration with and without dialysis in pediatric patients. ANNA J. 1996;23:35–9.
65. Foland JA, Fortenberry JD, Warshaw BL, et al. Fluid overload before continuous hemofiltration and survival in critically ill children: a retrospective analysis. Pediatr Crit Care. 2001;32(8):1771–6.
66. Michael M, Kuehnle I, Goldstein SL. Fluid overload and acute renal failure in pediatric stem cell transplant patients. Pediatr Nephrol. 2004;19:91–5.
67. Elbahlawan L, West NK, Avent Y, et al. Impact of continuous renal replacement therapy on oxygenation in children with acute lung injury after allogeneic hematopoietic stem cell transplantation. Pediatr Blood Cancer. 2010;55:540–5.
68. Tamburro RF, Thomas NJ, Pon S, et al. Pediatric acute lung injury and sepsis investigators (PALISI) network. Post hoc analysis of calfactant use in immunocompromised children with acute lung injury: impact and feasibility of further clinical trials. Pediatr Crit Care Med. 2008;9:459–64.

Chapter 12
Cardiac Dysfunction in Hematology Oncology and Hematopoietic Cell Transplant Patients

Saad Ghafoor, Marshay James, Jason Goldberg, and Jennifer A. McArthur

Introduction

There are approximately 14.5 million cancer survivors in the USA and approximately 16,000 new diagnoses of cancer in patients less than 20 years of age annually. In pediatric cancer patients, the 3-year survival rate is upward of 80% [1]. Cardiotoxicity is the leading cause of morbidity and mortality in long-term survivors of pediatric cancer. These patients are nine times as likely to have a cerebrovascular event, ten times

S. Ghafoor (✉)
Department of Pediatrics, Division of Critical Care Medicine,
St. Jude Children's Research Hospital, Memphis, TN, USA
e-mail: Saad.ghafoor@stjude.org

M. James
Vanderbilt University School of Nursing, Nashville, TN, USA
Department of Pediatrics, Division of Critical Care Medicine,
St. Jude Children's Research Hospital, Memphis, TN, USA

Department of Pediatrics, Division of Critical Care Medicine,
St. Jude Children's Research Hospital, Memphis, TN, USA
e-mail: Shay.james@stjude.org

J. Goldberg
Pediatric Cardiomyopathy and Heart Transplantation,
University of Tennessee School of Health Sciences, Memphis, TN, USA

Department of Pediatrics, Division of Critical Care Medicine,
St. Jude Children's Research Hospital, Memphis, TN, USA
e-mail: Jgoldbe4@uthsc.edu

J. A. McArthur
Department of Pediatrics, Division of Critical Care Medicine,
St. Jude Children's Research Hospital, Memphis, TN, USA

Medical College of Wisconsin, Milwaukee, WI, USA
e-mail: Jennifer.mcarthur@stjude.org

C. N. Duncan et al. (eds.), *Critical Care of the Pediatric Immunocompromised Hematology/Oncology Patient*, https://doi.org/10.1007/978-3-030-01322-6_12

more likely to have coronary artery disease, and fifteen times more likely to have heart failure than their siblings. Therefore, there is a need for providers with specialized knowledge to care for this unique population both in the acute and chronic setting [2]. Cardiac complications of sickle cell disease are also increasingly recognized [3].

Normal Heart Tissue Anatomy

The heart has three layers of tissue: endocardium, myocardium, and epicardium.

The epicardium is responsible for producing pericardial fluid for lubrication. The endocardium closely resembles the endothelial tissue and lines the inner surface of the heart, forming a vascular network to maintain the function of cardiac myocytes; the endocardium also contains the conduction system fibers. The myocardium is highly vascular and always open to perfusion. It relies on a complex arteriocapillary system as there are no major vessels to perfuse this tissue. Any damage to these myocardial capillaries results in poor perfusion and decreased contractility. The major blood supply to the heart is from the right and left coronary arteries. They originate from the root of the aorta, and the left divides into the left main and the left circumflex arteries.

Heart Failure and Therapy-Related Cardiotoxicity

Heart failure is a clinico-pathological syndrome of structural and functional defects of the heart, rendering it unable to maintain adequate cardiac output to meet the demands of vital organs and peripheral tissues. There are many definitions that describe cardiotoxicity in pediatric oncology patients, but none are comprehensive enough to account for baseline risk or to guide clinical outcomes. The National Cancer Institute (NCI) of the National Institutes of Health (NIH) has published standardized definitions for adverse events (AEs), known as the Common Terminology Criteria for Adverse Events (CTCAE). They define heart failure based on grades. Grade 1 is asymptomatic elevation of biomarkers or abnormalities on imaging. Grades 2 and 3 consist of grade 1 plus mild to moderate symptoms upon exertion. Grade 4 includes life-threatening symptoms requiring hemodynamic support, and Grade 5 involves death [4]. Common pathological causes of heart failure in oncology and hematopoietic cell transplant patients are discussed below.

Pathophysiology of Radiation-Induced Heart Damage (RIHD)

Tissue irradiation leads to fibrosis. Fibrosis is both an acute and late effect of tissue irradiation. Within minutes of radiation exposure, there is vasodilation, increased vascular permeability, and increased expression of adhesion molecules and growth factors. This prompts an acute inflammatory response and an influx of cytokines. The most commonly involved cytokines are tumor necrosis factor (TNF) and interleukins (IL-1, IL-6, and IL-8). After a few hours of radiation exposure, pro-fibrotic cytokines are released. The common ones are platelet-derived growth factor (PDGF), transforming growth factor B (TGF-B), basic fibroblast growth factor (bFGF), insulin-like growth factor (IGF), and connective tissue growth factor (CTGF). The expression of proto-oncogenes, including c-myc and c-jun, promotes fibrotic changes. Resulting endothelial damage triggers the coagulation cascade and results in fibrin deposition. The acute phase of radiation-induced damage can last for several days, after which there is usually a period with no obvious microvascular damage.

There are further pathways leading to fibrosis. Mediators such as chronic hypoxia and chronic oxidative stress can result in free radical production. In turn, this increases inflammatory mediators, proteases, and adhesion molecules and decreases nitric oxide. All of these mechanisms have the potential to further damage the endothelium. Upregulation of nuclear factor kappa B (NF-KB), a transcription factor, is a key link between oxidative stress and inflammatory pathways. Chronic hypoxia leads to upregulation of hypoxia-inducible factor (HIFIa), stimulating TGF-B and leading to fibrosis [5].

The microvasculature is more affected with subendothelial fibrosis than the large arteries, which are usually spared. Coronary arteries can develop endothelial damage, vasculopathy, and ischemia. Progressive fibrosis of myocardium leads to decrease in tissue elasticity and compliance resulting in diastolic and systolic dysfunction. A compensatory upregulation of beta-receptors preserves and stabilizes cardiac output, but as damage progresses, congestive heart failure can develop. Fibrotic valvular changes can also occur, though the exact mechanism of such is not well understood. Fibrosis of the pericardium results in a spectrum of pathologies ranging from mild constrictive physiology, severe restriction resulting in tamponade, to that of global pancarditis. Conduction system abnormalities are likely due to microvascular damage and damage to sinoatrial and atrioventricular nodes, typically presenting as heart block. Fibrosis of the left ventricle can lead to ventricular ectopy, such as premature ventricular contractions (PVCs) and ventricular tachycardia.

RIHD results in significant morbidity and mortality and requires further understanding of the pathophysiology for the development of therapeutic targets to prevent microvascular damage, inflammation and late fibrosis [6].

Pathophysiology of Renin Angiotensin-Aldosterone System (RAAS) Induced Cardiovascular Damage

The renin angiotensin-aldosterone system (RAAS) is an important physiological system that maintains intravascular blood volume and blood pressure. It involves various organ systems such as the central nervous system, kidneys, liver, lungs, and adrenal glands. When there is decreased cardiac output, poor renal perfusion, low blood pressure, or blood volume for any reason, RAAS becomes activated. This causes renin to be released into the bloodstream secondary to various mechanisms:

1. Afferent arteriole dilation (baroreceptors) in response to low blood pressure.
2. Increased sodium reabsorption due to reduced GFR (poor renal perfusion), sensing of low sodium load at the macula densa (chemoreceptors), which in turn release nitric oxide and prostaglandins to cause the release of renin.
3. Carotid bodies (baroreceptors) sensing low blood pressure cause an increased sympathetic outflow which directly stimulates beta-receptors on the juxtaglomerular apparatus and cause renin release.

Renin converts angiotensinogen into angiotensin I, which gets converted by pulmonary capillary endothelium into angiotensin II and inhibition of bradykinin (vasodilator). The overall result is very potent vasoconstriction.

Angiotensin II is subsequently responsible for:

1. Directly stimulating the sympathetic nervous system by decreasing reuptake of norepinephrine at the presynaptic motor endplate
2. Increasing expression of adrenergic receptors on vascular tissues
3. Stimulating receptors on venous and arteriolar surfaces to cause strong vasoconstriction
4. Increasing water and sodium reabsorption by stimulating the adrenal cortex to produce aldosterone, acting on the hypothalamus and the pituitary gland to cause release of ADH and increases thirst by acting on the thirst center

Chemotherapy, radiation, and bone marrow transplant individually or in combination can cause a significant inflammatory state, inciting endothelial damage which results in vasodilation and increased vascular permeability. Chronic inflammation and activation of RAAS leads to progressive pathological, morphological, and geometric changes in the heart. The consequence of this is persistent and chronic activation of the RAAS. Concurrent heart dysfunction promotes chronic sympathetic activation. Chronic pathological activation of the sympathetic system and RAAS causes angiotensin II and aldosterone to act on the myocardial cells and fibroblasts, stimulating proto-oncogenes. As a result, growth factors are produced by the myocardial cells, resulting in pathological hypertrophy and accumulation of excess connective tissue, extracellular matrix, and fibrotic tissue. The pathologic remodeling of the myocardium makes it poorly contractile and non-compliant.

Angiotensin II and aldosterone also act on vascular smooth muscle and cause pathological changes which result in vasculopathy and poor response to treatment. In turn, this leads to progressive hypertension and cardiovascular failure. Therefore, ACE inhibitors, angiotensin receptor blockers, and beta-blockers are key medications to be started preemptively to prevent or improve pathological remodeling and treat hypertension.

Pathophysiology of Chemotherapy-Induced Cardiovascular Damage

Conventional chemotherapy targets rapidly dividing cells, while targeted agents work on tumor specific pathways. Anthracyclines (i.e., doxorubicin, daunorubicin, epirubicin), alkylating agents (i.e., busulfan, cyclophosphamide), antimetabolites (i.e., 5 fluorouracil, cytarabine), anti-microtubule agents (i.e., vinca-alkaloids), targeted agents (i.e., trastuzumab), cisplatin, mitoxantrone, pyrimidine analogues, and several other known and suspected agents can affect the heart. Cancer drugs interact with cardiovascular signaling, particularly during times of increased stress.

Anthracyclines

The mechanism of anthracycline-induced toxicity is not completely understood. The drug enters the cardiac myocyte, intercalates into nuclear DNA, and impairs protein synthesis. Additionally, it forms reactive oxygen species through iron complex formation, which damages the mitochondria. As calcium homeostasis is initially affected, diastolic dysfunction may be the initial presentation of anthracycline-mediated cardiotoxicity. Diastolic dysfunction may be a harbinger of future systolic heart failure. Pathologic investigation has shown that as more anthracycline accumulates in cardiac cells, there is evidence of apoptosis and myocardial necrosis, which likely results in the observed myocardial dysfunction and clinical heart failure syndromes [7].

Anthracyclines and the anthracycline analogues are commonly used agents in many cancer protocols. They are known to be cardiotoxic and, in many instances, require a dose reduction or holding of the medication. There is a reported 2.8% incidence of heart failure in the first 6 years after a cumulative dose of 300 mg/m^2. A direct correlation exists between cumulative dosing and incidence of cardiotoxicity [8, 9]. Survivors have reduced LV systolic function and inadequate diastolic filling with larger LV dimension. This pathology is caused by a decrease in number of cardiomyocytes and stem cells capable of generating cardiac tissue [10].

Prolonged QTc intervals, sinus node dysfunction, PVCs, and decreased QRS voltage have been described after anthracycline administration in 10–30% of survivors [11]. Rhythm abnormalities associated with anthracyclines are usually transient and have been reported with a cumulative dose of 120 mg/m^2. There is also evidence of ischemic cardiac injury with doxorubicin and another anthracycline, pirarubicin. Genetic predisposition, arterial hypertension, previous or concurrent heart disease, and combination with radiation, alkylating agents, and anti-microtubule therapy increase sensitivity to anthracyclines. Currently, there are no evidence-based guidelines in pediatrics for treatment of heart failure secondary to anthracyclines.

Alkylating Agents

Alkylating agents (i.e., cyclophosphamide, ifosfamide, melphalan) inhibit DNA transcription and affect protein synthesis. Cardiovascular symptoms usually present within the first week to first month of therapy. Low doses are usually not associated with toxicity, but at higher doses, patients can present with severe symptoms.

Other Agents

Monoclonal antibodies may have deleterious effect on cardiovascular function, though the data is retrospective, and the sample size is small [12]. Trastuzumab is a monoclonal antibody that targets HER-2 receptor. In adults, it causes cardiotoxicity in approximately 4–7% of patients when taken alone and 27% when taken with anthracyclines. The effects are usually reversible after stopping treatment. It is hypothesized that the use of monoclonal antibodies inhibits repair processes of the damage caused by the anthracyclines [13]. Vascular endothelial growth factor (VEGF) plays an important role in myocardial and vascular homeostasis. Anti-VEGF medications disrupt myocardial metabolism, impairing myocardial function. Bevacizumab, an anti-VEGF monoclonal antibody, has been shown to decrease LV shortening fraction. As the use of monoclonal antibodies becomes more prevalent, it is crucial to watch for impaired cardiac function during treatment, particularly when treatment is combined with other cardiotoxic agents. Cardioprotective agents, such as dexrazoxane, may have benefit in these patients.

Tyrosine kinases catalyze the transfer of phosphate from ATP to tyrosine residues in polypeptides involved in growth receptor signal transduction. Tyrosine kinase inhibitors (TKIs) are frequently used in cancer therapy and are linked to left ventricular dysfunction, heart failure, and arrhythmias [12]. Imatinib and dasatinib are small molecule TKIs and have been described to cause cardiac failure. They are known to cause serositis. Patients may present with peripheral edema, pleural, and pericardial effusions [14].

Risk Factors for Cardiotoxicity

Treatment and Patient-Related Risk Factors

1. Cumulative anthracycline dose
2. Mantle field radiation
3. Cranial radiation
4. Inflammatory state during therapy
5. Cancer diagnosis
6. Female gender
7. Young children

8. Genetic factors
9. Preexisting cardiovascular disease
10. Traditional risk factors for coronary vascular disease

A high cumulative dose of anthracyclines is the biggest risk factor for cardiotoxicity, but there is no dose of anthracyclines where the risk is absent. Damage has been reported with doses <240 mg/m^2 [15]. Continuous infusions to reduce peak serum levels have been suggested but data does not support the practice in children. Patients treated with mantle field radiation are at higher risk for cardiac dysfunction than patients who never received radiation at all or received radiation outside of the mantle field [16]. Cranial radiation is described as a risk factor secondary to pituitary damage and growth hormone deficiency. Incidence of cardiac dysfunction after cranial radiation is 4% which increases to approximately 13% with concomitant use of anthracyclines. The female gender is more susceptible to anthracycline toxicity, most likely due to higher percentage of body fat affecting distribution of the drug [17].

A strong inflammatory response during therapy is felt to cause increased microvascular endothelial damage leading to increased risk of cardiac complications [18]. Cancer itself is a risk factor for cardiovascular damage as children who have not received cardiotoxic chemotherapy or radiation still have an increased risk for cardiovascular abnormalities [18]. Young children are at higher risk for LV wall thinning and dysfunction [17]. Mutations in the HFE gene and C282Y allele (hereditary hemochromatosis) carry a significantly increased risk for cardiovascular injury [19]. Patients with preexisting cardiovascular impairment are at much higher risk for progressive heart failure [18]. Traditional risk factors for coronary vascular disease such as physical inactivity, obesity, insulin resistance, vitamin D deficiency, and smoking increase the likelihood of cardiovascular damage post-therapy.

Clinical Manifestations of Cardiac Toxicity

Cardiac complications in children undergoing cancer-directed therapy or hematopoietic cell transplantation are increasingly appreciated in the ICU. The most common acute manifestations include cardiac dysfunction, pulmonary hypertension, and pericardial effusions. These will be discussed in more detail.

Cardiac Dysfunction

Acute cardiotoxic events happen within the first week of therapy and are usually reversible with dose reduction or in most cases discontinuation of the respective chemotherapy. The reversibility is not 100%, and there can be progression of left ventricular (LV) dysfunction. Early onset cardiotoxicity occurs within weeks to months and can present with restrictive cardiomyopathy and filling defects or dilated cardiomyopathy with LV wall thinning and systolic dysfunction. This is usually progressive. Late onset cardiotoxicity is more common, defined by cardiac dysfunction after 1 year of exposure to chemotherapy. This can be asymptomatic for several years before it is clinically evident, necessitating the need for surveillance echocardiograms. It most commonly manifests as LV wall thinning, dilation, and decreased function and is progressive [20].

Dilated cardiomyopathy can convert to a restrictive cardiomyopathy with diastolic dysfunction, or diastolic dysfunction can be an early marker or future systolic heart failure. The proposed mechanism causing this is that with LV failure, there is a limited number of normal cardiomyocytes and with somatic growth of children, there is inadequate and pathological hypertrophy leading to a restrictive cardiomyopathy [8]. Approximately 60% of children exposed to anthracyclines alone or in combination with other cardiotoxic agents have subclinical changes in their LV structure and function on echocardiography [21].

Cancer therapy-induced arterial hypertension is a well-described entity. This is most commonly associated with angiogenesis inhibitors but can present with other cancer drugs as well.

Hypertension can present at any time during therapy and cause complications such as heart failure, stroke, posterior reversible leukoencephalopathy, proteinuria, and thrombotic microangiopathy. In most cases, the hypertension is reversible and improves as treatment is withheld or stopped but may persist [22].

Cancer is a hypercoagulable state. Many cancer agents (i.e., hormonal therapy, cisplatin, bevacizumab, sunitinib, and sorafenib) have been known to increase the risk of thromboembolic events [23, 24]. Currently, no clear guidelines exist for thromboprophylaxis in these patients, but most cancer patients will benefit from prophylactic anticoagulation. In addition to the cancer-induced hypercoagulable state, coronary artery spasm and rhythm disturbances have been reported with pyrimidine analogues such as 5-fluorouracil. These mechanisms may partially explain the increased risk of early ischemic heart disease in pediatric cancer survivors.

QT prolongation is associated with a number of cancer agents, placing patients at risk for cardiac arrhythmias [25]. Physicians should exercise extreme caution when there is concomitant use of other QT-prolonging drugs (antiemetics, methadone, psychotropic agents) particularly in patients with ongoing electrolyte disturbances.

Pulmonary Hypertension

Pulmonary hypertension (PH) is defined as elevation in the pulmonary arterial pressure. It is rare in children, estimated to occur in <10 cases per 1 million children [26]. The etiology of pediatric pulmonary hypertension in the general population is varied. Over half of pediatric cases are idiopathic or familial, while the remainder are associated with other diseases, most commonly congenital heart disease or chronic lung disease. Endothelial cell damage seems to play a role in the development of PH. The inciting injury may be caused by hypoxia, increased blood flow, or toxins. This injury leads to smooth muscle cell proliferation in small peripheral pulmonary arteries which normally are not muscularized. There also seems to be evidence for a genetic predisposition, with mutations in the bone morphogenetic protein receptor type 2 (BMPR2) and TGF-B superfamily being associated with PH [26].

Diagnosis of pulmonary hypertension in critically ill children is primarily accomplished noninvasively by echocardiogram, though cardiac catheterization is the gold standard. The ECG may show changes suggesting right atrial enlargement right axis deviation, bundle branch block, or right ventricular hypertrophy in cases of chronic pulmonary hypertension. However, ECG is not sufficient to make a diagnosis. Chest X-ray is useful to look for lung disease as the etiology of the pulmonary hypertension. It may also show an enlarged right heart or pulmonary arteries, though many patients may not have any findings. The echocardiogram is what is most frequently used to make the diagnosis in critically ill oncology patients. Tricuspid valve regurgitant jet velocity can be used to estimate the pulmonary arterial pressure, with the use of the modified Bernoulli equation. However, in the setting of poor right ventricular function, this may be falsely low as a heart pumping without force is not able to generate as much velocity across the valve. Therefore, this number alone should not be the sole determination of the diagnosis. Other echocardiographic findings of pulmonary hypertension include septal wall flattening and right ventricular hypertrophy/dysfunction [26, 27].

Pulmonary hypertension is increasingly recognized as a complication of hematopoietic cell transplant and chemotherapy [28, 29]. It is also a recognized complication in patients with chronic hemolytic anemias such as sickle cell disease [30]. Early diagnosis and intervention are likely to provide improved outcomes. Therefore, it is important for hematologists, oncologists, and intensivists to consider this diagnosis in critically ill hematology, oncology, and stem cell transplant patients.

Pulmonary hypertension is not isolated to the pediatric oncology and hematopoietic cell transplant population. It is also prevalent in patients with sickle cell disease and is increasingly appreciated as an important complication impacting morbidity and mortality [3]. Thirty to forty percent of adults with sickle cell disease have echocardiographic evidence of PH. The incidence in children is variable, depending upon the publication, ranging from 8% to 47%. The risk for development of PH seems to be highest in patients with hemoglobin SS as opposed to other forms of sickle cell disease, those who were 13 or older and more anemic [3]. Other variables associated with PH in sickle cell patients include elevated serum creatinine, brain natriuretic peptide, cardiac troponin levels, history of sleep apnea, prolonged QTc, and short 6-min walk test [3, 30–32]. Pulmonary hypertension has also been described in other types of anemia. PH occurring several years after splenectomy has been described in patients with hereditary spherocytosis [33] and in patients with congenital dyserythropoietic anemia, a rare congenital macrocytic anemia [34].

Acute cardiac complications in HCT patients were once thought to be quite rare, reported to occur in less than 1% of pediatric HCT patients [35]. Newer data suggests cardiac abnormalities are more common. Cincinnati Children's Hospital reports a 30% incidence of abnormalities found on routine screening echocardiograms at day +7 after HCT [28]. In their study 13% of children had elevated right ventricular pressures on day +7 echocardiogram, and this was significantly associated with later development of thrombotic microangiopathy (TMA). Sixty percent of patients with elevated right ventricular pressures were diagnosed with TMA vs. 23% of patients with a normal day +7 echocardiogram ($p = 0.0003$). The incidence of TMA was even higher in HCT patients who had both a pericardial effusion and elevated right ventricular pressure at day +7. One hundred percent of these patients went on to develop TMA. The team at Cincinnati went on to broaden screening echocardiograms to include any HCT patient with respiratory distress, hypoxia, shock, or TMA on admission to the PICU and every 1–2 weeks thereafter [36]. In this population 50% of patients had echocardiographic findings warranting either intervention or further screening. Elevated right ventricular pressure was the most common abnormality seen in 34% of patients, 20% were deemed to be at risk for pulmonary hypertension, and 14% diagnosed with pulmonary hypertension. All patients diagnosed with pulmonary hypertension required treatment with pulmonary vasodilators. The majority of patients diagnosed with pulmonary hypertension did not have other physical exam or radiographic findings on CXR that would have clued clinicians into the diagnosis.

PH has also been described in specific populations undergoing HCT. Patients with malignant infantile osteopetrosis who undergo HCT appear to be at high risk for development of PH. The European Blood and Marrow Transplantation Group (EBMT) published a case series where 8 of 28 infants transplanted for malignant infantile osteopetrosis developed PH with a mortality rate of 62% [37]. A group from the USA also reported a case series where 5 of 12 infants transplanted for malignant infantile osteopetrosis developed PH with a mortality rate of 80% [38]. The reason for this association remains unclear. However, these patients warrant close monitoring and early intervention for PH.

Pulmonary veno-occlusive disease (PVOD) is a possible etiology for the development of pulmonary hypertension in HCT patients and should be considered in the differential. Patients with PVOD may present as either an early or late complications of HCT. Patients often present with increasing dyspnea. Their CXR may show cardiomegaly and pulmonary edema, while an echocardiogram shows pulmonary hypertension. If a biopsy is performed, characteristic findings are fibrosis of the small pulmonary veins and venules, while the larger pulmonary veins are normal [39, 40]. Lung biopsy had been the gold standard; however, it carries a high risk of complications. Mineo and colleagues looked at the accuracy of chest CT to make the diagnosis. They found that presence of two of three of the following findings, ground glass appearance, septal thickening, and mediastinal lymphadenopathy, was 95.5% sensitive and 89% specific for the diagnosis of PVOD [41]. PVOD is an important diagnosis to consider as these patients may respond to therapy much differently than other patients with PH. Defibrotide is a theoretically useful agent in this population, though there is little published data for use other than in hepatic VOD. Its use was described by the EBMT group in their case series of eight osteopetrosis patients with PH. Defibrotide was used in four of the eight patients for possible PVOD and/or documented liver VOD. Two of the four patients given defibrotide survived, while one of the four patients not given defibrotide survived [37]. The numbers are much too small to make any conclusions other than its use has been described in patients who may have had PVOD. The other potentially important aspect when considering treatment for PH due to PVOD is that traditional pulmonary vasodilators used for PH may cause pulmonary edema in patients with PVOD so should be used with caution [42].

PH has also been described in oncology patients. The majority of case reports have been in patients with neuroblastoma, particularly those undergoing autologous HCT [29, 43]. Patients who have received busulfan/melphalan conditioning may have the highest risk of developing PH [29], but PH has been described in patients who have received other chemotherapy [44]. PVOD was suspected as the cause of PH in two of the case reports of pulmonary hypertension in patients with neuroblastoma [43, 44]. Leukemic infiltrate in the lung has been suspected as a cause of PH in a case report of a patient with juvenile myelomonocytic leukemia [45]. There are case reports of PH as the cause of death in patients with hemophagocytic lymphohistiocytosis and idiopathic myelofibrosis [46, 47].

Treatment of pulmonary hypertension in the pediatric hematology/oncology/HCT population is the same as in other populations, with the caveat that PVOD should be considered in the differential as the cause of the PH, particularly if the patient's condition worsens with pulmonary artery vasodilator therapy. Acute management when patients present to the PICU acutely ill would include oxygen to maintain saturations at least 95%, inhaled nitric oxide (NO), diuretics if the patient is felt to be volume overloaded, or volume supplementation if the patient has a low right ventricular filling pressure [27]. Intravenous prostanoids such as epoprostenol may be used for their pulmonary vasodilatory effect. Patients need to be monitored closely for hypotension as they also decrease the systemic vascular resistance. Patients with hypotension and poor cardiac output may require inotropic and vasopressor support with milrinone being a particularly good choice for inotropy as it does not increase the heart rate. Vasopressor agents may be necessary to counteract the vasodilator effects of systemic prostanoids. Avoidance of hypotension is important to maintain adequate coronary perfusion. Oral agents such as sildenafil or bosentan can be added to help with weaning off of iNO [27, 48].

Pericardial Effusion (PCEF)

Pericardial effusion (PCEF) is a life-threatening complication among pediatric oncology patients [49, 50]. Reported incidence of PCEF in children with cancer ranges from 0.2% to 17% [51]. Knowledge continues to develop surrounding the incidence, risk factors, and outcomes associated with PCEF in children with oncologic disease. In the interim, it is incumbent upon clinicians to understand potential causal pathways, symptomology, and treatment considerations for PCEF in this population. PCEF in children is more frequently associated with hematopoietic stem cell or bone marrow transplant (HSCT or BMT). However, clinicians report, both in literature and anecdotally, occurrence of PCEF across all various types of pediatric oncological disease.

Risk Factors for PCEF

The population at highest risk for PCEF are patients who undergo HCT. Potentiating risk factors associated with incidence of PCEF include donor type, conditioning, infection, toxicity related to immunosuppressives, and graft-versus-host disease (GVHD) [51, 52]. Patients with high-risk disease status prior to HCT (e.g., active leukemia in relapse, active leukemia after induction failure, progressive solid tumor, and/or second allogeneic HSCT), myeloablative conditioning, and calcineurin inhibitor (CNI) (e.g., cyclosporine and tacrolimus) as well as other therapeutic agents (Fig. 12.1) are at relative increased risk for incidence of PCEF [53]. The literature varies on whether age, gender, and other factors are reliable predictors.

Oncological Pathways to PCEF

In normal physiology, the pericardium, a two-layered sac, protects the myocardium via the provision of a mechanical barrier, reducing friction between the heart and structures in close proximity [49]. The pericardial cavity lies between the visceral and parietal layers of the pericardium, containing a minute amount of plasma ultrafiltrate. In an acute pericarditis, the pericardium becomes inflamed, staging an effusive process that can lead to rapid accumulation of fluid in the pericardial cavity. The fluid can be serous, purulent, or sanguineous depending on the cause. Common pathways leading to occurrence of PCEF in pediatric oncology patients listed by frequency of occurrence (Fig. 12.2) [49]:

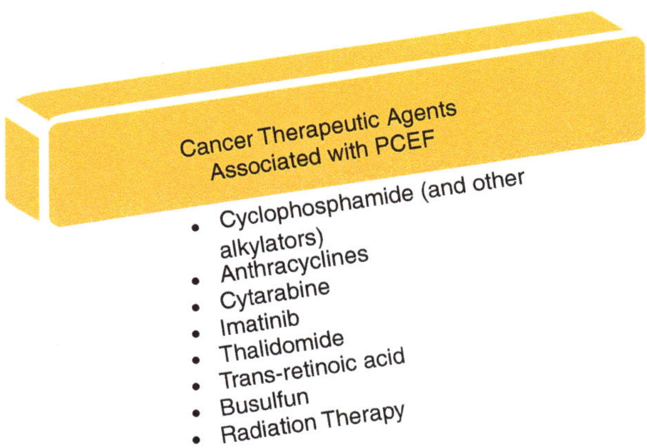

Fig 12.1 Cancer therapeutic agents widely known to have the adverse cardiac effect of pericardial effusion

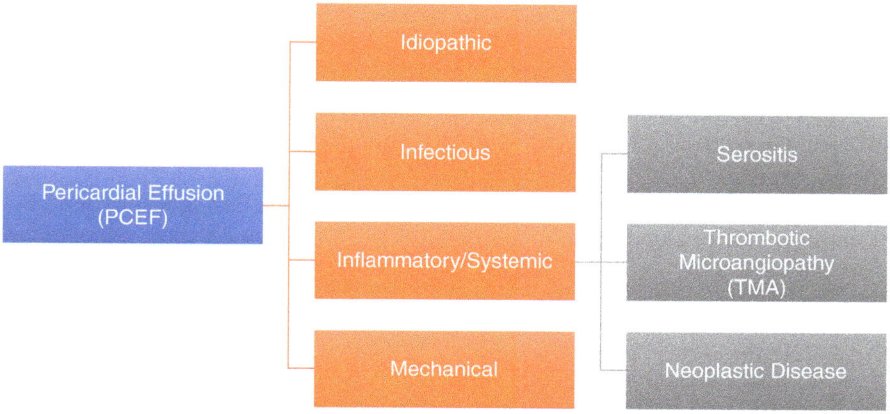

Fig. 12.2 Ordinal classification of common causes of pericardial effusion (PCEF) by frequency of occurrence in pediatric oncology patients

Subcategories of inflammatory or systemic-mediated occurrence of PCEF include global serositis, thrombotic microangiopathy (TMA), and pervasive neoplastic disease. The vast majority of PCEF in pediatric oncology patients is of uncertain origin. The notion of idiopathic PCEF is typically confirmed in the absence of significant diagnostic findings (i.e., negative cultures and pathology of PCEF fluid, nontoxic clinical presentation, no mechanical confounders, no known trauma history, etc.). Of the microorganisms attributed to infectious etiology of PCEF, the most frequent cause is viral infection (i.e., EBV, CMV, adenovirus, etc.); less common are bacterial, fungal, and parasitic infections [49].

Two specific inflammatory etiologies related to PCEF are worth highlighting. They are serositis and TMA. Serositis is an operational definition of a syndrome involving inflammation of serous tissues in the body, often resulting in fluid collections in the pericardial, pleural, and peritoneal cavities. Serositis is often considered in the absence of antimicrobial pathogenicity and in the setting of concurrent pleural effusions; it may or may not be indicative of underlying GVHD or immunosuppressive toxicity. Patients with TMA may present with pericardial effusions and pleural effusions in addition to thrombocytopenia, hemolytic anemia, acute kidney injury (AKI), altered mental status, severe pulmonary arterial hypertension (PAH), and dysfunction of other organs, leading to multi system organ failure (MSOF) [54].

Symptomology and Diagnosis of PCEF

A pattern of symptoms are often present in patients experiencing PCEF, including but not limited to:

- Tachycardia, accompanied by S3 (gallop), or pericardial friction rub on auscultation
- Narrow or decreased pulse pressure

- Dyspnea with or without oxygen desaturation
- Chest pain
- ECG changes, including low-voltage QRS complexes, electrical alternans, ST segment elevation, PR segment depression, and/or T-wave inversions
- Pulsus paradoxus (quantified as a systolic blood pressure (SBP) reduction of >10 mmHG)
- Kussmaul sign (i.e., elevation in jugular venous pressure during inspiration)
- In large PCEF, globular appearance of cardiac silhouette on chest radiography (CXR) [49, 52]

High-risk features such as fever, leukocytosis, elevated troponin, and history of PCEF or pericarditis are associated with poorer outcomes [49].

While awareness of symptomology is helpful, echocardiogram (ECHO) serves as the diagnostic gold standard. Of note, rarely do volumes quantified on ECHO match drained volumes upon intervention [51]. Perhaps counterintuitively, clinicians must be keenly aware that volume of effluent does not directly correlate with clinical presentation or allow for enhanced prognostication. In fact, "relatively small effusions may lead to important hemodynamic compromise," particularly in the small pericardial cavities of young children [50]. This appears especially true in the pediatric oncology population, where underlying diastolic dysfunction may contribute to hemodynamic instability even without classic markers of tamponade physiology.

Tamponade Physiology

By definition, cardiac tamponade occurs when the chambers of the heart are compressed as a result of increased intrapericardial pressure to the extent that systemic venous return to the right atrium (RA) is impaired; increased intrapericardial pressure decreases myocardial transmural pressure, and the chambers of the heart demonstrate reduced capacity and compliance, consequently reducing cardiac output and blood pressure. Typical ECHO findings in tamponade include diastolic collapse of the RA and right ventricle (RV) as intrapericardial pressure exceeds the intracavitary pressure [49].

In early tamponade, sinus tachycardia preserves cardiac output. Hypertension may also occur as part of a sympathetic response to pericardial annoyance. Atypical symptoms such as chest or shoulder discomfort and nausea may also be present [49]. Late signs of tamponade physiology may manifest as cardiogenic shock, hypotension, and pulsus paradoxus, and narrowing pulse pressure will progress to cardiac collapse without intervention.

Management of PCEF

Acute PCEF management is largely based on individual clinical presentation. Asymptomatic low-risk patients may be managed within a low-acuity setting. Management for stable PCEF should include serial ECHO follow-up, hemodynamic monitoring, and treatment of identifiable underlying causes. However, persistent and enlarging PCEF in the oncology patient may require more aggressive treatment, even despite evidence of hemodynamic compromise or tamponade physiology.

Diuretics are mostly ineffective, though often used. Infectious PCEF may be treated based on suspicion of pathogen. However, serologic testing and culturing of effluent are often low yield. Rituximab may be indicated in EBV-mediated PCEF. Immunosuppressive agents are often not helpful even with inflammatory etiologies. Discontinuation of CNIs has proven to be efficacious in ameliorating PCEF [51]. In TMA-associated PCEF, eculizumab and plasmapheresis have been used with some success [54]. If methotrexate has been used recently, leucovorin rescue may be helpful.

Large PCEF at risk for tamponade physiology, hemodynamic compromise, or rapidly increasing effusions necessitate critical care observation. Volume expansion may be required to optimize cardiac output, specifically in hypotension. Inotropic support is controversial as endogenous sympathetic output is typically maximal in tamponade [49]. Patients with concomitant respiratory distress may require noninvasive or invasive respiratory support with the caveat that positive-pressure ventilation (PPV) may worsen acute tamponade by impeding cardiac filling.

Evacuation of PCEF is achieved by ECHO-guided percutaneous pericardiocentesis, with or without drain placement. Recurrent PCEF may better be addressed by pericardial window or pericardectomy. Pericardiocentesis can be complicated in small children who have very little distance between the myocardium and the rim of the effusion [50]. Additionally, sedation in children with tamponade physiology is fraught with risk for hemodynamic compromise. Preprocedure tachypnea, cardiac tamponade, and hypoxia have proven to be reliable prognosticators for adverse events [55]. The preferred induction agent is ketamine. The transition from spontaneous respiration to positive-pressure ventilation carries risk of hemodynamic compromise and should be done with caution.

Monitoring for Cardiac Toxicity

Currently, there are no established evidence-based guidelines for monitoring cardiovascular structure and function during and posttreatment. It is widely recognized that it is necessary to do so, but there is no consensus on the modalities or their frequency of use.

EKG

There is evidence that prolonged QT interval can predict cardiac disease [25, 56]. Conduction abnormalities and cardiac hypertrophy are all associated with cancer-related therapy, whether drug induced or radiation induced. Therefore, an EKG is highly recommended for assessment and monitoring of cardiac dysfunction. EKG should be performed prior to initiation of therapy to establish baseline, periodically during therapy and after completion for comparison.

ECHO

Echocardiogram is a necessary tool in the evaluation of cardiac dysfunction during cancer therapy. Thorough echocardiographic protocols include assessment of diastolic dysfunction and myocardial strain as these abnormalities are often present before a decrease in systolic function is seen. Increased values of indexed left atrial volume are a direct result of impaired diastolic dysfunction, which is commonly seen in patients with early chemotherapy-induced cardiomyopathy [57]. Figure 12.3 shows a patient with a dilated left atrium, compared to a patient with a normal left atrial size. Specific Doppler velocities that are obtained during diastole can evaluate mitral valve inflow and cardiac wall deformation and have been shown to predict systolic heart failure in those who have received chemotherapy [58]. Figure 12.4 shows an elevated mitral valve inflow velocity, compared with a normal mitral valve

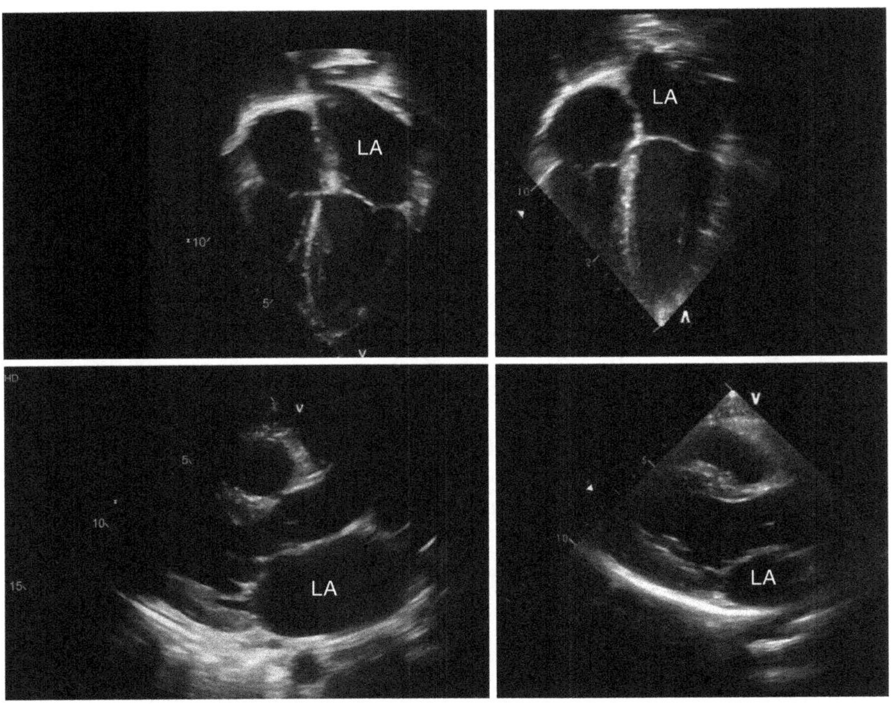

Fig. 12.3 Left panel shows dilated left atrium (LA), compared with normal LA size on the right panel

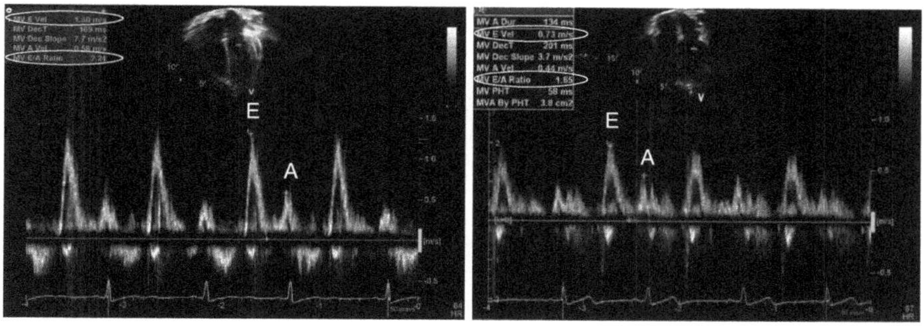

Fig. 12.4 Left panel shows tall, steep "E" (early diastolic) wave velocity and elevated E/A ratio, markers of diastolic dysfunction; compared with normal "E" wave velocity and normal E/A ratio on the right panel. E/A ratios greater than 2 are considered abnormal

inflow velocity. There has also been much attention given to evaluation of myocardial strain parameters, with a decrease in global longitudinal strain most reliably correlated with decreased cardiac function after chemotherapy [59]. Figure 12.5 shows an abnormal global longitudinal strain (GLS) profile, compared to a normal GLS profile. Figure 12.6 shows a patient with a large circumferential pericardial effusion.

Given the studied associations between cardiac toxicity and both anthracycline agents and chest radiotherapy, serial echocardiographic assessment has become an established part of these protocols. However, much is being learned about the acute hemodynamic alterations caused by bone marrow transplantation (BMT), with data suggesting cardiac dysfunction as a direct effect of hematopoietic cell transplantation and the need for serial echocardiography as part of these protocols as well [36].

Cardiac Magnetic Resonance Imaging

Cardiac MRI scans are superior to echocardiography to assess myocardial tissue structure. It is the gold standard for detection of ventricular volumes and function [60]. It provides a better assessment of myocardial edema, inflammation, and fibrosis and may identify cardiomyopathy more reliably than echocardiography. Cardiac MRI therefore has an important role in identification of early and late cardiotoxicity.

Positron Emission Tomography/Magnetic Resonance (PET/MR)

PET/MR is an emerging modality for assessment of cardiomyopathy. Imaging allows for determination of myocardial perfusion, glucose metabolism, and myocardial viability [61].

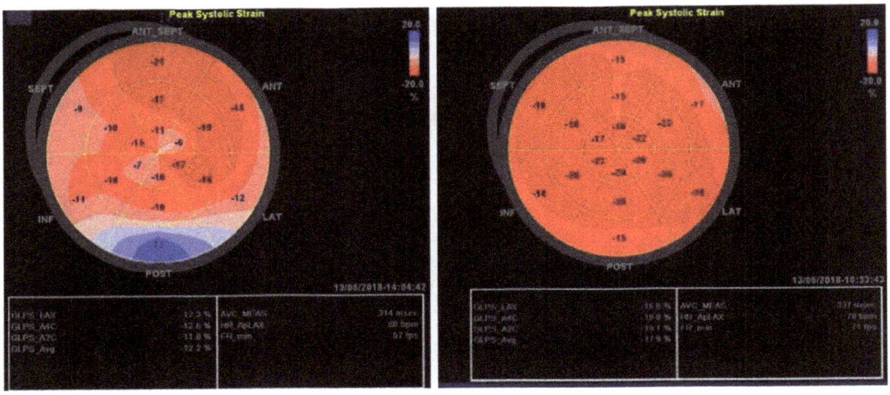

Fig. 12.5 Left panel shows abnormal global longitudinal strain, with dyssynchronous (blue) function mostly in the posterior basal segmental, compared with synchronous function throughout in the right panel

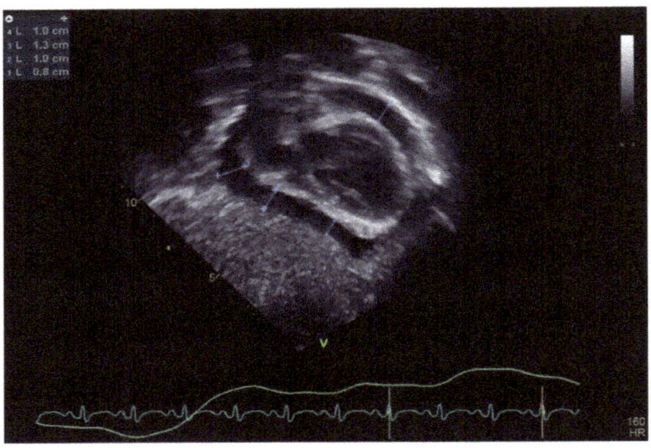

Fig. 12.6 Large, circumferential pericardial effusion

Biomarkers

Troponins

Cardiac troponins (troponin I and troponin C) present in the serum may indicate acute cardiac damage. Elevated troponins in the first 90 days of cancer therapy have been associated with reduced LV mass and thickness and function 5 years later [18]. Absence of troponin elevation has a high negative predictive value. Elevation has been described to predict diastolic dysfunction in approximately 35% of patients.

Elevation of troponin at the completion of therapy is predictive of subsequent left ventricular dysfunction. Cardinale et al. demonstrated a relationship between elevated troponin, anthracycline-induced cardiotoxicity, and patients who would benefit from ACE inhibitors [62].

Natriuretic Peptides

BNP and NT-pro BNP are elevated due to wall stress secondary to pressure or volume overload. These are elevated acutely in cardiac dysfunction but also predict LV remodeling in future years. As they are elevated in cardiac stress and do not necessarily indicate cardiomyocyte damage, they have the potential to detect early subclinical changes.

The elevation of NT-proBNP (natriuretic peptide), MR-pro ANP (mid-regional atrial natriuretic peptide, MR-proADM (mid-regional pro adrenomedullin), copeptin, and high-sensitivity troponin T prior to therapy is associated with higher mortality [23]. Elevation of BNP in the first 90 days is predictive of left ventricular dysfunction within 3, 6, 12 months, and 4 years [63, 64]. NT-proBNP is also shown to correlate with the increased cumulative exposure to anthracyclines.

High-Sensitivity C-Reactive Protein (CRP) and Myeloperoxidase (MPO)

High-sensitivity CRP predicts cardiotoxicity in patients treated with trastuzumab. MPO levels which rise early in therapy persist and are associated with cardiotoxicity [65].

Management

Cardiotoxicity causes a significant amount of morbidity and mortality and is progressive in nature. Therefore, early medical intervention is extremely important. Labs that help monitoring perfusion and guide acute heart failure management include lactic acid and mixed venous saturation. Volume status can be best predicted by pulse pressure variation, stroke volume variation, and IVC dynamics.

Milrinone (Phosphodiesterase 3 Inhibitors)

Milrinone is a commonly used infusion for acute heart failure. It increases the overall performance of the heart and decreases pulmonary vascular resistance. It is an ideal choice for systolic and diastolic dysfunction as per its inotropic, vasodilatory, and lusitropic effects.

As most patients with heart failure secondary to cancer therapy have hypertension, milrinone can decrease afterload while improving the contractility. There are times when other antihypertensives may be combined with milrinone specifically if there is persistent hypertension. Antihypertensives can be administered intermittently or as an infusion (beta-blockers or calcium channel blockers). The goal is to main borderline normal mean arterial pressure according to age.

Other Inotropes and Vasopressors

Low-dose epinephrine and inotropic dose of dopamine can be used alone or in combination with milrinone. This approach is especially beneficial in patients with poor contractility and hypotension. Vasopressin can be considered a vasopressor in addition to the inotropes to elevate the SVRI and improve organ perfusion. In patients with cardiac dysfunction and ongoing distributive shock as seen in sepsis or cytokine release syndrome, a short course of norepinephrine can be considered as the first line therapy. Low-dose epinephrine or dopamine may be added to provide more inotropic support. A calcium infusion may also be used as an inotropic and or vasopressor agent, specially in younger children.

Patients can present with poor contractility and high SVRI. In this case milrinone is the ideal choice. If the SVRI remains high even with titration of milrinone and patient is clinically symptomatic with evidence of poor perfusion, other vasodilators and positive-pressure ventilation should be considered to rest the patient and provide afterload reduction. Continuous measurement of systemic vascular resistance index, cardiac index, or regional oximetry may be useful for more informed titration of infusions in these very complicated and dynamic situations. Further study in this area is warranted.

Positive-Pressure Ventilation

Positive-pressure ventilation lowers the transmural pressure and off-loads the heart. This can be extremely beneficial in decreasing the metabolic demand by decreasing the work of breathing. Positive-pressure ventilation should be strongly considered in any patient with increased work of breathing and moderate to severe heart failure with down trending indicators of perfusion. Extreme caution is indicated when intubating these patients as their poor cardiac output puts them at high risk for decompensation with sedatives and the stress of intubation.

Angiotensin-Converting Enzyme (ACE) Inhibitors and Angiotensin Receptor Blockers (ARB)

ACE inhibitors reduce afterload, myocardial stress and show improvements in heart failure by preventing angiotensin I from converting into angiotensin II, a very potent vasoconstrictor and preventing abnormal remodeling in adults. Their efficacy still needs to be studied further in the pediatric population, particularly cancer survivors. A trial in pediatrics with enalapril showed improved LV function after doxorubicin use, but the improvement effect was transient and was lost after 10 years [66]. ARBs have similar to arguably better effects to that of ACE inhibitors and do not carry the risk for cough, a possible side effect of ACE inhibitors. However, caution is warranted in initiating these medications in the face of acute kidney injury as they lower the glomerular filtration rate by vasodilating the efferent arteriole.

Early initiation of ACE inhibitors may benefit cancer patients treated with cardiotoxic mediations or radiation therapy. This strategy warrants further study in the pediatric population.

Beta-Blockers

Beta-blockers prevent sympathetic stimulation of the heart by blocking beta-receptors. They have shown to be efficacious in adults and children with anthracycline use, as they control heart rate, lower sympathetic output response, and block renin release. Beta-blockers may be especially efficacious in the setting of diastolic dysfunction, which can be benefitted by reduction in heart rate. Improved LV function and ejection fraction were noted in children who received beta-blockers and anthracyclines. Children pretreated with beta-blockers show improved global peak systolic strain, LV shortening fraction, and a decrease in plasma troponin I and lactic dehydrogenase compared to controls [67].

Follow-Up

Proactive post treatment follow-up is of paramount importance. Recently the Children's Oncology group (COG) has published recommendations for long-term follow-up of childhood cancer survivors. These recommendations give detailed guidelines regarding frequency of monitoring based on anthracycline exposure, cumulative dose, and total dose of radiation received [68].

Future Directions

Prevention is key, and cardioprotective therapy (including dexrazoxane as well as ACE-inhibitors, ARBs, or beta-blockers) in the first 90 days of therapy should be a strong consideration [18]. All children with cancer are at higher risk regardless of the type of therapy, likely secondary to endothelial damage and remodeling. Further trials are needed to assess biomarker-guided therapy.

Current practice is to involve critical care and cardiology only when ventricular dysfunction or heart failure is clinically evident. This approach not only misses the opportunity for early recognition and intervention but also prevents risk assessment and therefore a lack of an individualized treatment plan.

An onco-critical care cardiac team working in unison should assess patients' risk factors, before and after therapy, and an individual-based strategy should be developed. The strategy may need modification as the clinical course dictates. A team approach is required to provide optimal management. There should be joint conferences, journal clubs, collaborative research, and continuous education for trainees and hospital staff. Adult colleagues should be consulted for uncommon pediatric issues such as early coronary artery disease. Heightened recognition, improved understanding of pathophysiology, and universally accepted definitions of cancer-related cardiotoxicity will allow for further advancement in the field.

References

1. Ward E, et al. Childhood and adolescent cancer statistics, 2014. CA Cancer J Clin. 2014;64(2):83–103.
2. Moller TR, et al. Decreasing late mortality among five-year survivors of cancer in childhood and adolescence: a population-based study in the Nordic countries. J Clin Oncol. 2001;19(13):3173–81.
3. Lilje C, et al. A modified noninvasive screening protocol for pulmonary hypertension in children with sickle cell disease-Who should be sent for invasive evaluation? Pediatr Blood Cancer. 2017;64(11)
4. Health, N.I.O. Cancer Therapy Evaluation Program Common Terminology Criteria for Adverse Events (CTCAE) v. 5.0. 2018 2018]; Available from: https://ctep.cancer.gov/protocol/Development/electronic_applications/CTC.htm
5. Yarnold J, Brotons MC. Pathogenetic mechanisms in radiation fibrosis. Radiother Oncol. 2010;97(1):149–61.
6. Taunk NK, et al. Radiation-induced heart disease: pathologic abnormalities and putative mechanisms. Front Oncol. 2015;5:39.
7. Nousiainen T, et al. Natriuretic peptides during the development of doxorubicin-induced left ventricular diastolic dysfunction. J Intern Med. 2002;251(3):228–34.
8. Lipshultz SE, et al. Chronic progressive cardiac dysfunction years after doxorubicin therapy for childhood acute lymphoblastic leukemia. J Clin Oncol. 2005;23(12):2629–36.
9. Kremer LC, et al. Anthracycline-induced clinical heart failure in a cohort of 607 children: long-term follow-up study. J Clin Oncol. 2001;19(1):191–6.
10. Lipshultz SE, Adams MJ. Cardiotoxicity after childhood cancer: beginning with the end in mind. J Clin Oncol. 2010;28(8):1276–81.
11. Bagnes C, Panchuk PN, Recondo G. Antineoplastic chemotherapy induced QTc prolongation. Curr Drug Saf. 2010;5(1):93–6.
12. Pansy J, et al. Add-on-therapy with bevacizumab in children and adolescents with poor prognosis non-CNS solid tumors. Anti-Cancer Drugs. 2013;24(2):198–203.
13. Force T, Krause DS, Van Etten RA. Molecular mechanisms of cardiotoxicity of tyrosine kinase inhibition. Nat Rev Cancer. 2007;7(5):332–44.
14. Quintas-Cardama A, et al. Pleural effusion in patients with chronic myelogenous leukemia treated with dasatinib after imatinib failure. J Clin Oncol. 2007;25(25):3908–14.
15. Trachtenberg BH, et al. Anthracycline-associated cardiotoxicity in survivors of childhood cancer. Pediatr Cardiol. 2011;32(3):342–53.

16. Mulrooney DA, et al. Cardiac outcomes in a cohort of adult survivors of childhood and adolescent cancer: retrospective analysis of the Childhood Cancer Survivor Study cohort. BMJ. 2009;339:b4606.
17. Lipshultz SE, et al. Female sex and higher drug dose as risk factors for late cardiotoxic effects of doxorubicin therapy for childhood cancer. N Engl J Med. 1995;332(26):1738–43.
18. Lipshultz SE, et al. Cardiovascular status of childhood cancer survivors exposed and unexposed to cardiotoxic therapy. J Clin Oncol. 2012;30(10):1050–7.
19. Lipshultz SE, et al. Impact of hemochromatosis gene mutations on cardiac status in doxorubicin-treated survivors of childhood high-risk leukemia. Cancer. 2013;119(19):3555–62.
20. Giantris A, et al. Anthracycline-induced cardiotoxicity in children and young adults. Crit Rev Oncol Hematol. 1998;27(1):53–68.
21. Lipshultz SE, et al. Late cardiac effects of doxorubicin therapy for acute lymphoblastic leukemia in childhood. N Engl J Med. 1991;324(12):808–15.
22. Maitland ML, et al. Initial assessment, surveillance, and management of blood pressure in patients receiving vascular endothelial growth factor signaling pathway inhibitors. J Natl Cancer Inst. 2010;102(9):596–604.
23. Ay C, et al. Prediction of venous thromboembolism in cancer patients. Blood. 2010;116(24):5377–82.
24. Choueiri TK, et al. Risk of arterial thromboembolic events with sunitinib and sorafenib: a systematic review and meta-analysis of clinical trials. J Clin Oncol. 2010;28(13):2280–5.
25. Nakamae H, et al. QT dispersion correlates with systolic rather than diastolic parameters in patients receiving anthracycline treatment. Intern Med. 2004;43(5):379–87.
26. McArthur J, Duncan C, Rajapreyar P, Talano J, Tamburro R. Critical illness involving children undergoing hematopoietic cell transplantation. In: Care PC, Fuhrman BZJ, editors. Fuhrman and Zimmerman's pediatric critical care. 5th ed. Philadelphia: Elsevier; 2017.
27. Kaestner M, et al. Pulmonary hypertension in the intensive care unit. Expert consensus statement on the diagnosis and treatment of paediatric pulmonary hypertension. The European Paediatric Pulmonary Vascular Disease Network, endorsed by ISHLT and DGPK. Heart. 2016;102(Suppl 2):ii57–66.
28. Dandoy CE, et al. Abnormal echocardiography 7 days after stem cell transplantation may be an early indicator of thrombotic microangiopathy. Biol Blood Marrow Transplant. 2015;21(1):113–8.
29. Desai AV, et al. Toxicities of busulfan/melphalan versus carboplatin/etoposide/melphalan for high-dose chemotherapy with stem cell rescue for high-risk neuroblastoma. Bone Marrow Transplant. 2016;51(9):1204–10.
30. Ambrusko SJ, et al. Elevation of tricuspid regurgitant jet velocity, a marker for pulmonary hypertension in children with sickle cell disease. Pediatr Blood Cancer. 2006;47(7):907–13.
31. Hebson C, et al. Elevated tricuspid regurgitant velocity as a marker for pulmonary hypertension in children with sickle cell disease: less prevalent and predictive than previously thought? J Pediatr Hematol Oncol. 2015;37(2):134–9.
32. Liem RI, et al. Tricuspid regurgitant jet velocity elevation and its relationship to lung function in pediatric sickle cell disease. Pediatr Pulmonol. 2009;44(3):281–9.
33. Das A, et al. Risk factors for thromboembolism and pulmonary artery hypertension following splenectomy in children with hereditary spherocytosis. Pediatr Blood Cancer. 2014;61(1):29–33.
34. El-Sheikh AA, et al. Congenital dyserythropoietic anemia type I presenting as persistent pulmonary hypertension with pigeon chest deformity. Pediatr Blood Cancer. 2014;61(8):1460–2.
35. Murdych T, Weisdorf DJ. Serious cardiac complications during bone marrow transplantation at the University of Minnesota, 1977–1997. Bone Marrow Transplant. 2001;28(3):283–7.
36. Dandoy CE, et al. Team-based approach to identify cardiac toxicity in critically ill hematopoietic stem cell transplant recipients. Pediatr Blood Cancer. 2017;64(10)
37. Steward CG, et al. Severe pulmonary hypertension: a frequent complication of stem cell transplantation for malignant infantile osteopetrosis. Br J Haematol. 2004;124(1):63–71.

38. Kasow KA, et al. Malignant infantile osteopetrosis and primary pulmonary hypertension: a new combination? Pediatr Blood Cancer. 2004;42(2):190–4.
39. Bunte MC, et al. Pulmonary veno-occlusive disease following hematopoietic stem cell transplantation: a rare model of endothelial dysfunction. Bone Marrow Transplant. 2008;41(8):677–86.
40. Trobaugh-Lotrario AD, et al. Pulmonary veno-occlusive disease after autologous bone marrow transplant in a child with stage IV neuroblastoma: case report and literature review. J Pediatr Hematol Oncol. 2003;25(5):405–9.
41. Mineo G, et al. Pulmonary veno-occlusive disease: the role of CT. Radiol Med. 2014;119(9):667–73.
42. Rowan CB, O; McArthur J. Non-infectious pulmonary complications of hematopoietic stem cell transplant. J Pediatr Intensive Care. 2014;3:133–46.
43. Ozyoruk D, et al. Pulmonary arterial hypertension in a child with stage-IV neuroblastoma after autologous hematopoietic stem cell transplantation and review of the literature. Pediatr Transplant. 2015;19(7):E185–8.
44. Yildirim ZK, et al. Resolution of pulmonary hypertension with low-molecular-weight heparin, steroid, and prostacyclin analogue therapy: could it be early-phase pulmonary veno-occlusive disease? Pediatr Hematol Oncol. 2011;28(6):529–34.
45. Alioglu B, et al. Pulmonary hypertension in a child with juvenile myelomonocytic leukemia secondary to pulmonary leukemic cell infiltration. Pediatr Hematol Oncol. 2006;23(8):667–75.
46. Zeilhofer U, et al. Pulmonary hypertension following haematopoietic stem cell transplantation for primary haemophagocytic lymphohistiocytosis. Pediatr Blood Cancer. 2013;60(3):521–3.
47. Shankar S, et al. Pulmonary hypertension complicating bone marrow transplantation for idiopathic myelofibrosis. J Pediatr Hematol Oncol. 2004;26(6):393–7.
48. Berger RM, et al. FUTURE-2: results from an open-label, long-term safety and tolerability extension study using the pediatric FormUlation of bosenTan in pUlmonary arterial hypeRtEnsion. Int J Cardiol. 2016;202:52–8.
49. Khandaker MH, et al. Pericardial disease: diagnosis and management. Mayo Clin Proc. 2010;85(6):572–93.
50. Law MA, et al. Novel, long-axis in-plane ultrasound-guided pericardiocentesis for postoperative pericardial effusion drainage. Pediatr Cardiol. 2016;37(7):1328–33.
51. Versluys AB, et al. Predictors and outcome of pericardial effusion after hematopoietic stem cell transplantation in children. Pediatr Cardiol. 2018;39(2):236–44.
52. Neier M, et al. Pericardial effusion post-SCT in pediatric recipients with signs and/or symptoms of cardiac disease. Bone Marrow Transplant. 2011;46(4):529–38.
53. Galderisi M, et al. Cancer therapy and cardiotoxicity: the need of serial Doppler echocardiography. Cardiovasc Ultrasound. 2007;5:4.
54. Dhakal P, Bhatt VR. Is complement blockade an acceptable therapeutic strategy for hematopoietic cell transplant-associated thrombotic microangiopathy? Bone Marrow Transplant. 2017;52(3):352–6.
55. Rawlinson E, Bagshaw O. Anesthesia for children with pericardial effusion: a case series. Paediatr Anaesth. 2012;22(11):1124–31.
56. Markman TM, et al. Electrophysiological effects of anthracyclines in adult survivors of pediatric malignancy. Pediatr Blood Cancer. 2017;64(11)
57. Nagueh SF, et al. Recommendations for the evaluation of left ventricular diastolic function by echocardiography: an update from the American Society of Echocardiography and the European Association of Cardiovascular Imaging. Eur Heart J Cardiovasc Imaging. 2016;17(12):1321–60.
58. Nagiub M, Nixon JV, Kontos MC. Ability of nonstrain diastolic parameters to predict doxorubicin-induced cardiomyopathy: a systematic review with meta-analysis. Cardiol Rev. 2018;26(1):29–34.
59. Hare JL, et al. Use of myocardial deformation imaging to detect preclinical myocardial dysfunction before conventional measures in patients undergoing breast cancer treatment with trastuzumab. Am Heart J. 2009;158(2):294–301.

60. Thavendiranathan P, et al. Cardiac MRI in the assessment of cardiac injury and toxicity from cancer chemotherapy: a systematic review. Circ Cardiovasc Imaging. 2013;6(6):1080–91.
61. Catana C, Guimaraes AR, Rosen BR. PET and MR imaging: the odd couple or a match made in heaven? J Nucl Med. 2013;54(5):815–24.
62. Cardinale D, et al. Prognostic value of troponin I in cardiac risk stratification of cancer patients undergoing high-dose chemotherapy. Circulation. 2004;109(22):2749–54.
63. Mackay B, et al. Assessment of anthracycline cardiomyopathy by endomyocardial biopsy. Ultrastruct Pathol. 1994;18(1–2):203–11.
64. Mitani I, et al. Doxorubicin cardiotoxicity: prevention of congestive heart failure with serial cardiac function monitoring with equilibrium radionuclide angiocardiography in the current era. J Nucl Cardiol. 2003;10(2):132–9.
65. Wassmuth R, et al. Subclinical cardiotoxic effects of anthracyclines as assessed by magnetic resonance imaging-a pilot study. Am Heart J. 2001;141(6):1007–13.
66. Lipshultz SE, et al. Long-term enalapril therapy for left ventricular dysfunction in doxorubicin-treated survivors of childhood cancer. J Clin Oncol. 2002;20(23):4517–22.
67. El-Shitany NA, et al. Protective effect of carvedilol on adriamycin-induced left ventricular dysfunction in children with acute lymphoblastic leukemia. J Card Fail. 2012;18(8):607–13.
68. Hudson MM, et al. Long-term follow-up guidelines for survivors of childhood, adolescent and young adult cancers version 3.0. 2008. Available from: http://www.survivorshipguidelines.org/pdf/LTFUGuidelines.pdf

Chapter 13
Acute Kidney Injury and Renal Replacement Therapy in Immunocompromised Children

Joseph Angelo and Ayse A. Arikan

Introduction

Acute kidney injury (AKI) is characterized by an abrupt decline in renal function with associated metabolic and fluid derangements. AKI occurs commonly in the pediatric intensive care unit (ICU) and can have significant impact on morbidity and mortality. Children developing AKI are at increased risk of death, longer time on mechanical ventilation, and longer ICU and hospital length of stay. While many children admitted to the ICU have few baseline comorbidities, those with oncologic diagnoses and with an immunocompromised state frequently have preexisting risk factors that predispose them to AKI such as prior renal injury, infection, sepsis, hematopoietic stem cell transplant, and nephrotoxic medication exposure. In addition, they are more likely to be admitted with shock or respiratory failure, increasing their AKI risk even further [1]. With this increased risk of AKI, and the association of AKI with poor outcomes, it is vitally important that patients at risk be identified early so that targeted and goal-directed therapy can be initiated. This chapter outlines current definitions of AKI, risk factors for the development of AKI in critically ill oncology patients, clinical features of AKI, and treatment of AKI in the pediatric ICU.

J. Angelo (✉)
Department of Pediatrics, Renal Section,
Texas Children's Hospital/Baylor College of Medicine, Houston, TX, USA
e-mail: jrangel1@texaschildrens.org

A. A. Arikan
Renal Section, Critical Care Section,
Texas Children's Hospital/Baylor College of Medicine, Houston, TX, USA

C. N. Duncan et al. (eds.), *Critical Care of the Pediatric Immunocompromised Hematology/Oncology Patient*, https://doi.org/10.1007/978-3-030-01322-6_13

Defining and Staging AKI

Current definitions of AKI are based on increases in serum creatinine (SCr) and decreased urine output over specified time periods. Until 2004 there was lack of a consistent definition of AKI, and more than 30 criteria for defining AKI were proposed [2]. In 2004 the Acute Dialysis Quality Initiative (ADQI) group created the Risk, Injury, Failure, Loss, End-stage (RIFLE) criteria in order to have a standardized definition to investigate the epidemiology and clinical outcomes associated with AKI as well as provide a framework for AKI severity. A pediatric adaptation called pRIFLE was proposed in 2007 and has been widely validated [3]. The Acute Kidney Injury Network (AKIN) criteria presented a modification to the original RIFLE criteria by adding a somewhat more stringent category of an absolute increase in SCr of ≥0.3 mg/dl in a 48 h period to meet the definition of AKI [4]. Most recently, in 2012, the Kidney Disease Improving Global Outcomes (KDIGO) classification system was developed as part of a clinical practice guideline for AKI. KDIGO defines AKI by integrating features from RIFLE, pRIFLE, and AKIN, applies to both pediatric and adult populations, and stages AKI into three stages based on severity of oliguria or rise in SCr. An outline of the above AKI classification schema is in Table 13.1. Of note, the KDIGO system is currently accepted as the gold standard for AKI diagnosis and staging and should be used when defining AKI and examining related outcomes.

An important concept highlighted by these classification systems is the staging of AKI, which has important clinical implications as severity of AKI has been associated with several patient outcomes. A recent large, prospective, multicenter study,

Table 13.1 KDIGO and pRIFLE criteria

	KDIGO			Pediatric modified RIFLE (pRIFLE)	
AKI Stage	Serum creatinine	Urine output	AKI Stage	Estimated creatinine clearance	Urine output
Stage 1	1.5–1.9 × baseline or ≥0.3 mg/dL increase	< 0.5 ml/kg/h for 6–12 h	R	eCrCl decrease by 25%	0.5 ml/kg/h for 8 h
Stage 2	2.0–2.9 × baseline	< 0.5 ml/kg/h for ≥12 h	I	eCrCl decrease by 50%	0.5 ml/kg/h for 16 h
Stage 3	3.0 × baseline or increase to ≥4 mg/dL or initiation of RRT or in <18 y/o eGFR <35 ml/min/1.73 m^2	< 0.3 ml/kg/h for ≥24 h or anuria ≥12 h	F	eCrCl decrease by 75% or <35 ml/min/1.73m^2	0.3 ml/kg/h for 24 h or anuria for 12 h

Refs. [3]; KDIGO clinical practice guideline for acute kidney injury. Kidney International Supplements, 2012; 2(1)

which defined severe AKI as KDIGO grade 2 or 3, showed that severe AKI conferred a nearly two times higher risk of 28-day mortality and also was associated with longer mechanical ventilator duration and likelihood of needing renal replacement therapy [1]. Even miniscule increases in SCr have important clinical implications and are associated with adverse outcomes [5, 6]. Additionally, reversal of even mild AKI still carries associations with adverse outcomes compared to children never developing renal injury [7]. Data such as this highlight the importance of identifying those children at risk for AKI, early recognition of the onset of AKI, and timely intervention to prevent the progression.

While establishing standardized AKI definitions has had an obvious impact both in terms of studying AKI and in the clinical setting, practitioners should keep in mind the potential shortcomings of using SCr as a functional biomarker of AKI. There can be significant lag time between a rise in SCr and the actual onset of AKI; therefore, SCr may not provide the earliest window for intervention [8]. In addition, SCr can be affected by patient-specific factors such as age, gender, nutrition status, muscle mass, and hydration status. Several of these confounders of SCr as a marker of AKI are particularly relevant to the pediatric oncology population who, owing to their underlying disease, can have relatively poor nutrition and muscle wasting. Similarly, small changes in SCr can represent a significant decline in renal function and have been shown to impact patient outcomes [9]. For example, a 2005 publication by Chertow et al. showed that an increase in SCr of as little as 0.3 mg/dl in adult patients was independently associated with increased mortality [10]. Heightened vigilance is needed as seemingly innocuous changes in SCr can have adverse patient outcomes [10, 6]. Regarding AKI progression, utilizing SCr to estimate glomerular filtration rate (GFR) also creates a potential problem since methods of estimating GFR are based on steady-state SCr levels, which does not account for the dynamic change in GFR when SCr is steadily rising and, thus, leading to an overestimation of GFR. This can be particularly problematic when dosing medications based on estimated GFR and presents the risk of further exacerbation of the progression of AKI. Finally, definitions of AKI utilize change in SCr relative to a baseline to identify AKI, thereby, presenting another problem, as this preadmission information might not be available. Despite these potential shortcomings, SCr remains a convenient and rapid way to identify AKI at the bedside, but awareness of potential limitations is important to consider when using it to guide clinical care.

Given some of the problems inherent when using SCr to detect AKI, other potential biomarkers have been investigated for the diagnosis of AKI. Cystatin C is an endogenous cysteine protease inhibitor that is secreted by all nucleated cells, is freely filtered through the glomerulus, metabolized completely by proximal renal tubular cells, is not secreted along the nephron, and does not undergo extrarenal clearance from the blood. Cystatin C is another filtration marker with a shorter half-life than SCr; thus, changes in cystatin C might be more sensitive and can detect AKI earlier than SCr. Additionally, cystatin C is not impacted by changes in body habitus, age, or fluid status [11, 12, 13]. Despite conflicting adult reports, cystatin C, and GFR estimation based on cystatin C, has shown promising results in children undergoing chemotherapy to detect changes in renal function; however, it has not been specifically tested in detection of AKI in the pediatric oncology population [14, 15]. A recent systematic review has shown good performance of serum cystatin C in monitoring changes in renal function in pediatric patients undergoing chemotherapy; however, cystatin C lacks the sensitivity to replace direct measurement of GFR for chemotherapy dose adjustment [16]. Other potential biomarkers fall into three broad categories: inflammatory markers (such as urinary and plasma neutrophil gelatinase-associated lipocalin (NGAL), urinary IL-18), tubular injury markers (such as urinary kidney injury molecule-1 (KIM-1), and, more recently, tubular stress markers (such as metalloproteinases) [17]. None have yielded consistently superior results to detection by SCr [18]. While each of these may have value in specific in clinical scenarios, a more robust utilization of such biomarkers might come in the form of an AKI panel similar to the use of troponins in the diagnosis of acute myocardial infarction [19]. Recently, a newer generation of biomarkers, called cell cycle arrest markers, has been shown to predict severe AKI in critically ill adults and in children after cardiac surgery but is yet to be tested in children with cancer [20, 21]. Another potential use for non-filtration-based markers is monitoring recovery of kidney function patients on renal replacement therapy (RRT) where SCr is no longer useful since it is cleared via dialysis. Inflammatory markers have shown promise in detection of nephrotoxicity, particularly chemotherapy-associated AKI; however, further study is needed for them to gain more widespread clinical use [18].

AKI Epidemiology

AKI is seen frequently in the pediatric ICU, and immunosuppressed patients can be particularly at risk. Prior to the development of more standardized definitions of AKI, the incidence of AKI in critically ill children was shown to range from 1% to as high as 80% [22]. In addition, the incidence of AKI can vary depending on the patient population examined and the timeframe over which AKI occurrence is tracked. For example, a 2007 study, using the pRIFLE criteria to define AKI in intubated PICU patients, found that 80% of patients developed AKI at some time during their ICU admission [3]. Other studies have shown rates of AKI of 32% in septic shock patients and 10% in children post stem cell transplant [23, 24]. Using more refined and standardized definitions, such as those outlined above, the incidence likely ranges from 30% to 60% depending on the risk factors of the group examined. Comparing the pRIFLE, AKIN, and KDIGO definitions of AKI, Sutherland et al. found the incidence of AKI to be 51% using pRIFLE, 37% using AKIN, and 40% using KDIGO criteria [25]. More recently, the AWARE study group examined 4683 pediatric ICU patients of which 1261 (26.9%) developed AKI of any stage. By stage, the incidence of AKI was 718 (15%), 294 (6%), and 249 (5%) for stages 1, 2, and 3, respectively. An important point demonstrated by this data is that nearly 12% of this group developed severe AKI defined as stage 2 or 3 [1]. The incidence of AKI in the oncology and bone marrow transplant group was almost 50%, nearly double the incidence in the general ICU population.

Another important aspect of AKI epidemiology is the transition that has been seen from AKI due to primary renal diseases to AKI that occur in association with other systemic illnesses or due to exposure to treatments for other diseases. For example, of 254 cases of AKI seen in a study by Hui-Stickle et al., only 17 (7%) were associated with primary renal disease; the most common causes were ischemic injury, nephrotoxic medications, and sepsis. Of note, 33 cases of AKI occurred in patients with an underlying hematologic/oncologic diagnosis [26]. The shift from AKI related to primary renal diseases to an entity in the context of systemic illness, often with coexisting multi-organ involvement, highlights the need to consider AKI in a more dynamic sense, with the kidney being a target of injury from external insults but also with AKI having independent influence on the function of other organs. Children with leukemia, particularly AML, have a high incidence of AKI, especially those with sepsis.

Bone marrow transplant patients are a particularly vulnerable population due to case mix and presence of risk factors. In a report from St Jude's including over 1000 BMT patients, AKI incidence was 50% within 1 month and 68% within 100 days of BMT [27].

Risk Factors for AKI Critically Ill Hematology/Oncology Patients

Children with cancer are a group particularly at risk for AKI secondary to exposure to chemotherapy and other potentially nephrotoxic medications, higher risk of infection and sepsis, hematopoietic cell transplantation, and direct effects from their primary malignancy. As noted above, for those becoming critically ill, the risk of AKI is increased further. Several risk factors for AKI are particularly prominent in the pediatric oncology population.

Volume depletion is a frequent confounder in the pathophysiology of AKI in oncology patients and, specifically, the HCT recipient. Nausea and vomiting associated with underlying disease or chemotherapy regimen, as well as increased insensible losses, and the fluid restriction commonly applied to HCT patients predispose to hypovolemia and functional AKI.

In HCT recipients, older age, total body irradiation (TBI), and calcineurin inhibitor-based graft versus host disease (GVHD) prophylaxis were risk factors for 100-day AKI development. In addition, unrelated donor, number of HCTs, and presence of veno-occlusive disease were strong predictors of renal replacement therapy (RRT) requirement [28]. Survival in stage III AKI was dismal, especially in patients requiring RRT, with less than 10% 1-year survival overall [27, 29].

As many as 90% of patients with sinusoidal obstruction syndrome (SOS) develop AKI, over half develop severe AKI [30]. Hepatorenal syndrome-like physiology and abdominal compartment syndrome with tight ascites may both contribute to onset of AKI due to perturbations in renal perfusion in this setting. GVHD prophylaxis and treatment can be associated with AKI, especially if it is based on calcineurin inhibitor use, which can lead to acute and chronic nephrotoxicity. Additionally, severe gut GVHD might lead to gastrointestinal bleeding and associated hypoperfusion-related AKI [31, 32]. The presence of GVHD has been independently linked to kidney injury [33]. In the HCT population, transplant-associated thrombotic microangiopathy (TA-TMA) also occurs commonly and is a significant risk factor for AKI [34, 28].

Many of the chemotherapeutic agents used to treat childhood cancer are nephrotoxic. Among the most frequent offenders are the platinum agents as well as cyclophosphamide, ifosfamide, and VP-16. Amount of radiation used and myeloablative conditioning regimens are associated with a higher risk of AKI in the 100 days following SCT. Cancer patients are frequently exposed to multiple other nephrotoxic medications for morbidity related to chemotherapy, such as antibiotics required for treatment of infections during immunosuppression [35].

Sepsis constitutes another significant risk factor for AKI in critically ill patients and in the pediatric oncology patient in particular. Almost half of patients with sepsis-associated severe AKI had neoplastic diagnoses or were transplant recipients in an international multicenter study of severe sepsis [36].

Implications of AKI in the ICU

AKI has been shown to be an independent predictor of several patient outcomes including increased hospital length of stay, increased ICU length of stay, need for and duration of mechanical ventilation, and mortality. For example, in a 2011 Canadian study of 2106 admissions to the PICU, those patients with AKI showed an increased number of days on mechanical ventilation, longer PICU length of stay, and 3.7 times increased risk of mortality [5]. Similar results were seen in the AWARE study with death occurring in 11% of patients with severe AKI compared to 2.5% of patients without severe AKI. The AWARE study also showed an incremental increase in mortality based on stage of AKI. Supporting data from prior studies, AKI was associated with increased risk of requiring mechanical ventilation, longer duration of mechanical ventilation, increased need for renal replacement therapy, and increased use of extracorporeal membrane oxygenation [1].

Fluid overload both in the setting of AKI and independently has also been associated with several negative outcomes in critically ill adults and children. Two populations that have been seen to be particularly affected by fluid overload are HCT patients and those with multi-organ dysfunction. A 2004 study showed that HCT patients with <10% fluid overload had improved survival compared to those that had >10% fluid overload during their ICU admission [24]. Considering those with multi-organ dysfunction, Foland et al. showed that survivors had a lower degree of fluid overload (9.2%) compared to non-survivors (15.5%) at initiation of continuous renal replacement therapy (CRRT) [37]. Fluid overload has also been associated with organ-specific outcomes, particularly lung function. A 2012 study by Arikan et al. showed that not only was peak level of fluid overload associated with peak oxygenation index value but also that incremental increases in percentage fluid overload correlated with similar increases in oxygenation index [38].

While available data does not necessarily support a causal relationship between AKI, fluid overload, and adverse outcomes, these studies do highlight the influence that the development of AKI and fluid overload can have in critically ill patients. This is particularly significant in immunosuppressed children with oncologic disease given that they frequently present to the ICU systemically ill with multiple organs affected by a primary disease process. Therefore, it is vitally important that the complex interplay between organ systems is addressed concurrently in order to maximize the implementation of a complete treatment plan.

AKI Evaluation

The potential etiologies of AKI fall into three broad categories: prerenal (now also called functional), intrinsic AKI, and post-renal obstructive etiologies. The classification of AKI into one of these categories can narrow the differential diagnosis and allow for therapeutic interventions that specifically target the underlying cause of AKI. Starting with a detailed initial medical history, information on the temporal relationship between inciting events and the onset of AKI, such as an episode of hypotension or the timing of administration of medications, needs to be gathered. The physical exam can provide other signs regarding systemic diseases with renal involvement, and also in terms of detailing the effects that changes in kidney function are having on the patient's overall status, particularly when fluid overload is present. Similarly, urinary volume output is a readily available data and an important marker in the setting of AKI since the management of non-oliguric and oligo-anuric AKI can be quite different. This basic history and physical exam data can then be integrated with other easily obtainable indices to distinguish which type of AKI is present.

Initial laboratory studies in the evaluation of AKI should include serum electrolytes, blood urea nitrogen (BUN), serum creatinine (SCr), and complete blood count. Urine studies should include urinalysis, urine-specific gravity, urinary sediment analysis, urine electrolytes, urine creatinine, urine protein, and urine osmolality. In addition to directly providing important pieces of data, these initial laboratory values can also be utilized to calculate additional indices for classifying AKI. These indices are fairly straightforward to compute and, thus, are readily available for use at the bedside. One very important step in assessing AKI is distinguishing between AKI from decreased renal perfusion (prerenal or functional) and AKI related to intrinsic renal tubular injury and dysfunction. Under conditions of hypoperfusion, the healthy kidney responds by increasing tubular reabsorption of both sodium and water through the actions of hormones such as aldosterone and antidiurectic hormone (ADH), and several indices are available to assess whether this mechanism is intact. The BUN/creatinine ratio can be used in this situation and typically is >20:1 in states of reduced renal perfusion. Similarly, the fractional excretion of sodium (FENa), based on the ability of the proximal and distal tubule to reabsorb sodium as renal perfusion falls, is another indicator of a decline in renal perfusion pressure. When the renal response to hypoperfusion is intact, sodium reabsorption by the renal tubule increases, urine sodium falls to <20 mEq/L, and the FENa is <1%, indicating the presence of prerenal/functional AKI. In contrast, the FENa in acute tubular necrosis (ATN) or intrinsic forms of AKI is typically >3% [39]. Calculation of the FENa requires simultaneous measurements of the serum sodium (SNa), serum creatinine (SCr), urine sodium (UNa), and urine creatinine (UCr); and then these values are entered into the formula:

$$\text{FENa} = (\text{UNa} \times \text{SCr}) / (\text{SNa} \times \text{UCr}) \times 100$$

In situations when urinary Na is affected by extrinsic factors, such as diuretic use, the fractional excretion of urea (FEurea) can be substituted for the FENa [39]. To calculate FEUrea, similar values are needed: serum urea (SUrea), urine urea (UUrea), serum creatinine (SCr), and urine creatinine (UCr). The formula for FEUrea is the same as FENa, substituting serum urea for serum sodium and urine urea for urine sodium:

$$\text{FEURea} = (\text{UUrea} \times \text{SCr}) / (\text{SUrea} \times \text{UCr}) \times 100$$

In prerenal AKI, the FEurea is typically <35%.

Examination of the urine with urinalysis and microscopic evaluation of the urinary sediment can also be useful in evaluating the underlying etiology of AKI. The presence of blood on urine dipstick without red cells in the sediment is usually indicative of other pigment – such as hemoglobinuria or myoglobinuria with risk of pigment nephropathy. Urinalysis in prerenal azotemia can show fine granular and hyaline casts, while renal tubular injury causes shedding of epithelial cells into the urine producing epithelial cell casts and coarse granular casts or muddy casts in severe AKI with tubular necrosis. Active inflammatory processes and glomerular processes, such as glomerulonephritis, can show the presence of white blood cells as well as albuminuria, red blood cells, and red blood cell casts.

Radiologic imaging of the kidney is also important, particularly if urinary obstruction is suspected. Of these, renal ultrasound (RUS) is the most commonly used, with typical findings in urinary obstructive processes including hydronephrosis, ureteral dilatation, and a dilated bladder. Retroperitoneal masses and the presence of mass effect on the urinary tract can also be detected using RUS. Changes in bladder wall contour can suggest cystitis. In children, RUS is also an effective modality to reveal any congenital renal anomalies, such as renal dysplasia, providing information on underlying chronic kidney disease as a risk factor for AKI. Further studies, such as a voiding cystourethrogram for urinary reflux, or nuclear medicine scans for examination of renal scarring or blood flow, can be based on initial RUS findings and increased index of suspicion for these specific problems.

Finally, although sometimes difficult to obtain in severally critically ill patients and oncology patients with underlying bleeding risk, renal biopsy can provide valuable information regarding the underlying pathogenesis of AKI. Due to these risks, biopsy should be reserved for situations in which the results will provide data that might change the treatment plan.

An important consideration when applying these diagnostic tools to evaluate AKI is that the results are not always specific to one etiology. There can be considerable overlap, and so each piece of data should be considered in the context of the patient's overall clinical picture in order to provide an integrated assessment, which will provide accurate guidance in developing a treatment plan. Additionally, as with other ICU conditions, AKI can be dynamic and progressive requiring that diagnostic tools and therapies be similarly adaptable to account for changes in a patient's current status. As noted previously, AKI now occurs most frequently as a multifactorial entity in the context of broader systemic disease rather than directly from isolated renal disease necessitating a multidisciplinary approach to diagnosis and management of AKI in the critically ill.

AKI Treatment

An attempt to uncover the main etiology underlying AKI must always be made in order to provide adequate treatment, as etiology will determine the specific treatment pathway. Early protocolized resuscitation bundle implementation is protective against development of sepsis associated AKI [40]. Restoration of intravascular volume is critically important in prevention of further AKI progression especially in volume-depleted states. Saline hydration is the cornerstone of tumor lysis-associated AKI and might garner some protection against contrast-induced AKI also. Rasburicase, recombinant urate oxidase, has favorably changed the pediatric tumor lysis syndrome (TLS)-associated AKI incidence. In overwhelming TLS, acute phosphate nephropathy can be seen with extensive calcium and phosphorus deposition in the tubulointerstitium and resultant tissue damage. Paracentesis might be necessary to restore optimal renal perfusion in abdominal compartment physiology; serial measurements of bladder pressure are useful to assess intra-abdominal pressure. SCr and/or cystatin C must be closely monitored, as well as urine volume as frequently oliguria is the earliest and most sensitive indicator of developing AKI. The risks of an indwelling urinary catheter must be balanced against the benefit of early detection. For oliguric AKI, renal reserve could be challenged with an adequate (at least 2 mg/kg) dose of furosemide, given circulatory stability. Non-oliguric AKI management largely rests on metabolic control with appropriate electrolyte supplementation and not infrequently urine output replacement in polyuric states. For oliguric patients, conservative management involves careful fluid administration (restriction to insensible losses of 400 cc/m2/day and urine output replacement) and potassium and phosphorus restriction. It is frequently necessary to start RRT in the oliguric patient, as the oncology patient often has ongoing needs of medication delivery and blood product replacement that surpasses the limits of fluid restriction. Continuous RRT is the dialytic therapy of choice and is discussed in detail below.

There are very few pharmacological options for AKI treatment. Nephrotoxic agents must be stopped when possible, and strict therapeutic drug monitoring must be instituted for those that are essential. Consultation with a clinical pharmacist is very beneficial and is highly recommended. Low-dose dopamine has not been shown to be renoprotective. Fenoldopam, a selective dopamine receptor agonist, has been shown to increase urine output in pediatric cardiac surgical patients but has not been tested in cancer or HCT population [41]. Diuretics do not prevent AKI but might assist in management of volume overload. In severely hypoalbuminemic patients with overt volume overload, albumin-assisted diuresis with infusion of concentrated albumin infusion followed by loop diuretics could be considered.

Renal Replacement Therapy

In general, indications for the initiation of renal replacement therapy (RRT) include correction of metabolic derangements, such as hyperkalemia and metabolic acidosis, and management of fluid overload and allow for provision of optimal nutritional in situations where this is limited by poor renal function. Several modes of RRT are available in the ICU: intermittent hemodialysis (IHD), peritoneal dialysis (PD), and continuous renal replacement therapy (CRRT). As many of the concepts and issues related to each modality have overlap, and as it has become the modality of choice in the ICU except for specific clinical scenarios, the following discussion will focus mainly on CRRT.

Several studies have supported the concept of early initiation of CRRT, particularly with respect to fluid overload. An initial study by Goldstein et al. in 2001 showed that children initiated on CRRT at lower percent fluid overload (%FO) of 16.4%, calculated as the difference of total fluid intake and output indexed to ICU admission weight, had increased survival compared to those initiated at higher %FO (34%) [42]. Subsequent studies have produced similar data regarding outcome and amount of FO at the time of CRRT initiation [37, 43, 44]. This fluid overload effect can be particularly prominent in specific patient populations, including those post HCT and children with MODS [24, 45].

While the definition of early initiation of CRRT is not clearly established, available data certainly supports the idea that with increasing accumulation of fluid, the implementation of CRRT should become more strongly considered. A suggested algorithm has been that at <10% FO to continue with medical therapy such as diuretics, at 10–15% FO CRRT should start to be considered, particularly in the HCT population, and at >15–20% FO CRRT should be initiated. Clearly, this pathway should be considered in the context of the patient's overall clinical status with a proactive approach to prevent emergent need for RRT and initiation as a controlled and planned procedure.

Once the decision to initiate CRRT has been made, there are several key steps that must take place. Obtaining good central venous access is the essential and frequently rate-limiting step in starting a pediatric patient on CRRT. In general, the minimum size of vascular catheters for optimal circuit survival is 7Fr for children less than 10 kg. However, emerging CRRT technology could allow for lower blood flows and, therefore, smaller catheter sizes, expanding the utility of CRRT in smaller children. Beyond this weight, catheter sizes should be selected that are appropriate to patient size. Appropriate catheter size during CRRT has been shown to increase circuit life-span with prolonged duration of circuit life favored by larger diameter catheters. Similarly, data supports internal jugular (IJ) location of dialysis catheters to optimize circuit life [46]. Typical CRRT circuit life is 72 h, and maximizing circuit life is an important aspect of CRRT as circuit downtime can contribute significantly to interruptions in therapy.

Regarding CRRT circuit anticoagulation, regional citrate has become the most commonly used for CRRT circuit anticoagulation and is generally a safe and effective method anticoagulation. Citrate infused on the access side of the CRRT circuit functions by interrupting the coagulation cascade via calcium chelation; thus, providing regional anticoagulation focused at the dialysis filter as opposed to the systemic anticoagulation with heparin. For patients with increased bleeding risk, the avoidance of systemic anticoagulation can lower the risk of bleeding events [47, 48]. When citrate is used, it is necessary to replete the patient's calcium stores, which is preferably done via a dedicated central line at a site away from the dialysis circuit tubing and dialysis catheter. Laboratory monitoring when using citrate includes systemic ionized calcium; post-dialysis filter ionized calcium, to insure adequate anticoagulation; and serum electrolytes. Coagulation parameters, such as prothrombin time, do not need to be monitored when using citrate. While citrate is the preferred agent for CRRT anticoagulation, there can be clinical situations in which the use of systemic heparin is more appropriate. For these cases, the risk/benefit ratio of citrate versus heparin anticoagulation should be considered. Protocols and lab monitoring when utilizing heparin are similar to those for heparin use in other clinical situations but will be unique to each institution and should be developed in conjunction with nephrology, hematology, and ICU teams.

As noted, one of the primary goals of CRRT is fluid balance regulation. Given this, high priority must be given to discussion of fluid removal goals prior to initiation of CRRT and at frequent intervals while therapy is ongoing, particularly when clinical changes occur. Achieving the agreed-upon goal is of utmost importance and requires accurate recording of fluid inputs and outputs which need to be readily available and clearly communicated to all members of the care team.

Several other specific aspects of CRRT also require consideration. Infants and younger children present unique issues in preparing for and while on CRRT. For children whose total blood volume (70 cc × Wt in kg) is <10% of the total volume of CRRT circuit, blood priming of the circuit will be needed. For example, for a 10 kg child with a total blood volume of 700 cc, a CRRT circuit volume of 200 cc would yield a 28% difference (200 cc/700 cc) and a blood prime with PRBCs would be required. Circuit volumes will be institution dependent depending on the brand of CRRT machine used and dialysis filter and tubing sizes available. CRRT circuit blood priming should get the same considerations as blood product infusions in other situations including transfusion reaction, changes in body temperature, and potassium load. In addition to these initial considerations, due to differences in metabolism and volume of distribution of drugs, small children can be more susceptible to toxicity related to citrate anticoagulation. Typical findings associated with this include hypocalcemia, manifested by falling ionized calcium levels despite stable or rising total calcium values. The majority of citrate infused is cleared by the CRRT circuit, and patients are only exposed to a residual amount. However, as citrate is metabolized to bicarbonate by the liver, prolonged use of citrate solutions can lead to metabolic alkalosis in CRRT patients. Patients with liver failure, such as those with veno-occlusive disease, are another group with increased risk of citrate lock and citrate toxicity due to alterations in citrate metabolism. Awareness of this potential complication is important to maintain safe delivery of CRRT in these groups. Consideration should be given to more frequent lab monitoring and possibly tailoring anticoagulation protocols for those with liver dysfunction. For example, tolerance of a higher post-filter ionized calcium allows for a decreased citrate load. This does need to be weighed against risk of circuit clotting because, as noted above, circuit downtime can have a significant impact on the delivery of adequate dialysis. Labs including electrolytes, ionized calcium, and blood gas may need to be followed more frequently, and abnormalities in these values should be discussed in conjunction with nephrology in order for appropriate adjustments to be made to the CRRT circuit, including citrate and calcium infusions.

Smaller children, particularly those who are severely ill, can also be less tolerant of fluid shifts associated with CRRT ultrafiltration. This highlights the need for establishing clear fluid removal goals among all teams, and even small hemodynamic changes should be monitored closely and changes in therapy made to prevent negative consequences. The potential for excessively rapid fluid removal to cause hemodynamic instability also emphasizes the importance of accurate recording of fluid balance on CRRT. Inaccurate fluid balance monitoring can manifest as increased fluid gain when ultrafiltration is not set appropriately to account for all fluid inputs. While this can be more of a problem in small children, it is the case for all patients on CRRT and is one of the most important discussions that care teams should have so that all are updated on the goals of dialysis.

Another important consideration for patients on CRRT, particularly relevant in the oncology population, is close monitoring of drug levels. Drug clearance on CRRT is highly variable depending on the properties of the drug molecule (e.g., size, charge, protein binding) and can also vary with changes in CRRT prescription, including when changes are made to volume of ultrafiltration. Both in vitro and in vivo studies highlight this concept [49, 50, 51]. For patients receiving chemotherapy or those on antibiotics for sepsis, potential changes in drug delivery can have significant consequences. When clinically available, levels of drugs, such as calcineurin inhibitors and antibiotics, need to be checked frequently to insure adequate drug delivery. Consultation with a pharmacist skilled in critical care and CRRT drug dosing is recommended.

As noted, another indication for the initiation of CRRT is in order to provide fluid regulation to allow for the provision of adequate nutrition. In general, a daily protein intake of ~3 mg/kg/day is a reasonable nutritional goal for children on CRRT. In order to avoid fluid and metabolic imbalances, close monitoring of total parental nutrition volume and electrolyte content is needed, and TPN or any electrolyte containing solutions should be held during circuit downtimes. Trace mineral and vitamin clearance can also occur on CRRT. One of particular note is carnitine [52]. As with drug dosing, nutrition consultation is recommended in order to optimally address specific nutritional needs.

Finally, hypothermia is common in patients undergoing RRT, and in-line circuit warmers should be used. For this reason, clinicians also need to be aware that the febrile response to infection can be masked while on CRRT. Therefore, monitoring of temperature trends and changes in hemodynamic stability should be used as indicators of a developing infection. There should be a low threshold for obtaining cultures from central catheters and for empirically starting or broadening antibiotic coverage.

Long-Term AKI Outcomes

Contrary to previous beliefs, AKI is not a completely reversible phenomenon and can result in decreased renal reserve and lead to chronic kidney disease over time. Childhood survivors of cancer are at particular risk, as decreased GFR has been reported in up to 50% of long-term survivors [53]. For patients who suffer from primary tumors that involve the kidney such as Wilm's tumor, nephron sparing surgery has been shown to have superior long-term outcomes [54]. Older age at nephrectomy is a risk factor for faster decline of GFR. These patients remain at high risk of renal functional decline and require close follow-up by a nephrologist. Patients who have received platin agents, ifosfamide, radiation therapy involving the kidney, and nephrectomy are at increased risk of CKD, hypertension, and proteinuria. Total body irradiation involving the renal fossae has also been linked to AKI and renal sequelae. Secondary malignancies are observed with increased frequency in childhood survivors of cancer and might involve the kidneys. End-stage renal disease has been reported to develop after HCT, most commonly in the setting of refractory TA-TMA but also after veno-occlusive disease. In addition, AKI has been shown to be a risk factor of new acquired disability or poorer functional outcome in pediatric critically ill patients with severe sepsis [36].

Conclusion

As treatments for hematologic and oncologic diseases have improved, survival for children with cancer has increased significantly. However, due to complications related to their primary disease, they remain a group at high risk for the development of AKI. The presence of AKI can have significant effects on other organ systems and complicates the care of critically ill children. In addition, AKI increases the likelihood of poor outcomes including mortality. This necessitates that caregivers be astute in order to facilitate early detection and treatment of AKI. AKI management also requires a multidisciplinary approach with effective communication between all teams involved in the care of these children. With further advancement of the science of AKI and the development of new therapies, survival for children with cancer will continue to improve.

References

1. Kaddourah A, et al. Epidemiology of acute kidney injury in critically ill children and young adults. N Engl J Med. 2017;376(1):11–20.
2. Kellum JA, et al. Developing a consensus classification system for acute renal failure. Curr Opin Crit Care. 2002;8(6):509–14.
3. Akcan-Arikan A, et al. Modified RIFLE criteria in critically ill children with acute kidney injury. Kidney Int. 2007;71(10):1028–35.
4. Mehta RL, et al. Acute Kidney Injury Network: report of an initiative to improve outcomes in acute kidney injury. Crit Care. 2007;11(2):R31.
5. Alkandari O, et al. Acute kidney injury is an independent risk factor for pediatric intensive care unit mortality, longer length of stay and prolonged mechanical ventilation in critically ill children: a two-center retrospective cohort study. Crit Care. 2011;15(3):R146.
6. Zappitelli M, et al. A small post-operative rise in serum creatinine predicts acute kidney injury in children undergoing cardiac surgery. Kidney Int. 2009;76(8):885–92.
7. Sanchez-Pinto LN, et al. Association between progression and improvement of acute kidney injury and mortality in critically ill children. Pediatr Crit Care Med. 2015;16(8):703–10.
8. Devarajan P. Emerging biomarkers of acute kidney injury. In: Ronco C, Bellomo R, Kellum JA, editors. Acute kidney injury. Basel: Karger Publishers; 2007. p. 203–12.
9. Samuels J, et al. Small increases in serum creatinine are associated with prolonged ICU stay and increased hospital mortality in critically ill patients with cancer. Support Care Cancer. 2011;19(10):1527–32.
10. Chertow GM, et al. Acute kidney injury, mortality, length of stay, and costs in hospitalized patients. J Am Soc Nephrol. 2005;16(11):3365–70.
11. Volpon LC, Sugo EK, Carlotti AP. Diagnostic and prognostic value of serum cystatin C in critically ill children with acute kidney injury. Pediatr Crit Care Med. 2015;16(5):e125–31.
12. Safdar OY, et al. Serum cystatin is a useful marker for the diagnosis of acute kidney injury in critically ill children: prospective cohort study. BMC Nephrol. 2016;17(1):130.
13. Inker LA, et al. Estimating glomerular filtration rate from serum creatinine and cystatin C. N Engl J Med. 2012;367(1):20–9.
14. Al-Tonbary YA, et al. Pretreatment cystatin C in children with malignancy: can it predict chemotherapy-induced glomerular filtration rate reduction during the induction phase? J Pediatr Hematol Oncol. 2004;26(6):336–41.
15. Barnfield MC, et al. Cystatin C in assessment of glomerular filtration rate in children and young adults suffering from cancer. Nucl Med Commun. 2013;34(6):609–14.
16. Whiting P, et al. Accuracy of cystatin C for the detection of abnormal renal function in children undergoing chemotherapy for malignancy: a systematic review using individual patient data. Support Care Cancer. 2017:1–10.
17. Nguyen MT, Devarajan P. Biomarkers for the early detection of acute kidney injury. Pediatr Nephrol. 2008;23(12):2151.

18. Sterling M, et al. Urine biomarkers of acute kidney injury in noncritically ill, hospitalized children treated with chemotherapy. Pediatr Blood Cancer. 2017;64(10)
19. Basu RK, et al. Incorporation of biomarkers with the renal angina index for prediction of severe AKI in critically ill children. Clin J Am Soc Nephrol. 2014;9(4):654–62.
20. Bihorac A, et al. Validation of cell-cycle arrest biomarkers for acute kidney injury using clinical adjudication. Am J Respir Crit Care Med. 2014;189(8):932–9.
21. Meersch M, et al. Validation of cell-cycle arrest biomarkers for acute kidney injury after pediatric cardiac surgery. PLoS One. 2014;9(10):e110865.
22. Fortenberry JD, Paden ML, Goldstein SL. Acute kidney injury in children: an update on diagnosis and treatment. Pediatr Clin. 2013;60(3):669–88.
23. Plötz FB, et al. Effect of acute renal failure on outcome in children with severe septic shock. Pediatr Nephrol. 2005;20(8):1177–81.
24. Michael M, Kuehnle I, Goldstein SL. Fluid overload and acute renal failure in pediatric stem cell transplant patients. Pediatr Nephrol. 2004;19(1):91–5.
25. Sutherland SM, et al. AKI in hospitalized children: comparing the pRIFLE, AKIN, and KDIGO definitions. Clin J Am Soc Nephrol. 2015;10(4):554–61.
26. Hui-Stickle S, Brewer ED, Goldstein SL. Pediatric ARF epidemiology at a tertiary care center from 1999 to 2001. Am J Kidney Dis. 2005;45(1):96–101.
27. Koh K-N, et al. Acute kidney injury in pediatric patients receiving allogeneic hematopoietic cell transplantation: incidence, risk factors, and outcomes. Biol Blood Marrow Transplant. 2018;24(4):758–64.
28. Hingorani S. Renal complications of hematopoietic-cell transplantation. N Engl J Med. 2016;374(23):2256–67.
29. Selewski DT, et al. Validation of the KDIGO acute kidney injury criteria in a pediatric critical care population. Intensive Care Med. 2014;40(10):1481–8.
30. Raina R, et al. Hematopoietic stem cell transplantation and acute kidney injury in children: A comprehensive review. Pediatr Transplant. 2017;21(4):e12935.
31. Krishnappa V, et al. Acute kidney injury in hematopoietic stem cell transplantation: a review. Int J Nephrol. 2016;2016:5163789.
32. Mori J, et al. Risk assessment for acute kidney injury after allogeneic hematopoietic stem cell transplantation based on Acute Kidney Injury Network criteria. Intern Med. 2012;51(16):2105–10.
33. Changsirikulchai S, et al. Renal thrombotic microangiopathy after hematopoietic cell transplant: role of GVHD in pathogenesis. Clin J Am Soc Nephrol. 2009;4(2):345–53.
34. Laskin BL, et al. Small vessels, big trouble in the kidneys and beyond: hematopoietic stem cell transplantation–associated thrombotic microangiopathy. Blood. 2011;118(6):1452–62.
35. Du Plessis L, Rassekh SR, Mammen C. High incidence of acute kidney injury during chemotherapy for childhood acute myeloid leukemia. Pediatr Blood Cancer. 2018;65(4):e26915.
36. Fitzgerald JC, et al. Acute kidney injury in pediatric severe sepsis: an independent risk factor for death and new disability. Crit Care Med. 2016;44(12):2241–50.
37. Foland JA, et al. Fluid overload before continuous hemofiltration and survival in critically ill children: a retrospective analysis. Crit Care Med. 2004;32(8):1771–6.
38. Arikan AA, et al. Fluid overload is associated with impaired oxygenation and morbidity in critically ill children. Pediatr Crit Care Med. 2012;13(3):253–8.
39. Varghese SA, et al. Identification of diagnostic urinary biomarkers for acute kidney injury. J Investig Med. 2010;58(4):612–20.
40. Arikan AA, et al. Resuscitation bundle in pediatric shock decreases acute kidney injury and improves outcomes. J Pediatr. 2015;167(6):1301–1305. e1.
41. Tumlin JA, et al. Fenoldopam mesylate in early acute tubular necrosis: a randomized, double-blind, placebo-controlled clinical trial. Am J Kidney Dis. 2005;46(1):26–34.
42. Goldstein SL, et al. Outcome in children receiving continuous venovenous hemofiltration. Pediatrics. 2001;107(6):1309–12.

43. Modem V, et al. Timing of continuous renal replacement therapy and mortality in critically ill children. Crit Care Med. 2014;42(4):943–53.
44. Choi SJ, et al. Factors associated with mortality in continuous renal replacement therapy for pediatric patients with acute kidney injury. Pediatr Crit Care Med. 2017;18(2):e56–61.
45. Goldstein SL, et al. Pediatric patients with multi-organ dysfunction syndrome receiving continuous renal replacement therapy. Kidney Int. 2005;67(2):653–8.
46. Hackbarth R, et al. The effect of vascular access location and size on circuit survival in pediatric continuous renal replacement therapy: a report from the PPCRRT registry. Int J Artif Organs. 2007;30(12):1116–21.
47. Fernández SN, et al. Citrate anticoagulation for CRRT in children: comparison with heparin. Biomed Res Int. 2014;2014:1–7.
48. Wu M-Y, et al. Regional citrate versus heparin anticoagulation for continuous renal replacement therapy: a meta-analysis of randomized controlled trials. Am J Kidney Dis. 2012;59(6):810–8.
49. Asín-Prieto E, et al. Population pharmacokinetics of piperacillin and tazobactam in critically ill patients undergoing continuous renal replacement therapy: application to pharmacokinetic/pharmacodynamic analysis. J Antimicrob Chemother. 2013;69(1):180–9.
50. Chaijamorn W, Wanakamanee U. Pharmacokinetics of vancomycin in critically ill patients undergoing continuous venovenous haemodialysis. Int J Antimicrob Agents. 2014;44(4):367–8.
51. Veltri MA, et al. Drug dosing during intermittent hemodialysis and continuous renal replacement therapy. Pediatr Drugs. 2004;6(1):45–65.
52. Sgambat K, Moudgil A. Carnitine deficiency in children receiving continuous renal replacement therapy. Hemodial Int. 2016;20(1):63–7.
53. Knijnenburg SL, et al. Early and late renal adverse effects after potentially nephrotoxic treatment for childhood cancer. Cochrane Libr. 2013;(10):1–197.
54. Mulder RL, et al. Glomerular function time trends in long-term survivors of childhood cancer: a longitudinal study. Cancer Epidemiol Prev Biomarkers. 2013;22(10):1736–46.

Chapter 14
Critical Care Management: Sepsis and Disseminated and Local Infections

Caitlin Hurley and Matt Zinter

Introduction

Children with malignancies, primary immunodeficiencies, prior solid organ or hematopoietic cell transplantation, and other immunocompromising conditions are at increased risk of becoming septic and dying from sepsis. Therefore, there are unique considerations for the management of sepsis in the immunocompromised child. First and foremost, fluid resuscitation and empiric broad-spectrum antibiotics covering opportunistic infections within the first 30 min of presentation are critical for reducing morbidity and mortality. This chapter will discuss available data that can be used to tailor the management of sepsis in this population.

Diagnostic Criteria

Initial management of presumed sepsis follows standard pediatric sepsis guidelines. According to the International Pediatric Sepsis Consensus Conference (IPSCC) of 2005, the spectrum of sepsis can be divided into systemic inflammatory response syndrome (SIRS), sepsis, severe sepsis, and septic shock [1]. Systemic inflammatory response syndrome describes an inflammatory state with immune activation that may have a variety of underlying etiologies. It is defined by two of the

C. Hurley
Division of Critical Care Medicine and Department of Bone Marrow Transplantation, St. Jude Children's Research Hospital, Memphis, TN, USA

M. Zinter (✉)
Department of Pediatrics, Division of Critical Care Medicine, UCSF Benioff Children's Hospitals, University of California, San Francisco, San Francisco, CA, USA
e-mail: matt.zinter@ucsf.edu

C. N. Duncan et al. (eds.), *Critical Care of the Pediatric Immunocompromised Hematology/Oncology Patient*, https://doi.org/10.1007/978-3-030-01322-6_14

SIRS

Presence of ≥ 2 of following 4 criteria (one must be abnormal temperature or leukocyte count)

- Core Temperature (rectal, bladder, oral or central catheter) >38.5 °C or <36 °C
- Leukocyte count elevated or depressed for age (not secondary to chemotherapy induced leukopenia) or >10% immature neutrophils
- Tachycardia – defined as a mean heart rate >2 standard deviations above normal for age in the absence of external stimuli, chronic drugs or painful stimuli; otherwise unexplained persistent elevation over a 0.5 to 4 hour time period; for children <1 year old: bradycardia, defined as a mean heart rate >10th percentile for age in the absence of external vagal stimuli, β-blocker drugs or congenital heart disease; or otherwise unexplained persistent heart rate depression over a 0.5 hour time period.
- Tachypnea, defined as a mean respiratory rate >2 standard deviations above normal for age, or the need for mechanical ventilation for an acute process not related to underlying neuromuscular disease or the influence of general of anesthesia.

SEPSIS
SIRS in presence of suspected or know infection

SEVERE SEPSIS
Sepsis plus one of the following criteria

- Cardiovascular organ dysfunction
- Acute respiratory distress syndrome
- Two or more other organ dysfunctions

SEPTIC SHOCK
Sepsis and cardiovascular organ dysfunction despite adequate fluid resuscitation

Fig. 14.1 Sepsis definitions. (Legend: Ref. [1])

following four criteria (Fig. 14.1). Sepsis is defined by SIRS with a suspected or proven underlying infection. The diagnosis can be escalated to severe sepsis if the patient has developed cardiovascular organ dysfunction or acute respiratory distress syndrome or two other organ system involvements. In cases where cardiovascular dysfunction is refractory to adequate fluid resuscitation, the diagnosis can be further escalated to septic shock.

In immunocompromised children, SIRS criteria alone may be present for a variety of infectious and noninfectious reasons (discussed in section "Considerations in High-Risk Patients"). Therefore, a high index of suspicion for infectious causes of SIRS physiology is mandatory. Importantly, the diagnosis of sepsis does not require a proven infection, but rather can be made with clinical suspicion for infection alone. Therefore, we and others advocate that the diagnosis of sepsis be made early, before progression from sepsis to severe sepsis and/or septic shock. [2, 3]

Initial Hemodynamic Management Strategies

The majority of data support that patients meeting the diagnostic criteria for sepsis should receive early empiric hemodynamic management. Interventions should aim to stabilize cardiovascular and respiratory systems, achieve adequate oxygen delivery by normalizing blood pressure and end-organ perfusion with initial fluid resuscitation, and maintain oxygenation and ventilation with supplementation oxygen support and possible advanced airway.

Early goal-directed therapy includes rapid intravascular volume re-expansion guided by hemodynamic monitoring and markers of organ dysfunction. Although initial reports demonstrated reduce mortality in adult emergency department populations by up to 15%, recent re-examination of these bundled interventions has not demonstrated reduction in mortality in adult populations [4–6]. Reports in pediatrics are not specific to immunocompromised patients, but demonstrate that early reversal of shock is associated with improved survival [7–10]. Therefore, the American College of Critical Care Medicine published the updated 2014 "Clinical Guidelines for Hemodynamic Support of Neonates and Children with Septic Shock" (Fig. 14.2), which advocates that recognition of fluid refractory shock should occur within the first 15 min [11, 12].

Strategies to Improve Oxygen Delivery

Fluid Resuscitation Early fluid resuscitation is critical to improving cardiac output and oxygen delivery during sepsis. Although some retrospective analyses have analyzed potential benefits for different types of resuscitation fluids, strong prospective data do not exist to favor the use of crystalloid over colloid or balanced over unbalanced fluids in this population [13–15]. The use of hydroxyethyl starches (HESs) is not recommended [16]. Rapid fluid resuscitation typically requires two large-bore peripheral intravenous catheters and should not rely solely on surgically implanted central venous catheters; in cases where difficult peripheral venous access delays fluid resuscitation, physicians should establish intraosseous access [17].

Although the ACCM guidelines advocate for early and aggressive fluid resuscitation of 20–60 mL/kg, the ideal volume of resuscitation fluids likely varies per patient and should be guided first and foremost by clinical exam. Resolution of hypotension, tachycardia, and impaired perfusion can be used to guide volume of resuscitation fluids [17]. Low central venous pressure (CVP) may be used to titrate volume resuscitation, but absolute measurements vary from child to child and thus require frequent or continuous measurement to establish patient-specific trends. Care should be taken when interpreting central venous pressure, as central venous pressure is related to both intravascular volume and right and left ventricular compliance. Further, children in septic shock with elevated central venous pressure frequently have diastolic dysfunction and left heart strain, which are associated with increased mortality [18–20]. Prediction of fluid responsiveness using other hemodynamic variables is an area of active interest, with some data supporting the use of aortic flow velocity and arterial pulse pressure variability with respiration [21, 22].

Oxygen-Carrying Capacity As arterial oxygen content = 1.36 (Hb g/dL) (% saturation) + 0.003 (PaO2), maintaining an adequate hemoglobin level is crucial for

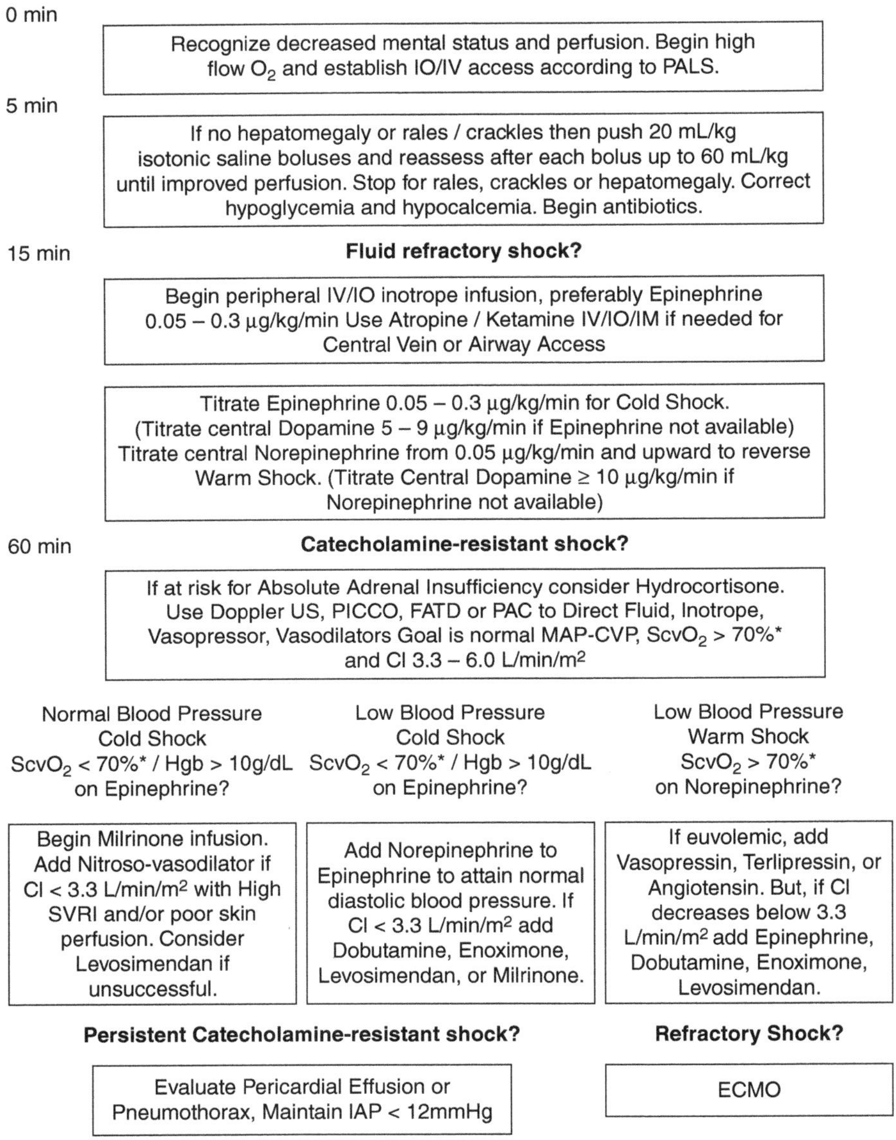

Fig. 14.2 Clinical guidelines for hemodynamic support of neonates and children with septic shock. (Legend: Ref. [11, 12])

maximizing the oxygen content in blood in sepsis physiology. In the general pediatric ICU population, thresholds of >7 g/dL and > 10 g/dL have been shown to be equally safe, with the advantage that a threshold of >7 g/dL resulted in fewer blood transfusions and potentially fewer nosocomial infections [23]. These results have been repeated in children with sepsis who have completed the resuscitation and stabilization period although sample size limitations precluded an appropriate analysis of mortality differences [24, 25]. However, the optimal transfusion threshold for patients with active septic shock has not been determined, and as of 2014, the majority of English- and French-speaking pediatric intensivists appear to use a transfusion threshold of >10 g/dL for children in active septic shock [26]. In a retrospective propensity score-adjusted study, more frequent RBC transfusions were associated with mortality in septic adults with hematologic malignancies, although whether this may be due to transfusion effects or underlying coagulopathy or hematologic failure is unknown [27]. As immunocompromised patients may have ineffective erythropoiesis and/or increased immune and nonimmune erythrocyte destruction, close attention to hemoglobin levels is warranted in sepsis [28].

Supplemental Oxygen Maintenance of hemoglobin saturation is critical for adequate arterial oxygen content and therefore is a principal component of managing sepsis physiology. Hence, early use of noninvasive supplemental oxygen, including nasal cannula, face mask, and non-rebreather masks, is warranted for pediatric immunocompromised patients with sepsis. Although pediatric data are lacking, among immunocompromised adults with infection-related acute respiratory failure, early application of noninvasive oxygen support can reduce progression to invasive mechanical ventilation [29, 30]. Data supporting the optimal timing of transition to noninvasive positive-pressure ventilation, and/or invasive mechanical ventilation, are limited in pediatrics. However, adult data suggest that patients who fail noninvasive ventilation should transition rapidly to endotracheal intubation, as prolonged failure of noninvasive ventilation is strongly associated with mortality [31]. A recent international sepsis point prevalence study identified that more than two-thirds of pediatric HCT patients with sepsis require endotracheal intubation during their course of sepsis [32]. Therefore we advocate that aggressive oxygenation support be offered to all critically ill immunocompromised children with sepsis.

Vasoactive Infusions Immunocompromised children with septic shock may require vasoactive infusions to improve their ability to meet the elevated metabolic demand of sepsis. Some patients may also have myocardial depression in the face of sepsis-induced hypercytokinemia [33, 34]. The choice of vasoactive infusions depends largely on clinical assessment of warm (vasodilatory) vs. cold (vasoconstricted) shock. Two separate double-blind, randomized controlled trial of dopamine vs. epinephrine for pediatric cold septic shock demonstrated clinical superiority of epinephrine over dopamine for multiple endpoints [35, 36]. Several other larger studies of adult and pediatric septic shock have demonstrated superiority of norepinephrine over dopamine for warm shock as well [37, 38]. Pediatric oncology patients with anthracycline exposure of any amount, particularly >300 mg/m^2 but even as low as 50 mg/m^2, are at increased risk for cardiotoxicity and may require significant attention to cardiopulmonary dynamics [39]. Additional vasoactive infusions including milrinone, terlipressin, levosimendan, and other agents may be required for refractory shock, although data are insufficient to recommend specific use in the pediatric immunocompromised population.

Extracorporeal Support (ECLS) Patients who are unable to meet systemic oxygen demand despite maximal medical management may benefit from venoarterial extracorporeal life support (VA-ECLS) to partially or completely augment cardiac output. The use of VA-ECLS is associated with approximately 50% mortality in pediatric septic shock [40]. Reports of ECLS use in immunocompromised children suggest approximately one third survive to hospital discharge [41]. The decision to initiate VA-ECLS for septic shock in immunocompromised children requires rapid but careful multidisciplinary discussion with informed parental consent where possible.

Strategies to Reduce Metabolic Demand

In addition to improving oxygen delivery, efforts to reduce metabolic demand may help balance tissue oxygen consumption and improve end-organ function. By reducing work of breathing and off-loading the left ventricle, invasive mechanical ventilation can reduce metabolic expenditure by up to 30% [42, 43]. Studies of timing of mechanical ventilation in adult sepsis suggest that delayed intubation may be associated with adverse outcomes and some patients may experience cardiopulmonary arrest due to decreased preload associated with vasodilation from sedation required for the procedure [44]. Of note, some data suggest that the use of etomidate during endotracheal intubation, particularly in patients receiving exogenous hydrocortisone, is associated with worse outcomes, potentially due to medication-induced adrenal suppression [45, 46].

Other strategies to reduce metabolic demand include control of fever with antipyretics, although data supporting the use of nonsteroidal anti-inflammatory drugs (NSAIDs) and acetaminophen are limited at this time [47–50]. Although sedation may play a role in reducing metabolic demand, current studies are inadequate to recommend an ideal sedation medication regimen at this time.

Hemodynamic Monitoring

In addition to measurement of central venous pressure and pulse pressure variability as described above, a variety of tools can be used to trend organ dysfunction over time. General biochemical markers of shock include lactate, base deficit, and anion gap, which show moderate-to-strong correlation with each other [51]. Several studies support the use of mixed venous oxygenation saturation measurements in the management of shock, wherein abnormally large arterial-venous saturation differential can suggest inadequate oxygenation and/or mitochondrial dysfunction prior to the rise of traditional markers such as serum lactate [52–56]. Data supporting the routine use of transpulmonary thermodilution are insufficient

Table 14.1 Vital sign abnormalities in pediatric sepsis

Age	Tachycardia	Bradycardia	Respiratory rate	Systolic blood pressure
0 days–1 week	>180	<100	>50	< 65
1 week–1 month	>180	<100	>40	<75
1 month–1 year	>180	<90	>34	<100
2–5 years	>140	N/A	>22	<94
6–12 years	>130	N/A	>18	<105
13–<18 years	>110	N/A	>14	<117

Legend: Adapted from Ref. [1]

at this time [57]. Continuous blood pressure transducing with arterial lines allows monitoring of arterial blood pressure and may be useful for rapid changes in hemodynamics. Although ideal blood pressure for each patient varies, the International Pediatric Sepsis Consensus Conference definitions of tachycardia, bradycardia, tachypnea, and hypotension in pediatric sepsis are listed in Table 14.1 (PMID 15636651) [1].

Anti-infective Strategies

Diagnostics

In patients with central catheters, it is recommended to obtain blood cultures both from peripheral venipuncture and from indwelling central catheters. A meta-analysis assessing the utility of paired central and peripheral blood cultures in both pediatric and adult cancer patients with suspected bloodstream infections demonstrated positive paired blood cultures in 17% of cases; 13% were only identified by peripheral blood and 28% only by central venous line samples [58]. Furthermore, a single center study of pediatric cancer patients demonstrated cases in which peripheral blood cultures were positive though central cultures were not. In this study of the 228 episodes of bacteremia, the peripheral blood culture was the only positive culture in 28 cases (12%). Therefore, obtaining both peripheral blood and central cultures could improve the sensitivity of bacteremia detection [59]. Additionally, obtaining both peripheral blood and central cultures and assessing the difference in time to detection in situations when both result in positive may assist with determination of catheter-related sepsis. A positive central line culture two or more hours prior to a positive peripheral culture has been associated with three times increased odds of catheter-related sepsis [60]. There was no direct evidence about the influence of peripheral blood cultures on clinical management decisions. Diagnostic yield can be increased by collecting two sets of blood cultures, and anaerobic cultures should be obtained as well. Blood cultures should be drawn prior to antibiotic administration if possible, but should not delay antibiotic administration [16].

Empiric Therapy

Careful attention to opportunistic organisms including bacteria, viruses, and fungi must be taken into consideration as well as individual patients' prior infectious history, specifically resistant organisms. Antibiotic administration should occur as early as possible and has been associated with reduced mortality in general pediatric septic shock [61, 62]. In the immunocompromised host, a third- or fourth-generation cephalosporin or carbapenem is frequently indicated for empiric gram-negative coverage, with the addition of vancomycin or other anti-methicillin-resistant *Staphylococcus aureus* (MRSA) therapy depending on patient and geographic risk factors. Furthermore, for patients presenting with shock, additional gram-negative bacterial coverage with a monobactam, fluoroquinolone, or aminoglycoside is frequently warranted for synergistic effect. Antimicrobial coverage for patients with suspected enteric sepsis or aspiration should include anaerobic coverage. Infectious disease subspecialty consultation is recommended to tailor coverage, review prior infectious history and patient-specific risk factors, recommend alternative therapies in the setting of medication allergy or intolerance, and guide dose adjustment in renal and hepatic injury. Removal of central lines should be strongly considered for refractory septic shock or recurrent positive blood cultures with differential time to positivity with consultation from infectious disease specialists [63].

Specific Pathogens

Bacterial Common gram-positive organisms include skin and mucosa-colonizing bacteria such as *Staphylococcus aureus* and *epidermidis* and *Streptococcus pyogenes* and the viridans group streptococci [64, 65]. *Streptococcus pneumoniae* and enterococci can cause disseminated disease from the upper/lower respiratory and gastrointestinal tracts and may present with antibiotic resistance requiring vancomycin, linezolid, ceftaroline, daptomycin, or other broad antibiotics. Common gram-negative organisms include respiratory colonizers (*Haemophilus*, *Moraxella*) as well as enteric and urologic organisms such as *Escherichia* and *Klebsiella*. These and other organisms such as *Pseudomonas* may present with multidrug resistance requiring carbapenem, fluoroquinolone, monobactam, and other extended spectrum therapies. Patients with severe *Clostridium difficile* enterocolitis may present with sepsis physiology as well.

Viral Community respiratory viruses including influenza, adenovirus, and enteroviruses can produce SIRS in immunocompromised children. Primary HSV-1 and 2 can cause liver failure, leading to a sepsis/shock overlap. Other herpesviruses such as CMV and EBV can also cause disseminated viremia with viral sepsis [66, 67].

Fungal Locally aggressive fungal infections or disseminated fungemia due to *Candida*, *Aspergillus*, zygomycoses of the *Mucorales* order, *Pneumocystis*, and endemic mycoses due to *Histoplasma* or *Blastomyces* can also cause sepsis physiology in immunocompromised children and require a high index of suspicion due to the frequent challenge in obtaining a microbiologic diagnosis [68, 69]. Due to the broad number of common and uncommon organisms that can cause sepsis in immunocompromised children, we strongly advocate close collaboration with infectious disease specialists to guide the diagnostic evaluation and treatment strategy.

Pharmacokinetic/Dynamic Considerations

Pharmacokinetic monitoring of drug levels is recommended where possible [16]. Vancomycin, gentamicin, tobramycin, and voriconazole levels should be followed when used for extended courses of therapy to ensure both therapeutic levels and avoidance of toxicity. Prudent attention to additional medications that may interact with anti-infectives in this high-risk population, specifically, the use of tacrolimus/cyclosporine for immunosuppression in the HSCT patient, is essential. Care should be paid to avoid drug-drug interactions, and hepatic and renal function should be assessed frequently, with dose adjustments as needed. Specialized clinical pharmacologists may assist in this role and reduce the frequency of deleterious drug-drug interactions [70, 71].

Immunomodulation

Patients with vasoplegia, refractory shock, adrenal insufficiency, long-term corticosteroid therapy, or short-term high-dose corticosteroid therapy may require stress-dose hydrocortisone; although steroids are used in nearly 50% of all children with septic shock, they have not been associated with improved outcomes, and some adult data suggest an association with mortality [72–79]. Although corticosteroids can modulate beta-adrenergic receptors, a growing body of evidence suggests they also may affect sepsis physiology through immunomodulation of innate immunity [78, 80]. The optimal patient selection, if any, for the use of corticosteroids in immunocompromised children with septic shock is unclear at this time. Minimal or absent cortisol increase in response to cosyntropin stimulation likely suggests adrenal insufficiency.

Granulocyte colony-stimulating factor (G-CSF) should be used in most neutropenic patients with nonmyeloid malignancies whose neutropenia is expected to respond to colony-stimulating factors [81]. Some centers perform granulocyte infusions to augment antimicrobial immunity, although studies do not support routine use in neutropenic sepsis and other immunocompromised states with infection [82]. Some centers have reported success in augmenting immunity with donor lymphocyte infusions (DLI), particularly with a cell source selected for anti-pathogen T cells [81, 83] or with engineered anti-pathogen cytotoxic T lymphocytes [84, 85]. Each of these therapies bear the risk of triggering inflammation, and clinicians should note that some patient may get worse due to intensified systemic inflammation prior to seeing clinical improvement in hemodynamics and metrics of end-organ function.

Standard use of IVIG in adult and pediatric sepsis has not demonstrated mortality benefit, although select patients with severe hypogammaglobulinemia may benefit [86]. Selective removal of inflammatory cytokines and bacterial endotoxin using customized pheresis membranes has been shown to affect cytokine levels in patients with septic shock, but data supporting a mortality benefit are lacking [87, 88]. Adult sepsis trials of activated protein C, immunomodulation in sepsis, and ARDS have not shown an overall survival benefit, but some subgroups may benefit [89–91]. Strong data supporting the use of antithrombin or thrombomodulin to control sepsis-related coagulopathy are not available at this time [16].

Management After the Acute Resuscitation

Systemic organ toxicities are common during and after the acute resuscitation of septic shock. For example, ARDS co-occurs with sepsis frequently. Pediatric allogeneic HCT patients with ARDS have <40% survival, and mechanical ventilation strategies differ widely by center and include high-frequency oscillatory ventilation (HFOV), inhaled nitric oxide, and veno-venous extracorporeal life support (VV-ECLS) [32, 92]. Secondary AKI is also strongly associated with mortality, and typical indications for continuous veno-venous hemodialfiltration (CVVHDF), including refractory fluid overload and uncontrollable electrolyte abnormalities, should be applied in immunocompromised patients [93]. Risk for secondary infections remains high due to a combination of indwelling invasive devices, altered intestinal and respiratory microbiomes, and sepsis-induced immunoparalysis, and thus care should be maintained to surveil for potential new infections [94]. As pediatric immunocompromised patients are at risk for prolonged PICU stay, they are also at high risk for immobilization-related weakness, and thus physical, occupational, speech, and rehabilitation therapies should be offered to maximize return of daily functional status [95, 96].

Considerations in High-Risk Patients

Immunocompromised patients, especially those with neutropenia, are at increased risk of infection and sepsis. The combination of fever and neutropenia warrants immediate medical attention. Several adult and pediatric studies have evaluated the risk of severe infection and sepsis in patients presenting with fever and neutropenia. An increase odds [OR = 1.80 (95% C.I. 1.43 to 2.26)] of severe infection was associated with severe neutropenia (defined as absolute neutrophil count <100/mm^3) in patients presenting with both neutropenia and fever [97–100]. Furthermore, a single center analysis of temperature as a continuous variable in pediatric cancer patients with neutropenia and fever and the associated need for critical care support demonstrated that children presenting with a one degree increase in temperature had a relative increase of the odds of receiving critical care within the first 24 h [1.74 (95% 1.25 to 2.43)] [101].

Predicting Patients at High Risk of Sepsis

Few studies have been published that offer predictive models of immunocompromised patients presenting with fever, neutropenia, and risk for mortality. Some data exist supporting the ability of laboratory markers, including CRP, lactate, and liver and kidney function tests to predict length of hospital stay in patients with fever and neutropenia; however, data are absent on the ability of these parameters to predict the need for critical care. In general, single center studies that have shown lactate, albumin, and creatinine levels have decent specificity though low sensitivity in predicting mortality [102, 103]. A multicenter study of adverse events in children with fever and neutropenia secondary to cancer therapy identified four predictive characteristics of adverse events. Adverse events were defined by either a serious medical complication as a result of infection, including death, complications necessitating critical care, an identified microbiological infection, and radiological confirmation of pneumonia. These four characteristics were an elevated hemoglobin level (>9 g/DL), WBC < 0.3 G/L, platelet count <50 G/L, and preceding chemotherapy with greater intensity than acute lymphoblastic leukemia maintenance therapy. Although a defined weighted score was able to predict an adverse event (as defined above) with an overall sensitivity of > 92%, a specificity of 45% and negative predictive value of 93%, the specific adverse event of intensive care admission or mortality was not predictive [104]. As a result, critical care physicians need to have a high index of suspicion for immunocompromised patients presenting with fever, neutropenia with any laboratory derangements, abnormal radiological findings suggestive of infections, and abnormal vital signs or toxic appearance as a definitive predictive model has not been well elucidated.

Leukemia Induction Therapy

Remission induction therapy for acute leukemia induces a profound immunosuppressive state with severe neutropenia and suppression of the innate immune system. Patients are extremely vulnerable to invasive bacterial and fungal infections. Treatment-related deaths have decreased dramatically with improved supportive care over the past several decades. In the United Kingdom, treatment-related deaths

(TRDs) in ALL patients dropped from 9% in 1980 to 2% in 1997 mostly attributable to decrease in measles and *Pneumocystis jirovecii* infections [105]. Similar results have been demonstrated worldwide with the Berlin-Frankfurt-Munster (BFM) group reporting approximately 1% TRDs in the ALL-BRM-95 trial. The St. Jude Total Therapy XIIIB trial showed grade 4 infections developing in 5% of patients during remission induction therapy, and disseminated fungal (grade 3 or 4) occurred in 4% of patients [106].

All patients receive sulfamethoxazole-trimethoprim (SMX-TMP) prophylaxis which offers coverage for *Pneumocystis jiroveci* as well as bacterial infections including gram-positive organisms such as *Streptococcus pyogenes*, *S. pneumoniae*, *Staphylococcus aureus*, and *S. epidermidis* as well as gram-negative organisms like *Escherichia coli*, *Klebsiella*, and *Salmonella*. SMX-TMP inhibits the formation of folinic acid in bacteria and blocks formation of purine, DNA, and RNA [107]. Additional bacterial and fungal prophylaxis during times of prolonged neutropenia with induction therapy may differ by institution, and it is prudent to know current institutional prophylaxis guidelines and understand what infections patient are more susceptible to, as well as appropriate expansion of antibiotic and antifungal coverage for patients undergoing induction who present with sepsis.

Post Hematopoietic Cell Transplant

HCT patients are at particularly high risk for sepsis and sepsis-related mortality [108, 109]. A clear understanding of the timing of immune reconstitution after allogeneic HSCT helps guide the clinician in anticipating which infectious pathogens patients are most at risk of developing during various time points after transplant. Initially, after conditioning therapy, patients develop an aplastic phase which involves severe neutropenia. This may also be termed a pre-engraftment phase. The innate immune system, consisting of neutrophils and NK cells, returns first over a time period of weeks, followed by adaptive immunity, T cells and B cells, over months to years. Specifically, neutrophils are the first cells to appear, followed by NK cells, then T cells and CD19+ B cells. The precise timing differs according to cell source, dose, and conditioning regimen. It is worth noting that even with return of cell counts, full function may be further delayed [110, 111].

With a clear understanding of immune reconstitution, the clinician may predict which infections patients are most vulnerable to in each phase. During the pre-engraftment phase, patients are most at risk of bacterial and fungal infections. Often prophylactic antibiotics and antifungal agents are given during this time with escalation to broader treatment dosing when acute infection is suspected. Following engraftment of neutrophils, the first 100 days, known as engraftment phase, is a time of cellular immunodeficiency as both NK cells from the innate immune system and T cells of the adaptive immune system are attenuated. Viral infections and/or reactivations predominate, including Epstein-Barr virus (EBV) and cytomegalovirus (CMV). Post-engraftment, after day 100, patients may still be vulnerable to viral infections. As B cells are the last to reconstitute, patients often have low levels of circulating immunoglobulins and as such are susceptible to infections with encapsulated bacteria including *Streptococcus pneumoniae* and *Haemophilus influenza* [110].

Sickle Cell Disease

Fever and Sepsis

Patients with SCD are at increased risk for bacterial infections, primarily due to impaired or absent splenic function. This often begins as early as 2 to 3 months of age as fetal hemoglobin levels begin to fall. As a result, children with SCD are at extremely high risk for disseminated bacterial infections causing septicemia or meningitis, predominantly with *Streptococcus pneumoniae*. Young children with HbSS are most at risk for pneumococcal infection and require prophylactic antibiotic coverage in the first 5 years of life with twice daily beta lactams as well as pneumococcal vaccination. Prophylactic antibiotics are discontinued at age 5 unless the child has undergone a splenectomy or has a history of pneumococcal infection [112]. Fever in a child with SCD warrants prompt assessment, blood cultures, and empiric antibiotics. Newborn screening for sickle cell disease is now universal in the United States, and all children with HbSS should be identified early with early initiation of pneumococcal prophylaxis; however, this does not entirely eliminate the risk, and invasive pneumococcal infection must be considered in pediatric patients with HbSS presenting with fever. Specific antibiotic regimens for patients with SCD presenting with fever may vary by institutional and hematology division guidelines; however, these often include ampicillin or third-generation cephalosporin with expansion to vancomycin for children who are toxic appearing, fever >39.5 degrees Celsius, leukopenia with WBC <5, or leukocytosis (WBC > 30).

Acute Chest Syndrome

Acute chest syndrome (ACS) is another common complication of SCD. It is defined by acute onset of respiratory symptoms (cough, hypoxia, rales) with a new infiltrate on chest X-ray, most commonly right upper or middle lobe in children. The etiology may vary but ACS often arises secondary to infection, usually associated with atypical bacteria, or to pulmonary fat embolism [113, 114]. T*he Management of Sickle Cell Disease Summary of the 2014 Evidence-Based Report by Expert Panel Members* published in JAMA identifies strong recommendations for the following: treatment with an intravenous cephalosporin, an oral macrolide antibiotic, supplemental oxygen to maintain oxygen saturation of >95%, and close monitoring for bronchospasm, acute anemia, and hypoxemia. Children developing critical illness with respiratory insufficiency or failure, worsening hypoxia with oxygen saturations <90% despite supplemental oxygen, progressive infiltrates, or acute anemia should receive urgent exchange transfusion in collaboration with the intensivist, hematologist, and apheresis teams. There is weak evidence for simple transfusion of 10 ml/kg of packed red blood cells to improve oxygen-carrying capacity for symptomatic children with ACS when hemoglobin concentration is >1 g/dL below baseline, with the exception of a baseline hemoglobin of ≥9 g/dL in which case transfusion may not be required. Lastly, the use of incentive spirometry while awake is strongly encouraged [115].

Conditions that May Mimic Sepsis

Several noninfectious conditions may mimic sepsis and warrant astute understanding and prompt recognition in an effort to offer appropriate targeted therapy. These conditions, often resulting in uncontrolled inflammation, have likely been present in pediatric critical care for years; however, they were previously diagnosed as "culture negative sepsis." Advancements in immunology, understanding of the inflammatory cascade, and genetics have improved the diagnosis of these diseases including hemophagocytic lymphohistiocytosis (HLH) and macrophage activation syndrome (MAS) and, subsequently, improved survival with the development of targeted therapies.

HLH and MAS fall on a spectrum of severe inflammatory disorders characterized by uncontrolled immune activation resulting from impaired cytotoxic T lymphocyte (CTLs) or natural killer (NK) cells. The dysfunctional CTLs and NK cells continually secrete cytokines with loss of normal negative feedback, resulting in further activation of macrophages, NK cells, and CTLs; an uncontrolled cytokine storm ensues [116, 117]. Diagnosis of HLH is clinical and often blurred with similar symptoms of severe sepsis. Signs of uncontrolled inflammation may include fever, distributive shock, and coagulopathy. Additionally, laboratory abnormalities may be present, including elevated liver enzymes, cytopenias, and renal failure. Patients may progress to acute respiratory distress syndrome, neurological impairment with encephalopathy, and seizures. HLH biology and treatment are discussed in detail in Chap. 9.

Additionally, other therapeutics used in the treatment of hematology/oncology and HSCT patients may cause immunosuppression and may elicit sepsis like clinical pictures. Notably, anti-thymoglobulin (ATG) is used as a therapy for severe aplastic anemia as well as for graft-versus-host disease prophylaxis and treatment in HSCT patients. Studies demonstrate elevations in circulating cytokines after the initiation of anti-T cell therapy with ATG, specifically IL-6, IL-8, IL-10 and granulocyte colony-stimulating factor (GCSF), IL4, IL13, TNFa, IFNg, interferon gamma-inducible protein-10 (IP-10), chemokine (C-C motif) ligand (CCL-2), and CCL-4 [118, 119]. Clinically, patients exposed to ATG (either rabbit or horse source) may develop acute hypersensitivity infusion reaction with fever, hypotension, as well as a delayed (approximately 10 days) serum sickness with fever, myalgias, arthralgias, and rash. Serum sickness results from host antibody responses to foreign proteins followed by formation and then deposition of immune complexes in tissues (skin, joints, and other organs) [118]. Careful attention to recent therapeutics may allow for quick and accurate diagnosis of underlying etiology of hematology/oncology patients presenting with signs and symptoms of sepsis.

Conclusion

In summary, immunocompromised children, including those with primary or acquired immunodeficiencies, malignancies, or hemoglobinopathies and those who have undergone solid organ or hematopoietic cell transplantation, are at particularly high risk for sepsis and sepsis-related mortality. Significant attention should be given to rapid initial hemodynamic resuscitation with empiric broad-spectrum antimicrobial coverage. Subsequent tailoring of care based on unique patient susceptibilities to infections and organ toxicity remains crucial to maximizing outcomes.

References

1. Goldstein B, Giroir B, Randolph A, et al. International pediatric sepsis consensus conference: definitions for sepsis and organ dysfunction in pediatrics. Pediatr Crit Care Med. 2005;6:2–8. https://doi.org/10.1097/01.PCC.0000149131.72248.E6.
2. Agulnik A, Mendez Aceituno A, Mora Robles LN, et al. Validation of a pediatric early warning system for hospitalized pediatric oncology patients in a resource-limited setting. Cancer. 2017;123:4903–13. https://doi.org/10.1002/cncr.30951.
3. Sano H, Kobayashi R, Iguchi A, et al. Risk factors for sepsis-related death in children and adolescents with hematologic and malignant diseases. J Microbiol Immunol Infect = Wei mian yu gan ran za zhi. 2017;50:232–8. https://doi.org/10.1016/j.jmii.2015.04.002.
4. Rivers E, Nguyen B, Havstad S, et al. Early goal-directed therapy in the treatment of severe sepsis and septic shock. N Engl J Med. 2001;345:1368–77. https://doi.org/10.1056/NEJMoa010307.
5. Kalil AC, Johnson DW, Lisco SJ, et al. Early goal-directed therapy for sepsis: a novel solution for discordant survival outcomes in clinical trials. Crit Care Med. 2017;45:607–14. https://doi.org/10.1097/CCM.0000000000002235.
6. Investigators P, Rowan KM, Angus DC, et al. Early, goal-directed therapy for septic shock – a patient-level meta-analysis. N Engl J Med. 2017;376:2223–34. https://doi.org/10.1056/NEJMoa1701380.
7. Han YY, Carcillo JA, Dragotta MA, et al. Early reversal of pediatric-neonatal septic shock by community physicians is associated with improved outcome. Pediatrics. 2003;112:793–9.
8. Inwald DP, Tasker RC, Peters MJ, et al. Emergency management of children with severe sepsis in the United Kingdom: the results of the Paediatric Intensive Care Society sepsis audit. Arch Dis Child. 2009;94:348–53. https://doi.org/10.1136/adc.2008.153064.
9. Oliveira CF, Nogueira de Sa FR, Oliveira DS, et al. Time- and fluid-sensitive resuscitation for hemodynamic support of children in septic shock: barriers to the implementation of the American College of Critical Care Medicine/Pediatric advanced life support guidelines in

a pediatric intensive care unit in a developing world. Pediatr Emerg Care. 2008;24:810–5. https://doi.org/10.1097/PEC.0b013e31818e9f3a.
10. Gelbart B, Glassford NJ, Bellomo R. Fluid bolus therapy-based resuscitation for severe sepsis in hospitalized children: a systematic review. Pediatr Crit Care Med. 2015;16:e297–307. https://doi.org/10.1097/PCC.0000000000000507.
11. Brierley J, Carcillo JA, Choong K, et al. Clinical practice parameters for hemodynamic support of pediatric and neonatal septic shock: 2007 update from the American College of Critical Care Medicine. Crit Care Med. 2009;37:666–88. https://doi.org/10.1097/CCM.0b013e31819323c6.
12. Davis AL, Carcillo JA, Aneja RK, et al. American College of Critical Care Medicine clinical practice parameters for hemodynamic support of pediatric and neonatal septic shock. Crit Care Med. 2017;45:1061–93. https://doi.org/10.1097/CCM.0000000000002425.
13. Akech S, Ledermann H, Maitland K. Choice of fluids for resuscitation in children with severe infection and shock: systematic review. Br Med J. 2010;341:c4416. https://doi.org/10.1136/bmj.c4416.
14. Emrath ET, Fortenberry JD, Travers C, et al. Resuscitation with balanced fluids is associated with improved survival in pediatric severe sepsis. Crit Care Med. 2017;45:1177–83. https://doi.org/10.1097/CCM.0000000000002365.
15. Weiss SL, Keele L, Balamuth F, et al. Crystalloid fluid choice and clinical outcomes in pediatric sepsis: a matched retrospective cohort study. J Pediatr. 2017;182:304–10 e310. https://doi.org/10.1016/j.jpeds.2016.11.075.
16. Rhodes A, Evans LE, Alhazzani W, et al. Surviving sepsis campaign: international guidelines for management of sepsis and septic shock: 2016. Crit Care Med. 2017;45:486–552. https://doi.org/10.1097/CCM.0000000000002255.
17. de Caen AR, Berg MD, Chameides L, et al. Part 12: pediatric advanced life support: 2015 American Heart Association guidelines update for cardiopulmonary resuscitation and emergency cardiovascular care. Circulation. 2015;132:S526–42. https://doi.org/10.1161/CIR.0000000000000266.
18. Choi SJ, Ha EJ, Jhang WK, et al. Elevated central venous pressure is associated with increased mortality in pediatric septic shock patients. BMC Pediatr. 2018;18:58. https://doi.org/10.1186/s12887-018-1059-1.
19. Sankar J, Das RR, Jain A, et al. Prevalence and outcome of diastolic dysfunction in children with fluid refractory septic shock—a prospective observational study. Pediatr Crit Care Med. 2014;15:e370–8. https://doi.org/10.1097/PCC.0000000000000249.
20. Lanspa MJ, Pittman JE, Hirshberg EL, et al. Association of left ventricular longitudinal strain with central venous oxygen saturation and serum lactate in patients with early severe sepsis and septic shock. Crit Care. 2015;19:304. https://doi.org/10.1186/s13054-015-1014-6.
21. Gan H, Cannesson M, Chandler JR, et al. Predicting fluid responsiveness in children: a systematic review. Anesth Analg. 2013;117:1380–92. https://doi.org/10.1213/ANE.0b013e3182a9557e.
22. Michard F, Boussat S, Chemla D, et al. Relation between respiratory changes in arterial pulse pressure and fluid responsiveness in septic patients with acute circulatory failure. Am J Respir Crit Care Med. 2000;162:134–8. https://doi.org/10.1164/ajrccm.162.1.9903035.
23. Lacroix J, Hebert PC, Hutchison JS, et al. Transfusion strategies for patients in pediatric intensive care units. N Engl J Med. 2007;356:1609–19. https://doi.org/10.1056/NEJMoa066240.
24. Karam O, Tucci M, Ducruet T, et al. Red blood cell transfusion thresholds in pediatric patients with sepsis. Pediatr Crit Care Med. 2011;12:512–8. https://doi.org/10.1097/PCC.0b013e3181fe344b.
25. Shieh HH, Barreira ER, Goes PF, et al. Mortality associated with restrictive threshold for red blood cell transfusion in pediatric patients with sepsis. Pediatr Crit Care Med. 2012;13:494–495; author reply 495. https://doi.org/10.1097/PCC.0b013e31824fbb29.

26. Du Pont-Thibodeau G, Tucci M, Ducruet T, et al. Survey on stated transfusion practices in PICUs*. Pediatr Crit Care Med. 2014;15:409–16. https://doi.org/10.1097/PCC.0000000000000121.
27. Mirouse A, Resche-Rigon M, Lemiale V, et al. Red blood cell transfusion in the resuscitation of septic patients with hematological malignancies. Ann Intensive Care. 2017;7:62. https://doi.org/10.1186/s13613-017-0292-3.
28. Shah N, Andrews J, Goodnough LT. Transfusions for anemia in adult and pediatric patients with malignancies. Blood Rev. 2015;29:291–9. https://doi.org/10.1016/j.blre.2015.02.001.
29. Azoulay E, Pickkers P, Soares M, et al. Acute hypoxemic respiratory failure in immunocompromised patients: the Efraim multinational prospective cohort study. Intensive Care Med. 2017;43:1808–19. https://doi.org/10.1007/s00134-017-4947-1.
30. Lemiale V, Resche-Rigon M, Mokart D, et al. High-flow nasal cannula oxygenation in immunocompromised patients with acute hypoxemic respiratory failure: a groupe de recherche respiratoire en reanimation onco-hematologique study. Crit Care Med. 2017;45:e274–80. https://doi.org/10.1097/CCM.0000000000002085.
31. Neuschwander A, Lemiale V, Darmon M, et al. Noninvasive ventilation during acute respiratory distress syndrome in patients with cancer: trends in use and outcome. J Crit Care. 2017;38:295–9. https://doi.org/10.1016/j.jcrc.2016.11.042.
32. Rowan CM, Smith LS, Loomis A, et al. Pediatric acute respiratory distress syndrome in pediatric allogeneic hematopoietic stem cell transplants: a multicenter study. Pediatr Crit Care Med. 2017;18:304–9. https://doi.org/10.1097/PCC.0000000000001061.
33. Antonucci E, Fiaccadori E, Donadello K, et al. Myocardial depression in sepsis: from pathogenesis to clinical manifestations and treatment. J Crit Care. 2014;29:500–11. https://doi.org/10.1016/j.jcrc.2014.03.028.
34. Fernandes CJ Jr, Akamine N, Knobel E. Myocardial depression in sepsis. Shock. 2008;30(Suppl 1):14–7. https://doi.org/10.1097/SHK.0b013e3181818617.
35. Ramaswamy KN, Singhi S, Jayashree M, et al. Double-blind randomized clinical trial comparing dopamine and epinephrine in pediatric fluid-refractory hypotensive septic shock. Pediatr Crit Care Med. 2016;17:e502–12. https://doi.org/10.1097/PCC.0000000000000954.
36. Ventura AM, Shieh HH, Bousso A, et al. Double-blind prospective randomized controlled trial of dopamine versus epinephrine as first-line vasoactive drugs in pediatric septic shock. Crit Care Med. 2015;43:2292–302. https://doi.org/10.1097/CCM.0000000000001260.
37. Vasu TS, Cavallazzi R, Hirani A, et al. Norepinephrine or dopamine for septic shock: systematic review of randomized clinical trials. J Intensive Care Med. 2012;27:172–8. https://doi.org/10.1177/0885066610396312.
38. Ranjit S, Natraj R, Kandath SK, et al. Early norepinephrine decreases fluid and ventilatory requirements in pediatric vasodilatory septic shock. Indian J Crit Care Med. 2016;20:561–9. https://doi.org/10.4103/0972-5229.192036.
39. Loar RW, Noel CV, Tunuguntla H, et al. State of the art review: chemotherapy-induced cardiotoxicity in children. Congenit Heart Dis. 2018;13:5–15. https://doi.org/10.1111/chd.12564.
40. Barbaro RP, Paden ML, Guner YS, et al. Pediatric extracorporeal life support organization registry international report 2016. ASAIO J. 2017;63:456–63. https://doi.org/10.1097/MAT.0000000000000603.
41. Gow KW, Heiss KF, Wulkan ML, et al. Extracorporeal life support for support of children with malignancy and respiratory or cardiac failure: the extracorporeal life support experience. Crit Care Med. 2009;37:1308–16. https://doi.org/10.1097/CCM.0b013e31819cf01a.
42. Roussos C, Macklem PT. The respiratory muscles. N Engl J Med. 1982;307:786–97. https://doi.org/10.1056/NEJM198209233071304.
43. Stock MC, Davis DW, Manning JW, et al. Lung mechanics and oxygen consumption during spontaneous ventilation and severe heart failure. Chest. 1992;102:279–83.

44. Delbove A, Darreau C, Hamel JF, et al. Impact of endotracheal intubation on septic shock outcome: a post hoc analysis of the SEPSISPAM trial. J Crit Care. 2015;30:1174–8. https://doi.org/10.1016/j.jcrc.2015.08.018.
45. Jung B, Clavieras N, Nougaret S, et al. Effects of etomidate on complications related to intubation and on mortality in septic shock patients treated with hydrocortisone: a propensity score analysis. Crit Care. 2012;16:R224. https://doi.org/10.1186/cc11871.
46. Dmello D, Taylor S, O'Brien J, et al. Outcomes of etomidate in severe sepsis and septic shock. Chest. 2010;138:1327–32. https://doi.org/10.1378/chest.10-0790.
47. Eisen DP. Manifold beneficial effects of acetyl salicylic acid and nonsteroidal anti-inflammatory drugs on sepsis. Intensive Care Med. 2012;38:1249–57. https://doi.org/10.1007/s00134-012-2570-8.
48. Aronoff DM. Cyclooxygenase inhibition in sepsis: is there life after death? Mediat Inflamm. 2012;2012:696897. https://doi.org/10.1155/2012/696897.
49. Janz DR, Bastarache JA, Rice TW, et al. Randomized, placebo-controlled trial of acetaminophen for the reduction of oxidative injury in severe sepsis: the Acetaminophen for the Reduction of Oxidative Injury in Severe Sepsis trial. Crit Care Med. 2015;43:534–41. https://doi.org/10.1097/CCM.0000000000000718.
50. Lee BH, Inui D, Suh GY, et al. Association of body temperature and antipyretic treatments with mortality of critically ill patients with and without sepsis: multi-centered prospective observational study. Crit Care. 2012;16:R33. https://doi.org/10.1186/cc11211.
51. Mallat J, Michel D, Salaun P, et al. Defining metabolic acidosis in patients with septic shock using Stewart approach. Am J Emerg Med. 2012;30:391–8. https://doi.org/10.1016/j.ajem.2010.11.039.
52. Deep A, Goonasekera CD, Wang Y, et al. Evolution of haemodynamics and outcome of fluid-refractory septic shock in children. Intensive Care Med. 2013;39:1602–9. https://doi.org/10.1007/s00134-013-3003-z.
53. Brierley J, Peters MJ. Distinct hemodynamic patterns of septic shock at presentation to pediatric intensive care. Pediatrics. 2008;122:752–9. https://doi.org/10.1542/peds.2007-1979.
54. Raimer PL, Han YY, Weber MS, et al. A normal capillary refill time of </= 2 seconds is associated with superior vena cava oxygen saturations of >/= 70%. J Pediatr. 2011;158:968–72. https://doi.org/10.1016/j.jpeds.2010.11.062.
55. Sankar J, Sankar MJ, Suresh CP, et al. Early goal-directed therapy in pediatric septic shock: comparison of outcomes "with" and "without" intermittent superior venacaval oxygen saturation monitoring: a prospective cohort study*. Pediatr Crit Care Med. 2014;15:e157–67. https://doi.org/10.1097/PCC.0000000000000073.
56. Boulain T, Garot D, Vignon P, et al. Prevalence of low central venous oxygen saturation in the first hours of intensive care unit admission and associated mortality in septic shock patients: a prospective multicentre study. Crit Care. 2014;18:609. https://doi.org/10.1186/s13054-014-0609-7.
57. Proulx F, Lemson J, Choker G, et al. Hemodynamic monitoring by transpulmonary thermodilution and pulse contour analysis in critically ill children. Pediatr Crit Care Med. 2011;12:459–66. https://doi.org/10.1097/PCC.0b013e3182070959.
58. Handrup MM, Moller JK, Rutkjaer C, et al. Importance of blood cultures from peripheral veins in pediatric patients with cancer and a central venous line. Pediatr Blood Cancer. 2015;62:99–102. https://doi.org/10.1002/pbc.25171.
59. Scheinemann K, Ethier MC, Dupuis LL, et al. Utility of peripheral blood cultures in bacteremic pediatric cancer patients with a central line. Support Care Cancer. 2010;18:913–9. https://doi.org/10.1007/s00520-009-0725-0.
60. Blot F, Schmidt E, Nitenberg G, et al. Earlier positivity of central-venous- versus peripheral-blood cultures is highly predictive of catheter-related sepsis. J Clin Microbiol. 1998;36:105–9.
61. Weiss SL, Fitzgerald JC, Balamuth F, et al. Delayed antimicrobial therapy increases mortality and organ dysfunction duration in pediatric sepsis. Crit Care Med. 2014;42:2409–17. https://doi.org/10.1097/CCM.0000000000000509.

62. Han M, Fitzgerald JC, Balamuth F, et al. Association of delayed antimicrobial therapy with one-year mortality in pediatric sepsis. Shock. 2017;48:29–35. https://doi.org/10.1097/SHK.0000000000000833.
63. Celebi S, Sezgin ME, Cakir D, et al. Catheter-associated bloodstream infections in pediatric hematology-oncology patients. Pediatr Hematol Oncol. 2013;30:187–94. https://doi.org/10.3109/08880018.2013.772683.
64. Slade M, Goldsmith S, Romee R, et al. Epidemiology of infections following haploidentical peripheral blood hematopoietic cell transplantation. Transpl Infect Dis. 2017;19 https://doi.org/10.1111/tid.12629.
65. Chang AK, Foca MD, Jin Z, et al. Bacterial bloodstream infections in pediatric allogeneic hematopoietic stem cell recipients before and after implementation of a central line-associated bloodstream infection protocol: a single-center experience. Am J Infect Control. 2016;44:1650–5. https://doi.org/10.1016/j.ajic.2016.04.229.
66. Sim SA, Leung VKY, Ritchie D, et al. Viral respiratory tract infections in allogeneic hematopoietic stem cell transplantation recipients in the era of molecular testing. Biol Blood Marrow Transplant. 2018; https://doi.org/10.1016/j.bbmt.2018.03.004.
67. Hiwarkar P, Gaspar HB, Gilmour K, et al. Impact of viral reactivations in the era of pre-emptive antiviral drug therapy following allogeneic haematopoietic SCT in paediatric recipients. Bone Marrow Transplant. 2013;48:803–8. https://doi.org/10.1038/bmt.2012.221.
68. Steinbach WJ, Roilides E, Berman D, et al. Results from a prospective, international, epidemiologic study of invasive candidiasis in children and neonates. Pediatr Infect Dis J. 2012;31:1252–7. https://doi.org/10.1097/INF.0b013e3182737427.
69. Wattier RL, Dvorak CC, Hoffman JA, et al. A prospective, international cohort study of invasive mold infections in children. J Pediatr Infect Dis Soc. 2015;4:313–22. https://doi.org/10.1093/jpids/piu074.
70. Alexander MD, Rao KV, Khan TS, et al. ReCAP: pharmacists' impact in hematopoietic stem-cell transplantation: economic and humanistic outcomes. J Oncol Pract. 2016;12:147–148, e118–126. https://doi.org/10.1200/JOP.2015.008797.
71. Lucena M, Bondarenka C, Luehrs-Hayes G, et al. Evaluation of a medication intensity screening tool used in malignant hematology and bone marrow transplant services to identify patients at risk for medication-related problems. J Oncol Pharm Pract. 2018;24:243–52. https://doi.org/10.1177/1078155217690923.
72. El-Nawawy A, Khater D, Omar H, et al. Evaluation of early corticosteroid therapy in management of pediatric septic shock in pediatric intensive care patients: a randomized clinical study. Pediatr Infect Dis J. 2017;36:155–9. https://doi.org/10.1097/INF.0000000000001380.
73. Markovitz BP, Goodman DM, Watson RS, et al. A retrospective cohort study of prognostic factors associated with outcome in pediatric severe sepsis: what is the role of steroids? Pediatr Crit Care Med. 2005;6:270–4. https://doi.org/10.1097/01.PCC.0000160596.31238.72.
74. Zimmerman JJ, Williams MD. Adjunctive corticosteroid therapy in pediatric severe sepsis: observations from the RESOLVE study. Pediatr Crit Care Med. 2011;12:2–8. https://doi.org/10.1097/PCC.0b013e3181d903f6.
75. Atkinson SJ, Cvijanovich NZ, Thomas NJ, et al. Corticosteroids and pediatric septic shock outcomes: a risk stratified analysis. PLoS One. 2014;9:e112702. https://doi.org/10.1371/journal.pone.0112702.
76. Weiss SL, Fitzgerald JC, Pappachan J, et al. Global epidemiology of pediatric severe sepsis: the sepsis prevalence, outcomes, and therapies study. Am J Respir Crit Care Med. 2015;191:1147–57. https://doi.org/10.1164/rccm.201412-2323OC.
77. Menon K, McNally JD, Choong K, et al. A cohort study of pediatric shock: frequency of corticosteriod use and association with clinical outcomes. Shock. 2015;44:402–9. https://doi.org/10.1097/SHK.0000000000000355.
78. Wong HR, Cvijanovich NZ, Allen GL, et al. Corticosteroids are associated with repression of adaptive immunity gene programs in pediatric septic shock. Am J Respir Crit Care Med. 2014;189:940–6. https://doi.org/10.1164/rccm.201401-0171OC.

79. Keh D, Trips E, Marx G, et al. Effect of hydrocortisone on development of shock among patients with severe sepsis: the HYPRESS randomized clinical trial. JAMA. 2016;316:1775–85. https://doi.org/10.1001/jama.2016.14799.
80. Zimmerman JJ. Adjunctive steroid therapy for treatment of pediatric septic shock. Pediatr Clin N Am. 2017;64:1133–46. https://doi.org/10.1016/j.pcl.2017.06.010.
81. Phillips R, Hancock B, Graham J, et al. Prevention and management of neutropenic sepsis in patients with cancer: summary of NICE guidance. Br Med J. 2012;345:e5368. https://doi.org/10.1136/bmj.e5368.
82. Price TH, Boeckh M, Harrison RW, et al. Efficacy of transfusion with granulocytes from G-CSF/dexamethasone-treated donors in neutropenic patients with infection. Blood. 2015;126:2153–61. https://doi.org/10.1182/blood-2015-05-645986.
83. Yoshihara S, Kato R, Inoue T, et al. Successful treatment of life-threatening human herpesvirus-6 encephalitis with donor lymphocyte infusion in a patient who had undergone human leukocyte antigen-haploidentical nonmyeloablative stem cell transplantation. Transplantation. 2004;77:835–8.
84. Bao L, Cowan MJ, Dunham K, et al. Adoptive immunotherapy with CMV-specific cytotoxic T lymphocytes for stem cell transplant patients with refractory CMV infections. J Immunother. 2012;35:293–8. https://doi.org/10.1097/CJI.0b013e31824300a2.
85. Roddie C, Peggs KS. Immunotherapy for transplantation-associated viral infections. J Clin Invest. 2017;127:2513–22. https://doi.org/10.1172/JCI90599.
86. Group IC, Brocklehurst P, Farrell B, et al. Treatment of neonatal sepsis with intravenous immune globulin. N Engl J Med. 2011;365:1201–11. https://doi.org/10.1056/NEJMoa1100441.
87. Kumagai T, Takeyama N, Yabuki T, et al. Apheresis of activated leukocytes with an immobilized polymyxin B filter in patients with septic shock. Shock. 2010;34:461–6. https://doi.org/10.1097/SHK.0b013e3181e14ca0.
88. Bengsch S, Boos KS, Nagel D, et al. Extracorporeal plasma treatment for the removal of endotoxin in patients with sepsis: clinical results of a pilot study. Shock. 2005;23:494–500.
89. Goldstein B, Nadel S, Peters M, et al. ENHANCE: results of a global open-label trial of drotrecogin alfa (activated) in children with severe sepsis. *Pediatr Crit Care Med.* 2006;7:200–11. https://doi.org/10.1097/01.PCC.0000217470.68764.36.
90. Dalton HJ, Carcillo JA, Woodward DB, et al. Biomarker response to drotrecogin alfa (activated) in children with severe sepsis: results from the RESOLVE clinical trial*. *Pediatr Crit Care Med.* 2012;13:639–45. https://doi.org/10.1097/PCC.0b013e318250ad48.
91. Ranieri VM, Thompson BT, Barie PS, et al. Drotrecogin alfa (activated) in adults with septic shock. N Engl J Med. 2012;366:2055–64. https://doi.org/10.1056/NEJMoa1202290.
92. Rowan CM, Gertz SJ, McArthur J, et al. Invasive mechanical ventilation and mortality in pediatric hematopoietic stem cell transplantation: a multicenter study. *Pediatr Crit Care Med.* 2016;17:294–302. https://doi.org/10.1097/PCC.0000000000000673.
93. Santiago MJ, Lopez-Herce J, Urbano J, et al. Clinical course and mortality risk factors in critically ill children requiring continuous renal replacement therapy. Intensive Care Med. 2010;36:843–9. https://doi.org/10.1007/s00134-010-1858-9.
94. Hall MW, Knatz NL, Vetterly C, et al. Immunoparalysis and nosocomial infection in children with multiple organ dysfunction syndrome. Intensive Care Med. 2011;37:525–32. https://doi.org/10.1007/s00134-010-2088-x.
95. Mehrholz J, Thomas S, Burridge JH, et al. Fitness and mobility training in patients with Intensive Care Unit-acquired muscle weakness (FITonICU): study protocol for a randomised controlled trial. Trials. 2016;17:559. https://doi.org/10.1186/s13063-016-1687-4.
96. Zinter MS, Holubkov R, Steurer MA, et al. Pediatric hematopoietic cell transplant patients who survive critical illness frequently have significant but recoverable decline in functional status. Biol Blood Marrow Transplant. 2018;24:330–6. https://doi.org/10.1016/j.bbmt.2017.10.036.

97. Ammann RA, Hirt A, Luthy AR, et al. Identification of children presenting with fever in chemotherapy-induced neutropenia at low risk for severe bacterial infection. Med Pediatr Oncol. 2003;41:436–43. https://doi.org/10.1002/mpo.10320.
98. Hakim H, Flynn PM, Srivastava DK, et al. Risk prediction in pediatric cancer patients with fever and neutropenia. Pediatr Infect Dis J. 2010;29:53–9. https://doi.org/10.1097/INF.0b013e3181c3f6f0.
99. Santolaya ME, Alvarez AM, Becker A, et al. Prospective, multicenter evaluation of risk factors associated with invasive bacterial infection in children with cancer, neutropenia, and fever. J Clin Oncol. 2001;19:3415–21. https://doi.org/10.1200/JCO.2001.19.14.3415.
100. Tezcan G, Kupesiz A, Ozturk F, et al. Episodes of fever and neutropenia in children with cancer in a tertiary care medical center in Turkey. Pediatr Hematol Oncol. 2006;23:217–29. https://doi.org/10.1080/08880010500506719.
101. West DC, Marcin JP, Mawis R, et al. Children with cancer, fever, and treatment-induced neutropenia: risk factors associated with illness requiring the administration of critical care therapies. Pediatr Emerg Care. 2004;20:79–84.
102. Ramzi J, Mohamed Z, Yosr B, et al. Predictive factors of septic shock and mortality in neutropenic patients. Hematology. 2007;12:543–8. https://doi.org/10.1080/10245330701384237.
103. Neutropenic sepsis: prevention and management of neutropenic sepsis in cancer patients. London; 2012. https://www.ncbi.nlm.nih.gov/pubmed/26065059
104. Ammann RA, Bodmer N, Hirt A, et al. Predicting adverse events in children with fever and chemotherapy-induced neutropenia: the prospective multicenter SPOG 2003 FN study. J Clin Oncol. 2010;28:2008–14. https://doi.org/10.1200/JCO.2009.25.8988.
105. Hargrave DR, Hann II, Richards SM, et al. Progressive reduction in treatment-related deaths in Medical Research Council childhood lymphoblastic leukaemia trials from 1980 to 1997 (UKALL VIII, X and XI). Br J Haematol. 2001;112:293–9.
106. Pui CH, Sandlund JT, Pei D, et al. Improved outcome for children with acute lymphoblastic leukemia: results of Total Therapy Study XIIIB at St Jude Children's Research Hospital. Blood. 2004;104:2690–6. https://doi.org/10.1182/blood-2004-04-1616.
107. Rungoe C, Malchau EL, Larsen LN, et al. Infections during induction therapy for children with acute lymphoblastic leukemia. The role of sulfamethoxazole-trimethoprim (SMX-TMP) prophylaxis. Pediatr Blood Cancer. 2010;55:304–8. https://doi.org/10.1002/pbc.22423.
108. Lindell RB, Gertz SJ, Rowan CM, et al. High levels of morbidity and mortality among pediatric hematopoietic cell transplant recipients with severe sepsis: insights from the sepsis PRevalence, OUtcomes, and therapies international point prevalence study. *Pediatr Crit Care Med.* 2017;18:1114–25. https://doi.org/10.1097/PCC.0000000000001338.
109. Tamburro R. Pediatric cancer patients in clinical trials of sepsis: factors that predispose to sepsis and stratify outcome. *Pediatr Crit Care Med.* 2005;6:S87–91. https://doi.org/10.1097/01.PCC.0000161288.00396.49.
110. Ogonek J, Kralj Juric M, Ghimire S, et al. Immune reconstitution after allogeneic hematopoietic stem cell transplantation. Front Immunol. 2016;7:507. https://doi.org/10.3389/fimmu.2016.00507.
111. Bosch M, Khan FM, Storek J. Immune reconstitution after hematopoietic cell transplantation. Curr Opin Hematol. 2012;19:324–35. https://doi.org/10.1097/MOH.0b013e328353bc7d.
112. Gaston MH, Verter JI, Woods G, et al. Prophylaxis with oral penicillin in children with sickle cell anemia. A randomized trial. N Engl J Med. 1986;314:1593–9. https://doi.org/10.1056/NEJM198606193142501.
113. Miller ST. How I treat acute chest syndrome in children with sickle cell disease. Blood. 2011;117:5297–305. https://doi.org/10.1182/blood-2010-11-261834.
114. Vichinsky EP, Neumayr LD, Earles AN, et al. Causes and outcomes of the acute chest syndrome in sickle cell disease. National Acute Chest Syndrome Study Group. N Engl J Med. 2000;342:1855–65. https://doi.org/10.1056/NEJM200006223422502.

115. Yawn BP, Buchanan GR, Afenyi-Annan AN, et al. Management of sickle cell disease: summary of the 2014 evidence-based report by expert panel members. JAMA. 2014;312:1033–48. https://doi.org/10.1001/jama.2014.10517.
116. Morimoto A, Nakazawa Y, Ishii E. Hemophagocytic lymphohistiocytosis: pathogenesis, diagnosis, and management. Pediatr Int. 2016;58:817–25. https://doi.org/10.1111/ped.13064.
117. Weitzman S. Approach to hemophagocytic syndromes. Hematol Am Soc Hematol Educ Program. 2011;2011:178–83. https://doi.org/10.1182/asheducation-2011.1.178.
118. Pihusch R, Holler E, Muhlbayer D, et al. The impact of antithymocyte globulin on short-term toxicity after allogeneic stem cell transplantation. Bone Marrow Transplant. 2002;30:347–54. https://doi.org/10.1038/sj.bmt.1703640.
119. Feng X, Scheinberg P, Biancotto A, et al. In vivo effects of horse and rabbit antithymocyte globulin in patients with severe aplastic anemia. Haematologica. 2014;99:1433–40. https://doi.org/10.3324/haematol.2014.106542.

Chapter 15
ECMO Use in the Pediatric Immunocompromised Hematology/Oncology Patient

Robert A. Niebler and Leslie E. Lehmann

Introduction

Any discussion of the use of extracorporeal membrane oxygenation (ECMO) in the pediatric immunocompromised hematology/oncology population must begin with a description of what ECMO is, what the mechanics/circuitry consist of, indications for ECMO, and procedure-associated complications.

A Brief History of ECMO

ECMO was developed out of the operating room as an extension of the use of cardiopulmonary bypass (CPB) and was initially used for surgical patients who did not tolerate separation from CPB [1]. The first successful report of prolonged use of what would now be termed venoarterial (VA) ECMO was in a victim of a traumatic aortic rupture by Hill et al. in 1972 [2]. Dr. Robert H. Bartlett is credited with expanding the use of ECMO to neonates with medically refractory respiratory failure in the early 1980s [3]. Dr. Bartlett further spearheaded an international collaboration of ECMO providers with the initiation of an annual meeting in 1982 and the organization of the Extracorporeal Life Support Organization (ELSO) in 1989. In addition to supporting regular scientific meetings and publishing several editions of

R. A. Niebler (✉)
Department of Pediatrics, Section of Critical Care,
Medical College of Wisconsin, Milwaukee, WI, USA
e-mail: rniebler@mcw.edu

L. E. Lehmann
Department of Pediatric Oncology,
Dana-Farber Cancer Institute/Boston Children's Hospital, Boston, MA, USA

C. N. Duncan et al. (eds.), *Critical Care of the Pediatric Immunocompromised Hematology/Oncology Patient*, https://doi.org/10.1007/978-3-030-01322-6_15

textbooks (aimed at guiding providers in the use of ECMO and the training of bedside personal), ESLO has also organized and supported a database of ECMO patients. This database contains data on 87,366 patients with a survival to hospital discharge rate of 55% as of July 2017 [4].

ECMO Physiology/Circuit Composition

The general principle of ECMO is the drainage of deoxygenated blood from the venous circulation through a pumping device which then pumps blood through an oxygenator and warmer before returning to either the arterial side as in VA ECMO or the venous side as in venovenous (VV) ECMO. Modern ECMO circuitry consists of cannulas, tubing, a pump, and an oxygenator.

Cannulas come in varying sizes and lengths depending on the vessel being cannulated and the type of ECMO support employed. Basic circuitry requires at least one lumen for the blood to flow out of the body into the ECMO circuit and one lumen for the blood to be delivered back to the body. VV ECMO can be accomplished with one double-lumen cannula in one vein, while VA ECMO requires separate cannulation of a vein to remove the blood from the body and an artery to deliver the blood from the circuit back to the body. The tubing diameter and total length of tubing are generally of low enough resistance that the flow-limiting factor through the circuit is the resistance within the smaller-diameter cannula(s). A larger-bore inflow cannula is necessary as the pressure is lower on the venous side of the circuit, while the arterial (the outflow side on a VV circuit) side can be smaller in diameter secondary to the higher pressures after the pump. Cannula selection is thus based on the size of the vessel being cannulated and calculated flow necessary to support the patient needs.

Roller head pumps and centrifugal pumps comprise the clear majority of current ECMO pumps. More traditional roller head technology consists of an area of tubing that is sequentially compressed by two rollers 180 degrees apart such that as one of the rollers loses contact with the tubing, the other comes into contact. The amount of blood propelled forward is proportional to the revolutions per minute (RPM) of the roller heads and the volume of blood pushed forward with each revolution. Roller head pumps typically operate between 60 and 120 RPM. Centrifugal pumps consist of a spinning rotor which converts rotational kinetic energy to the energy of blood flow. The blood enters the pump head near the center and is accelerated by the impeller flowing radially outward toward the exit. Centrifugal pumps rotate at thousands of RPMs, and the blood flow generated is dependent of the pump preload, RPM, and pump afterload.

Roller head pumps have the advantage of providing a guaranteed output for any given RPM provided a constant preload. Roller head pumps are not sensitive to afterload but are preload dependent and have the ability to create considerable negative pressure within the venous cannula if proper precautions are not undertaken. High negative pressure within the venous cannula has the potential of causing suction injury at the point of contact with the vessel or right atrium or causing cavitation resulting in bubble formation. In addition, the area of tubing compressed by the roller heads (the raceway) undergoes repeated stress and is at risk for rupture with prolonged ECMO support. Centrifugal pumps have the advantage of being more compact and are both preload and afterload sensitive, with varying outputs depending on the venous pressure supplying the pump and the pressure within the arterial cannula at the entrance into the bloodstream. As centrifugal pumps generally run in thousands of RPMs, there is a risk of heat generation near the rotor which resulted in hemolysis in older-generation pumps. Current-generation centrifugal pumps are magnetically levitated to prevent friction and limit the generation of heat, thus decreasing the damage to the blood cells traveling through the pump. Many programs have transitioned from the use of roller pumps to centrifugal pumps despite evidence of increased rates of complications including hemolysis and kidney injury [5, 6].

Modern oxygenator technology has evolved to be more compact, require a lower priming volume, and generate less resistance [7] while maintaining excellent gas exchange of carbon dioxide and oxygen. Carbon dioxide removal is accomplished by flowing a gas mixture (termed the "sweep gas," generally without carbon dioxide) countercurrent to the blood flow in the membrane. The gradient for removal is highest at the beginning and drops as carbon dioxide diffuses from the blood into the sweep gas, thus making the removal of carbon dioxide most dependent on the flow rate of the sweep gas. Oxygen diffusion is generally more efficient, and the concentration of oxygen in the blood and sweep gas equilibrates rapidly. This makes the effluent partial pressure of oxygen in the ECMO circuit more dependent on the partial pressure of oxygen contained within the sweep gas than the rate of the sweep gas flow.

VV Versus VA ECMO

The fundamental difference between VA and VV ECMO is the reliance on the function of the patient's heart for the entire cardiac output in VV ECMO as opposed to the hemodynamic energy delivered to the circulatory system by the ECMO pump in addition to any native cardiac output in VA ECMO. If direct cardiovascular support is required, VA ECMO must be employed.

While VV ECMO does not provide any direct circulatory energy to the patient, there are benefits to VV ECMO to the patient's cardiovascular system. Patients with severe respiratory failure being considered for ECMO generally require significant positive-pressure ventilation. This results in an increase intrathoracic pressure with a resultant decrease in right ventricular preload and increase in right ventricular afterload. Upon initiation of VV ECMO, the patient's gas exchange no longer depends on lung perfusion/ventilation, and the high positive-pressure ventilation settings can be decreased significantly. This decrease in intrathoracic pressure can provide relief to a right ventricle that may have been performing poorly under adverse loading conditions. Secondly, the VV ECMO circuit adds oxygen into the blood stream prior to the right ventricle, thereby increasing the oxygen content of pulmonary artery blood flow. Increased oxygen tension decreases pulmonary vascular resistance, thus decreasing right ventricular afterload. Finally, coronary blood flow is derived from the blood at the aortic root at the end of systole. As VV ECMO effectively increases the oxygen tension of the pulmonary artery blood, this also effectively increases the oxygen content of the pulmonary venous blood which returns to the left ventricle and is ejected into the aortic root to be perfused down the coronaries. On the contrary, during VA ECMO support, it is important to maintain some oxygenation to the lungs as coronary perfusion is derived from native left ventricular output when there is any native output from the aortic valve [8, 9].

The advantages of VV ECMO over VA ECMO include the possibility for single-vessel cannulation and removal of a source of systemic embolization. Dual-lumen cannulas are available in various sizes that can provide sufficient flow to support a VV ECMO circuit for patients as small as newborns through adulthood. Pediatric centers generally favor surgical cutdown implantation, but it is now common for adult institutions to place cannulas percutaneously by modified Seldinger techniques. As VV ECMO only delivers blood back to the venous side of the circulation, in the absence of a right-to-left intracardiac shunt, any embolus (air, particle, thrombus, etc.) produced by the circuit would not be delivered to the systemic circulation as it is in VA ECMO.

ECMO Indications

ECMO is a supportive, not curative, therapy. It can provide time for diagnosis and treatment of the underlying condition that led to the cardiopulmonary failure by supporting the function of the lungs and/or heart while those systems recover sufficiently to function without ECMO. In general, ECMO support is limited to weeks. Longer support times are generally associated with higher mortality [10]; as complications tend to occur, the longer ECMO support is necessary, and patients requiring longer support times likely have increased severity of cardiopulmonary failure [11]. Pediatric immunocompromised hematology/oncology patients are most likely to require ECMO support for sepsis, acute respiratory distress syndrome (ARDS), or sudden cardiac arrest (E-CPR).

Sepsis

Severe sepsis in a pediatric patient can lead to the need for ECMO support secondary to severe cardiac dysfunction, pulmonary dysfunction, or more commonly a combination of the two. Differentiation of the primary organ dysfunction can be difficult to discern in the acute situation leading many patients to be supported with VA ECMO when VV ECMO may be sufficient. Local practice, the individual practitioner's experience, and the patient's current condition are all reasonable factors to consider when deciding between support modalities.

ECMO is a valid support mechanism in sepsis as the underlying cause is generally time limited related to infection/inflammation. Sepsis is a multisystem disease by definition though, and supporting the heart and/or lungs with ECMO may not be sufficient to allow for recovery. Sepsis has been identified as a risk factor for survival in patients supported on ECMO, and survival rates are reported to be 36.8–82.4% [12–15]. The acute inflammatory milieu of sepsis results in impaired utilization of oxygen, disseminated intravascular coagulation (DIC), hepatic dysfunction, and renal dysfunction; all of which are not directly supported by ECMO. In particular, impaired utilization of oxygen is a problem frequently encountered in a patient with sepsis, and just supplying more cardiac output and oxygen via ECMO may not overcome this barrier. The group from Melbourne has theorized and shown some positive results with providing supraphysiologic cardiac output via central cannulation (cannulas placed directly in the right atrium and aorta via sternotomy) for ECMO [13, 14]. This technique allows for larger cannulas with shorter tubing lengths to decrease the resistance in the circuit, thereby allowing for higher flows. While central cannulation may allow for higher flows, others have been hesitant to pursue it given the additive hematologic impact of sepsis and ECMO with the need for anticoagulation and fears of increasing the high rate of hemorrhagic complications associated with ECMO with an open sternotomy.

ARDS

ARDS and other forms of acute respiratory failure have been the most successful applications of ECMO. Single organ system dysfunction which is mechanically supported by ECMO and can recover when allowed to rest (without further damage from aggressive positive-pressure ventilation) is the perfect disease state for ECMO to support. The ELSO database results bear this to be true as results for ECMO for pulmonary support are uniformly better than that for cardiac and E-CPR indications across all age groups [4].

As ARDS generally results in severe pulmonary dysfunction, VV ECMO is generally sufficient to support patients. Even patients requiring significant inotropic/vasopressor infusions prior to cannulation can be successfully managed with VV ECMO [16]. An initial trial in adult ARDS patients in 1979 did not show a significant survival benefit [17], but this trial has since been criticized by poor subject selection and poor management of ECMO in centers with very little experience prior to starting the trial. A more recent randomized trial in adult patients in the United Kingdom did show a survival and economic benefit which has reinvigorated the use of ECMO in the adult population [18]. While no equivalent randomized trial of ECMO vs. non-ECMO support has been or is likely to be done in pediatric age groups, current research efforts focus on when ECMO should be considered in an attempt to answer the questions of: (1) Does earlier ECMO initiation preserve lung function? and (2) When is consideration for ECMO support too late/futile?

E-CPR

ELSO defines E-CPR as the initiation of ECMO during an active cardiac or respiratory arrest. Most commonly this means ECMO is initiated during active chest compressions as the patient has failed conventional resuscitative efforts. Survival to discharge following E-CPR is generally reported around 40% [4, 19, 20]. Duration of cardiopulmonary resuscitation (CPR) prior to ECMO initiation would seem to be an intuitive determinant of outcome, but this has not been reliably shown [21]. Patients with good neurological outcomes have been reported with CPR durations as long as 280 min in extreme cases [22]. Neurological injury remains the paramount concern. Some neurological injury is identifiable in 22% of patients following E-CPR and accounts for the majority of the mortality [23]. In patients who survive to discharge following E-CPR, either no deficit or only mild dysfunction is seen in 79% [21]. All of these reports focus on in-hospital arrest and many specifically in patients with underlying cardiac disease. A recent review of the ELSO database attempted to look at patients without congenital heart disease receiving E-CPR and found a survival rate of 32% with a threefold increase in mortality in patients with sepsis [24].

Anticoagulation and Bleeding Complications

ECMO support requires the blood to travel outside the body and across the artificial surfaces of the pump and oxygenator. The blood interacts with these surfaces resulting in a consumptive coagulopathy [25]. Platelets and coagulation factors are activated and consumed. Anticoagulation during ECMO attempts to limit this consumption by preventing the coagulation system from interacting with the artificial surfaces. Modifications to ECMO circuits with bonding of heparin and albumin to plastic have been developed in an effort to limit the interaction [26, 27], but no clinical human study has shown this to be effective, and some have questioned the utility of these coatings [28]. While both coagulation factors and platelets are affected, traditionally only anticoagulants are used with few centers using platelet inhibitors [29]. Thromboembolic complications from clots within the circuit, particularly in VA ECMO, and thrombosis of the circuit with acute disruption of ECMO support are the primary complications resulting from inadequate anticoagulation.

The ideal anticoagulant would be fast acting, easy to monitor and titrate, and readily reversible in the event of bleeding. Unfractionated heparin (UFH) fits many of these characteristics and has been the mainstay of anticoagulation during ECMO. As UFH acts by enhancing the anticoagulant properties of antithrombin, antithrombin deficiency should be considered in patients unresponsive to standard doses of UFH. Some centers have advocated for more routine measurement and replacement of antithrombin [30, 31]. While most centers still use UFH primarily, there has been recent interest in the more routine use of direct thrombin inhibitors (argatroban, bivalirudin, and lepirudin) [29].

A whole blood activated clotting time (ACT) is the traditional method to monitor the level of anticoagulation. The ACT is a convenient test as it requires a small blood sample and can be done quickly at the bedside [32]. More recently, some centers have reported alternative anticoagulation strategies to include anti-Xa levels or thromboelastography [30, 31, 33, 34], but ACT monitoring remains the most utilized test [29].

Bleeding on ECMO is the most common patient complication. Transfusion support is the primary treatment to replace consumed platelets and coagulation factors. Each institution individualizes transfusion protocols to maintain adequate platelet numbers, coagulation factors (based traditionally on prothrombin times), and fibrinogen. Thromboelastography has been used by some centers to aid in the assessment of platelet and factor function [30, 35]. No hemostatic agent has been shown to reliably treat bleeding complications of ECMO. Several reports on the use of recombinant activated factor VII (rFVIIa) have shown some promise as a hemostatic agent, but thrombosis within the patient and circuit has also been reported [36, 37]. A general strategy for bleeding is (1) transfusion to correct coagulopathy and thrombocytopenia, (2) decrease or holding of anticoagulant infusion with lower anticoagulation test goals, (3) local control with consideration for surgical exploration and topical hemostatic agents, and (4) finally careful consideration for alternative therapies such as rFVIIIa.

Neurologic Complications and Monitoring

Neurologic complications including seizures, ischemic stroke from thromboembolism, and intracranial hemorrhage remain common and are potentially devastating complications of ECMO support [38–40]. The incidence of neurologic complications varies by age and definition of the complication. While VV ECMO may mitigate the risk of thromboembolic events and non-adjusted rates of neurologic injuries are greater in VA ECMO [38], no report has shown a risk-adjusted reduction in neurologic complications in VV ECMO. Not surprisingly, mortality and long-term morbidity are more common in patients with neurologic complications [38, 40, 41].

Monitoring of neurologic complications during ECMO varies by institution with no general consensus beyond the use of head ultrasound studies in infants with an open anterior fontanelle during the first few days of support [42, 43]. Real-time monitoring techniques including electroencephalograms, cerebral near-infrared spectroscopy, and transcranial Doppler ultrasound have been reported by single centers with a mixed ability to detect changes at the time of an event and poor correlation with more definitive neuroimaging techniques after ECMO support is completed [44]. With a high incidence in complications and lack of consensus regarding the best monitoring technique, the individual practitioner is left to decide what best techniques within any individual patient to employ. Monitoring should not place the patient at undue risk, but it is important to have a high index of suspicion as neurologic complications are common and have a profound effect on the outcome of ECMO support.

ECMO in Immunocompromised Hematology/Oncology Patients

The literature on patients receiving ECMO in the setting of an underlying malignancy comes from three large studies and multiple case reports. In 2010, Gow [45] reported the ELSO outcomes for 72 adult patients with solid tumors or hematologic malignancies (HM) receiving ECMO between 1992 and 2008. 39% of patients survived the ECMO run, and 32% survived to hospital discharge. Risk factors for mortality included requiring support for pulmonary versus cardiac failure and worse impairment of lung function prior to ECMO initiation. In 2014 the group from Vienna reported on fourteen adult HM patients requiring ECMO for ARDS [46]. Interestingly, the diagnosis of malignancy was made in four patients and five patients recieved their first chemotherapy while on ECMO support in this report. Survival to ICU and hospital discharge was 50%, and all survivors were alive at a median of 3 years of follow-up. The International ECMO Network (ECMONet) recently conducted a retrospective multicenter study and reported data from ten ICUs in seven countries on 203 immunocompromised patients greater than 15 years of age who underwent ECMO from 2008 to 2015 for severe ARDS [47]. 49% of patients had a HM or a solid tumor. In the entire cohort, 30% were alive at 6 months and 24%/20% in the HM/solid tumor subset, respectively, whereas 40% of solid organ transplant recipients were alive. A matched cohort analysis was performed between the entire group of immunocompromised patients and 94 non-immunocompromised patients receiving ECMO for ARDS. Six-month mortality was significantly higher (70 vs. 26%) in the immunocompromised patients. In an attempt to control for pre-ECMO severity of illness, 80 cases and controls were matched by PRESERVE mortality risk score; patients with an immunodeficiency diagnosis had an odds ratio of 5.7 for mortality when compared to the controls.

There is a paucity of data regarding outcomes of ECMO specifically in the pediatric oncology population. What literature exists is limited by small numbers and long reporting periods. Fourteen pediatric patients with malignancy received ECMO in Melbourne between 1993 and 2014, 9 of whom were neutropenic at the time of cannulation. Four children survived to discharge, and two (22%) from the most recent decade (2005–2014) are long-term survivors [48]. There are scattered recent individual case reports [49, 50] of successful short-term ECMO therapy for children with very specific indications: tumor lysis syndrome or support during induction chemotherapy to shrink a lymphoma-associated large mediastinal mass.

ECMO in Hematopoietic Stem Cell Transplant Patients

Whatever increased vulnerability exists for patients with malignancies in terms of ECMO candidacy would be expected to be even greater in patients undergoing hematopoietic stem cell transplantation (HSCT). Ablative conditioning, usually used in transplants for malignant diseases, involves the administration of extremely high doses of chemotherapy with or without radiation therapy. Children transplanted for nonmalignant conditions often receive reduced intensity approaches that rely on intense immunosuppression which delays robust immune reconstitution. Candidates for HSCT often have multiple preexisting comorbidities related to the underlying disease process. Examples include the end organ damage (cerebrovascular disease or pulmonary hypertension) seen in sickle cell disease or the incompletely controlled viral infections in patients with immunodeficiency disorders. Immune reconstitution is a process that generally takes months to accomplish and can be delayed even longer in the presence of graft versus host disease (GVHD), graft failure, relapse of malignancy, or uncontrolled infection.

The first series of pediatric HSCT patients receiving ECMO was reported by Gow in 2006 based on ELSO registry data spanning 1991–2004 [51]. In this cohort of 19 children, ECMO was initiated for pulmonary support in the majority (17/19). 79% died during the ECMO run, and only 1 of the 19 survived to hospital discharge. This dismal outcome led the HSCT/ICU community to question the role of ECMO in the treatment of HSCT patients. Di Nardo [52] updated this data to include 29 patients treated between 1991 and 2012. Notably 21% in this group were placed on ECMO for cardiac compromise in comparison to the primarily pulmonary indication in the earlier series. 21% were decannulated, and three patients (10%) survived to hospital discharge. Oxygenation index was the strongest predictor of survival. An oxygenation index (OI) less than 38 had 75% sensitivity and 81% specificity in differentiating survivors from non-survivors. In general, outcomes for children undergoing HSCT are superior to those in adults including in the subset of patients requiring ICU level care. There is insufficient data to know if this is true for the much smaller group of patients receiving ECMO. Wohlfarth reported the European experience in adult HSCT patients with ARDS from twelve ICUs between 2010 and 2015 [53]. 19% of the 37-patient cohort survived to hospital discharge, and all of these early survivors were alive in remission at a median of 18 months later. Interestingly this is the only group that assessed time post-HSCT as a predictor of outcome. Patients more than 240 days after HSCT had a survival of 46% vs. 4% (1 of 24 patients) for those less than 240 days after transplant. The authors hypothesize that in the early post-HSCT phase, patients have very poor immune function and are also at greater risk of developing multiple organ dysfunction syndrome, a known predictor of poor outcome in all critical patients. Despite the low likelihood of short- and long-term survival, there are, as in the oncology population, anecdotal reports describing novel indications and some successes. One child was placed on ECMO for respiratory support in the setting of fulminant adenoviral pneumonia; he ultimately recovered after receiving adenoviral-specific cytotoxic T lymphocytes, a recent advance in the therapy of severe viral infections [54]. ECMO was used as a bridge therapy to allow allogeneic HSCT in an infant with immunodeficiency syndrome who received conditioning and donor stem cells while on the circuit. He ultimately was removed from ECMO and expired in the setting of therapy refractory CMV pneumonia [55].

How Should We Decide?

It is impossible to draw firm evidence-based conclusions about the efficacy or toxicity of ECMO in the immunocompromised pediatric population from the existing literature. The combination of selection bias in terms of what patients are offered on ECMO and the reporting bias in terms of which cases are submitted for publication eventually published colors of any interpretation of the small body of literature that exists.

Given the medical intensity involved in initiating and continuing ECMO as well as the inherent risks associated with the procedure, there is understandable concern about the use of this modality in those receiving cancer therapy or undergoing HSCT. There is great heterogeneity in this group of patients, however, in terms of both the predicted efficacy and toxicity of ECMO therapy and in the ultimate prognosis. Thus, it may be helpful to have a standardized assessment tool for pediatric immunocompromised hematology/oncology/HSCT patients failing conventional support for whom ECMO is being considered (Fig. 15.1).

The first question, applicable to all ECMO candidates, is whether the cause of cardiorespiratory failure is treatable and potentially recoverable within the time that ECMO can provide heart/lung support. The next major consideration is the patient's status with regard to the underlying oncologic/HSCT diagnosis. In oncology patients,

<table>
<tr><th colspan="2">Is Cause of Cardiorespiratory Failure Treatable/Recoverable?</th></tr>
<tr><th>Oncology Population</th><th>Hematopoietic Stem Cell Transplant Population</th></tr>
<tr><td>Underlying Malignancy
• Remission Status
• Prognosis</td><td>Underlying Disease
Malignant
Non Malignant Disorder*
• Remission Status/Disease Control
• Prognosis</td></tr>
<tr><td>Place in therapy regimen</td><td>Time post-HSCT</td></tr>
<tr><td></td><td>Presence of graft vs. host disease</td></tr>
<tr><th colspan="2">Previous Organ Damage/Infections</th></tr>
<tr><td colspan="2">Current Comorbidities
• Marrow function
• Active infections
• Other organ dysfunction</td></tr>
<tr><th colspan="2">Input from parents, primary team, ICU, ECMO team</th></tr>
<tr><td colspan="2"></td></tr>
</table>

*Nonmalignant Disorders: Hemoglobinopathies, Bone Marrow Failure disorders, Immune Deficiencies

Fig. 15.1 Assessment tool when considering extracorporeal membrane oxygenation in immunocompromised/oncology/hematopoietic stem cell transplant pediatric patients

it is important to know the specific diagnosis and stage of disease, where the child is in the planned treatment course, whether the disease is currently responding to therapy, and the expected disease-free survival for this diagnosis. For example, a child with metastatic osteosarcoma who has not responded to initial therapy has a very different predicted outcome from a child with standard risk acute lymphoblastic leukemia (ALL) currently in complete remission. HSCT is rarely offered to patients for whom long -term survival is not possible. For these patients it is essential to know the underlying disease for which transplant was performed and whether the transplant has achieved the planned objective of cure. This would manifest as remission in children transplanted for malignant diseases and as good donor engraftment in those transplanted for bone marrow failure syndromes, hemoglobinopathies, and other nonmalignant conditions. A child several weeks after HSCT for high-risk leukemia not in remission at the time of transplant has a very different health status than a child transplanted 6 months previously for an underlying immunodeficiency disorder and who now has full donor engraftment. It is also important to know where the child is in the post-HSCT trajectory. Immediately following HSCT, patients have impairment in all hematopoietic lineages. They are neutropenic as well as platelet and red cell transfusion dependent. Neutrophil, platelet, and red cell counts usually improve 3–4 weeks following transplant, but lymphocyte function remains abnormal for months particularly in the setting of graft manipulation (T-cell depletion) or active GVHD. The information that must be obtained for all oncology/HSCT children includes previous infections/organ toxicities from the disease or treatment-related complications as well as current comorbidities. In all situations the goals of the parents and the primary medical team will be instrumental in the decision-making process and in delivering optimal care to these critically ill patients.

The existing data certainly suggests that oncology/HSCT patients requiring ECMO support have poorer outcomes as a group when compared to other populations receiving ECMO for similar indications. Schmidt et al. nicely reviewed some of the contributing factors, including underlying impairment in immune function increasing the risk of nosocomial infections, bleeding complications, and altered drug pharmacokinetics in a population receiving a myriad of medications [56]. However, it is also clear that ECMO can offer short- and long-term survival to some proportion of these vulnerable patients, approximately 30% of oncology and 5–20% of HSCT group. Notably, the majority of patients who are discharged from the ICU following ECMO are long-term survivors indicating that if ECMO can be successfully navigated, there is no unique long-term toxicity in these patients. Because of statistical limitations, most reports do not focus on the identification of risk factors that would allow candidate selection enriched for those predicted to gain the most benefit. The mortality score recently developed for children undergoing ECMO for respiratory failure [57] and based on ELSO data from 2001 to 2013 is a first step. In this cohort pre-ECMO factors shown to be predictive of outcome included the length of ventilation, severity of pulmonary disease, and presence of other organ dysfunction. Interestingly 4% of this group carried a cancer diagnosis as a comorbid condition, and this conferred two times the odds ratio of hospital mortality. This scoring system should be validated in immunocompromised children to ascertain whether the previously identified factors remain significant and to attempt to identify factors unique to this population (time from diagnosis or transplant, expected prognosis from underlying disease). Then a concerted effort must be made to develop consensus patient selection guidelines even in the absence of statistically robust data. This will allow the ICU/oncology/HSCT community to begin to determine whether the current poor survival is related to unique vulnerabilities in this population or reflects selection bias with ECMO only offered as a last resort to patients beyond the point where recovery is not feasible regardless of the intervention. A perspective piece from 2005 discusses the ethical dilemmas that arise when insufficient data exist yet decisions need to be made. They propose a possible approach in the context of describing the case of a 13-year-old autologous HSCT patient who required ECMO in the setting of neutropenic sepsis and was ultimately successfully weaned from ECMO with count recovery [58]. They raise many relevant issues including whether regulatory oversight and IRB approval are necessary and the difficulties in obtaining truly informed consent in this situation. They do not discuss other possible issues including resource utilization and staff discomfort when an intense procedure is predicted to fail more often than to succeed.

In conclusion the data that exists is not robust but does suggest across multiple studies in adult and pediatric populations that immunocompromised hematology/oncology/HSCT patients have an increased risk of ECMO failure compared to immunocompetent patients. The results seem to be improving in more recent eras, which mirrors the successes seen in outcomes for both immunocompromised patient populations in general and in other types of patients requiring ICU or ECMO support. Moving forward a reasonable goal would be to create and validate a predictive model for outcome in this specific population and to incorporate this into the development of consensus guidelines. Input from stakeholders caring for both pediatric immunocompromised hematology/oncology/HSCT patients and pediatric ICU patients is essential to address the combination of challenges presented by this heterogeneous critically ill patient population.

References

1. Baffes TG, Fridman JL, Bicoff JP, Whitehill JL. Extracorporeal circulation for support of palliative cardiac surgery in infants. Ann Thorac Surg. 1970;10(4):354–63.
2. Hill JD, O'Brien TG, Murray JJ, Dontigny L, Bramson ML, Osborn JJ, Gerbode F. Prolonged extracorporeal oxygenation for acute post-traumatic respiratory failure (shock-lung syndrome). Use of the Bramson membrane lung. N Engl J Med. 1972;286(12):629–34.
3. Bartlett RH, Andrews AF, Toomasian JM, Haiduc NJ, Gazzaniga AB. Extracorporeal membrane oxygenation for newborn respiratory failure: forty-five cases. Surgery. 1982;92(2):425–33.
4. Extracorporeal Life Support Organization. ECLS registry report-international summary. 2017.
5. Barrett CS, Jaggers JJ, Cook EF, Graham DA, Yarlagadda VV, Teele SA, Almond CS, Bratton SL, Seeger JD, Dalton HJ, Rycus PT, Laussen PC, Thiagarajan RR. Pediatric ECMO outcomes: comparison of centrifugal versus roller blood pumps using propensity score matching. ASAIO J. 2013;59(2):145–51.

6. O'Brien C, Monteagudo J, Schad C, Cheung E, Middlesworth W. Centrifugal pumps and hemolysis in pediatric extracorporeal membrane oxygenation (ECMO) patients: an analysis of extracorporeal life support organization (ELSO) registry data. J Pediatr Surg. 2017;52(6):975–8.
7. Stanzel RD, Henderson M. Clinical evaluation of contemporary oxygenators. Perfusion. 2016;31(1):15–25.
8. Kinsella JP, Gerstmann DR, Rosenberg AA. The effect of extracorporeal membrane oxygenation on coronary perfusion and regional blood flow distribution. Pediatr Res. 1992;31(1):80–4.
9. Secker-Walker JS, Edmonds JF, Spratt EH, Conn AW. The source of coronary perfusion during partial bypass for extracorporeal membrane oxygenation (ECMO). Ann Thorac Surg. 1976;21(2):138–43.
10. Gupta P, Robertson MJ, Beam B, Gossett JM, Schmitz ML, Carroll CL, Edwards JD, Fortenberry JD, Butt W. Relationship of ECMO duration with outcomes after pediatric cardiac surgery: a multi-institutional analysis. Minerva Anestesiol. 2015;81(6):619–27.
11. Schmidt M, Burrell A, Roberts L, Bailey M, Sheldrake J, Rycus PT, Hodgson C, Scheinkestel C, Cooper DJ, Thiagarajan RR, Brodie D, Pellegrino V, Pilcher D. Predicting survival after ECMO for refractory cardiogenic shock: the survival after veno-arterial-ECMO (SAVE)-score. Eur Heart J. 2015;36(33):2246–56.
12. Meyer DM, Jessen ME. Results of extracorporeal membrane oxygenation in children with sepsis. The extracorporeal life support organization. Ann Thorac Surg. 1997;63(3):756–61.
13. Maclaren G, Butt W, Best D, Donath S, Taylor A. Extracorporeal membrane oxygenation for refractory septic shock in children: one institution's experience. Pediatr Crit Care Med. 2007;8(5):447–51.
14. MacLaren G, Butt W, Best D, Donath S. Central extracorporeal membrane oxygenation for refractory pediatric septic shock. Pediatr Crit Care Med. 2011;12(2):133–6.
15. Smalley N, MacLaren G, Best D, Paul E, Butt W. Outcomes in children with refractory pneumonia supported with extracorporeal membrane oxygenation. Intensive Care Med. 2012;38(6):1001–7.
16. Roberts N, Westrope C, Pooboni SK, Mulla H, Peek GJ, Sosnowski AW, Firmin RK. Venovenous extracorporeal membrane oxygenation for respiratory failure in inotrope dependent neonates. ASAIO J. 2003;49(5):568–71.
17. Zapol WM, Snider MT, Hill JD, Fallat RJ, Bartlett RH, Edmunds LH, Morris AH, Peirce EC 2nd, Thomas AN, Proctor HJ, Drinker PA, Pratt PC, Bagniewski A, Miller RG Jr. Extracorporeal membrane oxygenation in severe acute respiratory failure. A randomized prospective study. JAMA. 1979;242(20):2193–6.
18. Peek GJ, Mugford M, Tiruvoipati R, Wilson A, Allen E, Thalanany MM, Hibbert CL, Truesdale A, Clemens F, Cooper N, Firmin RK, Elbourne D. CESAR trial collaboration. Efficacy and economic assessment of conventional ventilatory support versus extracorporeal membrane oxygenation for severe adult respiratory failure (CESAR): a multicentre randomised controlled trial. Lancet. 2009;374(9698):1351–63.
19. Tajik M, Cardarelli MG. Extracorporeal membrane oxygenation after cardiac arrest in children: what do we know? Eur J Cardiothorac Surg. 2008;33(3):409–17.
20. Thiagarajan RR, Laussen PC, Rycus PT, Bartlett RH, Bratton SL. Extracorporeal membrane oxygenation to aid cardiopulmonary resuscitation in infants and children. Circulation. 2007;116(15):1693–700.
21. Joffe AR, Lequier L, Robertson CM. Pediatric outcomes after extracorporeal membrane oxygenation for cardiac disease and for cardiac arrest: a review. ASAIO J. 2012;58(4):297–310.
22. Yu HY, Yeh HL, Wang SS, Tsai MK, Chen YS, Ko WJ, Lin FY. Ultra long cardiopulmonary resuscitation with intact cerebral performance for an asystolic patient with acute myocarditis. Resuscitation. 2007;73(2):307–8.
23. Barrett CS, Bratton SL, Salvin JW, Laussen PC, Rycus PT, Thiagarajan RR. Neurological injury after extracorporeal membrane oxygenation use to aid pediatric cardiopulmonary resuscitation. Pediatr Crit Care Med. 2009;10(4):445–51.

24. Conrad SJ, Bridges BC, Kalra Y, Pietsch JB, Smith AH. Extracorporeal cardiopulmonary resuscitation among patients with structurally normal hearts. ASAIO J. 2017;63(6):781–6.
25. Muntean W. Coagulation and anticoagulation in extracorporeal membrane oxygenation. Artif Organs. 1999;23(11):979–83.
26. Palmer K, Ehren H, Benz R, Frenckner B. Carmeda surface heparinization in neonatal ECMO systems: long-term experiments in a sheep model. Perfusion. 1995;10(5):307–13.
27. Urlesberger B, Zobel G, Rodl S, Dacar D, Friehs I, Leschnik B, Muntean W. Activation of the clotting system: heparin-coated versus non coated systems for extracorporeal circulation. Int J Artif Organs. 1997;20(12):708–12.
28. Silvetti S, Koster A, Pappalardo F. Do we need heparin coating for extracorporeal membrane oxygenation? New concepts and controversial positions about coating surfaces of extracorporeal circuits. Artif Organs. 2015;39(2):176–9.
29. Bembea MM, Annich G, Rycus P, Oldenburg G, Berkowitz I, Pronovost P. Variability in anticoagulation management of patients on extracorporeal membrane oxygenation: an international survey. Pediatr Crit Care Med. 2013;14(2):e77–84. PMCID: PMC3567253.
30. Agati S, Ciccarello G, Salvo D, Turla G, Undar A, Mignosa C. Use of a novel anticoagulation strategy during ECMO in a pediatric population: single-center experience. ASAIO J. 2006;52(5):513–6.
31. Urlesberger B, Zobel G, Zenz W, Kuttnig-Haim M, Maurer U, Reiterer F, Riccabona M, Dacar D, Gallisti S, Leschnik B, Muntean W. Activation of the clotting system during extracorporeal membrane oxygenation in term newborn infants. J Pediatr. 1996;129(2):264–8.
32. Green TP, Isham-Schopf B, Steinhorn RH, Smith C, Irmiter RJ. Whole blood activated clotting time in infants during extracorporeal membrane oxygenation. Crit Care Med. 1990;18(5):494–8.
33. Baird CW, Zurakowski D, Robinson B, Gandhi S, Burdis-Koch L, Tamblyn J, Munoz R, Fortich K, Pigula FA. Anticoagulation and pediatric extracorporeal membrane oxygenation: impact of activated clotting time and heparin dose on survival. Ann Thorac Surg. 2007;83(3):912–9; discussion 919–20.
34. O'Meara LC, Alten JA, Goldberg KG, Timpa JG, Phillips J, Laney D, Borasino S. Anti-Xa directed protocol for anticoagulation management in children supported with extracorporeal membrane oxygenation. ASAIO J. 2015;61(3):339–44.
35. Oliver WC. Anticoagulation and coagulation management for ECMO. Semin Cardiothorac Vasc Anesth. 2009;13(3):154–75.
36. Niebler RA, Punzalan RC, Marchan M, Lankiewicz MW. Activated recombinant factor VII for refractory bleeding during extracorporeal membrane oxygenation. Pediatr Crit Care Med. 2010;11(1):98–102.
37. Warren OJ, Rogers PL, Watret AL, de Wit KL, Darzi AW, Gill R, Athanasiou T. Defining the role of recombinant activated factor VII in pediatric cardiac surgery: where should we go from here? Pediatr Crit Care Med. 2009;10(5):572–82.
38. Cengiz P, Seidel K, Rycus PT, Brogan TV, Roberts JS. Central nervous system complications during pediatric extracorporeal life support: incidence and risk factors. Crit Care Med. 2005;33(12):2817–24.
39. Luyt CE, Brechot N, Demondion P, Jovanovic T, Hekimian G, Lebreton G, Nieszkowska A, Schmidt M, Trouillet JL, Leprince P, Chastre J, Combes A. Brain injury during venovenous extracorporeal membrane oxygenation. Intensive Care Med. 2016;42(5):897–907.
40. Nasr DM, Rabinstein AA. Neurologic complications of extracorporeal membrane oxygenation. J Clin Neurol. 2015;11(4):383–9. PMCID: PMC4596114.
41. Lorusso R, Gelsomino S, Parise O, Di Mauro M, Barili F, Geskes G, Vizzardi E, Rycus PT, Muellenbach R, Mueller T, Pesenti A, Combes A, Peek G, Frenckner B, Di Nardo M, Swol J, Maessen J, Thiagarajan RR. Neurologic injury in adults supported with veno-venous extracorporeal membrane oxygenation for respiratory failure: findings from the extracorporeal life support organization database. Crit Care Med. 2017;45(8):1389–97.

42. Heard ML, Clark RH, Pettignano R, Dykes FD. Daily cranial ultrasounds during ECMO: a quality review/cost analysis project. J Pediatr Surg. 1997;32(8):1260–1.
43. Khan AM, Shabarek FM, Zwischenberger JB, Warner BW, Cheu HW, Jaksic T, Goretsky MJ, Meyer TA, Doski J, Lally KP. Utility of daily head ultrasonography for infants on extracorporeal membrane oxygenation. J Pediatr Surg. 1998;33(8):1229–32.
44. Bembea MM, Felling R, Anton B, Salorio CF, Johnston MV. Neuromonitoring during extracorporeal membrane oxygenation: a systematic review of the literature. Pediatr Crit Care Med. 2015;16(6):558–64.
45. Gow KW, Lao OB, Leong T, Fortenberry JD. Extracorporeal life support for adults with malignancy and respiratory or cardiac failure: the extracorporeal life support experience. Am J Surg. 2010;199(5):669–75.
46. Wohlfarth P, Ullrich R, Staudinger T, Bojic A, Robak O, Hermann A, Lubsczyk B, Worel N, Fuhrmann V, Schoder M, Funovics M, Rabitsch W, Knoebl P, Laczika K, Locker GJ, Sperr WR, Schellongowski P. Arbeitsgruppe fur hamato-onkologische Intensivmedizin der Osterreichischen Gesellschaft fur Internistische und Allgemeine Intensivmedizin und Notfallmedizin (OGIAIN). Extracorporeal membrane oxygenation in adult patients with hematologic malignancies and severe acute respiratory failure. Crit Care. 2014;18(1):R20. PMCID: PMC4055976
47. Schmidt M, Schellongowski P, Patroniti N, Taccone FS, Reis Miranda D, Reuter J, Prodanovic H, Pierrot M, Dorget A, Park S, Balik M, Demoule A, Crippa IA, Mercat A, Wohlfarth P, Sonneville R, Combes A, International ECMO Network (ECMONet), the REVA Research Network and the IDEA Study Group. Six-month outcome of immunocompromised severe ARDS patients rescued by ECMO. An international multicenter retrospective study. Am J Respir Crit Care Med. 2018 Jan 3.
48. Smith S, Butt W, Best D, MacLaren G. Long-term survival after extracorporeal life support in children with neutropenic sepsis. Intensive Care Med. 2016;42(5):942–3.
49. Huang M, Owen E, Myers S, Raj A. Cardiopulmonary failure requiring ECMO bypass resulting from leukemia cell lysis in a patient with childhood acute myelomonocytic leukemia. Case Rep Hematol. 2015;2015:640528. PMCID: PMC4466370.
50. Lueck C, Kuehn C, Hoeper MM, Ganser A, Eder M, Beutel G. Successful use of extracorporeal membrane oxygenation during induction chemotherapy in a patient with mediastinal tumor mass of a T lymphoblastic lymphoma. Ann Hematol. 2016;95(10):1719–21.
51. Gow KW, Wulkan ML, Heiss KF, Haight AE, Heard ML, Rycus P, Fortenberry JD. Extracorporeal membrane oxygenation for support of children after hematopoietic stem cell transplantation: the extracorporeal life support organization experience. J Pediatr Surg. 2006;41(4):662–7.
52. Di Nardo M, Locatelli F, Palmer K, Amodeo A, Lorusso R, Belliato M, Cecchetti C, Perrotta D, Picardo S, Bertaina A, Rutella S, Rycus P, Di Ciommo V, Holzgraefe B. Extracorporeal membrane oxygenation in pediatric recipients of hematopoietic stem cell transplantation: an updated analysis of the extracorporeal life support organization experience. Intensive Care Med. 2014;40(5):754–6.
53. Wohlfarth P, Beutel G, Lebiedz P, Stemmler HJ, Staudinger T, Schmidt M, Kochanek M, Liebregts T, Taccone FS, Azoulay E, Demoule A, Kluge S, Svalebjorg M, Lueck C, Tischer J, Combes A, Boll B, Rabitsch W, Schellongowski P. Intensive Care in Hematologic and Oncologic Patients (iCHOP), Caring for critically ill immunocompromised patients Multinational Network (NINE-I). Characteristics and outcome of patients after allogeneic hematopoietic stem cell transplantation treated with extracorporeal membrane oxygenation for acute respiratory distress syndrome. Crit Care Med. 2017;45(5):e500–7.
54. Di Nardo M, Li Pira G, Amodeo A, Cecchetti C, Giorda E, Ceccarelli S, Brescia LP, Pirozzi N, Rutella S, Locatelli F, Bertaina A. Adoptive immunotherapy with antigen-specific T cells during extracorporeal membrane oxygenation (ECMO) for adenovirus-related respiratory failure in a child given haploidentical stem cell transplantation. Pediatr Blood Cancer. 2014;61(2):376–9.

55. Di Nardo M, Locatelli F, Di Florio F, Cecchetti C, Amodeo A, Rutella S, Bertaina A. Extracorporeal membrane oxygenation as a bridge to allogeneic T-cell depleted hematopoietic stem cell transplantation in infants with severe combined immune deficiency: is it feasible? Intensive Care Med. 2014;40(10):1600–1.
56. Schmidt M, Brodie D, Combes A. Patients with hematologic malignancies have many reasons to die during extracorporeal membrane oxygenation. Crit Care. 2014; 18(5): 522-014-0522-0. PMCID: PMC4163603.
57. Bailly DK, Reeder RW, Zabrocki LA, Hubbard AM, Wilkes J, Bratton SL, Thiagarajan RR. Extracorporeal life support organization member centers. Development and validation of a score to predict mortality in children undergoing extracorporeal membrane oxygenation for respiratory failure: pediatric pulmonary rescue with extracorporeal membrane oxygenation prediction score. Crit Care Med. 2017;45(1):e58–66. PMCID: PMC5532876.
58. Wolfson RK, Kahana MD, Nachman JB, Lantos J. Extracorporeal membrane oxygenation after stem cell transplant: clinical decision-making in the absence of evidence. Pediatr Crit Care Med. 2005;6(2):200–3.

Chapter 16
Pharmacy Implications

Stacey Albuquerque

Pharmacologic Principles

The immunocompromised patient often requires multiple medications in a critical care setting that are subject to changes in metabolism and clearance due to compromised organ dysfunction as a result of illness. Many drug classes of medications including anti-infective, analgesics, anxiolytics, neuromuscular blockers, antihypertensive, and inotropes are affected by pharmacokinetic and pharmacodynamic changes in these patients. The pharmacokinetic and pharmacodynamic properties of an agent may be influenced by developmental changes, interactions with drugs or nutrients, disease states, and genetics [1]. All these factors must be considered to manage these patients effectively. Refer to Fig. 16.1.

Pharmacokinetics

Pharmacokinetics describes the process of drug absorption, distribution, biotransformation, and excretion. Pharmacokinetics determines what the body does to the drug after administration. It is the determinant of the concentration at the site of action. The free concentration of drug in the plasma is available for distribution to the tissues to exert a pharmacologic effect and eventual biotransformation [1, 3].

S. Albuquerque (✉)
Boston Children's Pharmacy Department,
Dana Farber/Boston Children's Cancer and Blood Disorders Center,
Boston, MA, USA
e-mail: stacey.albuquerque@childrens.harvard.edu

C. N. Duncan et al. (eds.), *Critical Care of the Pediatric Immunocompromised Hematology/Oncology Patient*, https://doi.org/10.1007/978-3-030-01322-6_16

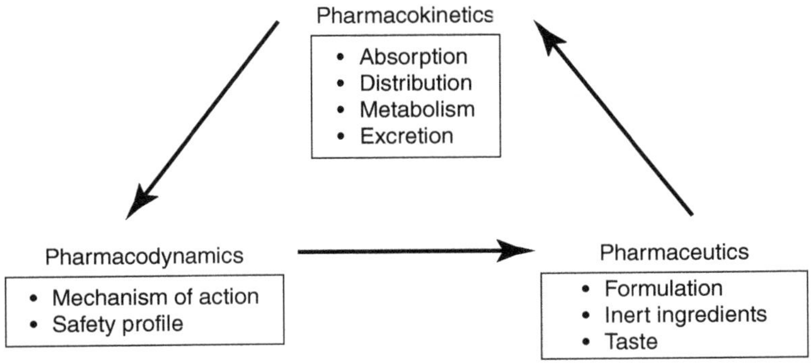

Fig. 16.1 Determinants of effective therapy. (Reproduced from [2])

Absorption

Absorption is the process of drug transfer from its site of administration to the bloodstream. Absorption of a drug when administered intravenously is the most efficient route with the entire drug reaching the circulation and is considered to be 100% bioavailable. When medications are administered by other routes (enteral, subcutaneous, rectal), the bioavailability is often less due to incomplete absorption, first-pass metabolism, and distribution to other tissues [1].

Distribution

Drug distribution describes the movement of drugs, active metabolites from the blood to tissues or body compartments. When drugs reach the tissues, they exert toxic and/or therapeutic effects [1]. Drug properties such as protein binding, lipid and water solubility, and pH, determine the extent and rate of distribution and are important in terms of their clinical implications [1, 3]. Protein binding is an important component of drug interactions and can rapidly change quantities of free drug in the circulation [1, 3]. Water solubility and lipophilicity determine distribution to tissue target sites such as the central nervous system and can have implications in determining drug dosing in obese patients [1]. The term volume of distribution (Vd) is a hypothetical volume which the drug is dispersed to help quantify the degree to which the drug is dispersed to various compartments (adipose tissue, plasma) [3].

Metabolism

The liver is the primary organ for drug metabolism. Other tissues such as the gastrointestinal tract, lungs, skin, and kidneys are also known to have substantial metabolic activity. The biotransformation of drugs may result in a weaker compound, an active metabolite, or a toxic metabolite depending on the drug. In other instances inactive parent compounds (prodrugs) may convert to active moiety. In the hepatocytes, there is a series of enzymatic processes [1]. Phase 1 reactions (nonsynthetic reactions) are catalyzed by enzymes of the cytochrome P450 system. The CYP3A4 pathway is a major metabolic pathway for almost 50% of the drugs, while CYP2D6 (31%) and CYP2C9 (10%) account for the majority of the remainder [1, 3]. These various enzymes and their isoforms result in characteristic inhibition and induction of activity of selected medications. Knowledge of which drugs are substrates for these various isoforms as well as their selective inducers/inhibitors allows for an understanding and anticipation of drug interactions. Phase II reactions (synthetic reactions) involve conjugation with glycine, glucuronide, or sulfate. Phase III enzyme reactions have recently been identified that involve P-glycoprotein (PGP) and related transporters [1, 3].

Elimination

Elimination is the process by which a drug is cleared from the body. The main organs responsible for elimination are the kidneys and liver. Often, clearance is a combination of renal and nonrenal clearance. Glomerular filtration and tubular secretion play roles in drug elimination, but clearance of a drug is also a function of molecular size, pH, and protein binding. Highly protein-bound drugs are less likely to be filtered and thus are unlikely to be removed by dialysis [3]. The liver also contributes to elimination through metabolism or excretion into the bile [1].

Pharmacodynamics

The pharmacodynamics of a drug is the effect of the drug on the body, the effects, or response to drug therapy [1]. It describes the relationship between a drug's concentration at its site of action and its effect. It also encompasses the mechanisms of action, therapeutic effects, and its safety profile [3]. The need for therapeutic drug monitoring becomes important as it can assess toxicity as well as efficacy. The reliance on a therapeutic effect often relies on a drug/dose response relationship [2].

Drug Effectiveness

When determining drug effectiveness, there must be clear expectations and therapeutic endpoints and expectations when initiating therapy. The target-effect strategy of treating a patient is a dose titration to various endpoints [2]. To use this strategy, a provider must understand the pharmacodynamic action of the drug as well as the side effect profiles to evaluate safety, efficacy, or toxicity. Alternatively, the target concentration strategy uses drug concentrations as a guide to drug dosing to see a pharmacodynamic effect, but does not allow for individual patient responsiveness. The reliance on a number goal is comforting for some, yet it must be understood that there may be pharmacokinetic influences and or additional influences related to the collection and processing of blood sampling. It is always recommended to evaluate the patient (drug effect on patient) and not necessarily a drug level [2].

Adverse Drug Reactions

Adverse drug reactions are a common indication for admission of an immunocompromised patient to the ICU. Other indications necessitating the need for ICU management include seizures, posterior reversible encephalopathy syndrome (PRES), respiratory failure, infections, and cardiovascular issues [4]. The Joint Commission on the Accreditation (JCAHO) defines an adverse drug reaction (ADR) as "an undesirable response associated with the use of a drug that compromises the therapeutic efficacy, enhances toxicity, or both." [5]

Patients in the ICU are more predisposed to the development of adverse drug reactions due to the increased incidence of hepatic and renal dysfunction [5]. Subsequent implications and manifestations are seen in areas that extend beyond the liver and kidneys. The affected organ systems and examples of pharmacologic agents that are often implicated are listed below.

Renal

Renal failure can affect the pharmacokinetics of many medications. Causes of renal dysfunction in critically ill immunocompromised patients include sepsis, nephrotoxic drugs, radiocontrast agents, chemotherapeutic agents, and post-HCT complications such as sinusoidal obstruction syndrome and hemolytic uremic syndrome [6]. Drugs that are more than 30% eliminated in the urine are likely to have diminished clearance in the presence of renal insufficiency [1]. Serum creatinine may not rise until the creatinine clearance has significantly fallen and clearance measurements may be unreliable in the critically ill [7]. Mechanisms by which nephrotoxins can cause kidney injury include hemodynamically mediated nephrotoxicity, tubular necrosis, interstitial nephritis obstructive neuropathy, and vascular toxicity [5].

Nephrotoxins
Aminoglycosides, amphotericin, carboplatin, cephalosporins, cisplatin, mannitol, pentamidine, radiocontrast agents, aminoglycosides, penicillins, sulfonamides, tacrolimus, thiazide and loop diuretics, vancomycin, angiotensin-converting enzyme inhibitors, nonsteroidal anti-inflammatory drugs [5]

Hepatic

Drugs that undergo extensive first-pass metabolism may have higher bioavailability in patients with liver failure. Slow gut motility may delay a peak response in these patients. Altered plasma protein concentrations may change the tissue distribution of drugs that are highly protein bound. The capacity of the liver to metabolize drugs depends on blood flow and hepatic enzyme activity which can be affected by liver disease. In addition, some P450 isoforms are more susceptible to liver disease than others impairing drug metabolism [1]. In a study by Carillo et al., it was concluded that CYP450-mediated drug metabolism was decreased in children with sepsis related in part due to the degree of inflammation and organ failure [8]. Drug-induced liver injury is often due to the accumulation of metabolites which can cause cell damage and trigger an inflammatory response. Drug-induced hepatic injury can be hepatocellular, cholestatic, or vascular in nature [5].

Hepatotoxins
Acetaminophen, erythromycin, isoniazid, ketoconazole, nitrofurantoin, phenobarbital, rifampin, sulfonamides, voriconazole

Cardiac

Circulatory shock and failure can alter the pharmacokinetics of drugs used in the intensive care setting. Decreased tissue perfusion combined with increased edema and total body water can unpredictably change the volume of distribution of medications causing unexpected changes including electrolyte disturbances [1]. Patients in the PICU may also require vasopressors that act on alpha adrenergic receptors which may result in arrhythmias. Unfortunately other classes of drugs used for immunocompromised patients have cardiac effects such as fluoroquinolones, antifungals, and some antiemetic medications (5HT-3 antagonists) can cause QT prolongation increasing potential for cardiac adverse effects especially when used concomitantly [5]. There is also the possibility that pediatric immunocompromised patients have been previously treated with cardiotoxic chemotherapy such as anthracyclines which are direct myocardial toxins; thus they may find themselves at higher risk due to multiple cardiac insults [5].

Cardiac Adverse Effects
Arrhythmias: dopamine, dobutamine, epinephrine
QT prolongation: fluoroquinolones, ondansetron
Cardiomyopathy: anthracyclines

Central Nervous System

Adverse effects associated with the central nervous system in the ICU include seizures, headache, and sedation. Drug-related seizures may be related to a characteristic of the drug itself, factors that influence drug levels, or a change in a patient's renal or hepatic condition causing decreased clearance.

Drug-induced seizure is an adverse effect of many antifective and immunosuppressive medications. Drug-induced headache is caused by vasodilators, chemotherapy agents, and immunosuppressants as well [5]. Posterior reversible encephalopathy syndrome (PRES), which is characterized by seizures and severe hypertension and headache, is thought to be associated with the use of cyclosporine and other calcineurin inhibitors.

Sedation is a well-known adverse effect of medications commonly used in the PICU. Commonly used medications with this effect include benzodiazepine and opioids. Clearance of these medications is affected by renal and hepatic function; thus close monitoring is essential to prevent central nervous system toxicities [7].

Drug Interactions

Risks for Drug Interactions

Drug interactions are associated with increased length of stay and/or admissions to PICU. When there is an interaction between two medications, the result can be an increase or decreased therapeutic effect (or adverse effect), or there will be a response that will not occur if each drug is given alone.

The Cytochrome P450 System

As was stated previously, the liver is the primary location of CYP 450 enzymes. In addition, some P450 enzymes, most notably CYP3A4 are located in the lining of the intestine and control the absorption of certain substrates into the portal circulation. Many drugs or their metabolites are induced or inhibited by the action of one or more of the CYP450 enzymes. These CYP450 enzymes and their various isoforms are the primary drivers of drug interactions [9].

> *Enzyme induction* occurs when a drug stimulates synthesis of that enzyme leading to increased activity of the enzyme. This process occurs over days to weeks; thus drugs that are substrates affected by this enzyme increase by threefold [9].

- An example of *enzyme induction* would be the administration of rifampin, a CYP3A4 inducer when it is added to the regimen of a patient receiving cyclosporine. The cyclosporine dose would need to be three to five times higher than the usual required dose to achieve the same therapeutic level before the rifampin was added.

Enzyme inhibition occurs immediately after drug administration, although maximal inhibition is not seen until steady-state levels are reached [9]. In most cases, steady state is defined as 4–5 half-lives of the drug.

- An example of *enzyme inhibition* would be the addition of voriconazole to the regimen of a patient on cyclosporine. The cyclosporine level would increase by over 50% approximately 3 to 5 days after the voriconazole was added to the regimen. Voriconazole requires about 5 days of doses before it reaches steady state.

Genetics and the Cytochrome P450 System

Levels of drug metabolizing enzymes may be influenced by the genetic makeup of each individual. For example, certain ethnic groups may be ultra-fast metabolizers of a particular isoform (CYP2D6) and require increased doses to achieve appropriate blood levels. Alternatively, slow metabolizers require smaller doses or longer intervals to avoid toxic drug levels [9]. This concept of the study of genetic makeup on drug metabolism is known as pharmacogenomics [1, 9].

The true impact of pharmacogenomics is yet to be seen but holds promise to be able to individualize therapy for an individual based on genetic makeup. In the meantime, it may be able to shed light on situations where drug dosing and therapeutic response/therapeutic levels cannot be explained [9].

Other Types of Drug Interactions

Other types of pharmacokinetic drug interactions must also be considered as they involve principles of absorption, distribution, and elimination. Many of these interactions may involve the use of other supportive care measures commonly addressed in patients in the ICU. For example, the use of proton-pump inhibitors for stress ulcer prophylaxis can change the absorption of some drugs by altering the pH of the stomach. In addition, it can delay the clearance of higher doses of methotrexate resulting in nephrotoxicity [9].

Management Principles of Immunocompromised Patients in the PICU

The admission of critically ill immunocompromised patients can be challenging to pediatric intensivists. However, admissions to the PICU have been shown to decrease mortality and improve outcomes [4]. Adherence to basic principles of drug therapy in immunocompromised patients regardless of their physical location is important. A sampling is listed below [4].

- Administration of anti-infective prophylaxis and treatment per accepted guidelines
- Early recognition of drug toxicity due to antineoplastic medications with appropriate reductions as needed
- Monitoring of drug interactions with oncology therapies
- Initiation or modification of appropriate supportive care medications where appropriate such as antiemetic and growth factors
- Initiation of drug antidotes when necessary for life-threatening toxicities related to antineoplastic therapy administration [4]

Future Drug Challenges in the Pediatric PICU Patient

As the oncology and stem cell transplant communities expand their use of novel chemotherapeutic agents and other targeted therapies to treat disease, the standards for addressing and recognizing toxicity are proceeding at a slower pace and are not fully standardized. Many of the new targeted therapies are thought to be less toxic than standard chemotherapy agents due to their specificity but can still necessitate an PICU admission in a heavily treated patient should the patient decompensate. The management of adverse effects often requires knowledge of the mechanism of action of the new unique oncology medication which can be challenging for a clinician [4].

Chimeric antigen receptor therapy (CAR-T) requires a collaboration of oncologists and intensivists to facilitate the management of unwanted side effects. Immunotherapy approaches such as monoclonal antibodies and manipulated T-cell therapies are well tolerated but can have potential life-threatening effects such as cytokine release syndrome (CRS). This syndrome is not fully understood, but there is activation of inflammatory cytokines and interleukin-6 which have some response anticytokine treatments [4].

In addition, the future role and applications of pharmacogenomics in drug therapy are still in their infancy. However, the field is rapidly expanding as the world of personalized medicine begins to progress in the treatment of oncologic disease.

References

1. Besunder JB, Pope J. Pharmacology in the PICU. In: Wheeler DS, Wong H, Shanley P, editors. Critical care medicine. London: Spriger; 2014. p. 55–73.
2. Reed MR, Blumer J. Therapeutic drug monitoring in the pediatric intensive care unit. Pediatr Clin N Am. 1994;41:1227–43.
3. Zuppa AF, Barrett JS. Pharmacokinetics and pharmacodynamics in the critically ill child. Pediatr Clin N Am. 2008;55:735–55.
4. Shimabukuro-Vornhagen AS, Boll B, Kochanek M, et al. Critical care of patients with cancer. CA Cancer J Clinic. 2016;66:496–517.
5. Benton WW, Brothers AW, Jefferis Kirk CC, et al. Adverse drug reactions and drug-drug interactions. In: Fuhrman BP, Zimmerman JJ, editors. Pediatric critical care. Philadelphia: Elsevier; 2011. p. 1569–89.
6. Benoit DD, Hoste E. Acute kidney injury in patients with cancer. Crit Care Clin. 2010;26:151–79.
7. Bodenham A, Shelly MP, Park GR. The altered pharmacokinetics and pharmacodynamics of drugs commonly used in critically ill patients. Clin Pharmacokinet. 1988;14:347–73.
8. Carcillo JA, Doughty L, Kofos D, et al. Cytochrome P450 mediated drug metabolism is reduced in children with sepsis-induced multiple organ failure. Intensive Care Med. 2003;29:280–4.
9. Blower P, deWit R, Goodin S. Drug-drug interactions in oncology: why are they important and how can they be minimized. Crit Rev Oncol Hematol. 2005;55:117–42.

Chapter 17
Psychosocial and Palliative Care

Sarah Tarquini, Candice Chow, and Christina Ullrich

Introduction

A life-threatening or life-limiting illness in childhood is universally stressful for patients, caregivers, and their families. At some point throughout the course of treatment for such conditions, patients may require care in a pediatric intensive care unit (PICU). By its very definition, care provided in the PICU is intensive; sophisticated medical technology helps monitor and support basic bodily functions, and nursing is available at the bedside 24 hours a day. While many admissions to the PICU are acute and unplanned, others are planned postoperatively to allow for close monitoring following a major procedure. Regardless of the reason for a PICU admission, pediatric patients and their families are coping not only with the medical acuity of such an admission but also with the far-reaching impact of the experience.

This chapter will address the psychosocial aspects of intensive care, specifically for immunocompromised patients and their caregivers. It will highlight the emotional needs of patients and families in the PICU and consider how psychological interventions and pediatric palliative care (PPC) aim to bolster adaptive adjustment and coping and maximize well-being. It is important to recognize the inherent diversity of the population of immunocompromised patients receiving critical care. There

S. Tarquini (✉) · C. Chow
Department of Psychosocial Oncology and Palliative Care,
Dana-Farber Boston Children's Cancer and Blood Disorders Center, Harvard Medical School, Boston, MA, USA
e-mail: sarah_tarquini@dfci.harvard.edu; candice_chow@dfci.harvard.edu

C. Ullrich
Department of Pediatric Oncology; Department of Psychosocial Oncology and Palliative Care, Dana-Farber Cancer Institute and Boston Children's Hospital, Harvard Medical School, Boston, MA, USA
e-mail: christina_ullrich@dfci.harvard.edu

C. N. Duncan et al. (eds.), *Critical Care of the Pediatric Immunocompromised Hematology/Oncology Patient*, https://doi.org/10.1007/978-3-030-01322-6_17

is a wide range in terms of their medical diagnoses, the duration and intensity of medical treatments experienced, and most fundamentally, in terms of the individual differences that exist across patients and their family systems. As such, the experience of admission to an intensive care unit for this population should be considered within the larger context of a patient and family's global experience of treatment.

Psychosocial Care

Patient Experience

PICU hospitalization results in significant distress and psychological sequelae for approximately 25% of youth admitted to the PICU, even up to a year after discharge [1–3]. Caregivers report many challenges for their children post-discharge, including a decrease in emotional well-being, confidence, and self-esteem; increased anxiety; sleep disturbance; social isolation; changes in memory, attention span, and cognitive functioning; and symptoms of posttraumatic stress disorder (PTSD) [2, 4, 5]. In an effort to mitigate some of the potential negative psychological effects of a PICU hospitalization, it is important to consider how children of different ages and developmental levels might make sense of their experiences.

Infants and Toddlers (Ages 0–2 Years)

Children in this age range are beginning to form strong bonds with their caregivers and are developing a sense of security within those relationships. Infants and toddlers experience separation from caregivers, pain, exposure to unfamiliar people, disruption of normal routines, and restriction of movement, as variables that may impede their development of security and trust. Although research points to the need for increased caregiver participation during a child's hospital stay, in reality, this may not always be feasible [6]. Ideally, interventions would include caregiver presence and interaction in the form of holding, soothing, and play whenever possible. Maintaining a consistent daily routine (i.e., for waking, feeding, naptime, bathing, and bed time) can help very young children build a sense of security, comfort, and trust in an otherwise unpredictable environment.

Preschool Children (Ages 3–5 Years)

Preschoolers who have spent time in intensive care settings have largely been excluded from psychological outcome studies, likely due to the fact that they are more challenging to assess and validated instruments for this age group are lacking [7]. The cognitive development of preschoolers is marked by egocentricity, the emergence of symbolic thought, and magical thinking – the notion that one's thoughts, desires, and wishes can have an effect on the external world. Providing simple, clear, and factual information about the child's illness, required medical care, the potential impact on the child's regular routine, and the anticipated expectations for caregiver presence are all important in facilitating adaptive adjustment and functioning. Pretend play, story books, music, videos, and drawing can be helpful ways to engage preschoolers around their illness and hospitalization experience and to encourage mastery of new routines and medical procedures.

School-Aged Children (Ages 6–12 Years)

Following a PICU hospitalization, a number of school-aged children report increased anxiety, fear of medical settings and interventions, delusional memories and hallucinations, and a negative impact on their friendships and sense of self [1]. This age group has the capacity for more logical thinking but continues to view the world in a fairly concrete way, with an emphasis on fairness and on cause and effect [8]. Some children may want to participate in discussions around their medical care, while others may shy away from medical discussions and decision-making opportunities. Encouraging communication between patients, caregivers, and medical providers is a critical step in determining how to best meet the unique needs of each patient [9].

Adolescents (Ages 13–18 Years)

This period marks the development of more complex thinking processes, including abstract thinking, the ability to consider multiple viewpoints, and the ability to reason and form new ideas. With this heightened capacity for abstract thought, adolescent patients are increasingly able to make informed decisions about their medical care. It is important to note that each child and adolescent's cognitive development progresses at varying rates and that emotional distress can sometimes interfere with one's ability to think with complexity about the intricacies of a situation. Providers should meet regularly with adolescent patients individually to provide them with opportunities for processing their emotions and talking about their decision-making processes without parental input.

Young Adults (Ages 19–25 Years)

Young adults are able to fully understand abstract concepts, consider the consequences of their decisions, and appreciate personal limitations. They have moved forward with the process of securing their autonomy and are likely more skilled in independent decision-making than they were in adolescence. This age group may also rely more on support from a romantic partner than on their parents. When in a medically compromised state, however, the role of parents may suddenly become more prominent again. This shift in independence may lead to emotional distress and regression. Identifying a healthcare proxy when appropriate and discussing preferences for care, communication, and decision-making will contribute to adaptive experiences for young adults in the PICU.

Caregiver Experience in the PICU

In the context of a PICU admission, particularly when such admissions are characterized by unexpected or particularly complicated medical circumstances, it is understandable and adaptive for patients, as well as their caregivers and loved ones to experience very strong emotions. The experience of caring for, bearing witness to, and recovering from the treatment of a critically ill child can be psychologically, socially, and financially overwhelming for family members. Perhaps not surprisingly, parents of critically ill patients are particularly vulnerable population who have been found to be at risk for anxiety, depression, and PTSD symptoms [10, 11]. In practical terms, it is important to understand that the manner in which such feelings are experienced, processed, and expressed are highly variable and dependent on a number of factors, including the specific medical circumstances, one's temperament, and one's ability to reliably access effective coping strategies and utilize social supports. Some caregivers may become more withdrawn or tearful, while others may become more irritable or angry. Some may feel most comfortable with a constant presence at the bedside, others may need more time away from the hospital setting.

The literature has increasingly recognized the impact of a child's critical illness on family functioning, and clinical practice has been expanding its focus from "patient"-centered care to "family"-centered care. This perspective highlights the significant role that the family plays in patient care, as well as the potential impact of family functioning on patient outcomes.

Clinical practice guidelines for the support of the family in critical care were originally published in 2007 by the American College of Critical Care Medicine and subsequently revised in 2017 [12]. An international, multidisciplinary team outlined 23 recommendations that focused on communication with family members, family presence, family support, consultations and ICU team members, and operational and environmental issues. Recommendations relevant for the pediatric immunocompromised patient are included in Table 17.1. Consistent with information provided throughout this chapter, the recommendations emphasize the importance of early and consistent access to psychosocial and palliative care as well as the importance of ongoing clear communication with patients and family members. Such interventions aim to maximize the effectiveness of team-family collaboration, maximize patient and family coping, and minimize patient and family distress.

Table 17.1 ICU family-centered care recommendations for pediatric patients

Family presence in the ICU
Family members of critically ill patients be offered open or flexible family presence at the bedside that meets their needs while providing support for staff and positive reinforcement for staff to work in partnership with families to improve family satisfaction
Family members of critically ill patients be offered the option of participating in interdisciplinary team rounds to improve satisfaction with communication and increase family engagement
Family members of critically ill patients be offered the option of being present during resuscitation efforts, with a staff member assigned to support the family
Family support
Family education programs be included as part of the clinical care as these programs have demonstrated beneficial effects for family members in the ICU by reducing stress, depression, posttraumatic stress, and generalized stress while improving family satisfaction with care
ICUs provide family with leaflets that give information about ICU setting to reduce family member anxiety and stress
ICU diaries be implemented in ICUs to reduce family member anxiety, depression, and posttraumatic stress
Validated decision-support tools for family members be implemented in the ICU setting when relevant validated tools exist to optimize quality of communication and medical comprehension and reduce family decisional conflict
Among surrogates of ICU patients who are deemed by a clinician to have a poor prognosis, clinicians use a communication approach such as the "VALUE" mnemonic (value family statements, acknowledge emotions, listen, understand the patient as a person, elicit questions), during family conferences to facilitate clinician-family communication
Communication with family members
Routine interdisciplinary family conferences be used in the ICU to improve family satisfaction with communication and trust in clinicians and to reduce conflict between clinicians and family members
Healthcare clinicians in the ICU should use structured approaches to communication, such as in the "VALUE" mnemonic when engaging in communication with family members, specifically including active listening, expressions of empathy, and making supportive statements around nonabandonment and decision-making. In addition, family members of critically ill patients who are dying be offered a written bereavement brochure to reduce family anxiety, depression, and posttraumatic stress and improve family satisfaction with communication
ICU clinicians receive family-centered communication training as one element of critical care training to improve clinician self-efficacy and family satisfaction
Use of specific consultations and ICU team members
Proactive palliative care consultation be provided
Ethics consultation be provided to decrease ICU and hospital length of stay among critically ill patients for whom there is a value-related conflict between clinicians and family
Social workers be included within an interdisciplinary team to participate in family meetings to improve family satisfaction
Family navigators (care coordinator or facilitator) be assigned to families throughout ICU stay to improve family satisfaction with physician communication, decrease psychological symptoms, and reduce costs of care and hospital stay
Spiritual support from a spiritual advisor or chaplain be offered to families of ICU patients to meet their expressed desire for spiritual care and the accreditation standard requirements

(continued)

Table 17.1 (continued)

Operational and environmental issues
Protocols be implemented to ensure adequate and standardized use of sedation and analgesia during withdrawal of life support
Nurses be involved in decision-making about goals of care and be trained to provide support for family members as part of an overall program to decrease ICU and hospital length of stay and to improve quality of communication in the ICU
Hospitals implement policies to promote family-centered care in the ICU to improve family experience
Given the evidence of harm related to noise, although in the absence of evidence for specific strategies, ICUs implement noise reduction and environmental hygiene practices and use private rooms to improve patient and family satisfaction
Family sleep be considered and families be provided a sleep surface to reduce the effects of sleep deprivation

Staff Experience

Providing care to seriously ill children and their families can be emotionally demanding. The intensity of the relationship that is often formed between providers and patients and their families in the PICU can be incredibly rewarding, but also stressful, physically demanding, and interpersonally challenging. The experience of observing very ill children at end of life can call into question accepted beliefs about life and death and contribute to feelings of helplessness, guilt, and failure. Repeated stress of this nature can lead to burnout, a syndrome characterized by emotional exhaustion, decreased work productivity and accomplishment, and a sense of detachment from one's job [13].

To prevent chronic distress and burnout, it is crucial for PICU staff to develop individualized coping strategies for managing stress, grief, and loss. These coping strategies can take many forms – maintaining professional boundaries, delegating tasks when appropriate, finding support through a peer consultation or supervision group, developing ways to process and grieve patient deaths, attending professional trainings, engaging in self-care activities, and carving out time in the workday to rest and recharge. Support staff, including psychologists, psychiatrists, social workers, and chaplains may have a role in providing guidance to multidisciplinary team members and devising interventions that may be implemented on a larger scale for staff. Staff members should never feel that they are navigating their experiences alone; consulting with colleagues and seeking support are important components to successfully managing the complex emotional experiences involved in caring for critically ill patients and their families.

An Integrated Model of Care

As highlighted above, psychosocial and palliative care supports can be helpful in supporting patients, their family members, and PICU staff providing care for critically ill children. The following sections of this chapter will describe an integrated model of care that incorporates psychosocial support as a core component of an interdisciplinary pediatric palliative care service. It should be noted though that it would not be possible for any one psychosocial provider or consulting service to adequately address the emotional, psychological, or spiritual needs of patients and families during this phase of medical care. Ideally, the support provided to patients and family members admitted on an PICU would afford them access to experts in all aspects of psychosocial care, as is clinically indicated. In addition to a PPC service, this may include the involvement of a child life specialist, resource specialist, chaplain, social worker, psychologist, and/or psychiatrist. While all members of the team work to minimize patient and family distress and maximize adaptive adjustment, each brings a unique, discipline-specific perspective and skill set. PICU providers should be aware of the supportive services available at their institutions and understand how to recruit such supports whenever necessary.

Palliative Care

According to the World Health Organization, "Palliative care for children is the active total care of the child's body, mind and spirit, and involves giving support to the family…Optimally, this care begins when a life-threatening illness or condition is diagnosed and continues regardless of whether or not a child receives treatment directed at the underlying illness." Rather than applying to a particular phase of care or life, pediatric palliative care (PPC) is a *philosophy* of care predicated on goal-concordant care, effective and compassionate communication, meticulous symptom management, and a focus on the well-being of the child and the child's family. There is nothing about PPC that is inherently at odds with intensive treatment aimed at sustaining or prolonging life. As such PPC should not be reserved for instances in which cure is no longer possible. And, while it is often mistakenly equated with end-of-life (EOL) care, it is highly relevant both before and at EOL and applies to seriously ill children throughout their illness trajectory. Thus, children with significant immunocompromise, including those who are critically ill, stand to benefit from pediatric palliative care, regardless of treatment goals or outcomes.

Primary and Subspecialty PPC

Palliative care is in effect oftentimes delivered by the primary (medical and psychosocial) team or critical care team, or both. This may be because a PPC team is not available, or because care for the seriously ill child does not require subspecialist PPC involvement. In this scenario, the primary team and critical care teams ensure the child's comfort, communicate with the child/family regarding prognosis and goals of care, and attend to the other aspects of palliative care while also overseeing ongoing therapy directed at the child's underlying medical condition. In such situations, they should possess basic palliative care skills, knowledge, and behaviors.

In other situations, such as challenging symptom management, complex communication or prognostication, goals of care that are challenging to navigate, or simply the need for added support for a child or family, the involvement of a subspecialty PPC team may be beneficial. Helpful strategies for introducing PPC to families are described in Box 17.1. In 2006, Hospice and Palliative Medicine (HPM) became a formal physician subspecialty, and board eligible physicians must now have completed a 1-year HPM fellowship.

The subspecialty practice of PPC is rooted in an interdisciplinary approach, in which nurses, physicians, social workers, and members of other disciplines see patients and provide care synchronously, as opposed to asynchronously (which would be a multidisciplinary approach). Such an interdisciplinary approach to patient care allows physical, emotional, and spiritual needs of the child and their family to be simultaneously addressed and permits a synergistic approach to the multidimensional needs of critically ill children and their families. While still a nascent subspecialty, PPC teams are increasingly available, especially in the inpatient setting. A 2013 survey of Children's Hospitals found that 69% had a PPC program [14]. When a PPC team is involved, it is often helpful to delineate the roles of each team and how they will work together collaboratively, thus minimizing confusion and duplication of roles.

Box 17.1 Strategies for Introducing Palliative Care to Families

1. Present PPC as a group of physicians, nurses, and social workers that partners with the child's current team(s) to maximize support for the child and family by
   - Focusing on quality of life for the child and family ("helping your child feel as well as possible")
   - Supporting the family's goals of care ("helping you to think about what is most important")
   - Helping them to think through options or the types of care that might make the most sense for them ("helping you to plan for now or the future")
   - Serving as an added layer of support
2. Refrain from equating PPC with there being "nothing left we can do," or a "redirection of care," as this framework does not accurately reflect PPC and is unlikely to resonate well with families.

Integration of Pediatric Palliative Care in the PICU

Early, integrated access to palliative care concepts (e.g., symptom assessment and intervention, effective communication) for children with cancer and their families is recognized as a standard of care in pediatric oncology [15]. Recognition that palliative care is an essential component of comprehensive care for critically ill adult and pediatric patients is also mounting [16, 17]. Moreover, there is increasing agreement that integration of palliative care during acute and chronic critical illness may benefit patients and families facing challenges post-discharge from the PICU [17]. While use of specific criteria prompting palliative care consultation may well increase access to palliative care for patients and families who would benefit from it [18], such criteria have not been delineated for the PICU population. Levine et al. have described strategies, including prompts, or "triggers," for early PPC consultation in the hematopoietic cell transplant (HCT) population [19], where palliative care is associated with less intensive care at end of life (e.g., intubation, receipt of CPR). Whatever the setting, strategies promoting early integration of PPC are determined by the specific population and its needs, available data, and the resources and support available.

Symptom Management

Intensive symptom management is a cornerstone of high-quality PPC. Critically ill, immunocompromised children may experience a range of pain and non-pain symptoms. For example, children with cancer experience multiple symptoms during the last month of life, with fatigue, pain, and dyspnea resulting in significant suffering. Palliative care services are associated with less child suffering from symptoms [20]. For all children, and especially those with advanced illness, intensive management of symptoms should be a top priority. Some of the most relevant symptoms are discussed below.

In all instances, integrative therapies should be part of the symptom management plan. Depending on the symptom and patient preferences, such integrative and mind/body therapies might include guided imagery, relaxation, hypnosis, art/pet/play therapy, massage, heat/cold, distraction, Reiki, acupuncture, clinical aromatherapy, prayer, nutritional supplements, and cannabidiol oil. Many families utilize such strategies though they do not share this information with their care team. It is therefore recommended that clinicians inquire about their use, and when permissible, support their use in the PICU.

Pain

Though triggered by tissue damage, pain is often greatly influenced by cognitive, behavioral, emotional, social, and cultural factors. Critically ill children experience pain that stems from a range of sources, including the physiology of their underlying condition, procedures, and other aspects of medical care. Effective pain relief is necessary to mitigate suffering and to prevent central sensitization, a central hyperexcitation response leading to escalating pain.

Routine assessment is a central component of effective pain relief. A range of behavioral and physiologic assessment and self-report tools exist. While self-report is considered the gold standard in symptom management, tools based on pain behaviors (e.g., grimacing, positioning) may be of particular utility in the PICU, when children may be unable to verbally self-report.

The WHO Pain guidelines were recently revised to contain two steps: step one for mild pain and step two for moderate/severe pain. For mild pain, acetaminophen ibuprofen, choline magnesium trisalicylate or celecoxib may be sufficient. Celecoxib, which has low antiplatelet activity, may be a good choice for children with thrombocytopenia. In the end, opioids are commonly needed to control pain in critically ill children.

A previously used intermediary step, the WHO pain guidelines proposed weak opioids, such as codeine, for moderate pain. However, codeine should be avoided when at all possible due to its potentially dangerous side effect profile and its lack of superiority over non-opioids. Its most dangerous side effects, oversedation and respiratory depression, are due to polymorphisms in the CYP2D6 gene in "ultrametabolizers" which rapidly convert codeine to its active form, morphine. At the other end of the spectrum are 10–40% of individuals with CYP2D6 polymorphisms that cause them to be "poor metabolizers" who cannot convert codeine to morphine and are therefore more likely to achieve inadequate analgesia. In addition, medications that are CYP2D6 inhibitors (e.g., bupropion, fluoxetine, paroxetine) can lessen the efficacy of codeine.

Many families hold misconceptions about opioids and worries about respiratory suppression, addiction, dependence, and the potential for opioids to hasten death. It is therefore important to explore concerns that they may hold. While opioids that are not carefully titrated against symptoms could theoretically cause life-threatening respiratory depression, no association *between administration or escalation of opioids and length of survival* has been found [21].

Non-pain Symptoms

Children also often experience a multitude of non-pain symptoms, including GI, hematologic, respiratory, and skin symptoms.

GI symptoms include *nausea and vomiting*, which may be common and may arise from a range of causes, including dysmotility, irritation or obstruction of the GI tract, medications, toxins, motion (i.e., motion sickness), and emotions (e.g., anxiety). Nausea is in fact frequently a result of several factors in this population (e.g., medications and dysmotility). Whenever possible, it is far preferable to prevent nausea than it is to treat it once started. A number of neurotransmitters are also associated with nausea, including dopamine, substance P, serotonin, acetylcholine, and histamine. Depending on the suspected underlying pathophysiology and neurotransmitters at play, drugs such as metoclopramide, olanzapine, aprepitant, 5-hydroxytryptamine antagonists, scopolamine, and meclizine may be used. Additional agents that relieve chemotherapy-associated nausea and vomiting include steroids and lorazepam. Nausea accompanied by retching is usually the most distressing form of nausea and should be prevented or treated intensively when present. Vomiting may also occur in the absence of nausea, such as with increased intracranial pressure.

Constipation is another common GI symptom, as many children receive medications that slow GI motility (vincristine, opioids). An assessment for potential constipation should take into account the child's usual bowel patterns. Treatment of constipation should address both stool consistency ("mush") and colonic motility ("push") by including a stool softener such as docusate in combination with a laxative such as Senna. Children on standing opioids should always be started on a bowel regimen, which can be titrated as needed. For children in need of treatment of opioid-induced constipation, parenteral methylnaltrexone is usually very effective. For *diarrhea*, loperamide (an opioid that does not cross the blood-brain barrier) may be helpful. For severe diarrhea, such as is seen in graft versus host disease, octreotide may be indicated.

Some children, such as those with solid tumors in the abdomen, may develop *bowel obstruction*. Symptoms of bowel obstruction include nausea, vomiting and abdominal pain (which may be continuous or colicky in nature). The primary treatment for malignant bowel obstruction is interventional – whether it be surgical correction, placement of a stent across the obstruction, or placement of a venting gastrostomy tube. Medical management to relieve symptoms may be most appropriate in the setting of advanced illness. Such management usually consists of a combination of analgesic (an opioid), antiemetic (haloperidol or ondansetron), and antisecretory agents. Antimuscarinic/anticholinergic drugs (e.g., atropine, glycopyrrolate) relieve colicky pain from smooth muscle spasm and bowel wall distention. Octreotide, a somatostatin analog, is also sometimes used. It exerts its effects of decreased secretions and peristalsis and a decrease in splanchnic blood flow, through several pathways.

Hematologic issues include *thrombocytopenia* (or bleeding) and *anemia*. For symptoms of bleeding, platelet transfusions may be considered if the platelet count is low or if platelet dysfunction is suspected. Fresh frozen plasma or cryoprecipitate may also be an option, if coagulation abnormalities are present. If life-threatening hemorrhage is a possibility, dark sheets and a fast-acting sedative should be at the ready, as such an event can be disturbing for all. Many children with hematologic/oncologic conditions encounter anemia. For those with symptoms (shortness of breath, fatigue, tachycardia, dizziness), red blood cells may be a consideration.

Respiratory symptoms: A subjective sensation of shortness of breath, or *dyspnea*, may arise from a range of sources, including respiratory causes (e.g., airway secretions, obstruction, infection) and cardiac causes, as well as psychological factors (e.g., anxiety). Dyspnea stems from a mismatch between afferent sensory input to the brain and the outgoing motor signal from the brain. The degree of dyspnea does not correlate reliably with respiratory parameters such as respiratory rate and oxygen saturation. It is for this reason that management of dyspnea in a child at end of life should be guided by self-report and clinical assessment, as opposed to vital sign values alone. Because opioids work *directly* on the brainstem to reduce the sensation of respiratory distress, they are the mainstay of dyspnea treatment. Contrary to popular belief, they do not work by causing sedation. The dose of opioid for dyspnea reduction is 25% of the amount that would be given for pain. Non-pharmacologic strategies can also alleviate dyspnea. They may include cool air flowing toward the face as well guided imagery or hypnosis to reduce anxiety can be effective. In contrast, oxygen is no more effective than blowing room air in reducing dyspnea. *Noisy breathing* at end of life is discussed below.

Some *neurologic symptoms*, such as *increased intracranial pressure* and *spinal cord compression*, are encountered in children with brain tumors or metastatic and solid tumors. The approach depends on the clinical situation and the goals of care and may involve radiation therapy, surgical interventions, and steroids. *Seizures* may also occur, particularly in children with brain tumors, and the incidence may increase at end of life. For children at risk of having a seizure at end of life, a plan for managing seizures should be made in advance, and anticonvulsants should be readily available. Children in the ICU are at especially increased risk for experiencing *delirium*, characterized by waxing and waning attention, confusion, and disorientation. While agitation and increased motor activity are often features of delirium, a hypomanic form occurs, which is particularly under-recognized. This brain disorder may have a range of causes, including medications (most notably anticholinergics and benzodiazepines), infection, electrolyte imbalances, and organ impairment. Environmental strategies (providing a calming environment) and orienting the child while addressing contributing factors are helpful. In some circumstances a neuroleptic medication may be indicated. For further discussion of delirium, refer to Chap. 18.

Skin care issues include prevention of problems by ongoing and timely assessment, frequent turning and repositioning, and alleviating pressure whenever possible. These measures are described in more detail in Chap. 16. Specific skin disorders include *pruritus*, which may be due to a systemic process or to medications. General approaches that may be helpful include using moisturizers and trimming fingernails. If the process is histamine-medicated, an antihistamine may be helpful. Other therapies such as topical or systemic steroids or specific therapies (e.g., cholestyramine or naloxone in biliary disease) may be indicated. Because most of the pruritus caused by opioids is not due to histamine release, antihistamines are rarely helpful for opioid-related itch. It is instead advisable to trial nalbuphine or alternatively a low dose of opioid antagonist or opioid rotation.

Psychological symptoms commonly experienced by children with advanced illness in the ICU include *depression* and *anxiety*. Diagnosing depression in either critical care setting or advanced illness may be a challenge because neurovegetative symptoms may not be reliable indicators. Relying on the expression of other emotions such as helplessness, hopelessness, worthlessness, and guilt may be of greater utility. Ongoing assessment and monitoring of depressive symptomatology is essential as one's medical course evolves. The most helpful strategy for child psychological distress in this context is to create opportunities for them to share and explore their concerns, worries, and hopes in an open and supportive setting. Members of the healthcare team representing psychology, social work, chaplaincy, child life, and palliative care may be well positioned to support children – and their families – in this way. Antidepressants may reduce depressive symptoms, though the downside to their use in advanced illness is that their effect is often preceded by a lag phase. When there is insufficient time for a typical antidepressant to take effect, methylphenidate, which has an immediately positive effect on mood, may be considered.

Communication, Decision-Making, and Goal-Concordant Care

At the heart of palliative care – whether primary PC or subspecialty – is the patient (or family's, depending on the situation) goals of care. Exploration of goals of care can occur in a variety of contexts, from intimate discussions at the bedside to larger family meetings and tends to occur over the course of several conversations. They may be indicated in a range of situations, such as consideration of tracheostomy, incorporation of new technology intended to sustain life outside the PICU (e.g., G-tube feedings or ventilatory support), initiation of new life-sustaining therapy (e.g., dialysis), or determination of resuscitation status.

When family goals are not clear and the next best step has not been defined, these conversations aim to elucidate patient/family preferences, values, and goals. Once these have been established, a plan of care can then be formulated. To explore a family's goals of care, it is most helpful to ask open-ended questions such as "What is most important to you?" and "What are you hoping for?" and "What worries you?" These types of questions tend to be far more productive than a narrower question focused on medical care such as "What do you want us to do?" A particularly helpful strategy is to offer a recommendation to the patient/family, which is founded on the patient/family's goals of care, takes the medical situation into account, and is formulated through clinician expertise. Such a recommendation is frequently appreciated by families, who commonly experience relief when the burden of a decision is lifted from their shoulders. Finally, the outcomes of goals of care communications should be documented in the medical record so that other members of the medical team who were not part of the conversation can understand the goals and rationale underlying a decision or the course of care predicated on these goals.

Clinician Language: More than Mere Words

> Similar to scalpels for surgeons, words are the palliative care clinician's greatest tools. Surgeons learn to use their tools with extreme precision, because any error can be devastating. So too should clinicians who rely on words. (Eric Cassell)

Our communications with patients and families about goals of care and medical treatment may have many aims. At the same time, we always hope to convey a message of compassion, respect, willingness to explore the patient/family's goals, hopes and fears, truthful expression of the medical situation and the care that can be provided, a commitment to continuing to take the very best care of them/their child, and a recognition that there may be multiple forms of caring. Use of words without full consideration of their impact can negatively impact how we think about our patients, the care we have to offer, and the decisions that are made. Careless communication is not without consequence; even unintentional messages can reinforce unspoken biases and assumptions. See Table 17.2 for concrete examples of unintended messages in the ICU environment, as well as recommended alternative communication strategies.

Advance Care Planning

In the setting of advanced illness, advance care planning allows the child's voice to be heard, even when they lose the capacity to express their own wishes. This is, in a sense, a way of preserving the child's autonomy. Consideration should be given to allowing the child to participate in such discussion if they have the developmental and cognitive capacity to participate. It has been shown that children with cancer as young as 10 years are able to understand and weigh risks, benefits, and burdens in end-of-life discussions such as those regarding phase I trial participation or resuscitation status [22].

A range of guides to facilitate advance care planning with children and adolescents are available (available at www.agingwithdignity.org). *My Wishes*, for children, helps them express how they would wish to be cared for in case they become seriously ill. *Voicing My Choices* is designed for adolescents and young adults and allows them to express how they wish to be comforted, supported, treated, and remembered. Both are available in English and Spanish and can be worked through with the child/adolescent, or alternatively as a guide to parents or other caregivers wishing to begin a conversation. Five Wishes guides adults through important considerations about their care and allows them to document them. Once completed and witnessed, it meets the legal requirements for an advance directive in 42 US states and the District of Columbia. It is available in 28 languages.

Considerations at the End of Life

Conversations at End of Life

In the last phase of a child's life, end-of-life discussions such as those regarding resuscitation status or life-sustaining treatment (LST) are of great importance and are a commonly encountered issue in the PICU. However, for children in the PICU, for those with cancer, and for pediatric HCT recipients, these conversations frequently occur late in the child's illness and sometimes do not occur at all. In a study of PICU and oncology physicians and nurses, 71% of all clinicians believed that such discussions happen too late in the child's clinical course [23]. In this study, the top three barriers were unrealistic parent expectations, differences between

Table 17.2 Considerations for clinician communications

Word or expression	Example	Unintended message	Alternative approach
Appropriate	*"The mother was completely appropriate when her baby died"*	Distinguishing "normal" from "pathological" requires a value judgment There is a suitable "right" way to be that is different from what is "wrong"	Reflect on the intended message Be more specific
Refused	*"The family refused tracheostomy"*	Patient is defiant and has taken a stance against something reasonable Puts the patient and clinician at odds	*"The family declined tracheostomy"* *"The family opted for…"* In addition, seek to understand the family's position
Use of "cases" or "diagnoses" to refer to a patient	*"The sickler in bedspace 18…."*	The person is reduced to a medical condition, ignoring their personhood	*"Jordan is a 16 year old boy with sickle cell disease"*
Use of "fail" with the patient as the subject	*"Sally failed first line chemotherapy"*	The patient is responsible for the outcome of treatment Assigns guilt to the patient	*"Sally's cancer was refractory to first line chemotherapy"*
"Nothing more can be done"	*"I'm afraid to say that nothing more can be done for your son"*	The only valid care for the patient is curative care Suggests the family and clinician are at odds We are "giving up" on the patient The clinician's only role is cure- this leaves patient/family feeling abandoned	Affirm that treatment options for the condition are limited but you remain able and available to care for the patient *"While there are no more treatments that can slow the growth of the cancer, we will continue to take the very best care of your son"*
"Do everything"	*"The parents said that they wanted everything to be done"*	Assumes all parties share the same definition of "everything" – Leaves much room for misunderstanding Precludes discussion of goals of care, treatment options	Use the opportunity to open a discussion: What is most important, what might we hope for, What the possible courses of action might be, how they would achieve those goals or hopes Use this opportunity to affirm commitment to caring for the patient and family.

(continued)

Table 17.2 (continued)

Word or expression	Example	Unintended message	Alternative approach
"*Withdrawing care/support*"	"*Because Emma's respiratory status continued to worsen the decision was made to withdraw care*"	The only (worthwhile) care is curative care We are "giving up" and will no longer care for the patient Suggests patient/family will be abandoned	"*Whether or not we continue chemotherapy, we will care for you, and will do our best to help you feel comfortable*"
Use of "do not resuscitate" to summarize a resuscitation status	"*Do not resuscitate*"	Focuses on what won't be done Implies that if resuscitation were attempted it would be successful	The term, "*Do not attempt resuscitation*" is preferable Some prefer "*Allow Natural Death*" though some feel this is too vague In any event, focus on the ways in which care will actively be provided to the child
Referring to parents as the signatories of a resuscitation status order	"*The parents signed the DNR*"	Erroneous because in most instances, the DNR order is a medical order, not signed by parents Moreover, this statement places the burden of the decision on parents.	"*The parents agreed to the team's recommendation regarding resuscitation status*"
Referring to a patient as "a DNR" when describing their resuscitation status	"*Jack is a DNR*"	The person is reduced to a status, ignoring their personhood Focuses on what will not be done for the patient, rather than on what will be done A vague statement that provides no information regarding goals of care or what interventions would be in line with those goals	*Jack and his team agreed that given the advanced state of his illness if his heart stopped it would signify the end of his natural life. The team would do everything possible to ensure his comfort, rather than attempting chest compressions*

clinician and patient/parent understanding of prognosis, and perceived lack of parent readiness to have the discussion. It is likely that clinician factors also play a role, since in this same study, less than half felt prepared to discuss resuscitation status with school-aged and adolescent patients and to conduct a family conference. The inherent nature of these high-stake conversations, frequently fraught with emotion and prognostic uncertainty, also adds to the challenge. These challenges suggest opportunities for collaboration between PICU and palliative care clinicians. An additional challenge is clinician desire to protect families from distress or loss of hope. However, most families can tolerate talking about their child's end of life and find relief when the care team opens to door to conversation about it. Moreover, parents value honesty, and honest, compassionate conversations can promote parent hopefulness, as well as trust and connection with the care team.

Despite the above challenges, clinicians should proactively create opportunities to have these conversations with patients/families, rather than deferring them until the last phase of life. Through earlier discussions that do not occur in the midst of a crisis, patients/families are much better positioned to consider these decisions. Earlier discussions also give them the opportunity to think and plan before a crisis arises.

Cancer-Directed Therapy

Provision of cancer-directed therapy in the absence of an agreed upon goal of cure warrants careful consideration, weighing the potential benefits with impact on child well-being. Even when there is no realistic hope for cure, it is not uncommon for families to choose continued cancer-directed treatment [24]. In fact, many families will seek out such treatment if it is not offered [25]. Reasons for this may include provision of hope and perceived increased attention and care from the medical team associated with receipt of treatment. Ongoing hope for cure/disease control is also prevalent. The majority of parents maintained a primary goal of extending life, in the last moments of a child's life [26, 27]. From the perspective of oncologists, parent preference for such continued treatment is a major contributing factor for its prescription [28].

Conversations regarding cancer-directed therapy at a child's end of life are in many ways similar to goals of care conversations about other treatments. Clinicians should be mindful of the fact that families often hold blended goals, and pursuit of cancer-directed therapy does not in and of itself mean that a family is unaware of the child's limited prognosis. Clinicians should also maintain nonjudgmental attitude if a family seeks to pursue cancer-directed therapy in the face illness deemed incurable by the medical team. While such therapy can present the risk of toxicity, there may be some benefits to the child and family beyond life extension. For example, Wolfe and colleagues found that in the child's last 12 weeks of life, receipt of mild cancer-directed therapy was associated with improved psychological quality of life [29]. Finally, it is helpful to avoid labeling cancer-directed therapy as either "curative" or "palliative." Such distinctions are usually artificial, and by equating "palliative" with "no hope for cure" undermine the term "palliative."

Resuscitation Status and Life-Sustaining Treatment

While resuscitation status and use of LST at EOL are highlighted as distinct topics, the overall approach to discussing them is the same as for other medical decisions. These conversations should be focused on the goals of care, as opposed to limitations of care. Instead of specifically discussing "withdrawing support" or a do-not-resuscitate (DNR) order, a discussion centered on goals of care will naturally lead to considering which interventions are in the child's best interests. And from there, clinicians can make recommendations based on these goals and medical knowledge of potential benefit and/or harm of these interventions. During these discussions with patients/families, what *will* be done to continue to care for them, such as continuing to be present and ensuring their comfort, should be reinforced. This is particularly important because families are often hesitant to limit resuscitation or LST as they fear it will also trigger limitation of other aspects of care. Clinicians should similarly not assume that having a DNR order in place or foregoing LST indicates that other types of care not specified have changed.

With regard to resuscitation status, many patients/families do not understand the legal mandate that resuscitation for cardiorespiratory arrest be attempted unless a DNR order is in place. This concept is important to explain particularly if discharge from the hospital is under consideration. In this case, most states have out-of-hospital DNR verification forms or physician orders for life treatment (POLST) forms. POLST forms (www.polst.org) are medical orders communicating patient preferences regarding resuscitation efforts and life-sustaining treatment across care settings. Both types of forms affirm that emergency response teams provide symptom management with comfort and relief of suffering when called to the scene, rather than initiating resuscitative efforts.

Feeding and Hydration

For children who can no longer feed by mouth, medical nutrition, either nasogastric or gastrostomy feedings, or intravenous nutrition or hydration may be options. Whether to proceed with these interventions for children approaching end-of-life requires careful evaluation of the risks and benefits, taking into account the family's goals, the medical circumstances, and the child's prognosis. Conversations around this topic must be approached with great sensitivity as it often evokes intense emotions in both family members and members of the care team alike.

Families often hold the misconception that medical nutrition and hydration are needed to prevent their child from experiencing hunger and thirst. However, clinical experience with patients able to articulate their experience tells us that they experience little hunger and that thirst may be alleviated with attentive mouth care and moistening. An honest and sensitive discussion about the potential harms of medical nutrition should be made with the family. Such potential harms include increased secretions and fluid overload (e.g., pulmonary edema), both of which can contribute to respiratory distress.

If possible, the optimal approach is to provide anticipatory guidance to families, describing how appetite and thirst wane, and the body's ability to handle medical nutrition/hydration decrease at end of life as well. Exploring the meaning that provision of nutrition and hydration that they may hold is helpful, as is identifying other ways in which they can continue to love and care for their child.

Other Considerations

Location of Care

For many children with advanced illness in the PICU, their final location of care may be the PICU. While much emphasis is placed on location of care (and location of death), with home deaths assumed to be the preferred location of death, the opportunity to plan for end of life may be what is most important. In a study of 140 parents who lost a child to cancer, the opportunity to plan location of death was associated with outcomes consistent with high-quality palliative care, even among nonhome deaths. It may therefore represent a more relevant outcome than actual location of death [30]. For children who do die in the PICU setting, technology may place distance between the parent and child. This highlights the importance of reconsidering and potentially discontinuing medical technology that is not of benefit to the child. Parents often also benefit from encouragement and assistance in touching, holding, or even sleeping alongside their child despite the surrounding tubes, lines, and technology.

For those families who express a desire for their child to spend their last moments in a non-ICU environment, transfer to the hematology-oncology unit is sometimes possible. Such a transfer may take some planning, to ensure adequate staffing (e.g., additional nursing, respiratory therapy). Palliative care teams may be helpful in coordinating such efforts and in providing additional support for the hematology-oncology in caring for the child. In some institutions, palliative transport and discontinuation of LST (e.g., extubation) is possible, logistical and clinical circumstances permitting. Families view this opportunity as positive and meaningful, with memories of the experience bringing them comfort and a sense of fulfillment [31].

Autopsy and Organ Donation

Postmortem examinations (autopsies) may yield important information furthering clinical and research efforts. For example, Sirkia found that of 40 children who died of progressive cancer, autopsy afforded new information in 20% of cases and important additional information in 55% [32].

Families also value new information that may be discovered about their child, often viewing the contribution to medical knowledge as part of their child's ongoing legacy. Return of autopsy results may also provide an opportunity for families to return for follow-up discussions, which in and of themselves are often helpful during bereavement [33]. Many families appreciate the opportunity to consider autopsy in advance of the child's death, when possible. Some have in fact been considering it, are unsure how to bring it up with the medical team, and are relieved when the door is opened to conversation about it. In support of this, Wiener found that most bereaved parents feel that autopsy should be introduced when it becomes clear that cure is no longer possible [34].

Like autopsy, families often appreciate the opportunity to discuss in advance of their child's death. While some families find the option of organ donation meaningful, the array of factors influencing their decision is complex. Representatives from organ procurement organizations are available to speak with families about the possibility of organ donation, which frequently facilitates a decision to pursue organ donation. A shared approach in which medical teams and organ procurement organizations' representatives partner to provide families with the support and information needed when considering this topic may be particularly helpful to families.

Palliative Sedation

Many children in the PICU are sedated at end of life. Among those who are not, some experience symptoms or suffering that is refractory to the most intensive efforts. For these children, palliative sedation may relieve their suffering by reducing their level of consciousness. Prior to embarking on such sedation, its indication, goals, endpoints, and potential effects on the child should be discussed with the family and members of the interdisciplinary care team. These issues should be revisited as sedation is ongoing as well. Open and ongoing communication is particularly important as moral distress may emerge. Agents such as midazolam, pentobarbital, dexmedetomidine, or propofol most commonly used for palliative sedation should be administered via continuous infusion with a bolus dose available and dose escalation undertaken as needed. Previously started opioids should be continued for the purposes of analgesia and withdrawal prevention, though opioids alone should never be used for palliative sedation per se.

Supporting the Child and Family at End of Life

Anticipatory Guidance

A critical aspect of supporting families in the last moments of the child's life is provision of anticipatory guidance. If death is imminent, families should be informed of this, even if the time frame is uncertain. Even letting them know that it may range from hours to days (or longer) is often helpful to them. Families also appreciate anticipatory guidance with regard to physical changes that may become evident, such as decreases in child responsiveness, and changes in circulation and breathing pattern. For some children, breathing may become noisy, due to pooling of secretions. At the point when this occurs, children are not sufficiently conscious enough to be disturbed by this. For family members at the bedside, however, such noisy breathing may be distressing. Anticipatory guidance around this can oftentimes mitigate such distress. When this is not the case, an anticholinergic agent such as atropine ophthalmologic drops, scopolamine, L-hyoscyamine drops, or or glycopyrrolate can be helpful in drying secretions, as can gentle suctioning.

As medical management is increasingly guided by symptom control as opposed to physiologic derangements, monitoring of vital signs may be less relevant. Open conversation with families about ongoing intensive care of the child now guided by clinical cues from the child as opposed to monitoring of vital signs may help them to know that possible removal from monitoring does not indicate lessening of care.

Family Togetherness and Memory Making

Families may not know what is permissible or acceptable, particularly in the high-tech environment of the PICU. As above, they may benefit from encouragement and assistance in maintaining close physical contact. Bereaved parents also describe the importance of opportunities to care for their child, as well as privacy, and access to professional and personal support [35]. Attention should also be paid to spiritual needs, whether it be through visits from hospital chaplaincy or leader of their faith community, as well as prayer and ritual [36, 37].

The family should also be offered the opportunity for siblings to spend time with the child. Child Life Specialists are often invaluable in talking with siblings and preparing them for changes they may see. Such times of family togetherness are often opportunities for memory-making including taking photographs, making molds of family members' hands together. Additional memory-making activities that might be offered include locks of the child's hair and recording of the child's heartbeat (sometimes done by music therapists). These memories and mementoes are an important way for families to maintain a sense of connection to their child in the moment and moving forward.

On some occasions, resuscitative efforts may be made at the end of a child's life, either because they experience an unplanned cardiopulmonary decompensation or because such efforts were part of the plan of care. While witness resuscitative efforts are controversial, parents should have the opportunity to decide for themselves whether to be present for the resuscitation. If they do, the presence of a seasoned clinician dedicated to supporting the parents is essential. Parents describe it as distressing, but for many, it also provides benefits. One study found that the vast majority of bereaved parents who had witnessed resuscitative efforts for their child would do so again [38].

Bereavement

Families who have lost a child face enormous challenges. The support they received prior to their child's death should continue into bereavement, as families often describe a double loss – the loss of their child and the loss of the care team whom they have known, trusted, and traversed a very traumatic time in their lives [39]. Clinicians can both commemorate the child and express support for the family in a number of ways, including attending the funeral or memorial service, sending a condolence note, or making a phone call. Family members place great importance on these expressions of support and commemoration, appreciate them when they occur, and may be disappointed if they do not occur [40]. Many families also appreciate an opportunity to review the child's illness course and end of life. If an autopsy has been conducted, results can be shared during the visit. Families may hold difficult or confusing misconceptions or questions in need of answers. Addressing these allows them to undertake the difficult psychological work lying ahead. Staff, including trainees, may similarly hold lingering thoughts and unanswered questions about caring for the child. Debriefing sessions for staff may allow them to review the child's story and remember remember him/her. They may be particularly helpful to hematology/oncology or PICU staff who cared for the child during part but not all of the illness course and wish to hear the story in its entirety.

References

1. Colville G, Kerry S, Pierce C. Children's factual and delusional memories of intensive care. Am J Respir Crit Care Med. 2008;177(9):976–82.
2. Rees G, Gledhill J, Garralda ME, Nadel S. Psychiatric outcome following paediatric intensive care unit (PICU) admission: a cohort study. Intensive Care Med. 2004;30(8):1607–14.
3. Rennick JE, Rashotte J. Psychological outcomes in children following pediatric intensive care unit hospitalization: a systematic review of the research. J Child Health Care. 2009;13(2):128–49.
4. Carnevale FA. The experience of critically ill children: narratives of unmaking. Intensive Crit Care Nurs. 1997;13(1):49–52.
5. Connolly D, McClowry S, Hayman L, Mahony L, Artman M. Posttraumatic stress disorder in children after cardiac surgery. J Pediatr. 2004;144(4):480–4.
6. Just A. Parent participation in care: bridging the gap in the pediatric ICU. Newborn Infant Nurs Rev. 2005;5(4):179–87.
7. Davydow DS, Richardson LP, Zatzick DF, Katon WJ. Psychiatric morbidity in pediatric critical illness survivors: a comprehensive review of the literature. Arch Pediatr Adolesc Med. 2010;164(4):377–85.
8. Perrin EC, Gerrity PS. There's a demon in your belly: children's understanding of illness. Pediatrics. 1981;67(6):841–9.
9. Brand SR, Tarquini S, Mack JW. Communication in the pediatric oncology setting. Cham: Springer International Publishing; 2016.
10. Davidson JE, Jones C, Bienvenu OJ. Family response to critical illness: postintensive care syndrome-family. Crit Care Med. 2012;40(2):618–24.
11. Tunick RA, Meyer EC. Pediatric critical care. In: DeMaso RJSDR, editor. Textbook of pediatric psychosomatic medicine. Washington, DC: American Psychiatric Publishing; 2010.
12. Davidson JE, Aslakson RA, Long AC, et al. Guidelines for family-centered care in the neonatal, pediatric, and adult ICU. Crit Care Med. 2017;45(1):103–28.
13. Maslach C, Leiter MP. Understanding the burnout experience: recent research and its implications for psychiatry. World Psychiatry. 2016;15(2):103–11.
14. Feudtner C, Womer J, Augustin R, et al. Pediatric palliative care programs in children's hospitals: a cross-sectional national survey. Pediatrics. 2013;132(6):1063–70.
15. Weaver MS, Heinze KE, Kelly KP, et al. Palliative care as a standard of care in pediatric oncology. Pediatr Blood Cancer. 2015;62(Suppl 5):S829–33.

16. Boss R, Nelson J, Weissman D, et al. Integrating palliative care into the PICU: a report from the improving palliative care in the ICU advisory board. Pediatr Crit Care Med. 2014;15(8):762–7.
17. Aslakson RA, Curtis JR, Nelson JE. The changing role of palliative care in the ICU. Crit Care Med. 2014;42(11):2418–28.
18. Nelson JE, Curtis JR, Mulkerin C, et al. Choosing and using screening criteria for palliative care consultation in the ICU: a report from the improving palliative care in the ICU (IPAL-ICU) advisory board. Crit Care Med. 2013;41(10):2318–27.
19. Levine DR, Baker JN, Wolfe J, Lehmann LE, Ullrich C. Strange bedfellows no more: how integrated stem-cell transplantation and palliative care programs can together improve end-of-life care. J Oncol Pract. 2017;13(9):569–77.
20. Wolfe J, Hammel JF, Edwards KE, et al. Easing of suffering in children with cancer at the end of life: is care changing? J Clin Oncol. 2008;26(10):1717–23.
21. Sykes N, Thorns A. The use of opioids and sedatives at the end of life. Lancet Oncol. 2003;4(5):312–8.
22. Hinds PS, Drew D, Oakes LL, et al. End-of-life care preferences of pediatric patients with cancer. J Clin Oncol. 2005;23(36):9146–54.
23. Durall A, Zurakowski D, Wolfe J. Barriers to conducting advance care discussions for children with life-threatening conditions. Pediatrics. 2012;129(4):e975–82.
24. Tomlinson D, Bartels U, Hendershot E, Maloney AM, Ethier MC, Sung L. Factors affecting treatment choices in paediatric palliative care: comparing parents and health professionals. Eur J Cancer. 2011;47(14):2182–7.
25. Bluebond-Langner M, Belasco JB, Goldman A, Belasco C. Understanding parents' approaches to care and treatment of children with cancer when standard therapy has failed. J Clin Oncol. 2007;25(17):2414–9.
26. Wolfe J, Klar N, Grier HE, et al. Understanding of prognosis among parents of children who died of cancer: impact on treatment goals and integration of palliative care. JAMA. 2000;284(19):2469–75.
27. Ullrich CK, Dussel V, Hilden JM, Sheaffer JW, Lehmann L, Wolfe J. End-of-life experience of children undergoing stem cell transplantation for malignancy: parent and provider perspectives and patterns of care. Blood. 2010;115(19):3879–85.
28. Kang TI, Hexem K, Localio R, Aplenc R, Feudtner C. The use of palliative chemotherapy in pediatric oncology patients: a National Survey of Pediatric Oncologists. Pediatr Blood Cancer. 2013;60(1):88–94.
29. Wolfe J, Orellana L, Ullrich C, et al. Symptoms and distress in children with advanced cancer: prospective patient-reported outcomes from the PediQUEST study. J Clin Oncol. 2015;33(17):1928–35.
30. Dussel V, Kreicbergs U, Hilden JM, et al. Looking beyond where children die: determinants and effects of planning a child's location of death. J Pain Symptom Manag. 2009;37(1):33–43.
31. Nelson H, Mott S, Kleinman ME, Goldstein RD. Parents' experiences of pediatric palliative transports: a qualitative case series. J Pain Symptom Manag. 2015;50(3):375–80.
32. Sirkia K, Saarinen-Pihkala UM, Hovi L, Sariola H. Autopsy in children with cancer who die while in terminal care. Med Pediatr Oncol. 1998;30(5):284–9.
33. Bates C, Burgess H. A case for autopsy in palliative medicine. Palliat Med. 2004;18(7):652–3.
34. Wiener L, Sweeney C, Baird K, et al. What do parents want to know when considering autopsy for their child with cancer? J Pediatr Hematol Oncol. 2014;36(6):464–70.
35. Meert KL, Briller SH, Schim SM, Thurston CS. Exploring parents' environmental needs at the time of a child's death in the pediatric intensive care unit. Pediatr Crit Care Med. 2008;9(6):623–8.
36. Meert KL, Thurston CS, Briller SH. The spiritual needs of parents at the time of their child's death in the pediatric intensive care unit and during bereavement: a qualitative study. Pediatr Crit Care Med. 2005;6(4):420–7.

37. Maxton FJ. Parental presence during resuscitation in the PICU: the parents' experience. Sharing and surviving the resuscitation: a phenomenological study. J Clin Nurs. 2008;17(23):3168–76.
38. Shaw K, Ritchie D, Adams G. Does witnessing resuscitation help parents come to terms with the death of their child? A review of the literature. Intensive Crit Care Nurs. 2011;27(5):253–62.
39. Contro N, Larson J, Scofield S, Sourkes B, Cohen H. Family perspectives on the quality of pediatric palliative care. Arch Pediatr Adolesc Med. 2002;156(1):14–9.
40. Macdonald ME, Liben S, Carnevale FA, et al. Parental perspectives on hospital staff members' acts of kindness and commemoration after a child's death. Pediatrics. 2005;116(4):884–90.

Chapter 18
Delirium

Chani Traube

Learning Objectives
1. Define delirium
2. Describe the short- and long-term effects of delirium
3. Discuss the epidemiology of pediatric delirium
4. Identify delirium in critically ill children
5. Plan an approach to treat and prevent delirium in the pediatric immunocompromised hematology/oncology patient

What Is Delirium?

Delirium is the behavioral manifestation of brain dysfunction that can occur due to an underlying serious illness or as an unwanted side effect of treatment for that illness. Delirium is an acute event and represents a change from the child's neurologic baseline. It is characterized by altered cognition and awareness. Delirium is not a static process but rather fluctuates over the course of a day. Generally, delirium is reversible and will improve when the underlying trigger resolves [1–3].

There are three subtypes of delirium described in pediatrics: hypoactive, hyperactive, and mixed. Hyperactive delirium is the most easily recognized, as it presents with refractory agitation, emotional reactivity, and restlessness. These children are often incorrectly labeled as "impossible to sedate." Hypoactive delirium is characterized by decreased reactivity, emotional withdrawal, and lethargy. It may be inappropriately dismissed as "sickness behavior" or confused with depression. Mixed

C. Traube (✉)
Department of Pediatrics, Division of Pediatric Critical Care Medicine,
Weill Cornell Medical College, New York, NY, USA
e-mail: chr9008@med.cornell.edu

C. N. Duncan et al. (eds.), *Critical Care of the Pediatric Immunocompromised Hematology/Oncology Patient*, https://doi.org/10.1007/978-3-030-01322-6_18

delirium involves symptoms of both hypoactive and hyperactive delirium over the course of a day. Hypoactive and mixed delirium are far more common than hyperactive delirium in children [4–7].

In all subtypes of pediatric delirium, there is a marked disruption of sleep cycles. In younger children, the motoric symptoms may be quite notable, with frequent purposeless movements. Adolescents may describe auditory, visual, or tactile hallucinations. Although hallucinations are not necessary in order to diagnose delirium, hallucinations are diagnostic of delirium when they do occur. Oftentimes, a parent or caregiver will be one of the first to note the symptoms of delirium: "something is wrong; this behavior is not characteristic of my child" [8–10].

Etiology of Delirium

The underlying pathophysiology of delirium is multifactorial and complex. Inflammation is thought to play a significant role (particularly in pediatric delirium), with modification of blood-brain barrier permeability and alteration in neurotransmitter release. Irrespective of the specific underlying trigger for delirium, the final common pathway involves a disruption to brain network connectivity, which manifests as altered cognition and awareness [11–13].

Clinically, delirium in critically ill children occurs as a result of three interconnected problems: the underlying illness, side effects of medications given to treat that illness, and the disruptive environment in the pediatric intensive care unit (PICU) [2, 14] (Fig. 18.1). As an example, consider a child undergoing treatment for

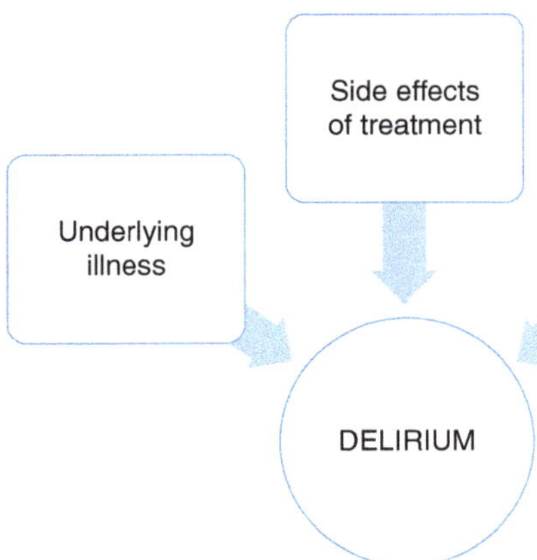

Fig. 18.1 Delirium triggers. A child with delirium displays an acute and fluctuating change in awareness and cognition, generally as a result of serious illness, iatrogenic factors, and/or the abnormal environment in the critical care unit

leukemia, with sepsis and associated respiratory insufficiency. This child is at risk for delirium due to the inflammatory process that accompanies her infection and the oxidative stress and cytokine release that result from hypoxia. She is further predisposed to delirium by the chemotherapy she recently received and the sedatives that are prescribed to facilitate her tolerance of respiratory support. Finally, this preschool-age child is situated in a PICU where she is exposed to lights and noise 24 h a day and confined to bed without much opportunity for cognitive stimulation or physical activity. It is highly probable that this child will develop delirium during her critical illness.

Delirium-Associated Morbidity and Mortality

Delirium is a cause of considerable distress to the patient, family, and clinical care team [15]. Evidence confirms that pediatric delirium is independently associated with substantial short-term morbidity. Children with delirium have lengthier stays in the intensive care unit (adjusted relative length of PICU stay 2.3 × (CI 2.1–2.5), after controlling for severity of illness and need for mechanical ventilation) [7]. Delirium is associated with increased hospital length of stay in the noncritically ill child as well (median 10 vs. 5 days ($p < 0.01$) in a cohort of children with cancer) [16]. Delirious children are more difficult to wean from invasive mechanical ventilation; a single-center study showed a 3-day increase in duration of mechanical ventilation in children with delirium ($p < 0.001$) [7]. Delirious children are more difficult to care for, and are more resource-intensive, often requiring one-to-one nursing. Children with delirium also have an increased number of radiologic and laboratory studies. Data shows that annual hospital costs attributable to delirium exceed 500 million dollars each year [17]. Most importantly, even after controlling for underlying severity of illness, delirium in critically ill children is independently associated with in-hospital mortality (adjusted odds ratio 4.4, $p < 0.001$) [7]. Similarly, in adults with cancer, data shows a tight link to excess mortality [18, 19], with one study reporting a mortality odds ratio of 14 when comparing age- and diagnosis-matched patients with and without delirium for up to 5 years after initial delirium diagnosis [20].

Even after recovery from critical illness, delirium is thought to have long-term psychological and behavioral effects on children and their families. Children describe distressing delusional memories of their ICU stay, and parents of children with delirium may experience posttraumatic stress symptoms [2, 5, 21, 22]. There is an extensive literature in adults clearly linking delirium to long-term cognitive impairment [23–26]. Adults with cancer who experienced delirium during their hospital stay had decreased performance status upon discharge when compared to those who did not experience delirium; this population was also shown to have a higher frequency of anxiety disorders and neurocognitive deficits up to 1 year after discharge [27, 28]. Further research is needed to investigate the long-term effects of pediatric delirium on cognitive and emotional health [29].

Epidemiology and Risk Factors for Pediatric Delirium

Delirium frequency varies significantly between institutions and based upon the pediatric population studied [30]. A large multi-institutional point prevalence study including 25 separate pediatric critical care units showed that delirium occurred in approximately one out of every four critically ill children; this translates into more than 60,000 children with delirium in the United States each year. The delirium prevalence rate increased to 38% in children who were in the PICU for more than 5 days [30]. Higher delirium rates were reported in cardiac (49%) and postsurgical (65%) pediatric critical care units [31, 32]. Most studies demonstrate that younger patients (less than 2 years old), and children with underlying developmental disabilities, are both at higher risk for developing delirium [7, 30, 31, 33]. Delirium rates are also higher in children who require invasive mechanical ventilation [7, 30, 33].

There are few studies describing delirium rates specifically in children with cancer, hematologic diseases, and immunodeficiency. A case series described four children with neuroblastoma who all developed delirium [34]. A single-center retrospective study (n = 70) using a chart review to diagnose delirium reported a 10% incidence. The authors acknowledged that this was likely a gross underestimation, as without routine screening delirium often goes unnoticed [35]. In a study of 319 consecutive admissions to an inpatient pediatric cancer service, with prospective daily screening for delirium, the incidence was 18.8%. In these children, risk factors independently associated with a delirium diagnosis included brain tumor, age less than 5 years, and recent surgery (Table 18.1) [16].

Medications represent a possible modifiable risk factor for pediatric delirium. Specifically, benzodiazepine-based sedation has been strongly associated with delirium in children. A single-center study including 1547 children used a multivariable logistic regression analysis to show an odds ratio for delirium of 5.2 (CI 3.7–7.5) in children who were prescribed benzodiazepines [7]. A multi-institutional study (n = 994) demonstrated an odds ratio of 2.2 (CI 1.5–3.3) for delirium diagnosis in children receiving benzodiazepines [30]. Another single-center study (n = 300) showed that greater benzodiazepine exposure was associated with longer delirium duration (incident rate ratio 2.5, p = 0.005) [36]. In a cohort of 319 children with cancer, multivariable regression showed that receipt of benzodiazepines nearly quadrupled delirium rates (OR = 3.7, $p < 0.001$) [16]. The relationship between benzo-

Table 18.1 Risk factors for delirium in the immunocompromised child

Risk factors for delirium in the immunocompromised child:
Age < 5
Benzodiazepines
Brain tumor
Do not resuscitate status
Poor nutrition
Postoperative status

Adapted from Traube et al. [16]

diazepines and delirium is not merely an association; a recent study showed a causal link between receipt of benzodiazepines and the development of pediatric delirium (OR 3.3, CI 1.4–7.8), with a dose-response effect (43% increase in risk for delirium with every one-log increase in benzodiazepine dose, $p < 0.001$) [37].

Delirium Timing and Duration

Prospective longitudinal studies, where children are screened for delirium throughout their PICU stay, have enabled us to describe patterns of delirium. In the largest cohort of delirious children ($n = 267$), delirium often developed early in the ICU course, with nearly 80% of children developing delirium by PICU day 3. 27% of this cohort experienced repeated episodes of delirium. Median duration of delirium was 2 days (IQR 1–5 days) [7]. Similarly, in a cohort of 61 delirious children admitted to a German PICU after surgery, 50% had an early short-lasting delirium (24 h) [32]. Consistent with these reports, a study involving 95 children with delirium after cardiac bypass surgery showed that delirium most often developed before hospital day 3 and lasted a median of 2 days (SD +/− 6.5 days) [31]. In the cohort of hospitalized children with cancer, delirium also generally occurred early in the hospital course (median hospital day 2, IQR days 1–4) and was often of short duration (median 2 days, range 1–18 days) [16]. Frequent onset of delirium early in the PICU course underscores the need for early screening.

Duration of delirium described in these longitudinal studies suggests two phenotypes of pediatric delirium: a milder form (of short duration) and a more severe form (lasting >2 days). It is important to note that even delirium of short duration is associated with poor outcome, with a "dose – response" effect on excess mortality, ICU length of stay, and hospital costs [7, 17, 32]. In a prolonged hospitalization, a frequent pattern described in pediatrics begins with hyperactive delirium, is followed by mixed delirium, and may then develop into hypoactive delirium which is considered the most severe phenotype [2].

Delirium Detection

Traditionally, the diagnosis of pediatric delirium required a comprehensive psychiatric interview and exam, with establishment of an acute and fluctuating change in awareness and attention [4, 38]. This labor-intensive and time-consuming approach was not feasible for widespread screening in the PICU. As a result, recognition of delirium in children lagged until the recent development of well-validated, reliable tools feasible for the nonpsychiatrist to use at the child's bedside [39]. There are two types of pediatric delirium screening tools available: a point-in-time interactive tool (the pediatric and preschool versions of the Confusion Assessment Method for the ICU (CAM-ICU)) and a longitudinal observational tool (the Cornell Assessment for

Pediatric Delirium (CAPD)) [33, 40, 41]. Both can be used in any child arousable to verbal stimulation, and both are designed for use by the bedside nurse. The CAPD has been found to be user-friendly, as it does not require the child's cooperation and can be applied to children of all ages and developmental stages. Feasibility of use was demonstrated in a multi-institutional study, where 25 PICUs of varying cultures were able to easily use the tool in 84% of patients [30]. The European Society of Pediatric and Neonatal Intensive Care has released clinical practice guidelines calling for use of the CAPD as standard of care to screen all critically ill children for delirium [42].

The CAPD (Fig. 18.2) consists of eight questions, scored on a Likert-type scale by the child's nurse; in most instances, this occurs toward the end of the nurse's shift in order to take into account the greatest period of observation. The tool uses observable behaviors to test for cognition and awareness (assessing for eye contact, purposefulness, awareness, communication, restlessness, consolability, underactivity, and delayed responses) [41]. For preverbal children, a developmental anchor point chart is available

Cornell Assessment of Pediatric Delirium (CAPD) revised						
RASS Score___(if -4 or -5 do not proceed) Please answer the following questions based on your interactions with the patient over the course of your shift:						
	Never 4	Rarely 3	Sometimes 2	Often 1	Always 0	Score
1. Does the child make eye contact with the caregiver?						
2. Are the child's actions purposeful?						
3. Is the child aware of his/her surroundings?						
4. Does the child communicate needs and wants?						
	Never 0	Rarely 1	Sometimes 2	Often 3	Always 4	
5. Is the child restless?						
6. Is the child inconsolable?						
7. Is the child underactive—very little movement while awake?						
8. Does it take the child a long time to respond to interactions?						
					TOTAL	

Fig. 18.2 Cornell assessment of pediatric delirium. A score of >8 is consistent with delirium. (Reproduced from: Traube et al. [41]; p. 657)

to use as a point-of-care reference when needed [43]. A score of nine or higher on the CAPD is consistent with a psychiatric diagnosis of delirium (sensitivity 94%, specificity 86%, interrater reliability kappa = 0.94). A child's score can be trended from day to day to assess delirium trajectory and response to interventions [2, 30, 44].

Treatment of Delirium

When a child is diagnosed with delirium, the clinician's approach should be multimodal (Table 18.2) [2, 9, 45]. It is essential to begin with an evaluation of potential underlying triggers. Is the delirium a result of new-onset hypoxemia? Or has the child acquired an infection (for example, a urinary tract infection or occult peritonitis)? If that is the case, approach to delirium requires treatment of the underlying trigger – oxygen for hypoxemia or antibiotics for infection.

Oftentimes, delirium may result from iatrogenic factors. Minimizing sedation as much as feasible, particularly limiting exposure to benzodiazepines, will often lead to improvement in delirium [26]. Conversely, recognizing and treating opiate withdrawal are essential, as opiate withdrawal can precipitate a very particular form of hyperactive delirium. A careful review of the child's medication list is warranted so as to minimize exposure to unnecessary medications. In particular, many delirium researchers believe that anticholinergics play a significant role in delirium development, specifically in very young patients [2, 14].

Table 18.2 Approach to treatment of delirium

Illness related	Iatrogenic	Environmental	Pharmacologic[a, b]
Identify and address potential triggers	Minimize sedation (particularly benzodiazepines)	Physical mobilization	If risk-benefit ratio is favorable, consider
Acidosis Dehydration Fever	Optimize pain control	Cognitive stimulation	Atypical antipsychotic
Hypoxia Infection Inflammation	Identify and treat opiate withdrawal	Family involvement	Clonidine
New central nervous system pathology Seizure Stroke	Discontinue unnecessary Medications Invasive lines Catheters Remove restraints	Day-night routine Natural light during day Quiet, dark night- time environment Cluster care to allow for consolidated sleep	Dexmedetomidine Valproic acid

[a]Please note that these agents have never been labeled by the Food and Drug Administration for the treatment of pediatric delirium
[b]For catatonic delirium only, high-dose benzodiazepines have been successfully used as treatment

Finally, attention should be paid to optimizing the PICU environment. It is important to try to improve opportunities for sleep – a delirious child will have difficulty sleeping, and sleep deprivation will further potentiate delirium [26]. The most effective way to promote sleep in a critically ill child appears to be establishing a day-night routine. A well-lit space during the day, with cognitive and physical stimulations (and as much mobilization as possible), will set the stage for sleeping at night [46]. Parents should be reminded to bring in eyeglasses (when appropriate) and familiar objects from home. A bedtime schedule should be established, with incorporation of as much of the home routine as is feasible, followed by "lights out" and clustering of care to allow for consolidation of sleep [47].

In most cases delirium will improve when underlying medical, iatrogenic, and environmental factors are addressed. On occasion, when symptoms of hyperactive delirium are severe, pharmacological management may be indicated [26]. Intensivists and oncologists have found success using clonidine, dexmedetomidine, valproic acid, and the atypical antipsychotics [2, 9, 48–50]. These drugs have not been labeled by the Food and Drug Administration (FDA) for treatment of pediatric delirium, and to date, there have been no randomized controlled trials proving efficacy of the pharmacologic management of pediatric delirium. A retrospective review of the use of quetiapine (an atypical antipsychotic with a favorable side effect profile) as treatment for delirium in 50 critically ill children ranging in age from 2 months to 20 years found no serious adverse events [51]. As this is an off-label use of quetiapine, it should only be used when the risk-benefit analysis is favorable.

Although delirium is generally reversible, there is a specific delirium subtype – terminal delirium – that is not. Terminal delirium occurs near the end of life, and goals of treatment are not to reverse the delirium but rather to palliate the symptoms in order to minimize patient – and caregiver – distress [52, 53]. The terminally ill pediatric hematology-oncology patient will benefit from a comprehensive palliative care team consultation to help with the symptom management of terminal delirium.

Delirium Prevention

Many pediatric intensive care units around the country are embracing a comprehensive approach to delirium prevention. The cornerstone of all delirium prevention programs involves multidisciplinary unit-wide education, including nurses, physicians, housestaff, pharmacists, and therapists (physical, occupational, respiratory, and child life) [26]. PICUs are establishing routine screening for delirium and adopting a minimalist attitude to sedation. They are encouraging early mobilization and modifying the PICU environment to create opportunities for consolidated sleep [54]. As proof of principle, a single academic PICU consecutively rolled out three bundles of care: first, universal delirium screening; second, protocolized sedation; and third, an early mobilization program. Delirium rates in this PICU decreased 39% over the course of the initiative [44].

Conclusions

Delirium occurs frequently in the critically ill pediatric immunocompromised hematology-oncology patient and has measurable effects on outcomes. Without routine screening early delirium is often missed. It is vital to implement routine screening for all critically ill children with underlying immunodeficiency, as early delirium detection allows for recognition of underlying triggers, prompt intervention, and decreased delirium burden. When PICU staff begin to identify delirium and recognize the deleterious effects of delirium on their patients, culture change ensues and delirium prevalence decreases in these high-risk children.

References

1. Diagnostic and statistical manual of mental disorders. 5th ed. Arlington: American Psychiatric Association; 2013.
2. Patel AK, Bell MJ, Traube C. Delirium in pediatric critical care. Pediatr Clin N Am. 2017 Oct;64(5):1117–32.
3. Silver G, Traube C, Gerber LM, Sun X, Kearney J, Patel A, et al. Pediatric delirium and associated risk factors: a single-center prospective observational study. Pediatr Crit Care Med. 2015;16(4):303–9.
4. Silver G, Traube C, Kearney J, Kelly D, Yoon MJ, Nash Moyal W, et al. Detecting pediatric delirium: development of a rapid observational assessment tool. Intensive Care Med. 2012;38(6):1025–31.
5. Smith HAB, Fuchs DC, Pandharipande PP, Barr FE, Ely EW. Delirium: an emerging frontier in the management of critically ill children. Anesthesiol Clin. 2011;29(4):729–50.
6. Peterson JF, Pun BT, Dittus RS, Thomason JWW, Jackson JC, Shintani AK, et al. Delirium and its motoric subtypes: a study of 614 critically ill patients: delirium subtypes in the critically ill. J Am Geriatr Soc. 2006;54(3):479–84.
7. Traube C, Silver G, Gerber LM, Kaur S, Mauer EA, Kerson A, et al. Delirium and mortality in critically ill children: epidemiology and outcomes of pediatric delirium. Crit Care Med. 2017;45(5):891–8.
8. Turkel SB, Trzepacz PT, Tavare CJ. Comparing symptoms of delirium in adults and children. Psychosomatics. 2006;47(4):320–4.
9. Schieveld JNM, Leroy PLJM, Os J, Nicolai J, Vos GD, Leentjens AFG. Pediatric delirium in critical illness: phenomenology, clinical correlates and treatment response in 40 cases in the pediatric intensive care unit. Intensive Care Med. 2007;33(6):1033–40.
10. Schieveld JN, Staal M, Voogd L, Fincken J, Vos G, Os J. Refractory agitation as a marker for pediatric delirium in very young infants at a pediatric intensive care unit. Intensive Care Med. 2010;36(11):1982–3.
11. Maldonado JR. Neuropathogenesis of delirium: review of current etiologic theories and common pathways. Am J Geriatr Psychiatry. 2013;21(12):1190–222.
12. Ritter C, Tomasi CD, Dal-Pizzol F, Pinto BB, Dyson A, de Miranda AS, et al. Inflammation biomarkers and delirium in critically ill patients. Crit Care. 2014;18(3):R106.
13. Cerejeira J, Firmino H, Vaz-Serra A, Mukaetova-Ladinska EB. The neuroinflammatory hypothesis of delirium. Acta Neuropathol (Berl). 2010;119(6):737–54.
14. Smith HAB, Brink E, Fuchs DC, Ely EW, Pandharipande PP. Pediatric delirium: monitoring and management in the pediatric intensive care unit. Crit Care Pediatr Patient. 2013;60(3):741–60.

15. Breitbart W, Gibson C, Tremblay A. The delirium experience: delirium recall and delirium-related distress in hospitalized patients with cancer, their spouses/caregivers, and their nurses. Psychosomatics. 2002;43(3):183–94.
16. Traube C, Ariagno S, Thau F, Rosenberg L, Mauer EA, Gerber LM, et al. Delirium in hospitalized children with cancer: incidence and associated risk factors. J Pediatr. 2017;191:212–7.
17. Traube C, Mauer EA, Gerber LM, Kaur S, Joyce C, Kerson A, et al. Cost associated with pediatric delirium in the ICU. Crit Care Med. 2016;44(12):e1175–9.
18. Lawlor PG, Bush SH. Delirium in patients with cancer: assessment, impact, mechanisms and management. Nat Rev Clin Oncol. 2014;12(2):77–92.
19. Caraceni A, Nanni O, Maltoni M, Piva L, Indelli M, Arnoldi E, et al. Impact of delirium on the short term prognosis of advanced cancer patients. Cancer. 2000;89(5):1145–9.
20. van Hemert A. Excess mortality in general hospital patients with delirium. J Psychosom Res. 1994;38(4):339–46.
21. Colville G, Kerry S, Pierce C. Children's factual and delusional memories of intensive care. Am J Respir Crit Care Med. 2008 May;177(9):976–82.
22. Schieveld JNM, van Tuijl S, Pikhard T. On nontraumatic brain injury in pediatric critical illness, neuropsychologic short-term outcome, delirium, and resilience. Crit Care Med. 2013;41(4):1160–1.
23. Girard TD, Jackson JC, Pandharipande PP, Pun BT, Thompson JL, Shintani AK, et al. Delirium as a predictor of long-term cognitive impairment in survivors of critical illness. Crit Care Med. 2010;38(7):1513–20.
24. Pandharipande PP, Girard TD, Jackson JC, Morandi A, Thompson JL, Pun BT, et al. Long-term cognitive impairment after critical illness. N Engl J Med. 2013;369(14):1306–16.
25. Morandi A, Rogers BP, Gunther ML, Merkle K, Pandharipande P, Girard TD, et al. The relationship between delirium duration, white matter integrity, and cognitive impairment in intensive care unit survivors as determined by diffusion tensor imaging: the VISIONS prospective cohort magnetic resonance imaging study. Crit Care Med. 2012;40(7):2182–9.
26. Barr J, Fraser GL, Puntillo K, Ely EW, Gélinas C, Dasta JF, et al. Clinical practice guidelines for the management of pain, agitation, and delirium in adult patients in the intensive care unit. Crit Care Med. 2013;41(1):278–80.
27. Basinski JR, Alfano CM, Katon WJ, Syrjala KL, Fann JR. Impact of delirium on distress, health-related quality of life, and cognition 6 months and 1 year after hematopoietic cell transplant. Biol Blood Marrow Transplant. 2010;16(6):824–31.
28. Fann JR, Alfano CM, Roth-Roemer S, Katon WJ, Syrjala KL. Impact of delirium on cognition, distress, and health-related quality of life after hematopoietic stem-cell transplantation. J Clin Oncol. 2007;25(10):1223–31.
29. Pandharipande PP, Ely EW, Arora RC, Balas MC, Boustani MA, La Calle GH, et al. The intensive care delirium research agenda: a multinational, interprofessional perspective. Intensive Care Med. 2017;43(9):1329–39.
30. Traube C, Silver G, Reeder RW, Doyle H, Hegel E, Wolfe HA, et al. Delirium in critically ill children: an international point prevalence study. Crit Care Med. 2017;45(4):584–90.
31. Patel AK, Biagas KV, Clarke EC, Gerber LM, Mauer E, Silver G, et al. Delirium in children after cardiac bypass surgery. Pediatr Crit Care Med. 2017;18(2):165–71.
32. Meyburg J, Dill M-L, Traube C, Silver G, Von Haken R. Patterns of postoperative delirium in children. Pediatr Crit Care Med. 2017;18(2):128–33.
33. Smith HAB, Gangopadhyay M, Goben CM, Jacobowski NL, Chestnut MH, Savage S, et al. The preschool confusion assessment method for the ICU: valid and reliable delirium monitoring for critically ill infants and children. Crit Care Med. 2016;44(3):592–600.
34. Traube C, Augenstein J, Greenwald B, LaQuaglia M, Silver G. Neuroblastoma and pediatric delirium: a case series: neuroblastoma and delirium. Pediatr Blood Cancer. 2014;61(6):1121–3.
35. Combs D, Rice SA, Kopp LM. Incidence of delirium in children with cancer: delirium in children with cancer. Pediatr Blood Cancer. 2014;61(11):2094–5.

36. Smith HAB, Gangopadhyay M, Goben CM, Jacobowski NL, Chestnut MH, Thompson JL, et al. Delirium and benzodiazepines associated with prolonged ICU stay in critically ill infants and young children. Crit Care Med. 2017;45(9):1427–35.
37. Modi K, Kaur S, Mauer E, Gerber L, Greenwald B, Silver G, et al. Benzodiazepines and development of delirium in critically ill children: estimating the causal effect. Crit Care Med. 2018;46:1486–91.
38. Silver G, Kearney J, Traube C, Atkinson TM, Wyka KE, Walkup J. Pediatric delirium: evaluating the gold standard. Palliat Support Care. 2014;24:1–4.
39. Schieveld JN, Janssen NJ. Delirium in the pediatric patient: on the growing awareness of its clinical interdisciplinary importance. JAMA Pediatr. 2014;168(7):595–6.
40. Smith HAB, Boyd J, Fuchs DC, Melvin K, Berry P, Shintani A, et al. Diagnosing delirium in critically ill children: validity and reliability of the pediatric confusion assessment method for the intensive care unit. Crit Care Med. 2011;39(1):150–7.
41. Traube C, Silver G, Kearney J, Patel A, Atkinson TM, Yoon MJ, et al. Cornell assessment of Pediatric delirium: a valid, rapid, observational tool for screening delirium in the PICU. Crit Care Med. 2014;42(3):656–63.
42. Harris J, Ramelet A-S, van Dijk M, Pokorna P, Wielenga J, Tume L, et al. Clinical recommendations for pain, sedation, withdrawal and delirium assessment in critically ill infants and children: an ESPNIC position statement for healthcare professionals. Intensive Care Med. 2016;42(6):972–86.
43. Silver G, Kearney J, Traube C, Hertzig M. Delirium screening anchored in child development: the Cornell assessment for pediatric delirium. Palliat Support Care. 2014;15:1–7.
44. Simone S, Edwards S, Lardieri A, Walker LK, Graciano AL, Kishk OA, et al. Implementation of an ICU bundle: an interprofessional quality improvement project to enhance delirium management and monitor delirium prevalence in a single PICU. Pediatr Crit Care Med. 2017;18(6):531–40.
45. Breitbart W, Alici Y. Evidence-based treatment of delirium in patients with cancer. J Clin Oncol. 2012;30(11):1206–14.
46. Wieczorek B, Ascenzi J, Kim Y, Lenker H, Potter C, Shata NJ, et al. PICU up!: impact of a quality improvement intervention to promote early mobilization in critically ill children. Pediatr Crit Care Med. 2016;17(12):e559–66.
47. Kudchadkar SR, Yaster M, Punjabi NM. Sedation, sleep promotion, and delirium screening practices in the care of mechanically ventilated children: a wake-up call for the pediatric critical care community. Crit Care Med. 2014;42(7):1592–600.
48. Sher Y, Cramer ACM, Ament A, Lolak S, Maldonado JR. Valproic acid for treatment of hyperactive or mixed delirium: rationale and literature review. Psychosomatics. 2015;56(6):615–25.
49. Aydogan MS, Korkmaz MF, Ozgül U, Erdogan MA, Yucel A, Karaman A, et al. Pain, fentanyl consumption, and delirium in adolescents after scoliosis surgery: dexmedetomidine vs midazolam. Anderson B, editor. Pediatr Anesth. 2013;23(5):446–52.
50. Carrasco G, Baeza N, Cabré L, Portillo E, Gimeno G, Manzanedo D, et al. Dexmedetomidine for the treatment of hyperactive delirium refractory to haloperidol in nonintubated ICU patients: a nonrandomized controlled trial. Crit Care Med. 2016;44(7):1295–306.
51. Joyce C, Witcher R, Herrup E, Kaur S, Mendez-Rico E, Silver G, et al. Evaluation of the safety of quetiapine in treating delirium in critically ill children: a retrospective review. J Child Adolesc Psychopharmacol [Internet]. 2015 Oct 15 [cited 2015 Oct 18]; Available from: http://online.liebertpub.com/doi/10.1089/cap.2015.0093
52. Gagnon P, Allard P, Gagnon B, Mérette C, Tardif F. Delirium prevention in terminal cancer: assessment of a multicomponent intervention. Psychooncology. 2012;21(2):187–94.
53. Breitbart W, Alici Y. Agitation and delirium at the end of life: "we couldn't manage him.". JAMA. 2008;300(24):2898–910. E1
54. Traube C, Greenwald BM. "The times they are A-Changin": universal delirium screening in pediatric critical care. Pediatr Crit Care Med. 2017;18(6):594–5.

Chapter 19
Nursing Considerations

Brienne Leary, Barbara Cuccovia, and Colleen Nixon

Overview: A Nursing Perspective

Introduction

Hematologic, immunologic, and oncologic diagnoses can be devastating to a child and their family [1]. Many of the current treatment options have complex potential side effect profiles. While any one of these diagnoses is potentially life-threatening, almost 85% of all children with cancer will survive [2, 3]. Advances in treatment protocols and marked improvements in supportive care have resulted in pediatric cancer becoming, more often than not, a chronic condition versus a life-threatening illness [2, 3]. It is estimated that between 25% and 40% of children living with this vast scope of diagnoses will, at some point in their disease and treatment course, require an escalation in their supportive care beyond the means of their hematology/

B. Leary (✉)
Pediatric Medical-Surgical Intensive Care Unit,
Boston Children's Hospital,
Boston, MA, USA
e-mail: Brienne.Leary@childrens.harvard.edu

B. Cuccovia
Pediatric Stem Cell Transplant Unit, Boston Children's Hospital,
Boston, MA, USA
e-mail: Barbara.Cuccovia@childrens.harvard.edu

C. Nixon
Pediatric Hematology/Oncology Unit, Boston Children's Hospital,
Boston, MA, USA
e-mail: Colleen.Nixon@childrens.harvard.edu

C. N. Duncan et al. (eds.), *Critical Care of the Pediatric Immunocompromised Hematology/Oncology Patient*, https://doi.org/10.1007/978-3-030-01322-6_19

oncology/hematopoietic cell transplant (HCT) units and require some form of intensive care support [4, 5].

Throughout the child's disease and treatment continuum, nurses provide direct, hands-on nursing care and coordination, education, advocacy, and holistic psychosocial support. Ensuring excellent nursing care is an essential component in the effort to improve and optimize outcomes.

Framework for Categorizing Patients

Given the complexity of this patient population, it is helpful to systematically categorize the patients in order to anticipate nursing care needs. The following framework places patients into three categories (Fig. 19.1): (1) planned pediatric intensive care unit (PICU) admissions, (2) episodes of acute decompensation, and (3) chronically critically ill.

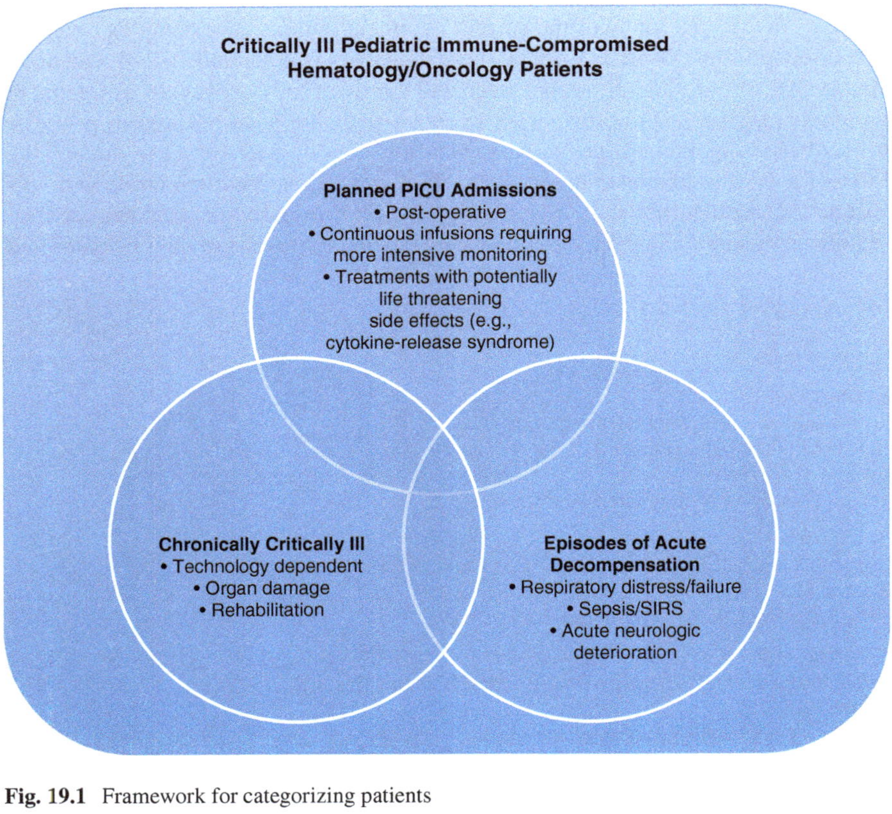

Fig. 19.1 Framework for categorizing patients

Category One: Planned Admissions

The first category encompasses children whose admission to the PICU is planned. Surgery is an essential component of diagnosis and treatment for many patients with an oncologic disease. Children may require postoperative care in the PICU following a surgical procedure as a part of their treatment course or workup for a complication related to their disease or treatment (e.g., tumor debulking, lung biopsy, or bronchoscopy). Also encompassed in this category are children who are predicted to require nursing care needs beyond those possible on the pediatric hematology/oncology/HCT ward for a finite amount of time. An example may be a child receiving a chemotherapy regimen for treatment of a brain tumor that triggers a transient need for a vasopressin infusion to manage diabetes insipidus (DI) not able to be controlled with oral DDAVP.

Children may also require treatments that trigger significant, but expected, side effects, such as cytokine release syndrome (CRS). It may be necessary to preemptively transfer the patient to a higher level of care, such as the PICU. These side effects are typically an expected part of treatment and often time-limited with appropriate supportive therapy.

With planned admissions, there is a more predictable trajectory, and the nursing staff can be educated on specific care needs required for the patient. For example, patients admitted postoperatively after undergoing surgical resection might temporarily require intubation to titrate fluid balance and pain control. These are conditions that are anticipated, managed successfully and expeditiously, and have an expected treatment and outcome course.

Category Two: Episodes of Acute Decompensation

The second category includes children whose clinical condition is acutely deteriorating as a result of complications related to either disease process or treatment course. This is the most complex, acutely ill, and unstable category of patients. Common conditions necessitating transfer to the PICU include, though are not limited to, respiratory distress/failure, sepsis and/or systemic inflammatory response syndrome (SIRS), neurologic deterioration, bleeding issues and/or altered coagulation, and multi-system organ failure [5–12]. Patients admitted for acute decompensation differ from planned admissions in that they are less predictable and the pace of their decline can be rapid. Despite treatment interventions being guided by evidence, no universally accepted guidelines and/or protocols exist, leading to variation in management strategies. This results in unique, nuanced care decisions that make patient care more challenging.

Category Three: The Chronically Critically Ill Child

The third category of patients is the chronically critically ill patient. The 5-year survival rate for children diagnosed with cancer before the age of 20 in the United States is greater than 80% [2, 3]. Despite the high likelihood of survival, modalities used in treatment can result in long-term effects. Many are significant enough to cause chronic cardiac, pulmonary, and renal toxicities [13]. This group of children who develop chronic critical illness related to complications of treatment is a relatively new phenomenon resulting from the changing landscape in pediatric hematology/oncology/HCT and impacts nursing care and resource allocation. Pediatric hematology/oncology/HCT programs need to consider the long-term disposition and implications of the potential future expansion of this population.

Technology Dependence Advances in technology allow many children with chronic conditions to live with the support of various machines at home [14, 15]. The term "technology dependent" has been accepted since the 1980s [15]. This describes the chronic use of machines in conjunction with nursing care to prolong life while optimizing quality [15]. In the context of pediatric cancer, this may refer to a child who becomes technology dependent due to their disease process and/or side effects of treatment. A growing number of diseases, such as mucopolysaccharidosis type I (MPS I, aka Hurler syndrome), are considered treatable by HCT [16]. Diseases such as MPS I can cause primary respiratory failure [17]. Children with MPS I and similar diseases may require tracheostomy and long-term ventilator support before even receiving a HCT.

When Categories Collide

The aforementioned categories should not be thought of as mutually exclusive. Rather, there may be times when children drift back and forth across the categories (Fig. 19.1). For example, an episode of acute decompensation may overtake a child who is chronically critically ill. This is often referred to as "acute-on-chronic" illness. Simply defined, this is a chronic condition exacerbated by an acute illness [18]. Numerous factors should be considered when arranging for how and where nursing care can be delivered to the patient. The interdisciplinary team must remain fluid in their thinking as they consider the evolving needs of the patient.

Box 19.1 Case Study: When Categories Collide

Jonathan underwent a matched, unrelated allogeneic HCT for a rare combined immunodeficiency. Eighteen months post HCT, he is admitted to the inpatient unit for increased work of breathing. As a part of his workup, Jonathan undergoes a lung biopsy. Unfortunately, he fails to extubate postoperatively and is admitted to the PICU for recovery. Jonathan develops worsening respiratory distress that progresses to respiratory failure and is diagnosed with chronic pulmonary graft-versus-host disease (cGVHD). After 6 weeks, Jonathan is unable to wean off of the ventilator despite numerous interventions. Multiple extensive discussions occur between the family, the HCT team, and the PICU team regarding goals of care. The family's priority is to bring Jonathan home. Once stabilized, Jonathan's family chooses to place a tracheostomy as a means to provide long-term ventilation and rehabilitation, with a goal to be considered for a lung transplant.

Describing the Complexity: High Acuity-Low Frequency

Conceptually speaking, the pediatric hematology/oncology/HCT patient's baseline condition is complex. Nevertheless, most treatment occurs on general inpatient units and in the ambulatory setting. If the patient decompensates to a point of requiring critical care, the expertise of a pediatric critical care specialist (i.e., pediatric intensivist) becomes a necessary addition to the child's care team to create an effective management plan designed to support the patient through their critical illness. The evolving *direct patient care needs* are those most commonly provided and performed by *nurs*es. These include (though are not limited to) noninvasive and/or invasive mechanical ventilation, vasopressor support, renal replacement therapies (intermittent and/or continuous), and physiologic monitoring and nursing care needs beyond those possible on a standard pediatric hematology/oncology/HCT unit. The complexity of these patients requires extensive resource utilization, multidisciplinary expertise, and high-level care coordination.

On average, less than 40% of children with a hematology/oncology diagnosis will require admission need to the PICU [2, 4, 5]. Estimates range from 15% to 45% for the pediatric HCT population [10, 12, 19]. Compared to other PICU admissions, children with cancer and undergoing HCT account for less than 10 % of all patients in medical-surgical PICUs [5, 11, 20]. As a result, these patients represent a *high acuity-low frequency* patient population potentially placing the continuity of their care at risk. Ensuring excellent collaboration and communication can combat this phenomenon [21]. See section "Developing a Collaborative Interdisciplinary Care Model", for an in-depth discussion.

Managing the Complexity: Nursing Care Issues

Introduction: Improved Critical Care Outcomes

As recently as the early 1990s, controversy existed over whether or not to offer intensive care support to pediatric hematology/oncology/HCT patients [22–24]. These concerns stemmed from abysmal outcomes, both perceived and published, in the 1970s–1980s, most of which were extrapolated from adult studies [25–31]. Advanced understanding of disease nuances has allowed the development of targeted therapies and a decrease in patient toxicities, while simultaneously, advances in pediatric critical care were made. Improved critical care outcomes have allowed children to survive to PICU discharge that previously never would have [5].

General Considerations: Balancing Competing Priorities

The complexities surrounding the care of the critically ill pediatric hematology/oncology/HCT patient are vast and often overlapping. The child's condition often creates competing demands, requiring nursing expertise to balance a delicate scale of priorities. Precedence must be given to acute life-saving measures, such as intubation, volume resuscitation, or emergency medications, without losing sight of the primary disease process and treatment. The child's ongoing immune-compromised state must continuously be considered. These competing priorities can often be achieved simultaneously but, at other times, may require difficult decisions (Fig. 19.2).

When caring for these patients in the PICU, it is essential for the interdisciplinary team to coordinate with the nursing staff in prioritizing care. For example, fluid overload may be a cause of concern for the patient with pulmonary issues, but ensuring hyperhydration during a chemotherapy infusion known to cause acute kidney injury or hemorrhagic cystitis may be necessary. Patients on continuous renal replacement therapies (CRRT) also require attention to both dialysis settings and the patient's physiologic response to therapy. Timing of medication administration, blood product transfusions, and/or other supportive care needs must also be taken into consideration. It is also common for children receiving cancer therapy to be enrolled in clinical trials [32]. This often necessitates pharmacokinetic samples to be obtained at precise time points. This may be misinterpreted as superfluous at a time when a child is critically ill, but these laboratory results bear significant weight in ensuring the child stays compliant with their protocol. These and other similar scenarios necessitate a cohesive and

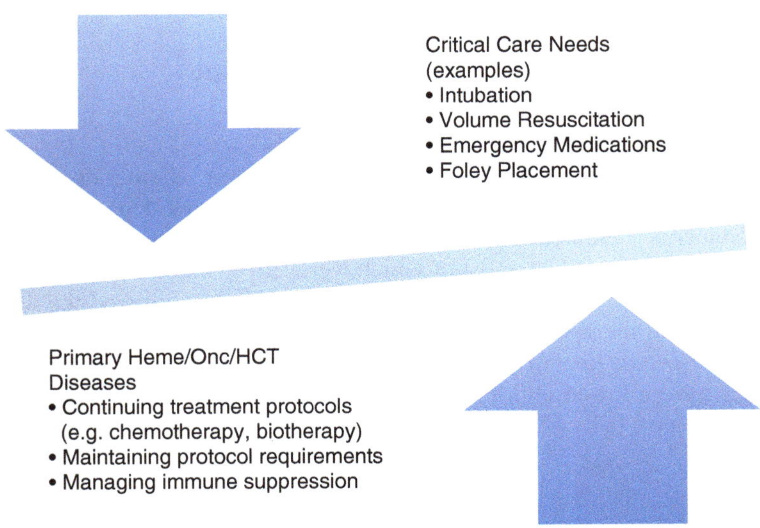

Fig. 19.2 Balancing competing priorities

dynamic conversation between the hematology/oncology/HCT teams and the PICU nurses and providers to determine which factors take precedence to minimize risk and optimize healing.

Nuances in Nursing Care: Considerations for the Immune-Compromised Patient

Patients with compromised immune systems present specific concerns. Their complex needs and vulnerability to infections, both common and rare, along with the medications being used to treat and prevent infections should be considered in their care plan.

Medications and Monitoring Devices: Neutropenic Considerations

It is considered standard of care to avoid suppositories, enemas, digital rectal exams, and/or rectal thermometers in neutropenic patients [33], particularly those undergoing HCT [34]. Axillary, oral, tympanic, or temporal thermometers are preferred. Alternatives to rectal medications should be sought, and oral substitutes are often available. If the patient is NPO or unable to tolerate oral medications, consider placement of an enteral feeding tube for administration of enteral medications if platelet count/bleeding risk allows. It is necessary to educate staff on the rationale behind these interventions to improve adherence and ensure best practice.

Indwelling Urinary Catheters (IUCs)

Indwelling urinary catheters (IUCs) are important devices used to monitor urine output. IUCs can provide essential information pertaining to a child's end-organ perfusion, renal function, hydrations status, and signs of bleeding. The longer an IUC is in place, the higher the risk of developing a catheter-associated urinary tract infection (CAUTI) [35, 36].

Preventing hospital-acquired infections (HAIs) is a priority [37]. CAUTIs are responsible for the majority of HAIs and are associated with patient morbidity, mortality, secondary bloodstream infections [35], and increased cost [38]. Critically ill pediatric hematology/oncology/HCT patients are at an increased risk to develop a CAUTI secondary to their compromised immune state [35, 39]. There are circumstances when placement of an IUC is necessary, such as with severe sepsis or sinusoidal obstruction syndrome (SOS). Other indications may include severe hemorrhagic cystitis requiring bladder irrigation [40], urinary retention due to opioid side effects, or liquid stools that cannot otherwise be easily delineated from urine output.

Strategies to protect these patients from a potential infection focus on narrowing indications for placement to those of absolute necessity; ensuring vigilant aseptic technique during insertion and manipulation of the IUC; maintaining free-flowing drainage (i.e., drainage bag maintained below the patient's waist); and the implementation of evidence-based algorithms that promote early removal and prevent premature replacement [35, 36, 39]. Weighing the risks and benefits in each circumstance is essential to providing optimal care for each patient.

Sepsis, Systemic Inflammatory Response Syndrome (SIRS), and Shock

Sepsis is a leading cause of death in children nationally and internationally [41, 42]. Pediatric immune-compromised hematology/oncology/HCT patients are at greater risk for morbidity and mortality secondary to sepsis [43–45]. Chapter 11 presents a comprehensive discussion of sepsis. The focus here will be on nursing recognition, intervention, and ongoing assessment and monitoring of the critically ill immune-compromised child with sepsis.

Sepsis is defined as systemic inflammatory response syndrome (SIRS) that is associated with the presence of a known or suspected infection. Sepsis in combination with cardiovascular (CV) organ dysfunction *or* acute respiratory distress syndrome (ARDS) *or* two or more other organ dysfunctions describes *severe sepsis*. If severe sepsis goes untreated or is unresponsive to therapy, septic shock can develop. *Septic shock* is sepsis in the presence of cardiovascular dysfunction despite 40 ml/kg IV fluid resuscitation in <60 min (Fig. 19.3) [46].

Gram-negative organisms are often the cause of septic shock, resulting in a higher mortality rate. *Escherichia coli* is the most common gram-negative organism identified in sepsis, although *Pseudomonas aeruginosa* is identified in more sepsis-related mortality cases than any other bacteria in neutropenic and immune-compromised patients [47].

Risk Factors

Nurses must be aware of the factors that put immune-compromised patients at higher risk to develop and potentially succumb to sepsis [48]. These include

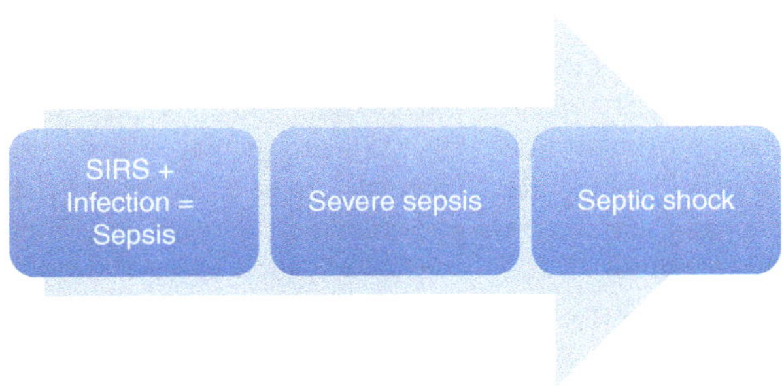

Fig. 19.3 Sepsis continuum

neutropenia, generalized immune suppression, altered body defenses, endocrine abnormalities, and pre-existing organ damage.

1. *Neutropenia*: Children with cancer, hematologic disorders, primary immune deficiency syndromes, and undergoing HCT are at risk for neutropenia and thus sepsis. Neutropenia may be the result of disease infiltration in the bone marrow or related to treatment side effects from chemotherapy and/or radiation. Neutropenia is a decrease in the number of circulating neutrophils. Any child having an absolute neutrophil count (ANC) <500/mm^3 is at risk for serious infection. Periods of prolonged neutropenia (i.e., >7 days) place children at a higher risk for the development of sepsis. When a child has fever and is neutropenic, this is called fever and neutropenia (i.e., "F & N"). The risk of infection is determined by the ANC, which is calculated by multiplying the total white blood cell (WBC) count by the percentage of neutrophils (also referred to as "polys" or "segs") and bands present in the blood [49].

Box 19.2 Calculating Absolute Neutrophil Count (ANC)

$$\text{Absolute neutrophil count}(\text{ANC}) = \text{WBC} \times (\%\text{neutrophils} + \%\text{bands})$$

$$\text{Example: WBC of 1.5 with 60\% neutrophils and 10\% bands}$$

$$0.60(\%\text{neutrophils}) + 0.10(\%\text{bands}) = 0.70$$

$$1.5 \times 0.70 = 1.05$$

$$\text{ANC} = 1050$$

2. *Generalized Immune Suppression*: Hematologic/oncologic disease processes, and/or the therapies used to treat them, can impact all cell lines. HCT, for example, in addition to eliminating neutrophils, destroys the host's T and B cell lines, creating a total loss of immunity. Allogeneic HCT patients remain on immune-suppressing medications, such as steroids and calcineurin inhibitors, to prevent graft-versus-host disease. Consequently, these patients remain at risk for months after their transplant [50]. Children with primary immune deficiencies, such as severe combined immunodeficiency (SCID), may have a significantly or entirely compromised ability to respond to pathogens (viral, bacterial, fungal, and protozoa). It is important to consider a child's place in diagnosis and treatment to fully understand the severity of their immune compromise.
3. *Altered Body Defenses*: Radiation and chemotherapy are common treatment modalities. Both can alter skin integrity, impacting one of the body's most important natural defenses – the integumentary system. In addition, the presence of indwelling lines and tubes, both common in these patients, creates pathways for pathogens to enter the body and is a known risk factor for sepsis, regardless of

the patient's ANC [45, 47, 49, 51]. Invasive procedures such as biopsies, bone marrow aspirations, and lumbar puncture are also opportunities for exposure to pathogens.

4. *Endocrine Abnormalities*: The use of steroids remains a mainstay of some pediatric oncology treatment. Chronic steroid use may predispose a child to adrenal insufficiency and/or catecholamine resistance which may inhibit a child's ability to respond to sepsis. However, the exact impact of prior steroid therapy on a child's response to sepsis is not fully understood and continues to be investigated [47]. Exposure to previous steroid therapy should be considered when deciding on a treatment plan for a child with sepsis [52].
5. *Pre-Existing Organ Damage*: Children may have organ damage from the therapy they received or their underlying disease. This may make them more susceptible to further organ damage if they develop septic shock.

Early Recognition and Treatment In 2002, the Centers for Disease Control (CDC) launched a joint initiative with the Society of Critical Care Medicine (SCCM) and the European Society of Intensive Care Medicine (ESICM) known as the "Surviving Sepsis Campaign," aimed at improving outcomes related to sepsis [53]. Additionally, the World Federation of Pediatric Intensive and Critical Care Societies (WFPICCS) (http://www.wfpiccs.org/projects/sepsis-initiative/) is committed to reducing mortality in children related to sepsis. These initiatives advocate for early recognition and treatment of sepsis and shock in all patients through the use of early recognition tools and clinical guidelines focused on goal-directed therapies.

Nurses fulfill an essential role in these initiatives, as they are often the ones in closest proximity to the patient and perform the most frequent assessments. These initiatives have had an impact on reducing deaths related to sepsis [53–55]. One intervention that has proven successful in pediatrics is the use of an early recognition tool, or "sepsis trigger tool," aimed at identifying patients with potential risk of sepsis earlier to ensure rapid treatment [54] (Fig. 19.4). Some institutions have had preliminary success with electronic medical record (EMR)-based tools [55]. The primary goal of these tools is to alert the interdisciplinary team of the potential developing sepsis and begin early treatment. Algorithms that guide care decisions based upon the patient's score should accompany these tools.

Box 19.3 Clinical Pearl

In immune-compromised children, fever may be the first sign of infection and/or sepsis. Infection should be considered the presumed cause of a fever in a neutropenic or immune-compromised patient until proven otherwise. The nurse notifies the medical team immediately to initiate a "sepsis huddle" for a new fever in these patients. Fever in a neutropenic patient is defined as a single oral temperature ≥38.3 °C (101 °F) or a temperature ≥38 °C (100.4 °F) sustained over a 1 hour period. The above temperature criteria are meant to guide practice, in conjunction with clinical judgment, to determine which patients should receive antibiotic therapy [56, 57].

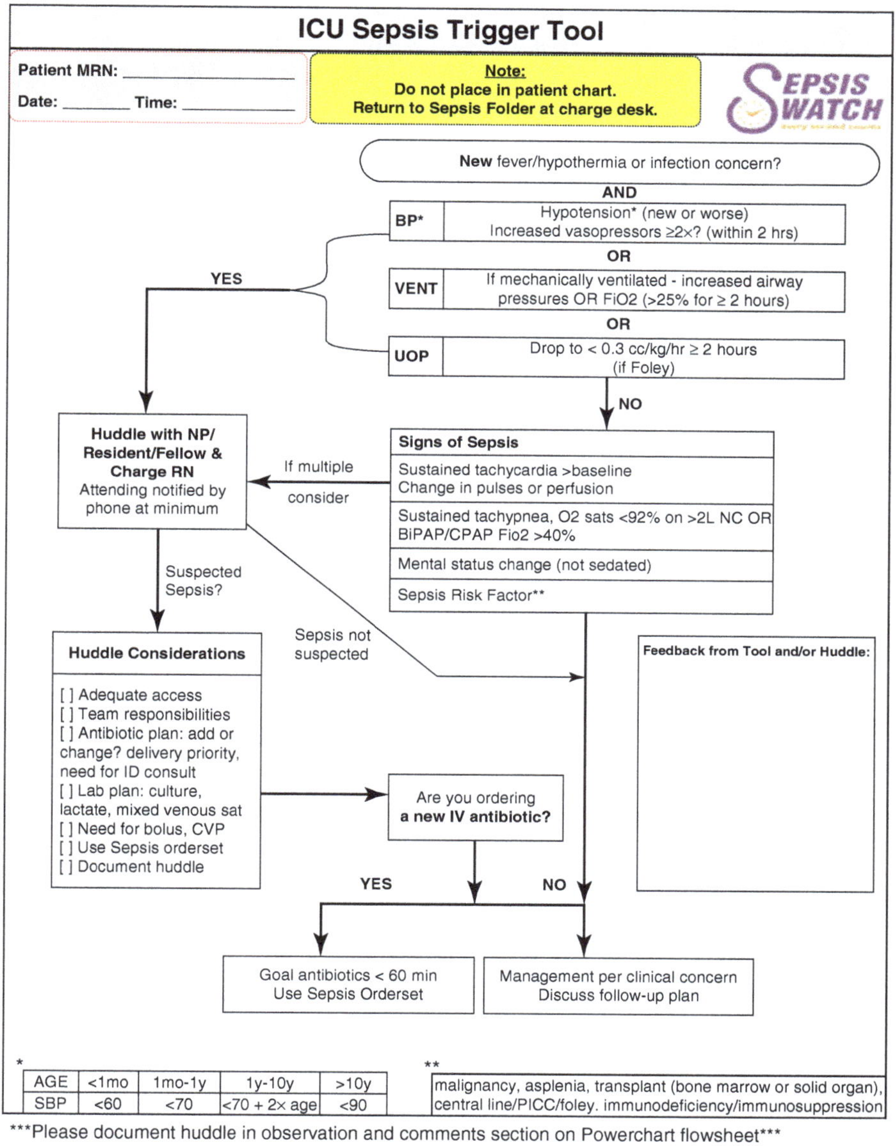

Fig. 19.4 Example of sepsis trigger tool. (Adapted from Boston Children's Hospital, Boston, MA)

Box 19.4 Nursing Assessment and Monitoring for Children with Sepsis
Therapy for sepsis is goal-directed. Frequent reassessment is essential to evaluate the efficacy of interventions as they are implemented and advocate for rapid escalation in therapy as needed.

- New fever/hypothermia or infection concern.
- Tachycardia (>2 standard deviations [SD]) or bradycardia (<2 SD normal HR).
- Age-based tachypnea.
- Age-based hypotension.
  - Clinical Pearl: Early signs of sepsis may be subtle. Decreased blood pressure is a late sign of shock and is associated with negative outcomes.
- Laboratory values
  - Elevated C-reactive protein (CRP) and/or erythrocyte sedimentation rate (ESR).
  - Elevated lactate/lactic acid.
  - Decreased central venous oxygen saturation ($ScvO_2$).
  - Increased or decreased WBC (may or may not be pertinent in children with immune-compromised state).
  - Blood cultures of all indwelling lines; consider also obtaining a peripheral blood culture sample.
- Signs of decreased perfusion and compromised end-organ perfusion
  - Altered mental status.
  - Delayed capillary refill (>3 sec).
  - Decreased urine output.
  - Cold versus warm shock.
    - Cold shock: cool/cold extremities, diminished/absent peripheral pulses, delayed capillary refill, and pallor
    - Warm shock: warm/hot extremities, bounding peripheral and/or central pulses, and normal to slightly delayed capillary refill

Quality measures for sepsis outcomes include administration of antibiotics within one hour, immediate and adequate fluid resuscitation, and appropriately timed initiation of vasopressor/inotropic support. It becomes essential for all nurses who care for hematology/oncology/HCT patients to be aware of early signs of sepsis, anticipate the treatment plan, and initiate the necessary care and resources (See Table 19.1).

Vasoactive/Inotrope Support in Pediatric Sepsis Selection of an inotropic agent(s) for a child in septic shock is complex. An individualized plan should be made in consult with the bedside nurse and the PICU providers. Recommendations regarding inotrope support have evolved. Epinephrine is now the recommended

Table 19.1 Intervention priorities for septic shock [57]

• Identify shock (i.e., altered level of consciousness (LOC), changes in perfusion, tachycardia/bradycardia, etc.)
• Provide high concentration, humidified oxygen
• Establish IV/IO access
• IV push volume repletion with crystalloid fluids in 20 ml/kg increments up to and over 60 ml/kg, monitoring for improvement in vital signs and perfusion
• Obtain blood cultures if it does not cause significant delay of antimicrobial treatment
• Antimicrobial administration STAT <60 min
• Initiate inotropic infusions for fluid refractory shock
• Frequent monitoring
• Consider administration of corticosteroids in fluid refractory patients or for those with concern for adrenal insufficiency

Adapted from: Dellinger et al. [57]

first-line inotrope therapy for children with cold shock [52, 57–59]. Vasodilators (such as milrinone) may be considered in conjunction with the epinephrine infusion to reduce afterload/peripheral vascular resistance if the child is in a low cardiac output state. With the addition of a vasodilator, the child must be closely monitored for potentially worsening hypotension [52, 57, 59].

If the child is experiencing warm shock, norepinephrine is often accepted as the first-line agent first for its potent alpha vasoconstrictor effect and B_1 agonist properties for improved cardiac output [58, 59]. Doses can be titrated quickly to achieve optimal effect.

Continuous vasoactive infusions are high-risk medications that come in a variety of concentrations. Policies should be in place to ensure correct dosing is established and infusion pumps are programmed correctly. If nurse-driven titration of vasoactive infusions is practiced within the institution, the provider must order clear physiologic parameters (i.e., systolic blood pressure [SBP], diastolic blood pressure [DBP], and/or mean arterial pressure [MAP]) and the allowable dose range. Reasons to notify the provider should also be specified. The nurse is responsible for ongoing monitoring of the patient's hemodynamic response and clinical exam as well as for titration of the infusion(s) accordingly. The nurse plays an instrumental role in identifying any changes in the patient's condition (e.g., the patient evolves from warm shock to cold shock) and is responsible to alert the critical care team immediately to reevaluate the inotropic management plan whenever necessary.

The nurse should be prepared to administer corticosteroids in the event the child suffers shock refractory to fluid resuscitation and inotropic agents. Children undergoing treatment for cancer have often been exposed to steroid therapy and are at risk for adrenal insufficiency. The nurse needs to be aware of this and must advocate for evaluation of the patient's need for stress-dose steroid therapy [45, 57, 59].

Invasive Mechanical Ventilation

Critically ill immune-compromised children requiring invasive mechanical ventilation are at an increased risk of mortality [60]. As with all critically ill patients, these children require meticulous nursing care to optimize outcomes. The nurse should [61, 62]:

- Monitor and record routine ventilator settings and parameters, including:
  - Tidal volume (TV), minute ventilation (MV), inspiratory time (I-time or Ti), mean airway pressure (MAP), end-tidal carbon dioxide ($ETCO_2$), peak inspiratory pressure (PIP), positive end-expiratory pressure (PEEP), fraction of inspired oxygen (FiO_2), and flow loops
- Promote ongoing airway management and clearance as tolerated with judicious use of pulmonary toilet methods balanced with risk of bleeding.
- Monitor for signs and symptoms of developing pneumonia including fever, tachypnea, increased work of breathing, and decreased tidal volume.

Ventilator-associated pneumonia (VAP) is one potential complication related to mechanical ventilation that can have significant morbidity [63]. Preventing a VAP during mechanical ventilation requires diligence. Preventative strategies include [64]:

- Whenever possible, use noninvasive positive pressure ventilation.
- Evaluate daily for extubation readiness.
- Optimize sedation to avoid unplanned extubation while targeting lowest effective dosing.
  - Consider scheduled sedation interruptions.
- Provide routine oral care with sterile water and mechanical tooth brushing.
- Maintain head of bed (HOB) at 30–45 degree angle.
- Avoid unnecessary ventilator circuit changes.
- Use cuffed endotracheal tubes.
- Monitor for development of condensate in ventilator tubing; drain away from patient.

Lung-Protective Strategies Historically, children who required positive pressure invasive mechanical ventilation suffered barotrauma as a result of toxic settings. The evolution of lung-protective ventilation techniques following the landmark acute respiratory distress syndrome (ARDS) network study in 2000 [65] has markedly decreased long-term effects related to mechanical ventilation and is the accepted standard of care when treating children with pediatric acute respiratory distress syndrome (ARDS) [65, 66]. Lung-protective strategies are designed to allow for permissive hypercapnia to achieve an arterial blood pH goal of 7.25–7.3, allowing for lower tidal volumes (TVs) of 4–6 ml/kg and a liberal target SpO_2 range (generally >/88%) [61, 62, 65, 66].

Immune-compromised patients can be at increased risk for pulmonary injury directly related to their underlying disease, but more commonly, to specific therapies, and infectious or idiopathic processes. Ongoing research is investigating the safety and application of hypercapnia and low tidal volume (TV) ventilation strategies specifically in immune-compromised pediatric patients with promising results [67].

Nurses can serve as advocates to minimize barotrauma by understanding the inherent risks of mechanical ventilation. See Chap. 11: *Acute Respiratory Failure and Ventilatory Management*, for a more detailed discussion of ventilation strategies in this population.

Tracheostomy and Long-Term Ventilation For children who require longer-term ventilation, tracheostomies are a mainstay therapy in the setting of pulmonary rehabilitation. Tracheostomy may also be performed for anatomic challenges such as a solid tumor threatening airway patency. Historically, it was uncommon to perform a tracheostomy in a child who is immune compromised and/or thrombocytopenic or to allow a child with a tracheostomy to undergo HCT.

General opinion supported concerns that the risks of infection, poor wound healing, and bleeding would outweigh any potential benefits. While there is a paucity of research in the pediatric population, adult studies suggest that neither a HCT nor a hematologic/oncologic/immune-compromised condition should be a limiting factor to performing a tracheostomy [68, 69]. The option for tracheostomy placement to provide long-term ventilation has improved survival and should be considered in this patient population in appropriate circumstances [70].

Intravenous (IV) Access Considerations

General Concepts

It is well documented that needle-related pain remains a source of anxiety and discomfort in the pediatric oncology population [71–74] and for children in the PICU [75]. If venipuncture is necessary for an alert and awake child, topical anesthetics should be considered [73, 75, 76]. These have proven to be effective in minimizing pain during the procedure as well as reducing future anxiety related to needle procedures [75]. The need for stable, reliable, long-term intravenous (IV) access for repeated lab draws as well as frequent and caustic infusions is well established [76]. For these reasons, children undergoing treatment for most hematologic/oncologic diseases and HCT often have a semipermanent central intravenous access point such as a peripherally inserted central catheter (PICC), tunneled external central venous catheter (CVC) (e.g., Broviac®, Hickman®, etc.), or implanted ports (e.g., Mediport® or Port-a-Cath®) placed. This central IV access is typically adequate for routine monitoring and medications throughout a child's treatment course [76, 77].

Children that require transfer to the PICU will often have a condition that necessitates supplementary IV access in the form of peripheral intravenous (PIV) catheters and/or arterial lines. Despite physiologic necessity, placement of new IV access can cause additional stress for patients and parents in an already challenging scenario [75, 78]. It is essential to thoughtfully evaluate the necessity of additional IV access and explain the procedure and rationale to the child and family.

Physical challenges to successfully obtaining peripheral IV access may also be present. Vasculature may be damaged from repeated venipuncture attempts, connective tissue disorders (such as skin GVHD), or other inflammatory changes (rash). Gross edema can also compress the blood vessels making it challenging to successfully cannulate the vein with an IV catheter [79]. Altered skin integrity may also present challenges in stabilizing IV access. Staff should consider the patient's sensitivities to certain dressings and select a specialty product if the child's condition necessitates it.

Venous Thromboembolism (VTE)

Venous thromboembolism (VTE) is of growing concern among children admitted to the PICU with prevalence significantly higher than in the general pediatric population [80]. Research is ongoing about specific risk factors, although a pediatric cancer diagnosis or immunologic disorder and the presence of a central venous catheter have been implicated in studies [81]. The consensus from the Subcommittee on Hemostasis and Malignancy and the Subcommittee on Pediatric/Neonatal Thrombosis and Hemostasis [81] recommends that all children in the PICU be screened for VTE risk to ensure appropriate monitoring. Prophylaxis (medical and mobility) is considered in consultation with hematologists for children identified as high-risk.

Signs and symptoms of a VTE include changes in patency or loss of blood return from an indwelling CVC as well as any redness, swelling, or pain in the extremity with an indwelling line [80, 81]. Acute-onset respiratory distress in a child with a central line should be evaluated immediately, and the risk of a pulmonary embolism should be considered.

Bloodstream Infections (BSIs)

A bloodstream infection (BSI) is the presence of an infectious pathogen identified in a patient's bloodstream by blood culture or other appropriate microbiologic testing methods [82]. BSIs are clinically significant events to the hematology/oncology/HCT patient population as they carry significant risk of morbidity and mortality [83, 84] and may originate from a variety of sources.

Central Line-Associated Bloodstream Infections Central lines can become infected and are the most common cause of BSIs [85]. When a BSI is identified in the presence of an indwelling central line, it is known as a central line-associated bloodstream infection (CLABSI). CLABSIs are considered preventable but remain a leading cause of morbidity and financial cost among critically ill pediatric patients [82,

83]. PICUs have some of the highest CLABSI rates in acute care facilities [86]. CLABSIs are reportable events and are monitored by the CDC's National Healthcare Safety Network (NHSN) as an indicator of patient safety and quality [82, 83, 87]. This metric affects both public and private insurance reimbursement [88]. For the purposes of CLABSI identification and infection rate surveillance, "central lines" include [82]:

- Permanent tunneled catheters, such as Broviac®, and implanted ports
- Temporary non-tunneled catheters such as a peripherally inserted central catheter (PICC) or percutaneous internal jugular (IJ) catheters
- Arterial and venous umbilical catheters

Central lines are clinically necessary for many pediatric hematology/oncology/HCT patients for prolonged periods of time as their treatment requires multiple medications, frequent lab draws, and blood product administration. Unfortunately, these factors [89, 90], along with young age and compromised immune systems [86, 90], place this population at an increased risk to develop a CLABSI as compared to other patients.

Mucosal Barrier Injury Laboratory-Confirmed Bloodstream Infections In addition to their risk of a CLABSI, these patients are also at risk to develop a BSI secondary to altered gastrointestinal/mucosal integrity potentially resulting in translocation of gut microorganisms [91–93]. The most commonly implicated bacteria are viridans group streptococci, *Enterobacteriaceae (E. coli, Klebsiella* spp., *Enterobacter* spp.), and enterococci (*E. faecium* and *E. faecalis*) [94]. Recognition of this phenomenon in immune-compromised patient populations led the NHSN to reevaluate how CLABSIs are defined and monitored [95]. In 2013, the CDC/NHSN first defined mucosal barrier injury (MBI) bloodstream infections as a subset of CLABSIs [95]. In 2018, MBI-LCBSIs were *differentiated* from CLABSIs and are now reported separately [82]. Mucosal barrier injury laboratory-confirmed bloodstream infections (MBI-LCBSIs) account for almost half of the healthcare-associated bloodstream infections (BSIs) in oncology patients [91].

Since its origination, the surveillance definition of MBI-LCBSI has undergone multiple revisions [91, 95, 96]. To qualify as an MBI-LCBSI, the patient and BSI event must meet specific surveillance definition criteria. The patient must be neutropenic (two separate ANC and/or WBC values less than 500 cells/mm^3) within the patient's infection window period (i.e., day of the positive blood culture collection date and the three calendar days before and after). If the patient is not neutropenic, he/she must be an allogeneic HCT recipient with (1) grade III or IV gastrointestinal graft versus host disease (GVHD) or (2) have ≥20 ml/kg of diarrhea in a 24 hours period which began within the 7 days prior to the collection date of their positive blood culture. The patient must have at least one blood specimen with *only* intestinal organisms from a qualifying NHSN list *or* at least *two* blood specimens with *only* viridans group streptococci. Infants must have at least *two* blood specimens with nothing except viridans group streptococci *and* qualifying clinical symptoms [82]. Specific surveillance definition criteria can be found in

Chap. 5 of the 2018 National Healthcare Safety Network (NHSN) Patient Safety Component Manual [97].

Secondary Infections Bloodstream infections (BSIs) can also be caused by a pre-existing source of infection such as pneumonia, urinary tract infection, or abscess [82]. These are referred to as secondary BSIs and are accounted for separately from CLABSIs and MBI-LCBSIs in infection surveillance.

Clinical Implications While these surveillance definitions are useful in tracking the incidence and prevalence of different types of BSIs, the clinical presentation is often similar. Patients undergoing chemotherapy treatment or HCT are at risk for all types of BSIs and may or may not present with the typical signs of infection. It is imperative to continually assess for hypo-/hyperthermia, subtle vital sign changes, flushing, and rigors. Establishing strict blood culture criteria is essential for early BSI identification. In these cases, early treatment with appropriate antibiotics and supportive care are necessary to avoid devastating outcomes (see section "Sepsis, Systemic Inflammatory Response Syndrome (SIRS), and Shock").

Prevention of BSIs, particularly CLABSIs, is of utmost importance in minimizing morbidity and mortality. Extensive and successful prevention efforts have reduced the rate of CLABSIs in intensive care units by 58% since 2001 [83]. The separation of MBI-LCBSIs from CLABSIs has revealed that the overall BSI rate is higher than the CLABSI rate alone. Infection prevention interventions need to address all BSIs, not just CLABSIs [84, 94]. Similarly, surveillance techniques will need to account for these changes in definition to accurately monitor BSI incidence, prevalence, and efficacy of prevention strategies [84]. It is important to recognize that the differentiation of CLABSI from MBI-LCBSI may also impact approaches to prevention of BSIs. While standard CLABSI bundles may help reduce MBI-LCBSI rates [98], MBI-BSI targeted prevention initiatives should also be considered. However, efficacy of current strategies remains to be seen [98].

Nurses caring for patients with central lines must be diligent in their management and follow a standardized approach for line maintenance. Prevention "bundles" are an effective tool in decreasing CLABSI rates in PICU patients [99, 100], particularly when coupled with multicenter quality improvement collaboratives [85, 99, 100]. There are a number of professional and national recommendations/guidelines that drive facility-based policy. One example is the Centers for Disease Control and Prevention (CDC) Checklist for Prevention of Central Line-Associated Bloodstream Infections which can be found at https://www.cdc.gov/hai/pdfs/bsi/checklist-for-clabsi.pdf. The Society for Healthcare Epidemiology of America (SHEA) led a collaborative effort with the Infectious Diseases Society of America (IDSA), the American Hospital Association (AHA), the Association for Professionals in Infection Control and Epidemiology (APIC), and The Joint Commission and produced similar guidelines [90]. The Children's Hospitals' Solutions for Patient Safety (SPS) also offers recommendations specific to pediatrics [101]. While each has its own nuances, common recommendations include [90, 101, 102]:

A. General

(i) Ensure all healthcare professionals (HCPs) involved with central line insertion and care are educated on indications, insertion procedures, and maintenance. Intermittently assess knowledge and compliance with established practices.
(ii) Only trained personnel should insert and maintain central lines.
(iii) Ensure appropriate nurse staffing in the PICU, and minimize the use of float pool nurses.

B. Insertion

(i) Carefully assess indication for central venous catheters (CVCs); ensure that the reason is in alignment with recommended indications.
(ii) Perform hand hygiene prior to insertion.
(iii) Use chlorhexidine scrub for patient's skin preparation.
(iv) Provide prepackaged insertion cart, tray, or box to ensure standardized and sterilized supplies are readily available.
(v) Perform insertion checklist; empower staff to interject with concerns about sterile/aseptic technique and/or contamination.
(vi) For providers trained in the technology, use ultrasound to guide placement to minimize access attempts.
(vii) Utilize maximum sterile barrier during insertion.

C. Maintenance

(i) Daily team discussion of line necessity.
(ii) Daily chlorhexidine baths should be performed on patients older than 2 months unless contraindicated.
(iii) Regular assessment of dressing to ensure it is clean/dry/occlusive; use chlorhexidine-impregnated dressing in patients older than 37-week gestational age.
(iv) Standardize access procedure (i.e., via needless connectors) using alcohol/chlorhexidine gluconate mixture, povidone-iodine, or 70% alcohol, with a focus on friction and >15 second cleansing time.
(v) Standardize dressing, cap, and tubing change procedures/timing:

    (i) Change dressing every 7 days unless risk of dislodgment outweighs benefit.
    (ii) Cap and administration tubing are changed no more frequently than every 96 hours with the exception of administration tubing used to administer blood, blood products, or fat emulsions. These should be changed every 24 hours.

(vi) Remove any nonessential central lines as soon as possible.

Infection Control: Practical Issues

For patients requiring ICU care, it is often disconcerting to leave the perceived isolated environment of the hematology/oncology/HCT unit. However, by following national infection control standards, immune-compromised children can be safely cared for in the PICU (see Table 19.2) [103, 104].

Specifically for children admitted to the PICU while undergoing *allogeneic HCT*, a "protective environment" (PE) should be maintained for patients during the first 100 days posttransplant or longer if the patient has graft-versus-host disease (GVHD) [34]. A *protective environment (PE)* is defined as a "specialized patient-care area, usually in a hospital…[that] creates an environment which can safely accommodate patients who have undergone allogeneic hematopoietic stem cell transplant (HSCT)" (CDC [107], p. 4). Components from five categories contribute to ensuring a protective environment: (1) the patient, (2) precautions, (3) engineering/hospital design, (4) surfaces, and (5) others. HCT units are typically designed and constructed according to these criteria. When caring for allogeneic HCT recipients outside of the HCT unit, such as in the PICU, certain components may present challenges, while many are easily transferrable. See Table 19.2.

Appropriate Use of Isolation Precautions

The Centers for Disease Control (CDC) does not recommend or promote the use of "reverse precautions." "Reverse precautions" are defined as the empiric use of isolation precautions (i.e., gowns, gloves, and masks worn by health care providers and/or visitors) to protect neutropenic patients from infection [103]. Terminating the use of reverse precautions within an institution results in cost savings and improved nurse/patient interactions [105, 106]. For critically ill immune-compromised pediatric hematology/oncology/HCT patients, focus should be on implementing transmission-based isolation precautions for known or suspected communicable and antibiotic-resistant organisms [34, 103], maintaining standard precautions, and promoting hand hygiene [103, 104]. Nurses should continue to educate families to avoid interactions with potentially infectious contacts [104].

Visitor and Staff Considerations

All staff should feel well and be free of signs or symptoms of infection and be fully vaccinated per institutional policy. Staff should avoid caring for an immune-compromised patient, particularly those undergoing allogeneic HCT, if they recently received a live attenuated vaccine. All visitors should be screened for communicable diseases and encouraged to postpone visitation if they recently received a live vaccine such as varicella or measles-mumps-rubella (MMR) [34, 103].

Table 19.2 Maintaining a protective environment (PE) in the PICU

Component	Protective environment guidelines	Implications in the PICU
(1) Patient	– Patient to remain in PE except when travel is necessary for tests, procedures, etc. – Patient should wear a mask outside of PE – Avoid areas with construction	– Procedures are often done within the PICU, reducing the necessity of travel outside of the unit. If travel is necessary, follow standard recommendations (see left) – A mask is not necessary if the patient is intubated on closed ventilator circuit – Consider traveling back to PE (i.e., HCT unit) for activities such as physical therapy when able, or remain in patient's individual room with doors closed – Patients should not ambulate within the PICU outside of their room
(2) Precautions	– Perform hand hygiene before/after patient contact – Empiric use of gown/gloves/mask by healthcare workers is not necessary without evidence or suspicion of infection in patient – Employ appropriate transmission-based precautions for children with known or suspected infection – Continue standard precautions for all patients	– Continue these recommendations in the PICU – Institutions must establish surveillance policies to monitor for pertinent infections – Implement transmission-based precautions for suspected infection(s). Viral precautions for immune-compromised patients may need to be extended given a prolonged period of viral shedding – Establish a clear algorithm to discontinue precautions once infection is ruled out
(3) Engineering and hospital design	– Use of high-efficiency particulate air (HEPA) filtration – Rooms with doors that fully close and well-maintained seals at construction joints – Unit/room constructed with directed, clean airflow through patient room – Positive pressure out of room in relation to hallway – Self-closing doors – If patient requires airborne precautions, use room with anteroom, and add portable HEPA filtration if available	This may be the least transferrable category in the PICU dependent on the institution's design. Effective interventions: (1) Place patient in a *private room* with a door that is able to completely close (2) Avoid *shared* or open bays (3) Keep *door closed* to patient's room whenever possible (4) Select room with *positive pressure* if possible
(4) Surfaces	– No carpeting or fabric/upholstered furniture – Use wet dusting methods	– Often standard throughout an institution
(5) Other	– Flowers or live plants are not allowed on the unit – Cleaning equipment such as vacuums should be equipped with HEPA filtration	– Flowers or live plants are not allowed on the unit – Often standard equipment throughout an institution

Adapted from Siegel et al. [103]

Personal Care Considerations

Hand Hygiene

Hand hygiene remains the leading intervention in preventing [103] HAIs, and vigilance by all is essential [104]. Ensure alcohol-based sanitizers are readily available throughout the unit. Soap and water is recommended (1) after contact with patients with known or suspected infectious diarrheal illness, such as *Clostridium difficile* (*C. difficile*) or norovirus, (2) when hands are visibly soiled, (3) after eating/drinking, and (4) after using the bathroom [34, 103, 104]. Gloves are changed between patients and when soiled or contaminated. Standard precautions should be followed at all times [34, 102, 103, 107–109].

Diet

Neutropenic patients are often "prescribed" a "low-bacteria" or "neutropenic diet" as a way to reduce the risk of exposure to bacteria found in certain foods. Literature supporting any specific type of diet and/or dietary restrictions required for neutropenic patients is inconsistent and lacks evidence to support that these types of diets have any benefit to patients [104, 108, 109]. Despite the lack of randomized controlled trials (RCTs), low-bacteria diet restrictions are often still recommended for neutropenic patients, and the degree of restriction varies among institutions [104, 108, 109]. Guidelines for safe handling and preparation of food are of utmost importance in decreasing the risk of infection [34, 108, 109].

However, for patients undergoing allogeneic HCT who are not yet engrafted, current guidelines recommend a low-bacteria diet [34]. In addition, patient drinking water sources should be limited to bottled water guaranteed to have *Cryptosporidium* removed by filtration through a 1 μmm filter, reverse osmosis, or distillation [34]. See section "Nutritional Considerations" for a discussion of general nutritional considerations for all immune-compromised hematology/oncology/HCT patients.

Skin Care

The first line of defense against infection is the skin. The risk for alteration in skin integrity in pediatric hematology/oncology/HCT children is multifactorial. These factors include, but are not limited to, the treatment the child is receiving, the presence of surgical incisions, nutritional status, impaired mobility, incidence of GVHD, and/or the use of medical devices [110]. Hospital-acquired pressure injuries (HAPIs) are a potential risk for any hospitalized patient, potentially leading to increased hospital costs and length of stay [111–113]. Patients in the PICU are at an even higher risk for developing HAPIs than the general population [114].

Risk factors that may impact pediatric hematology/oncology/HCT patients include:

- Decreased mobility due to acute and chronic illness
- Decreased sensory perception related to sedation and/or neurotoxicities as treatment side effects
- Friction/shear secondary to their deconditioned state
- Inadequate nutrition and protein deficiency related to decreased oral intake and/or nausea/vomiting/diarrhea necessitating enteral and/or intravenous supplemental nutrition
- Altered tissue perfusion and oxygenation related to decreased hemoglobin levels and/or potentially altered hemodynamics
- Increased skin and linen moisture related to fever, diaphoresis and incontinence
- Medical devices that may or may not be able to be repositioned [111, 115]

Any skin breakdown can be a source of infection [34, 116]. Consequently, the prevention of skin breakdown is a nursing care priority. All children should have a thorough baseline skin assessment documented upon hospital admission and daily thereafter to assess for any open sites that could become portals for infectious pathogens [34]. The skin should be routinely screened using a pressure ulcer risk assessment tool validated for pediatric patients [114], such as the Braden Q [115] or Braden QD Scales [111]. Patients should be repositioned at minimum intervals of every 2–4 h, particularly those who are sedated, deconditioned, have localized or generalized edema, and/or are on a ventilator [114]. Nurses should take care to avoid medical device associated pressure ulcers by using blanket rolls and padding to support devices and/or provide a protective barrier between the device and the patient's skin when feasible [114].

Evidence suggests that immune-compromised patients can become systemically infected with pathogens endogenous to the patient. Diligent and meticulous skin cleansing is a priority to minimize contamination and prevent skin breakdown. Daily baths with gentle soap are encouraged for all patients, and for those with a central venous catheter (CVC), daily chlorhexidine baths should be performed on patients older than 2 months unless contraindicated [34, 90, 101, 102]. Fragrance- and allergen-free emollients should be routinely used on dry or cracked skin, such as with skin GVHD, to promote and maintain skin integrity [34].

Oral Hygiene

Maintaining good oral hygiene is imperative for children who are immune compromised and undergoing cancer therapies [104, 108, 109]. Children should have a dental exam prior to initiation of cancer treatment as recommended by the American Academy of Pediatric Dentistry [108]. Routine mechanical brushing of the teeth, gums, and tongue with a soft toothbrush is recommended in the absence of moderate to severe mucositis regardless of ANC or platelet count [108]. In cases of moderate or severe mucositis, oral care with a super soft brush and normal saline is adequate. Mouth care with saline remains the single evidence-based intervention proven to prevent and improve mucositis [104, 108]. Oral solutions containing chlorhexidine are not effective in preventing mucositis and should be avoided as they have sometimes proven harmful to patients [104, 108]. In the PICU, using sterile water to provide oral care and mechanical debridement (i.e., toothbrushing) is an essential component of ventilator-associated pneumonia (VAP) prevention in intubated patients [63].

Oral fungal infection (i.e., thrush) can develop in the immune-compromised patient. Oral nystatin is ineffective for routine oral fungal/thrush prophylaxis [104, 108]. If prophylaxis is required, specific antifungal medications absorbed by the gastrointestinal tract have proven effective [104, 108]. Decisions regarding oral cavity fungal prophylaxis should be individualized by the patient's care team.

Box 19.5 Summary

PICU nursing education should encourage prioritization of practices that are proven to reduce the risk of infection in the critically ill pediatric immune-compromised hematology/oncology/HCT patient. These include [34, 104, 108, 109]:

- Frequent hand hygiene.
- Keeping doors closed as much as possible to maintain a protective environment and positive pressure when available.
- High-efficiency particulate airflow (HEPA) filtration for allogeneic HCT patients if possible.
- No fresh flowers/plants.
- Educate patients and families; enlist them as champions in infection prevention/control.
- Continue isolation precautions as indicated for known infections, but avoid "reverse precautions" or "protective isolation" (i.e., prophylactic gowns/gloves/masks).
- Screen visitors for infectious diseases and symptoms (i.e., fever, cough, sore throat, rhinorrhea).
- Visitors do not need to wear protective coverings.

Nutritional Considerations

Pediatric hematology/oncology/HCT patients can present with nutritional issues ranging from malnutrition to obesity at the time of their diagnosis, during therapy, and as a survivor. Approximately 8–60% of pediatric cancer patients have cancer-related malnutrition at the time of diagnosis or during therapy [117]. Patients who are malnourished are at risk for treatment-related challenges including increased infection rates, decreased tolerance of therapy, and reduced quality of life [118]. Obesity is a growing concern in the United States and cannot be overlooked when patients are undergoing cancer therapy. Clinical providers are continuing to study and understand the pharmacokinetics of chemotherapy in the obese patient population [118].

At the time of diagnosis and throughout the care continuum, a patient's nutritional status should be continually assessed. Nutritional assessment should include patient history, cancer therapy treatment plan, height, weight, body mass index (BMI) (age >2), dietary history, and albumin/prealbumin [118]. Utilizing growth charts during therapy to plot a patient's height and weight will help providers identify patients at risk. In addition, the Centers for Disease Control and Prevention website has a BMI percentile calculator that can be easily accessed [119]. During cancer therapy, the multidisciplinary team's aim should be to sustain and promote normal growth and development for the pediatric patient population. During phases of acute illness, monitoring weights on a more frequent routine basis may be helpful in understanding fluid balance as well as nutritional status.

Oral intake is the preferred route for nutrition, but is not always feasible for pediatric hematology/oncology/HCT patients, particularly when they are critically ill. Enteral tube feeding is the preferred route when patients have a functioning gastrointestinal tract and has been found to maintain gut integrity and reduce bacterial translocation [118, 120]. Variability in practice exists across and within institutions regarding the use of enteral feedings, despite a growing body of literature to support enteral feedings as the first line of nutritional support [117, 118, 120]. Total parenteral nutrition (TPN) is supported when the gastrointestinal tract is nonfunctional or when patients are completely unable to tolerate oral or enteral feedings [118] but comes at a higher cost and is resource intensive. TPN therapy also places the patient at higher risk for complications. This includes an increased risk of infection secondary to long-term central intravenous (IV) access and potential electrolyte imbalances requiring frequent monitoring [118, 121].

Nurses can support initial and ongoing nutritional assessment for patients and should work closely with registered dietitians to ensure patients receive adequate nutrition (See Table 19.3). Managing treatment-related side effects such as controlling nausea, vomiting, and pain with pharmacologic and non-pharmacologic interventions is essential to promoting oral/enteral feeds whenever possible. Nurses and registered dietitians can provide patients and families with age-appropriate education regarding

Table 19.3 Nursing interventions

• Obtain height and weight on admission, and calculate BMI
• Monitor weight daily
• Record patient's daily intake and output
• Offer frequent small meals/snacks if able to tolerate oral ingestion
• Monitor electrolytes as ordered
• Optimize nausea/vomiting/pain symptom management to promote oral/enteral intake
• Educate and support patient/family: – Nutritional status – Nasogastric/nasojejunal tube – TPN

nutritional supplements, enteral feedings, and the role of TPN if needed. Cancer treatment is a stressful time, and food intake can be a source of tension between parents and their children leading to unpleasant meal times. Providing psychosocial support and guidance around food intake and nutrition is helpful to patients and families [122].

Blood Product Administration

General Concepts

Transfusion of blood and blood products is fundamental in supportive care for hematology/oncology/HCT patients. Myelosuppression is a common side effect of chemotherapy necessitating the need for transfusion therapy. The decision to administer blood products must incorporate evidence-based clinical practice guidelines, as well as careful patient assessment. The need for patient education about the risks and benefits of blood transfusions is essential. There are several blood product manipulations that can be performed prior to transfusion to provide a safer transfusion to this patient population. See Table 19.4 for specifics related to different blood products.

All blood components, including plasma, contain large numbers of leukocytes. Leukocyte reduction, or the removal of white blood cells in blood products, reduces the risk of transfusion-associated reactions such as febrile transfusion reactions, cytomegalovirus (CMV) transmission, and platelet alloimmunization [123]. The advantage of preventing transfusion-transmitted (TT) CMV is well documented. However, the financial cost is controversial [130]. Countries such as Canada have instituted universal leukoreduction (ULR) at collection, in an effort to eliminate transfusion reactions. In 2010, nearly 85% of respondents from children's hospitals in the United States reported that leukocyte reduction of RBCs is performed [131]. Patients with childhood cancer should receive leukocyte-reduced blood products [124].

Irradiation of red blood cells (RBCs) and platelets causes a depletion of T lymphocytes resulting in prevention of transfusion-associated graft-versus-host disease (TA-GVHD). This can occur when donor T lymphocytes replicate and engraft in an immune-compromised recipient [124]. Patients who are immune-compromised should receive irradiated blood products [132].

Washing RBCs uses normal saline to remove remaining plasma. This may be indicated for patients who have experienced severe allergic or anaphylactic transfusion reactions. Washed RBCs have a shelf life of no more than 24 h, and 20% of the red cells may be lost in the process [123].

Nursing Implications for all Blood and Blood Product Transfusions [123, 124, 126, 127, 133]

- Evaluate signs and symptoms closely before decision is made to transfuse the patient.
- Verify order.
- Provide appropriate patient and family education.

Table 19.4 Blood component guide for children with cancer and hematologic diseases and recipients of hematopoietic cell transplants (HCTs)

	Indications	Dose	Administration	Nursing implications
Packed red blood cells (PRBCs) Pathophysiology and etiology: Decreased RBC production due to impaired erythropoiesis or infiltration of marrow by disease Hemolysis, infection, shortened cell survival due to chemotherapy and/or radiation therapy Increased RBC loss as a result of surgery, gastrointestinal bleeding, and/or blood loss through diagnostic phlebotomy	Goal: Increase oxygen-carrying capacity Transfusion guidelines: Patient with a hemoglobin <7 and/or clinically symptomatic Indicated in exchange transfusions for: Sickle cell disease Severe methemoglobinemia Severe hyperbilirubinemia in infants	PRBCs are irradiated and leukocyte reduced 10–15 ml/kg over 3–4 hours Hemoglobin level ↑ approximately 2–3 g/dl for each 10 ml/kg transfused	The patient and donor's blood must be ABO and Rh compatible Blood administration set with in-line filter (170–260 micron) Compatible fluid = isotonic saline (0.9% sodium chloride) Infusion rate dependent on the level of anemia, amount of blood loss, and cardiovascular status **Note**: Slower transfusion rates may be indicated in patients at risk for congestive heart failure	Monitor clinical signs and symptoms of anemia (tachycardia, tachypnea, pallor, headache, lethargy, hypotension, and dizziness) Rapid infusion of RBCs in patients who are chronically transfused or have a hemoglobin level of <5 g/dl should be observed for signs/symptoms of congestive heart failure. Patients with active bleeding or acute blood loss may receive 20 ml/kg, which can be infused rapidly Patients with hyperleukocytosis must be monitored closely if receiving RBCS, as this can further increase blood viscosity

(continued)

Table 19.4 (continued)

	Indications	Dose	Administration	Nursing implications
Platelets Pathophysiology and etiology of thrombocytopenia can be due to: Decreased platelet production due to treatment or infiltration of marrow by disease Increased platelet destruction (sepsis, DIC)	Goal: Prevent or stop bleeding **Prophylactic platelet transfusion guideline**: • Patient thrombocytopenic with a platelet count <10,000 per mm^3 • Patient undergoing lumbar puncture or other invasive procedures >50,000 per mm^3 **Therapeutic platelet transfusion guidelines**: Administered in the presence of bleeding (epistaxis, menstrual bleeding, hemorrhagic cystitis, mucosal bleeding) and before surgery Platelet count, clinical manifestations, and the child's diagnosis and therapy schedule guide the decision to transfuse for treatment of bleeding and/or prophylactic transfusion	Platelets are irradiated, leukocyte reduced Infuse platelets rapidly (30–60 min). The faster they are infused, the more effective the transfusion	ABO/Rh compatibility preferred, not required Cross matching is not needed Leukocyte reduction helps to decrease the rates of platelet alloimmunization, CMV transmission, and febrile transfusion reactions Blood administration set with in-line filter (170–260 micron) Compatible fluid = isotonic saline (0.9% sodium chloride) Irradiate to prevent transfusion-associated-GVHD (TA-GVHD)	Evaluate reasons for thrombocytopenia before transfusion decision is made Determine platelet transfusion thresholds for critically ill children

Granulocytes	Goal: Treatment for patients with prolonged neutropenia with severe infections who are not responding to conventional antimicrobial medications and expected to have delayed bone marrow count recovery Patient with granulocyte dysfunction who has an overwhelming infection	Presently there are no guidelines on the optimal dose, frequency, and duration of granulocyte transfusion exits. The literature suggests: • Typically administered over 1–2 h • Treatment occurring daily x 5 days or as patient condition changes Infuse as soon as possible after collection (ideally within 24 h of collection)	The patient and donor's blood must be ABO compatible and cross matched Irradiate granulocytes to prevent TA-GVHD Do not administer using a leukocyte- depleting filter Blood administration set with in-line filter (170–260 micron)	Premedicate with acetaminophen and antihistamines; consider corticosteroids if reaction is severe Assess for reactions • Chills, febrile reactions, acute respiratory distress (dyspnea, chest pain, hypoxia), rash, graft-versus-host disease (granulocytes) Administration of amphotericin B and granulocytes should be administered at least 4 h apart to decrease the risk of severe pulmonary reactions
Fresh frozen plasma (FFP)	Goal: Replace coagulation factor deficiencies in bleeding or expected bleeding (surgery, disseminated intravascular coagulation (DIC), liver failure) Therapeutic plasma exchange	Typically 10–20 ml/kg, although dose is determined by patient size and clinical condition	Plasma products must be ABO compatible Rh not required Do not need to be leukocyte reduced or irradiated due to WBC destruction during freezing process Blood administration set with in-line filter (170–260 micron)	Monitor coagulation studies If only volume expansion is required, consider administering saline or colloids (albumin) • Plasma can transmit most of the infections present in whole blood and can also cause transfusion reactions

(continued)

Table 19.4 (continued)

	Indications	Dose	Administration	Nursing implications
Cryoprecipitate	Bleeding associated with rare fibrinogen deficiency disorders such as dysfibrinogenemia, hypofibrinogenemia, or afibrinogenemia Factor XIII deficiency with active bleeding and/or invasive procedures	1 unit per 5–10 kg should increase fibrinogen by 60–100 mg/dL Fibrinogen concentration needed to support hemostasis is approximately 50–100 mg/dl	ABO compatibility is not required, but preferred Rh not required Does not need to be leukocyte reduced or irradiated. Blood administration set with in-line filter (170–260 micron)	Factor VIII (hemophilia A) factor XIII, and Von Willebrand factor are found in cryoprecipitate; this should not be used as replacement treatment for patients with these disorders

Adapted from Weinstein [123], Andrews et al. [124], Carson et al. [125], Conte [126], Burke and Salani [127], Slichter [128], Nester et al. [129]

- Obtain blood sample for blood typing and antibody screening per institutional guidelines.
- Confirm consent for blood/blood product has been obtained and is current (per institutional guidelines).
- Assess IV patency.
- Premedicate with acetaminophen and antihistamine if indicated. Consider history of previous reactions.
- Verify specific processing requirements (leukocyte reduced/irradiated); all component and transfusion information remains attached to product.
- Verify patient identification per institutional policy.
- Obtain vital signs prior to and during transfusion per institutional policy.
- Wear personal protective equipment according to standard precautions.
- Use blood administration set with filter (unless otherwise indicated).
- Start transfusion within 30 min after product has left blood bank, and complete infusion within 4 h.
- Only 0.9% normal saline may be infused through the same line when blood products are infusing.
- Monitor for signs and symptoms of potential adverse reactions.
- Document per institutional policy.

Transfusion Complications [123–125, 127, 132–134]

Any blood or blood product transfusion can potentially result in an adverse consequence. Signs and symptoms that can indicate a reaction range from low-grade fever or nausea and vomiting to life-threatening emergencies such as anaphylaxis and shock. Transfusion reactions require immediate recognition, laboratory evaluation, and clinical management.

Treatment of transfusion reactions includes:

- Stop the transfusion.
- Maintain IV patency. Keep line open with 0.9% normal saline.
- Support the airway.
- Notify MD/NP/PA.
- Assess vital signs.
- Activate emergency response if needed.
- Administer medications (epinephrine, diphenhydramine, hydrocortisone, if applicable).
- Follow institutional policies for blood transfusion reaction.
  - Notify blood bank.
  - Recheck the blood bag for compatibility and patient identification.
  - Return untransfused blood and IV tubing to blood bank for further evaluation (per institutional policy).
  - Obtain blood and urine samples as required.
  - Document reaction in patient's medical record.

Acute Hemolytic Transfusion Reactions

Acute hemolytic transfusion reactions (AHTRs) occur as a result of ABO incompatibility or mismatch between patient and donor [123]. This results in hemolysis of the donor red blood cells. Signs and symptoms which can occur almost immediately [134] include fever spike of >1 °C (2 °F), chills, nausea, anxiety, abdominal, chest, flank or back pain, hemoglobinuria, disseminated intravascular coagulation (DIC), renal failure, hypotension, shock, and death. The amount of incompatible blood infused is related to the severity of the symptoms [133, 134].

If AHTR is suspected:

- Stop the infusion.
- Administer vigorous hydration to maintain urine output (UOP) >1 cc/kg/h.
- Possible diuretic administration to enhance UOP.
- Symptom management (treat DIC, vasopressors if needed).
- Consider transfer to higher level of care if indicated.

Febrile Nonhemolytic Transfusion Reactions

The most common type of transfusion reaction is a febrile nonhemolytic transfusion reaction (FNHTR), characterized by fever, frequently accompanied by chills, as well as increased respiratory rate, and potentially hypotension. FNHTR should be considered with a fever spike of >1 °C (2 °F) from baseline within 2 h of start of transfusion and not associated with any other cause [123]. Any fever occurring during a transfusion needs to be evaluated, particularly in neutropenic patients. The occurrence of FNHTRs is diminished with leukocyte reduction [132]. The management is symptomatic. Patients may benefit from premedication with acetaminophen or antihistamines before future transfusions [134].

Allergic Reactions

An allergic reaction occurs when the recipient experiences a hypersensitivity reaction to allergens in the donor's blood. Severe allergic reactions (i.e., anaphylaxis) tend to occur within minutes of the infusion starting, but patients can develop a less severe reaction during, or several hours following, the completion of the transfusion. Clinical signs include urticaria, pruritus, irritability, vomiting, wheezing, swollen lips, anxiety, hypotension, and/or progression to anaphylaxis [123, 132–134].

Allergic reactions to blood transfusions can vary in severity. Mild reactions typically begin during the first hour of the infusion, and anaphylaxis occurs during the first few minutes. With complaints of itch or rash, the transfusion must be stopped immediately, IV status maintained, and an antihistamine administered [133]. In the absence of fever and resolution of symptoms, the infusion should be re-started and the patient should be closely monitored [134]. Systemic symptoms indicate a more serious allergic reaction. Emergency management including oxygen, epinephrine, steroids, or fluid boluses may be needed if life-threatening symptoms of anaphylaxis develop [123, 127, 133]. Any allergic reaction needs to be reported to the blood bank.

Transfusion-Related Acute Lung Injury

Transfusion-related acute lung injury (TRALI) is a rare, but potentially life-threatening, transfusion complication. TRALI is the leading cause of transfusion-related mortality in the United States [124]. Critically ill immune-compromised patients are at particular risk for TRALI due to their transfusion requirements and risk factors from their underlying malignancies. The development of TRALI is typically characterized by an acute onset of non-cardiogenic pulmonary edema with hypoxemia, dyspnea, fever, chills, and hypotension [124, 133, 134]. Hypertension occurring before the hypotension is not uncommon [134]. Clinical symptoms of TRALI develop within 1 to 2 h after completion of transfusion and can be observed within 6 h following transfusion of any plasma-containing components (whole blood, red blood cells, platelets, cryoprecipitate, and fresh frozen plasma) [134].

The development of TRALI is hypothesized to occur in the context of two independent clinical events [135]. The first event occurs because of recipient risk factors such as sepsis, recent surgery, cytokine administration, and need for transfusions [124, 133, 134]. These risk factors increase the propensity for neutrophil activation in the pulmonary endothelium, which leads to the sequestration of neutrophils in the lungs [134]. The second clinical event occurs with the administration of blood products that contain anti-HLA antibodies and biologic response modifiers (BMRs). This process triggers the already activated neutrophils in the lungs. This activation results in endothelial damage, capillary leakage, and subsequent development of pulmonary edema [134].

If TRALI is suspected during the transfusion, the transfusion is immediately stopped. The treatment of TRALI is supportive care that often necessitates patients receiving supplemental oxygen and potentially mechanical ventilator support. The ensuing hypotension will have minimal if any response to fluid resuscitation. Vasopressors may be required [124, 134]. The majority of patients who develop TRALI will have symptom resolution within 48–96 h. As TRALI is a diagnosis of exclusion, there are clear predictors, but diagnosis is made primarily on clinical and radiological findings [124, 134, 136]. The American Association of Blood Banks (AABB) standards now prohibit the production of plasma from women with a history of pregnancy unless they have been screened and found negative for anti-HLA antibodies [137].

Transfusion-Associated Graft-Versus-Host Disease

Transfusion-associated graft-versus-host disease (TA-GVHD) occurs when a severely immune-compromised patient receives a transfusion from a HLA-similar donor (typically a family member). Given their immune-compromised state, the recipient is unable to identify the donor cells as foreign, and the immune system does not destroy the donor lymphocytes as it typically would. As a result, an immune reaction is mounted by the donor lymphocytes against the recipient (graft vs. host). Symptoms of TA-GVHD are similar to GVHD (rash, diarrhea, maculopapular rash) except pancytopenia develops and death almost always occurs [124].

Prevention of TA-GVHD can be prevented by administering only irradiated cellular components (RBCs and platelets) particularly to patients treated with high-dose, intensive chemotherapy such as recipients of hematopoietic cell transplants (HCT) and patients treated with purine analog drugs (e.g., fludarabine) [123, 124, 127].

Transfusion-Associated Circulatory Overload (TACO)

Rapid administration of fluid/volume may be required to maintain or recover a patient's hemodynamic function. This may include rapid infusion of blood products for a patient in shock, with frank bleeding, or in DIC. The nurse should understand the risk of circulatory overload potentially associated with transfusion of any blood products, particularly with RBCs, plasma products, and 25% albumin. Patients who are chronically transfused or have a hemoglobin level of <5 g/dl, infants, young children, and older adults (especially with pre-existing cardiac or pulmonary comorbidities) are at greatest risk. Symptoms such as dyspnea, cough, tachycardia (or gallop), hypertension, and severe headache can develop suddenly and quickly. Early recognition is imperative to treat circulatory overload. If symptoms do occur, consult with the PICU care team, stop the transfusion, transition to a crystalloid fluid if additional volume repletion is required, optimize oxgyenation, elevate the head of bed, and administer diuretics if indicated [123, 127].

Chemotherapy and Biotherapy Safety Considerations in the Pediatric Intensive Care Unit

Oncologic emergencies may develop when patients are first diagnosed, as a result of therapy or if there is disease relapse. The severity of symptoms and patient acuity may require care in a PICU and the need for administration and management of chemotherapeutic and biotherapeutic agents in this setting. A fundamental aspect in the care of children, adolescents, and young adults with cancer is the safe administration and management of chemotherapeutic and biotherapeutic agents. These agents have a narrow therapeutic window. This means there is a thin margin of difference between the desired dose and doses that are too high and cause devastating side effects, or too low to be beneficial [138].

The complexity of chemotherapy/biotherapy administration and management, as well as the risk of adverse effects, makes it imperative to develop and adhere to consistent, evidence-based standards to ensure safe patient and staff outcomes. All members of the healthcare team share responsibility in assuring patient safety by adhering to error prevention strategies throughout chemotherapy/biotherapy ordering, prescribing, preparation, administration, and management. This process is challenged when patients need to receive chemotherapy/biotherapy outside of an area where chemotherapy is typically administered, such as in the PICU.

In 2016, chemotherapy safety administration standards were updated to include pediatric specific safety considerations. These standards are divided into four domains and describe the minimum expectations for ordering, preparing, administering, and monitoring chemotherapy/biotherapy across treatment locations [139, 140]. The complete standards are available here: https://www.ons.org/sites/default/files/2016%20ASCO_ONS%20Chemo%20Standards.

These standards should be reviewed in full and incorporated as the basis for policy and procedure development to promote an environment of safety. The fundamental concepts pertinent to pediatric oncology patients in the intensive care unit are highlighted.

Domain 1: Creating a Safe Environment – Staffing and General Policy
Nurses must be knowledgeable about treatment regimens and chemotherapeutic agents, together with the indications for each agent, safe dosage, the route of administration, side effects, proper administration, and safe handling techniques, in addition to patient response and family education. In any setting where chemotherapy/biotherapy is administered, comprehensive education, preparation, and training are required for all nurses who administer and/or monitor systemic cancer therapies and should be reassessed annually. This standard further specifies the education program needs to be "comprehensive," such as the Association of Pediatric Hematology/Oncology Nurses (APHON) Chemotherapy and Biotherapy Provider course and the Provider Renewal program. This education is essential to ensure safe care for the patient and the individual administering the agents [141]. This standard also reviews the necessary elements to determine if a patient has met specific criteria to receive chemotherapy/biotherapy.

Another important element in creating a safe environment is incorporating a system for safe patient handoff between all sites of care. This includes timely, accurate information about a patient's plan of care, the treatment being administered, including chemotherapy and supportive care schedule, and specific monitoring for any safety concerns. Identified error prevention strategies and the commitment from individuals and organizations to practice these can reduce the potential for patient harm [142, 143].

Domain 2: Treatment Planning, Patient Consent, and Education
Principles in this section emphasize the standardization of obtaining and documenting the patient and guardian's chemotherapy treatment consent and assent. The consent includes information about the patient's diagnosis, goals of treatment (cure, disease, prolong life, or reduce symptoms), treatment options and duration, as well as common and rare side effects. An assessment of health literacy is essential in order to offer education based on learning needs, abilities, and readiness to learn.

Domain 3: Ordering, Preparing, Dispensing, and Administering Chemotherapy

The role of the PICU nurses in chemotherapy administration is dependent on the policies of individual hospitals. Institutions determine what deems an individual to be chemotherapy competent as there is no nationally recognized certification for chemotherapy/biotherapy administration [141]. Cancer therapy involves drugs that are considered by the Institute of Safe Medication Practices (ISMP) to be "high alert medications", meaning if any error occurs, even when used as intended, these drugs are more apt to cause patient harm [144]. Key points in this section include the need for the provider to communicate to other team members and the caregiver, risks of the therapy, as well as document any treatment changes, including dose modifications. If the patient is to receive chemotherapy, it is essential that this information is communicated and coordinated with the bedside nurse in the PICU. Before each agent is administered, at least two practitioners determined by the institution to administer chemotherapy verify the following (Fig. 19.5):

It is essential that the nurses and physicians caring for hematology/oncology/HCT patients are aware of the chemotherapeutic and biotherapeutic agents that are part of their patient's treatment plan. This information can be found in various locations such as the institution's formulary, within a patient's treatment plan, or in consultation with the oncology team. Important nursing considerations include [145]:

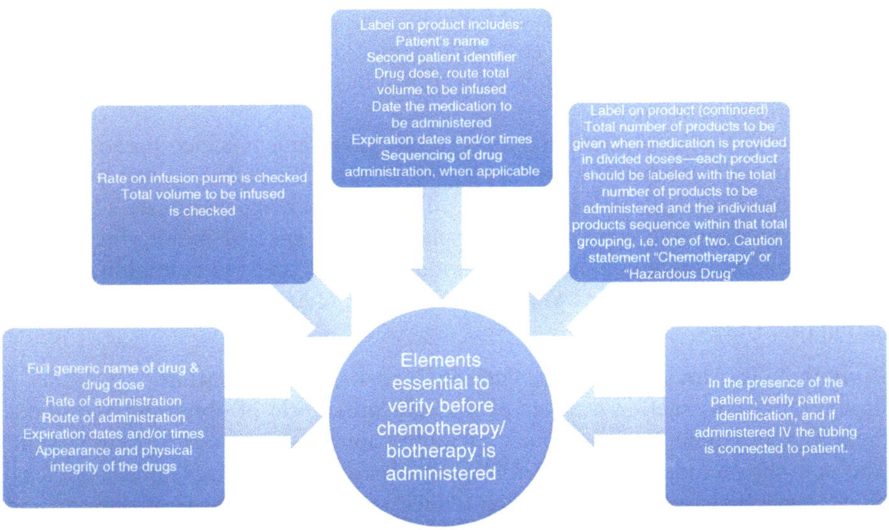

Fig. 19.5 Essential components to review prior to administration of chemotherapy/biotherapy

- The emetogenic potential of the agent being administered
- Specific hydration guidelines
- Any agents that need to be protected from the light
- Pertinent laboratory monitoring
- Timing of administration

Box 19.6 Nursing Pearls
- Verbal orders are not accepted on chemotherapy orders.
- Vinca alkaloids (e.g., vincristine and vinblastine) are *fatal* if administered intrathecally.
- National safety measures include:
  - Vinca alkaloids to be administered via a small-volume "mini" bag.
  - Chemotherapy agents administered via the central nervous system are delivered from pharmacy to the procedural area.

Domain 4: Monitoring After Chemotherapy Is Administered Including Adherence, Toxicity, and Complications
Participation in clinical trials is a driving force in the development of new treatments for pediatric cancers. Approximately 60% of children, adolescent, and young adults are enrolled in a clinical trial [146]. Compliance with the protocol and its treatment delivery is paramount in obtaining the clinical data that will demonstrate the safety and efficacy of the new treatment/therapy. To assure this compliance, the bedside nurse must receive education and demonstrate an understanding of the treatment administration, adhering to the protocol monitoring schedule and observation of adverse effects. Education specific to all aspects of chemotherapy/biotherapy administration and monitoring is essential to ensure a safe level of care for patients receiving the agents, as well as for the nurses who are administering the drugs. Additional support must be provided to the PICU staff to ensure continuity when the patient is off the general hematology/oncology/HCT unit. These standards should be used as a guide to develop policies and procedures to support and promote a safe environment for patients.

Promoting Comfort: Population-Specific Considerations in Managing Pain and Agitation and Providing Sedation

Pain and Agitation Assessment

Critically ill pediatric immune-compromised hematology/oncology/HCT patients require thorough and frequent pain assessments at regular intervals. This assessment includes location, quality, and severity of pain using a developmentally appropriate, validated pain scale. Commonly used self-report scales in pediatrics include (1) the FACES pain scale for children ages 4 years and older [147, 148]; (2) the numeric rating scale (NRS), for children older than 8 years [149]; and (3) the visual analog scale (VAS) for children older than 8 years [150]. Self-report is often viewed as the gold standard for pain assessment in children who are verbally communicative and are developmentally able to comprehend the scale [151]. In children less than 3 years and those with limited verbal or cognitive skills, observation of behaviors and caregiver reports are valid assessment strategies [151]. The FLACC pain scale is a behavior observation tool used for children less than 7 years of age [152, 153]. It has also been shown to have some application in children with cognitive impairment [154] and in older critically ill children [155] with limited ability to communicate. For a child with developmental delays or limited verbal communication, an individualized pain scale should be created in collaboration with a primary caretaker based on behavioral signs that indicate pain [75, 151, 156, 157].

Also important to consider is how pain is assessed in children whose ability to verbally communicate is hindered [75, 158]. This includes patients receiving long-term sedation and/or chemical paralysis to tolerate noxious life-sustaining treatments such as invasive mechanical ventilation via endotracheal tube or those with debilitating acute or chronic diseases. Instead of relying solely on self-report tools, clinicians need to integrate clinical indicators of pain and discomfort such as vital sign (VS) changes, dilated pupillary exam, and behavioral cues such as grimacing/facial expression, tearing/crying, or thrashing [75, 158] with validated pain scales.

For patients receiving continuous sedation, their level of comfort and sedation must be continually assessed in addition to pain. A number of validated sedation scales exist to guide titration of sedative and pain medications in the PICU. The COMFORT and State Behavioral Scales (SBS) are two of the most clinically useful tools in pediatrics [158]. The SBS is a validated tool for intubated patients less than 18 years old which assigns a degree of sedation ranging from unresponsive (−3) to agitated (+2) with zero (0) being awake and calm. It cannot be applied to patients who are chemically paralyzed [159]. The COMFORT scale was originally proposed in 1992 as a means of assessing pain- and non-pain-related distress in mechanically ventilated patients [160] and has been further validated in multiple studies [158]. The COMFORT-behavioral (Comfort-B) scale [161] was created to adjust for the possibility that the physiologic parameters of the original COMFORT tool may be affected by the patient's disease state or side effects of treatment [158, 162]. It should be noted that while both the SBS and COMFORT scales assess sedation, they are limited in that they do not provide a pain-specific assessment for procedural or intermittent pain episodes [158, 162]. Pain should continue to be evaluated with an appropriate pain scale for the patient.

Principles of Treatment

Children with cancer have many causes of pain including the disease itself, treatment side effects, and/or diagnostic and therapeutic procedures [74]. A stepwise approach should be applied to pain management [151]. Interventions should correlate with the severity of pain beginning with enteral non-opioid medications for mild pain, escalating to enteral opioid medications for moderate pain and further to intravenous (IV) opioid medications for moderate to severe pain or when unable to tolerate enteral medications [151]. Attempts should always be made to understand the cause of the child's pain and minimize any contributing factors [75, 164, 165].

Patients may require ongoing sedation in order to tolerate noxious stimuli. Sedation involves intermittent and/or continuous infusions, most commonly of opioids and benzodiazepines, with or without other adjunct medications [75, 166]. It is essential to ensure pain continues to be adequately treated once sedation is administered [165]. Chronic pain medications or their IV equivalent must also be continued in order to avoid withdrawal symptoms and to ensure that pain does not become a contributing factor to preventing adequate sedation [165].

Given the potential for adverse effects from long-term analgesia and sedation in children, ensuring optimal comfort at the lowest possible doses is a nursing priority [167, 168]. Nurse-driven sedation protocols in the PICU show promise in achieving optimal sedation levels while reducing potential complications. Further research is needed to establish a new standard of care [167–169].

Adequately managing pain throughout a child's treatment course is essential to long-term physical and mental health/recovery. The consequence of untreated pain is now better understood. While it used to be thought that children would become more tolerant to pain the more they were exposed, the reverse is actually true. Instead, repeated exposure to inadequately treated pain results in multiple adverse effects including hyperactive stress responses, increased anxiety, fear, and hopelessness and may result in chronic pain syndromes [75, 76, 170]. Unmanaged needle pain can lead to phobia and anxiety as well as more significant pain responses to future treatments [171].

Pharmacologic Interventions

Non-opioid Analgesics

Critically ill children frequently use non-opioid medications such as acetaminophen and nonsteroidal anti-inflammatory drugs (NSAIDs) to optimize pain management [75, 162, 170]. However, these medications must be used judiciously in patients with primary hematology/oncology diagnoses and/or undergoing HCT. Both categories of medications can mask fever, which may be the only early sign of infection in an immune-compromised child. Obscuring this red-flag finding by administering these medications without routinely assessing for fever can have ominous implications. There should be a discussion with the provider prior to their administration and prophylactic dosing. NSAIDs present additional challenges to children with thrombocytopenia as they act as platelet inhibitors [165]. NSAIDs can also be nephrotoxic [162] and therefore raise concern as children receiving chemotherapy are at risk for renal insufficiency and acute kidney injury [172]. Ketorolac (Toradol®) is an NSAID commonly used in the PICU to help manage short-term, moderately severe acute pain [162] as it is the only NSAID available to administer via IV or IM route and is useful for children who are NPO. If a child is permitted to receive NSAIDs, the nurse should monitor for decreased platelet counts, abnormal coagulation studies, and any clinical signs of increased bleeding such frank bleeding or occult blood in stool, urine, or gastric output.

Other adjuvant medication categories include corticosteroids (e.g., dexamethasone), anticonvulsants (e.g., gabapentin), anxiolytics (e.g., diazepam), antidepressants (e.g., amitriptyline), or others (e.g., clonidine) [164]. Dexamethasone can be useful in relieving chemotherapy-induced nausea or increased intracranial pressure, such as from a brain tumor. However, caution should be exercised if dexamethasone is prescribed for comfort as many children undergoing cancer therapy are already receiving corticosteroids as a part of their disease treatment plan. Additional dosing may cause safety risks and/or protocol violations.

Dexmedetomidine (Precedex®) is a medication growing in popularity in the PICU given both its analgesic and sedative properties [173, 174]. Dexmedetomidine is an $alpha_2$ adrenergic agonist that promotes sedation without causing significant respiratory depression, potentially allowing for a reduction in the use of other sedatives [173–175]. It is typically administered as a continuous infusion with or without a loading dose [175]. The patient requires careful monitoring for potential side effects, particularly bradycardia, hypotension, and hypertension [175]. Many institutions require a patient to be in an intensive care or procedural unit during administration [162, 173, 175].

Low-dose ketamine infusions for pain management are being explored with great success [176–180]. Ketamine is a powerful N-methyl-D-aspartate (NMDA) receptor antagonist and dissociative anesthetic. When used in certain doses and in conjunction with lower-dose opioids, it may help to decrease opioid usage and subsequent tolerance [176, 177]. Institutional policies dictate if low-dose ketamine infusions are administered on a regular unit or require admission to the PICU for monitoring [75, 178].

Opioid Therapy for Pain

Pain treatment for children with cancer is complex, but the foundation of management for moderate to severe pain in pediatric cancer continues to be opioid medications [74]. Children with hematologic/oncologic diagnoses or those undergoing HCT may have previous exposure to opioids prior to PICU admission. Healthcare providers must have a thorough knowledge of the child's history of opioid use to determine if the patient is naïve or at risk for physiologic tolerance due to past exposure [165, 170].

Tolerance Children with chronic pain, such as patients with sickle cell disease (SCD), may have a history of opioid use requiring doses significantly higher than standard starting dosing to achieve effective pain management [179]. Acute pain, if coupled with the underlying chronic pain, may necessitate a dose escalation and/or the addition of another pain medication.

Children requiring critical care may necessitate prolonged periods of sedation to tolerate invasive mechanical ventilation [75, 158, 159, 165]. Over time, these patients can become more tolerant of the infusions, requiring close monitoring for diminishing efficacy of their current dosing. Opioid doses should be titrated to the patient's response, and thus there is no maximum daily dose.

In cases where the patient's pain is not adequately controlled with opioids, adjuvant medications such as dexmedetomidine (Precedex®), ketamine, barbiturates (e.g., pentobarbital), or intermittent methadone and lorazepam may become necessary additions to the patient's care plan [75].

Side Effects Respiratory depression is the most serious potential side effect of opioid therapy. However, when dosed appropriately and according to physiologic need, patients typically tolerate these medications well. The PICU is an ideal location to provide intravenous opioid therapy if the patient's pain necessitates it, given the availability of continuous monitoring and assessment [165]. Children who are opioid-naïve should be monitored closely with initial doses. If given for sedation purposes to a child who is intubated, respiratory depression may be an expected and tolerable side effect.

Certain patients have other risk factors that make them more vulnerable to even mild respiratory depression related to opioid use. For example, a patient may present with a tumor burden that compromises their airway, such as a mediastinal mass secondary to T-cell acute lymphoblastic leukemia or a solid tumor near or around the upper or lower airways. Once given an opioid, the child may experience mild to moderate subsequent respiratory depression and/or drowsiness that may further compromise the child's ability to maintain their natural airway. While receiving opioid or sedative therapy, patients with these or similar risk factors may benefit from close monitoring in an ICU to allow for rapid intervention if needed.

Mucositis is a common complication of chemotherapy and often identified as a significant source of pain [74]. Mucositis results in swelling, increased mucous production, and potential bleeding in a patient's airway. Moderate to severe mucositis often requires opioid therapy to effectively mitigate the pain. Typically, this treatment complication can be managed with routine care and monitoring in the general ward. However, in cases of particularly severe mucositis, a child's airway may become swollen and narrowed as a result. This is particularly plausible in infants as their normal airway diameter is notably smaller than an older child's. In extreme cases, intubation may be required to support the child through the healing course to ensure patient safety while allowing for adequate pain control.

Constipation can be a side effect of opioid therapy as well as cancer treatment regimens. Preemptive, preventative, anticipatory management is necessary. Children should be initiated early on a prophylactic bowel regimen [181, 182]. Methylnaltrexone is an opioid receptor antagonist that is used to treat opioid-induced constipation (OIC). It is the only medication currently available to treat OIC that can be administered by intravenous (IV) or subcutaneous (SQ) routes. Thus, it can be given to patients who are NPO without risk of counteracting the efficacy of the opioids in reducing pain [182–184].

Methadone is a long-acting opioid used to treat chronic, complex, and neuropathic pain and pain uncontrolled by other high-dose opioids or in order to wean patients off of opioid therapy [185, 186]. Methadone has been shown to cause corrected QT (QTc) prolongation on electrocardiogram in adults that, if left untreated, can lead to lethal arrhythmias. However, it is generally well tolerated in pediatrics and, infrequently, if at all, associated with QTc prolongation in children less than 18 years of age being treated for cancer [186, 187]. If experienced, it is typically in the setting of comorbid conditions [187].

Organ Dysfunction Children undergoing treatment for hematologic/oncologic diagnoses are at risk for hepatic and renal insufficiency. The nurse should monitor for acute changes in sedation status that are inconsistent with patient history and may be symptoms of medication buildup, or "stacking," from reduced hepatic and renal clearance. Laboratory values measuring hepatic and renal dysfunction should also be monitored. In addition to oversedation, buildup of by-product from some opioids and benzodiazepines can have neurotoxic effects such as myoclonus [165].

Withdrawal Management As patients recover from critical illness, technological support is weaned and, with it, the patient's sedation infusions. When administered for more than 5 days, opioids, benzodiazepines and barbiturates are known to have high risk for withdrawal symptoms with rapid discontinuation [75]. Dexmedetomidine (Precedex®) given over prolonged periods has also been shown to cause signs and symptoms of withdrawal that may look slightly different than those associated with opioids and benzodiazepines [188]. Given the risk of prolonged periods of invasive mechanical ventilation, the hematology/oncology/HCT patient should be monitored closely for signs and symptoms of withdrawal at regular intervals using a validated scale, such as the Withdrawal Assessment Tool – Version 1 (WAT-1) [189]. Nurses are instrumental in facilitating optimal and efficient weaning schedules. A baseline score is established at the start of the weaning process, and as weaning commences, a clear goal score should be established among the multidisciplinary care team. Families should be educated about what signs and symptoms of withdrawal to look for, and reassured that some amount of withdrawal may be unavoidable and safely tolerated. Reassure families that the child will return to their baseline. Consulting with pain treatment experts is often helpful in ensuring a safe and efficient weaning plan.

Non-pharmacologic Interventions

While pharmacologic intervention is an integral part of pain and comfort management, non-pharmacologic interventions can be powerful additions to a child's regimen. Preparing a child physically, psychologically and emotionally for painful procedures is essential in helping to minimize anxiety and reduce pain. Child life specialists can be instrumental in facilitating preparation and distraction when appropriate. Hypnosis, aromatherapy, Reiki, massage, acupuncture, relaxation techniques, and behavioral therapy are all feasible options and can be offered to reduce a patient's pain [75, 170].

Anxiety is not an uncommon experience for hematology/oncology/HCT patients. It is important to decipher what symptom(s) are afflicting the patient and utilize the most appropriate therapies. Partnering with psychosocial clinicians and child life specialists can be useful in developing alternative non-pharmacological approaches to care [75, 76, 170].

Managing Procedure-Related Pain

Achieving optimal sedation during invasive procedures is important to reduce anxiety and eliminate emotional and physical trauma related to procedural pain. Children undergoing cancer therapy often cite invasive procedures as some of the most distressing experiences they endure. Recommendations are to use appropriate procedural sedation when general anesthesia is not necessary or plausible [71, 75, 170].

While in the PICU, the patient may require procedures as a part of their diagnostic workup and/or treatment [190], such as a lumbar puncture or placement of a peritoneal drain for ascites related to sinusoidal obstruction syndrome (SOS). In the PICU, these children are often intubated and can safely and easily receive additional sedation to facilitate procedures. Sometimes, however, these children may not be intubated yet still require sedation to undergo a procedure. When a child is breathing spontaneously while maintaining a natural airway and receives sedation, it is known as "procedural sedation." Procedural sedation is defined as altering the patient's level of consciousness to allow for procedures to safely and comfortably take place [190–192]. A patient can be sedated along a continuum of sedation from minimal to moderate to deep sedation before finally progressing to general anesthesia [191, 192]. Use of moderate sedation can promote patient cooperation and safety during a procedure, as well as reduce anxiety and fear for future interventions [162, 190–193].

Nursing Implications and Monitoring

Procedural sedation monitoring should follow national guidelines consistent for all patients [190, 192, 193]:

- Ensure consent is obtained
- Ensure procedure is explained to the patient and family
- Assess for aspiration risk and last known oral/enteral intake. Ensure NPO status according to established institutional policies in accordance with national guidelines
- Ensure emergency equipment is readily available
- Obtain baseline vital signs
- Place patient on continuous cardiorespiratory monitoring including HR, RR, SpO2, and end-tidal CO_2 ($ETCO_2$) (if available) for duration of the procedure
- A goal sedation level is to be determined by the licensed provider prior to beginning of procedure
- Perform a time-out
- Document vital signs according to institutional policy
- Document a recovery score

Any provider who is caring for a patient receiving procedural sedation must be aware of the appropriate reversal agents for commonly used sedation medications. *Naloxone (Narcan)* is the reversal agent for opioids, and *flumazenil* is the reversal agent for benzodiazepines [192, 193]. These medications should be readily available in the location where the patient is undergoing the procedure [193]. If reversal agents are administered for respiratory depression, the patient needs to be monitored for a sufficient amount of time following administration to ensure complete recovery of adequate spontaneous breathing [192–194]. It is imperative to understand the risk of recurrent respiratory depression following administration of a reversal agents. Doses of one or both reversal agents may need to be repeated if the patient has recurrent episodes of respiratory depression due to the short half-life of reversal agents as compared to the longer half-life of sedatives. The patient should also be closely monitored for rebound pain, tachycardia, hypertension, and flash pulmonary edema with the administration of reversal agents [193, 194]. In addition, reversal of benzodiazepines should be avoided in children with a history of seizures or long-term benzodiazepine use as this may put the child at a higher risk for seizure activity.

Providing developmentally appropriate psychological preparation and support is paramount to minimizing distress from pain in children during painful procedures by optimizing their coping abilities. Medical play can be helpful, as can involving parents or family members when appropriate and in accordance with their wishes. Utilizing non-threatening language provides rationale(s) for any procedure(s) and accurate information about what to expect. Distraction, self-talk, guided imagery, and behavioral coping strategies may all be helpful in supporting patients through procedures [195].

End-of-Life (EOL) Symptom Management Considerations

Successful pain management at the end of life (EOL) may require a more intensive approach when children are critically ill. The fear of, or actual, inadequate pain control can put unnecessary stress on patients and families, further intensifying their pain [196]. When formulating a multidisciplinary plan for EOL symptom management, the following factors must be considered:

1. Explore and understand family goals and wishes so that medical EOL strategies can be aligned accordingly, focusing on [196–198]:
   - Relief of suffering.
   - Assuring the child is as comfortable as possible in terms of pain, agitation, and anxiety.
   - Having the child be awake and able to relate whenever possible. Depending on the child's clinical status, this may not always be feasible, but must be addressed and considered. If it is not possible, rationale should be explained to the family and alternative forms of memory making offered such as photographs, hand/foot prints, or story-telling and reminiscing. Families should still be encouraged to speak to the child and reassured that their presence is meaningful.
2. Pain is a "crisis" and must be treated as quickly as possible.
   - Avoid promising the child can be "pain-free."
   - Continually assess pain, and ensure that all attempts are made to relieve pain and suffering.
3. Consider previous pain management history and patient's response, including:
   - Opioid and sedative history and potential for high tolerance levels
   - Other agents previously administered to the patient and his/her response to them

4. Evaluate current pain management regimen, including:
   - Total hourly doses of opioids, benzodiazepines, and other agents being administered by both continuous infusions and scheduled intermittent doses
   - Current PRN bolus doses
   - Duration of treatment on current sedation infusions
5. Assure family of careful titration of comfort medications. Educate the family that this will likely include continuous infusion(s) of pain medication with bolus doses available for optimal symptom management.
6. For children in the PICU, invite the primary hematology/oncology/HCT team members to be a part of EOL discussions and planning. This can facilitate more effective and efficient clarification of goals of care and promote feelings of trust and collaboration.
7. Perform a huddle daily, or more frequently as needed, with the multidisciplinary team *and* then the family. This is essential to ensure a cohesive and clear plan to promote symptom relief at end-of-life. When the mode of death will be a terminal wean of life-sustaining technologies, a huddle should be held just prior to the event, including contingency planning for comfort medications in the event non-traditional strategies are unsuccessful [199].
8. Discuss with the family the role of palliative sedation if symptoms cannot be controlled with typical comfort medications.
   - Medications such as propofol and/or ketamine are considered for children at end of life with intractable pain or incredibly high tolerance levels to traditional medications to relieve their burden of pain [198–200].

Emphasize the power of presence for a child facing EOL [196–198]. Often, caregivers simply need reminding and reinforcing of the importance of "being with" their child; holding, reading to, playing music, sharing memories, and praying are tools that may bring calmness and relieve existential as well as physical pain. Utilize all members (child life specialists, chaplaincy, psychosocial clinicians) of the multidisciplinary team in caring for family. Each member can bring a unique contribution to patients and families through this difficult time [196–198]. *See* Chap. 17: *Psychosocial Aspects of Care and Palliative Care* for a comprehensive and multidisciplinary discussion of EOL considerations.

Developing a Collaborative Interdisciplinary Care Model

Introduction

Advances in supportive and intensive care have improved the outcomes of critically ill pediatric immune-compromised hematology/oncology/HCT patients. However, the transition of care from the inpatient unit to the PICU can be challenging for patients, families, and healthcare providers. The complexity of this patient population's physical and emotional care needs demands a free flow of information both across disciplines and across specialties. Thus, interdisciplinary communication and collaboration remain the foundation for successful care of these patients in the PICU [201–203]. Throughout the patient's care continuum, these principles should be applied on both the individual and institutional levels.

Optimizing Transfer of Care

Pediatric hematology/oncology/HCT patients are transferred to the PICU for a multitude of reasons that can be classified into one of the three categories: planned admissions, episodes of acute decompensation, and chronically critically ill (see section "Framework for Categorizing Patients"). Regardless of the reason for a patient's PICU admission, it is essential to ensure there is comprehensive communication between the various members of the patient's care team.

Criteria for Escalation in Level of Care

Variability exists among institutions about when a patient should be transferred to a PICU for a higher level of care [204, 205]. Individual institutional policies and procedures determine these criteria and are based on a multitude of factors including staffing, nursing education and expertise, patient monitoring capabilities, and availability of supportive care measures [204, 206]. When a child develops a condition that is immediately life-threatening or potentially life-threatening, or there is an acute change in their stability, transfer to the PICU is necessary [204]. Each institution should have policies in place, including physiologic parameters, to distinguish what the acceptable level of care for the general ward is and what care must be provided in the PICU [204, 207]. As pediatric hematology/oncology/HCT care advances with newer therapies such as immunotherapy, the location of care for the patient may become less clear. The pediatric oncology nurse has the most knowledge and expertise about the patient's disease and therapy, but the potential risks of the therapy may be so significant that care is best provided in the intensive care unit. Approaches to these types of scenarios are ideally addressed in advance of administering a new or potentially high-risk therapy with patient safety being the main priority.

Whenever possible, the care for a critically ill pediatric hematology/oncology/HCT patient should be provided in an intensive care unit specific to pediatrics. Outcomes are better when this specialized patient population is cared for in a PICU versus an adult ICU [208].

Early Warning Systems

Early intervention and transfer to the PICU for the pediatric hematology/oncology/HCT patient population with respiratory failure and shock have been shown to improve outcomes [5, 6, 11, 202, 209]. Additionally, early initiation of noninvasive ventilation (NIV) has shown promise in avoiding endotracheal intubation for immune-compromised children who develop acute respiratory distress syndrome (ARDS) [210, 211]. However, success depends on early referral and treatment.

Institutions should consider implementing an early warning scoring tool to aid in identifying those patients at risk for potential clinical deterioration. Algorithms that guide care decisions based upon the patient's score should accompany these tools. Identifying patients who are clinically deteriorating and transferring them to an intensive care unit prior to a cardiopulmonary arrest is a priority for acute care institutions [212, 213]. Approximately 8.5–14% of all cardiopulmonary arrests in hospitalized pediatric patients occur in non-intensive care unit settings, and outcomes for these patients are poor [213]. Upon review of patient events, there are often physiologic changes and/or abnormalities documented within 8–12 h of the patient's deterioration [214]. Staff members from inpatient units have concentrated on developing effective and efficient bedside assessment tools that provide an early warning for patient deterioration [214].

Early warning scores were first implemented in the adult population in the late 1990s and found to be helpful in identifying patients at risk for clinical deterioration [215]. An early warning tool specific to pediatric patients was developed in 2005 known as the Pediatric Early Warning Score (PEWS) [216]. PEWS was based on three clinical components: the patient's behavior, cardiovascular status, and respiratory status. PEWS calculated an aggregate score ranging from 0 to 13 [217].

Since the development and implementation of early warning scoring systems, several institutions have modified the tools. There are four validated tools in pediatrics: the PEW tool, the PEW System Score, the Bedside PEW System Score [218], and the Children's Hospital Early Warning System (CHEWS) [219]. Each uses a set of variables that are summed to give the patient a score, which is then applied to an intervention algorithm identifying tiers of monitoring and a set of responses [218–220]. The identified score and interventions support communication between the nurse and provider, allow for timely ICU consultation, and prompt management of a deteriorating patient [219, 220]. These tools have been validated in the pediatric hematology/oncology/HCT patient and are appropriate and essential to use for this population [213, 220].

Box 19.7 Considerations for Patient Transfer to a Higher Level of Care

- Hemodynamic instability
- Vasopressor support
- Escalating respiratory needs
- Increasing pain/comfort management
- Acute changes in mental or neurological status
- Frequent lab monitoring requiring electrolyte replacement
- Medication administration traditionally restricted outside of an intensive care unit
- A feeling something is wrong with the patient

Standardized Exchange of Patient Information

A leading cause of medical errors and patient harm is poor communication among healthcare professionals [221]. Any time a patient's care is transferred, it is essential that there is clear communication between the clinical care providers. This exchange of information may be known as patient handoff, sign-out, patient report, or shift report. The handoff period is a high-risk event and errors that have occurred during this critical exchange of information have been linked to sentinel patient events [222]. Standardizing the communication of information during patient handoff can help mitigate the risk for loss of information. One method is to utilize a structured handoff tool, such as I-PASS. I-PASS is a mnemonic that stands for *I*llness severity, *P*atient summary, *A*ction list, *S*ituation awareness and contingency planning, and *S*ynthesis by the person receiving the information [223]. See Fig. 19.6 for an example.

In addition to the exchange of clinical information, it is also essential for the pediatric hematology/oncology/HCT patient population to communicate non-physiologic information, including input from psychosocial clinicians and child life therapists. This information may be overlooked, particularly if the transfer of care was unexpected or urgent. Time is needed to understand a patient's prior history, their family unit, and other pertinent psychosocial history. This information is necessary to support the patient and family's transition to a higher level of care and promote their adaptation to the new, potentially unfamiliar setting. During urgent transfers, this information may need to be communicated at a later date/time versus in the acute moment of transfer in order to expedite the transition. Complete exchange of all pertinent information requires ongoing communication between the multidisciplinary PICU and hematology/oncology/HCT teams.

Collaboration Throughout the PICU Admission

Promoting Continuity

Communication and collaboration are two of the six tenets that contribute to a healthy work environment [224]. The PICU bedside nurses provide the majority of the hands-on care to the patient and are responsible for the continuous monitoring of a patient's condition. A collaborative relationship with clear and respectful communication between the nurse and interdisciplinary team is essential to maintaining a healthy work environment (HWE) [201, 206, 225]. A HWE has been shown to positively impact patient outcomes.

Hull and O'Rourke (2007) propose five opportunities to improve the continuity of care provided for hematology/oncology/HCT patients in the ICU [206]:

1. Relationship building: Use of open communication to develop a trusting relationship between both nursing specialties.
2. Collaborative relationships: Highlights the importance of a free-flow exchange of information between the two units.

I-PASS Handoff:
Transfer from HCT Unit to Pediatric Intensive Care Unit (PICU)

Patient name: ______________________________ MRN: __________________

Age: _____ Weight: _____ kg Allergies: ________________________________

I	**Illness Severity**	• Diagnosis/Type of HCT/Transplant Day (ex: ALL, Allogeneic MURD, Day +40) • ICU Admission Route: Code, ICU Stat, ICU Consult, Post Operative, Other • Assessment of Current Condition: Stable/Unstable; Mild/Moderate/Severe Distress • CHEWS (or other early warning system) score

P	**Patient Summary**	• Reason for admission to PICU (e.g. respiratory distress/failure, hypotension, sepsis, altered mental status/seizures, other)
		• Significant events leading to transfer
		• PMH/Co-Morbidities
		• Review of Systems
		  o Neurological and Pain/Comfort
		  o Respiratory
		  o Cardiovascular
		    ▪ Total Fluid Resuscitation Given: ______________ ml/kg
		    ▪ Vasopressor Requirements
		    ▪ Access: ______________________________
		  o Infectious disease
		    ▪ Pending Cultures/Last Blood Cultures
		    ▪ Current Antibiotics
		    ▪ Precautions
		  o Graft/Hematology;
		    ▪ Immunosuppression: ______________
		    ▪ Designated Lumen: ______________
		    ▪ Transfusion parameters: ____________
		    ▪ Current Blood Counts
		    ▪ Pre-Medications for Blood Pruducts?
		  o GI/GU
		    ▪ Anti-Emetic Plan; Next Dose Due
		  o FEN
		    ▪ Nutrition
		    ▪ Fluid Balance
		    ▪ Weight Trend? Last Weight: __________
		  o Skin
		  o Musculoskeletal
		• Psychosocial Needs
		• Other Special Care Needs

A	**Action List**	• Plan for Time of Transfer
		• Patient Needs that Require Follow Up:
		  o Cultures/Labs to be Sent
		  o Outstanding/Overdue/Newly Ordered Medications
		  o Fluid Boluses/Blood Products to be given
		  o Diagnostic Tests to be done (i.e. CXR, ultrasound)
		  o Upcoming Procedures

S	**Situational Awareness**	Red flag issues (i.e. decompensating hemodynamics; outstanding chemotherapy/biotherapy; pre-medication for blood products, SOS Watch etc.)
S	**Synthesis (by receiver)**	Close loop communication: PICU Receiving RN synthesizes and summarizes the patient's status and plan to HCT RN. Provide opportunity to ask clarifying questions.

Abbreviations: HCT = hematopoietic cell transplant; PICU = pediatric intensive care unit; MRN = medical record number; ALL = acute lymphoblastic leukemia; CHEWS = Children's Hospital Early Warning System; PMH = past medical history; MURD = matched unrelated donor; GI/GU = gastrointestinal/genitourinary; FEN = fluid, electrolytes and nutrition; CXR = chest xray; SOS = sinusoidal obstruction syndrome

Fig. 19.6 Example of I-PASS tool. (Adapted from Boston Children's Hospital)

3. Continuing education: Successful care of the patient is reliant on ongoing and real-time education between the two nursing specialties.
4. Scheduled reviews: Multidisciplinary collaborative efforts should be evaluated on a regular basis to assess impact on patient outcomes.
5. Enhanced baccalaureate curriculum: Critical care and hematology/oncology education and experience should be offered in the undergraduate, nursing curriculum.

These principles should be applied throughout a patient's course in the PICU. Specific interventions and practices should be tailored to each institution. Successful and ongoing collaboration between specialties is essential. Often, additional consulting teams are involved, such as infectious disease specialists, pain treatment experts, or nephrologists, in addition to the hematology/oncologist/HCT team(s). One technique to optimize communication is adopting a joint rounding practice. This involves collecting, at a minimum, the PICU bedside nurse, intensive care providers, and representative(s) from the hematology/oncology/HCT team, for daily or twice daily rounds. A nursing liaison from the hematology/oncology/HCT team should also be included [206]. This may be the patient's primary nurse from the ward, a charge nurse, advanced practice nurse, or nurse in a designated liaison position [206]. Additional consulting services may also be invited. It is important to schedule a mutually agreed-upon time and for both teams to be mindful and respectful of the other's time. A commitment from both the PICU and hematology/oncology/HCT team must be made to adhere to the agreed-upon schedule and optimize success.

Nursing Education

Exposure to pediatric hematology/oncology and pediatric critical care is limited if not absent in the traditional baccalaureate nursing curriculum. Nursing orientation in the critical care environment is multifaceted and must cover a wide range of diseases. It is important that staff have access to resources such as clinical nurse specialists, unit educators, and current policies and procedures. Critical care staff educators need to work closely with their hematology/oncology/HCT colleagues to develop a comprehensive education plan for orientation as well as on-demand, as therapies are constantly evolving. Opportunities such as scheduled education days and just-in-time education at the point of care provide great opportunities for learning [201, 206]. Institutions should also consider providing cross-training or shadowing experiences for nurses across the units [201, 203, 226, 227].

Providing Patient- and Family-Centered Care (PFCC)

Overview of Patient- and Family-Centered Care (PFCC)

The concept and practice of family-centered care came about in the latter half of the twentieth century as awareness increased regarding the positive impact of families and the role families play in their child's development [228]. A patient- and family-centered care approach is based on a shared relationship between the patient, family, and clinician that values the importance of the family and their role in ensuring overall patient health and well-being [228]. A patient- and family-centered care model includes sharing of information in a clear, complete, and honest manner with minimal medical terminology; mutual listening; and shared decision-making when appropriate [229]. Individualization of the patient- and family-centered approach should be based on the unique needs of each patient and family [229]. Nurses play a key role in information sharing, often translating the messages from the physician groups [201, 227].

Box 19.8 Examples of Patient/Family Inclusion

- Allowing the parent to stay overnight at the bedside
- Including patient (age appropriate) and/or caregivers to participate in daily rounds
- Actively involving the patient/parent in decision-making and goal setting
- Allowing the patient/parent to participate and assist with care when appropriate

Engaging the Psychosocial Care Team

Providing care to pediatric hematology/oncology/HCT patients requires a team approach, inclusive of various disciplines. Social workers, psychologists, psychiatrists, chaplaincy, and child life specialists each bring a unique set of knowledge and are able to support patients and families in a multitude of ways. Patients and families struggle when they have a sick child in the ICU and need emotional support. Social workers are able to provide emotional support, as well as help to facilitate communication among the patient, family, and clinical team [230]. Hospital chaplaincy should be available to support patients' and families' spiritual and religious needs. Child life specialists are integral team members and ensure the developmental needs of patients are being met with age-appropriate play and environmental accomodations. They are also a great resource in supporting parents and staff in ensuring communication to patients is provided at an appropriate-age level.

Combating Compassion Fatigue, Burnout, and Distress in the Bedside Nurse

Background: Resilience in the Face of Compassion Fatigue, Burnout, and Distress

Caring for pediatric hematology/oncology/HCT patients, particularly when they are critically ill, can be physically and cognitively demanding, stressful, and sad [227, 231–235] but also greatly fulfilling [232, 235, 236]. Nurses who work with this patient population find great meaning and satisfaction in their work [232, 234, 236–238]. Often, meaning is derived from the relationships built with their patients and families [232, 238, 239] in combination with the nurse's personal and professional development [238]. Finding meaning in their work is an essential component to nurses experiencing satisfaction in their job [232, 236, 238–240]. PICU nurses report similar feelings of satisfaction [235] and value the therapeutic relationships built with patients and families. In both fields, nurses describe the privilege and honor of being present to support the child and their family through their experience undergoing cancer therapy and/or critical illness [232, 236, 238]. These positive effects contribute to two important concepts: *compassion satisfaction* [241] and *compassionate presence* [232] (See Box 19.9). These effects promote resilience and serve as the positive balance to negative experiences that can contribute to burnout and compassion fatigue [240, 242]. Resilience appears to strengthen over time, as a nurse gains more experience in the profession [235].

Box 19.9 Definitions

- *Compassion satisfaction* describes the joy and meaning one gains from competently providing care to another person. This helps to balance, or combat, compassion fatigue [235, 241].
- *Compassionate presence* is achieved when the nurse is present, physically and existentially, with a patient and family, to freely provide care while sharing in their experience with total compassion. During the experience, the nurse shares in the entirety of the patient/family experience, including the pain, sorrow, and resulting emotions, thereby achieving fulfillment and enlightenment, in spite of the pain and suffering being witnessed [232].
- *Compassion fatigue*, sometimes called "secondary traumatization," is the emotional toll taken by caring for people who are suffering or undergoing a traumatic experience(s) [243]. Symptoms of compassion fatigue can include, but are not limited to [244]:

• Mood swings	• Loss of objectivity	• Increased use of sick days
• Restlessness	• Memory issues	• Headaches, digestive problems (nausea, vomiting, diarrhea), muscle tension, altered sleep patterns, chest pain/palpitations, fatigue
• Irritability	• Poor concentration, focus, and judgment	

• Oversensitivity	• Avoidance or dread of working with certain patients	
• Anxiety	• Decreased ability to feel empathy toward patients	
• Excessive use of substances: nicotine, alcohol, illicit drugs	• Lack of joyfulness	
• Depression		
• Anger and resentment		

- *Burnout* is a constellation of symptoms representing a care provider's (i.e., nurse's) disengagement from their work, often driving them to depart a once beloved and meaningful profession. Three of the most common signs are emotional exhaustion, depersonalization, and a decreased sense of personal accomplishment [240].
- *Moral distress* is a complex phenomenon with a multitude of environment-specific nuances. Generally speaking, however, *moral distress* refers to the scenario of an individual making a judgment as to what the morally right thing is to do yet perceives institutional, social, or procedural factors that prevent them from proceeding with the right thing and instead force them to engage in perceived moral wrongdoing [245–247]. This scenario leads to moral distress within the provider.
- *Distress* is a general term that is different than moral distress. Distress simply implies discomfort and concern over a hard situation [248].

Nurses frequently bear witness to suffering [232, 235, 239]. Nurses who work with chronically ill hematology/oncology/HCT patients, particularly those who are dying, report struggling to complete the complex and numerous tasks required to provide ongoing physical and emotional care while simultaneously preparing for the patient's decline or death [227, 232, 249]. Often, they report feeling too busy with tasks to perform the emotional and spiritual support they recognize patients and families need [227, 238, 250]. Similar phenomena are described in pediatric intensive care [227, 251]. In addition, caring for patients with complex, chronic illnesses and those at the end of their life has been identified as a risk factor for moral distress [240, 252, 253].

This multifaceted stress experienced by nurses can contribute to the development of *burnout* and *compassion fatigue*. Both compassion fatigue and burnout are well-known concepts to pediatric hematology/oncology/HCT and pediatric critical care and can have a detrimental effect on nursing job satisfaction, staff turnover rates, and cost and subsequently negatively impact patient outcomes [254].

Moral distress is a separate but related phenomenon. Moral distress is a well-documented risk factor to developing burnout and compassion fatigue in nurses and is also implicated in negatively impacting patient outcomes [240, 253, 254]. Maintaining a HWE, however, is shown to *lower* the levels of moral distress [224, 253]. Nurses who care for the pediatric critically ill hematology/oncology patient are at particularly high risk to experience moral distress and develop burnout and compassion fatigue [231, 239].

Raising Awareness

In order to combat compassion fatigue, burnout, and moral distress, both the individual(s) experiencing the phenomena and their nurse leaders must identify their presence [243, 247, 252, 255]. A number of different tools are available to assist in screening for these effects. Ongoing research is working to validate these scales for nurses working in pediatrics (Table 19.5).

Table 19.5 Assorted selection of screening tools for compassion fatigue, burnout, and moral distress

Tool	What it measures	Description
a. Professional Quality of Life (ProQOL) Elements Theory and Measurement for Compassion Satisfaction and Compassion Fatigue, Burnout, Secondary Traumatic Stress. Vicarious Traumatization and Vicarious Transformation [241]: http://proqol.org/Home_Page.php	Measures compassion satisfaction and compassion fatigue	A comprehensive 30-item self-report questionnaire that can be administered to an individual or group
b. Moral Distress Thermometer [256]	Moral distress	Simple self-report tool with visual and numeric cues to quantify the amount of moral distress being experienced
c. The Maslach Burnout Inventory (MBI) [257]	Aspects of burnout/compassion fatigue (e.g., emotional exhaustion, depersonalization, and personal accomplishment)	Self-administered 22-question survey
d. Moral Distress Scale – Revised (MDS-R) [258]	Frequency and intensity of moral distress	Self-administered 21-item questionnaire

Strategies to Combat Compassion Fatigue, Burnout, and Moral Distress

Guiding Principles

Suggested strategies to combat compassion fatigue, burnout, and all facets of distress are presented below. The following guiding principles apply to the planning of any intervention(s):

1. It is imperative to recognize signs and symptoms of moral distress early in order to implement effective change [252].
2. Self-awareness is important, and the ability to identify signs of burnout and compassion fatigue is essential [255].
3. Successful interventions *require* proactive institutional support from the senior leadership level [239, 252].
4. The American Association of Critical Care Nurses (AACN) Healthy Work Environment initiative offers helpful guiding principles when framing strategies [224].
5. Fostering meaning making and compassion satisfaction can balance out compassion fatigue, burnout, and moral distress [232, 240, 242].
6. No single intervention can or will be successful in isolation. Successful management of staff distress relies on multidimensional and varied strategies tailored to the staff and their specific patient population and needs [237].
7. Reassessment of interventions is required and should be followed to evaluate the efficacy of implemented programs [231].

Suggested Strategies

1. Provide opportunities for nurses to develop moral resilience by promoting self-awareness and self-regulatory strategies, supporting nurses in voicing concerns professionally and confidently, searching for meaning in spite of sadness, fostering therapeutic relationships, and promoting ethics involvement [259].
2. Apply AACN's "the four A's": *Ask* – *Affirm* – *Assess* – *Act* [260].
    - *Ask* – Is moral distress being experienced?
    - *Affirm* – Confirm with colleagues that moral distress is present.
    - *Assess* – Evaluate the type of distress, obstacles to intervention, and preparation to intervene.
    - *Act* – Develop possible intervention for the bedside nurse to use.
3. Consider setting "boundaries" between nurse and patients/families. "Boundaries" carry a wide variety of meaning for all nurses [233]. While some describe it negatively as "disconnecting" [233], others find that it helps to maintain a sense of being a nursing "professional," without closing off [233, 238].
4. Encourage and implement creative methods of meaningful recognition [261]. This may include:
    - The Daisy Award®
    - Unit-based recognitions/awards

- Peer-to-peer acknowledgments
- Personalized "thank you" notes

5. Offer mindfulness training [237].
6. Provide workshops in relaxation, self-care, and stress reduction [239].
7. Seek early ethics consults [252, 262]. Consider providing educational programs designed to develop nurses' competency [259, 263].
8. Refer nurses to institution-based clinician support programs.
9. Ensure opportunities to talk about episodes of moral distress in order to debrief and learn from them [262, 264].
10. Provide updates to PICU staff about patient success stories at discharge and beyond [227].
11. Consider early palliative care team involvement to support not only the family but the nurses at the bedside [233].
12. Foster healthy coping skills [238]:

    (a) Allow for humor.
    (b) Share experiences and feelings with others who are familiar with and/or understand your situation/experiences [233].
    (c) Maintain a life outside of the hospital to balance the experiences at work.

Acknowledgments We are grateful to the following individuals for the insight, guidance, and knowledge they shared with us throughout the development of this chapter: Robyn Blacken, Peggy Brill-Conway, Celeste Chandonnet, Janet Duncan, Colleen Gerrity, Steven Sloan, and Lindsay Weir.

References

1. Kendall S. Witnessing tragedy: nurses' perceptions of caring for patients with cancer. Int J Nurs Pract. 2007;13(2):111–20. https://doi.org/10.1111/j.1440-172X.2007.00615.x.
2. Howlader N, Noone AM, Krapcho M, Miller D, Bishop K, Kosary CL, Yu M, Ruhl J, Tatalovich Z, Mariotto A, Lewis DR, Chen HS, Feuer EJ, Cronin KA, editors. SEER cancer statistics review, 1975–2014. Bethesda, MD: National Cancer Institute. https://seer.cancer.gov/csr/1975_2014/, based on November 2016 SEER data submission, posted to the SEER web site, April 2017
3. National Cancer Institute. Cancer in children and adolescents. In: Childhood cancers. 2017. https://www.cancer.gov/types/childhood-cancers/child-adolescent-cancers-fact-sheet
4. Rosenman MB, Vik T, Hui SL, Breitfeld PP. Hospital resource utilization in childhood cancer. J Pediatr Hematol Oncol. 2005;27(6):295–300.
5. Dalton HJ, Slonim AD, Pollack MM. Multicenter outcome of pediatric oncology patients requiring intensive care. Pediatr Hematol Oncol. 2003;20:643–9.
6. Dursun O, Hazar V, Karasu GT, Uygun V, Tosun O, Yesilipek A. Prognostic factors in pediatric cancer patients admitted to the pediatric intensive care unit. J Pediatr Hematol Oncol. 2009;31:481–4.
7. Heying R, Schneider DT, Körholz D, Stannigel H, Lemburg P, Göbel U. Efficacy and outcome of intensive care in pediatric oncologic patients. Crit Care Med. 2001;29(12):2276–80. https://doi.org/10.1097/00003246-200112000-00007.

8. Maude S, Fitzgerald J, Fisher B, Li Y, Huang YS, Aplenc R, et al. Outcome of pediatric acute myeloid leukemia patients receiving intensive care in the United States. Pediatr Crit Care Med. 2014;15:112–20. https://doi.org/10.1097/PCC.0000000000000042.
9. Balit CR, Horan R, Dorofaeff T, Frndova H, Doyle J, Cox PN. Pediatric hematopoietic stem cell transplant and intensive care: have things changed? Pediatr Crit Care Med. 2016;17(3):e109–16. https://doi.org/10.1097/PCC.0000000000000607.
10. Chima RS, Daniels RC, Kim M, Li D, Wheeler DS, Davies SM, Jodele S. Improved outcomes for stem cell transplant recipients requiring pediatric intensive care. Pediatr Crit Care Med. 2012;12(6):e336–42. https://doi.org/10.1097/PCC.0b013e318253c945.
11. Hallahan AR, Shaw PJ, Rowell G, et al. Improved outcomes of children with malignancy admitted to a pediatric intensive care unit. Crit Care Med. 2000;28(11):3718–21. http://www.ncbi.nlm.nih.gov/pubmed/11098979
12. Duncan CN, Lehmann L, Cheifetz IM, Greathouse K, Haight AE, Hall MW, McArthur J, et al. Clinical outcomes of children receiving intensive cardiopulmonary support during hematopoietic stem cell transplant. Pediatr Crit Care Med. 2013;14(3):261–7. https://doi.org/10.1097/PCC.0b013e3182720601.
13. Herring RA, Hesselgrave J, Norville R, Madsen LB. Toxicity and symptom management. In: Kline N, editor. The pediatric chemotherapy and biotherapy curriculum. 3rd ed. Chicago: APHON; 2011. p. 105–51.
14. Murphy G. The technology-dependent child at home part 1: in whose best interest? Paediatr Nurs. 2001;13:14–8.
15. Wagner J, Power E, Fox H. Technology-dependent children: hospital versus home care. 1987. Congress of the United States: Office of Technology Assessment.
16. National Marrow Donor Program, a contractor for the C.W. Bill Young Cell Transplantation Program operated through the U.S. Department of Health and Human Services, Health Resources and Services Administration, Healthcare Systems Bureau. Growth in number of registry transplants. 2013. http://bloodcell.transplant.hrsa.gov/images/transplants_growth_lg.gif. Accessed 18 Jan 2018.
17. U.S. National Library of Medicine. Mucopolysaccharidosis type I. https://ghr.nlm.nih.gov/condition/mucopolysaccharidosis-type-i# (2012). Accessed 1 Jan 2018.
18. Douglas IS, Schmidt GA, Hall JB. Acute-on-chronic respiratory failure. In: Hall JB, Schmidt GA, Wood LDH, editors. Principles of critical care. 3rd ed. New York: The McGraw-Hill Companies; 2005.
19. Chima RS, Abulebda K, Jodele S. Advances in critical care of the pediatric hematopoietic stem cell transplant patient. Pediatr Clin of North Am. 2013;60(3):689–707. https://doi.org/10.1016/j.pcl.2013.02.007.
20. Zinter MS, Dvorak CC, Spicer A, Cowan MJ, Sapru A. New insights into multicenter PICU mortality among pediatric hematopoietic stem cell transplant patients. Crit Care Med. 2015;43:1986–94. https://doi.org/10.1097/CCM.0000000000001085.
21. Shannon E. How can oncology and ICU nurses work together to treat critically ill patients with cancer? ONS Voice. 2017;32(7):19.
22. Lo B, Jonsen AR. Clinical decisions to limit treatment. Ann Intern Med. 1980;93:764.
23. Schuster DP, Marion JM. Precedents for meaningful recovery during treatment in a medical intensive care unit: outcome in patients with hematologic malignancy. Am J Med. 1983;75:402.
24. Schapira DV, Studnicki J, Bradham DB, Wolff P, Anne JA. Intensive care, survival, and expense of treating critically ill cancer patients. JAMA. 1993;269:783–6.
25. Lloyd-Thomas ART, Dhaliwal HS, Lister TA. Intensive therapy for life-threatening complications of hematologic malignancy. Intens Care Med. 1986;12:317–24.
26. Torrecilla C, Corte's JL, Chamorro C. Prognostic assessment of the acute complications of bone marrow transplantation requiring intensive therapy. Intens Care Med. 1988;14:393–8.
27. Butt W, Barker G, Walker C, et al. Outcome of children with hematologic malignancy who are admitted to an intensive care unit. Crit Care Med. 1988;16:761–4.

28. DeNardo SJ, Oye RK, Bellamy PE. Efficacy of intensive care for bone marrow transplant patients with respiratory failure. Crit Care Med. 1989;17:4–6.
29. Sivan Y, Schwartz PH, Schonfeld T, et al. Outcome of oncology patients in the pediatric intensive care unit. Intensive Care Med. 1991;17:11–5.
30. Todd K, Wiley F, Landaw E, et al. Survival outcome among 54 intubated pediatric bone marrow transplant patients. Crit Care Med. 1994;22:171–6.
31. Nichols DG, Walker LK, Wingard JR, et al. Predictors of acute respiratory failure after bone marrow transplantation in children. Crit Care Med. 1994;22:1485–91.
32. Adamson P. Developing drugs for pediatric malignancies. Clin Adv Hematol Oncol. 2011;11:227–9.
33. Baggot C. Neutropenia. In: Kline NE, editor. Essentials of pediatric hematology/oncology nursing: a core curriculum. 4th ed. Glenview: Association of Pediatric Hematology/Oncology Nurses; 2014. p. 95–6.
34. Tomblyn M, Chiller T, Einsele H, Gress R, Sepkowitz K, Storek J, Wingard JR, Young JH, Boeckh MA. Guidelines for preventing infectious complications among hematopoietic cell transplantation recipients: a global perspective. Biol Blood Marrow Transplant. 2009;15:1143–238. https://doi.org/10.1016/j.bbmt.2009.06.019.
35. Lo E, Nicolle L, Classen D, Arias KM, Podgorny K, Anderson DJ, et al. Strategies to prevent catheter-associated urinary tract infections in acute care hospitals. Infect Control Hosp Epidemiol. 2008;29(Suppl 1):S41–50. https://doi.org/10.1086/591066.
36. Gould CV, Umscheid CA, Agarwal RK, Kuntz G, Pegues DA, the Healthcare Infection Control Practices Advisory Committee (HICPAC). Guideline for prevention of catheter-associated urinary tract infections 2009: Centers for Disease Control; 2017. https://www.cdc.gov/infectioncontrol/pdf/guidelines/cauti-guidelines.pdf
37. Joint Commission. National patient safety goals effective January 1, 2013. 2012. http://www.jointcommission.org/assets/1/18/NPSG_Chapter_Jan2013_HAP.pdf. Accessed 1 Dec 2017.
38. Scott DR. The direct medical costs of healthcare-associated infections in U.S. hospitals and the benefits of prevention: Centers for Disease Control; 2009. https://www.cdc.gov/HAI/pdfs/hai/Scott_CostPaper.pdf
39. McCoy C, Paredes M, Allen S, Blackey J, Nielsen C, Paluzzi A, Jonas B, Radovich P. Catheter-associated urinary tract infections: implementing a protocol to decrease incidence in oncology populations. Clin J Oncol Nurs. 2017;21:460–5. https://doi.org/10.1188/17.CJON.460-465.
40. Riachy E, Krauel L, Rich B, McEvoy M, Honeyman J, La Quaglia M, et al. Risk factors and predictors of severity score and complications of pediatric hemorrhagic cystitis. J Urol. 2014;191(1):186–92. https://doi.org/10.1016/j.juro.2013.08.007.
41. Angus DC, Linde-Zwirble WT, Lidicker J, Clermont G, Carcillo J, Pinsky MR. Epidemiology of severe sepsis in the United States: analysis of incidence, outcome, and associated costs of care. Crit Care Med. 2001;29(7):1303–10.
42. Centers for Disease Control. Preventing infections in cancer patients. 2017. https://www.cdc.gov/cancer/preventinfections/. Accessed 1 Jan 2018.
43. Novosad SA, Sapiano MR, Grigg C, et al. Vital signs: epidemiology of sepsis: prevalence of health care factors and opportunities for prevention. MMWR Morb Mortal Wkly Rep. 2016;65:864–9. https://doi.org/10.15585/mmwr.mm6533e1.
44. Lindell R, Gertz S, Rowan C, McArthur J, Beske F, Fitzgerald J, et al. High levels of morbidity and mortality among pediatric hematopoietic cell transplant recipients with severe sepsis: insights from the Sepsis PRevalence, OUtcomes, and Therapies International Point Prevalence Study. Pediatr Crit Care Med. 2017;18(12):1114–25. https://doi.org/10.1097/PCC.0000000000001338.
45. Singer K, Subbaiah P, Hutchinson R, Odetola F, Shanley TP. Clinical course of sepsis in children with acute leukemia admitted to the pediatric intensive care unit. Pediatr Crit Care Med. 2011;12:649–54. https://doi.org/10.1097/PCC.0b013e31821927f1.

46. Goldstein B, Giroir B, Randolph A, et al. International Consensus Conference on Pediatric Sepsis. International pediatric sepsis consensus conference: definitions for sepsis and organ dysfunction in pediatrics. Pediatr Crit Care Med. 2005;6:2–8. https://doi.org/10.1097/01.PCC.0000149131.72248.E6.
47. Simmons ML, Durham SH, Carter CW. Pharmacological management of pediatric patients with sepsis. AACN Adv Crit Care. 2012;23(4):437–48. https://doi.org/10.1097/NCI.0b013e31826ddccd.
48. Weiss SL, Fitzgerald JC, Pappachan J, Wheeler D, Jaramillo-Bustamante JC, Salloo A, Singhi SC, Erickson S, Roy JA, Bush JL, Nadkarni VM, Thomas NJ. Sepsis Prevalence, Outcomes, and Therapies (SPROUT) study investigators and Pediatric Acute Lung Injury and Sepsis Investigators (PALISI) network. Global epidemiology of pediatric severe sepsis: the sepsis prevalence, outcomes, and therapies study. Am J Respir Crit Care Med. 2015;191(10):1147–57.
49. Burke ML, Salani D. Hematologic and oncologic emergencies requiring critical care. In: Hazinski MF, editor. Nursing care of the critically ill child. 3rd ed. St. Louis: Elsevier; 2013. p. 825–50.
50. Norville R, Staton S. Hematopoietic stem cell transplantation. In: Kline N, editor. Essentials of pediatric hematology/oncology nursing: a core curriculum. 4th ed. Chicago: APHON; 2014. p. 160–80.
51. Secola R, Reid D. Oncologic emergencies. In: Kline N, editor. Essentials of pediatric hematology/oncology nursing: a core curriculum. 4th ed. Chicago: APHON; 2014. p. 252–9.
52. de Caen AR, Berg MD, Chameides L, et al. Pediatric Advanced Life Support 2015 American Heart Association guidelines update for cardiopulmonary resuscitation and emergency care. Pediatrics. 2015;136:S176. https://doi.org/10.1542/peds.2015-3373F.
53. Society of Critical Care Medicine. History: Surviving Sepsis Campaign. 2016. http://survivingsepsis.org/About-SSC/Pages/History.aspx
54. Davis A, Carcillo J, Aneja R, Deymann A, Lin J, Zuckerberg A, et al. American College of Critical Care Medicine clinical practice parameters for hemodynamic support of pediatric and neonatal septic shock. Crit Care Med. 2017;45(6):1061–93. https://doi.org/10.1097/PCC.0000000000001259.
55. Balamuth F, Alpern E, Abbadessa M, Hayes K, Schast A, Zorc J, et al. Improving recognition of pediatric severe sepsis in the emergency department: contributions of a vital sign-based electronic alert and bedside clinician identification. Ann Emerg Med. 2017;70(6):759.e2–68.e2. https://doi.org/10.1016/j.annemergmed.2017.03.019.
56. Freifeld AG, Bow EJ, Sepkowitz KA, Boeckh MJ, Ito JI, Mullen CA, et al. Clinical practice guideline for the use of antimicrobial agents in neutropenic patients with cancer: 2010 update by the Infectious Diseases Society of America. Clin Infect Dis. 2011:52(4). https://doi.org/10.1093/cid/cir073.
57. Rhodes A, Evans LE, Alhazzani W, Levy MM, Antonelli M, Ferrer R, et al. Surviving sepsis campaign: international guidelines for management of sepsis and septic shock: 2016. Intensive Care Med. 2017;43(3):304–77. https://doi.org/10.1007/s00134-017-4683-6.
58. Ventura AM, Shieh HH, Bousso A, et al. Double-blind prospective randomized controlled trial of dopamine versus epinephrine as first-line vasoactive drugs in pediatric septic shock. Crit Care Med. 2015;43:2292–302. https://doi.org/10.1097/CCM.0000000000001260.
59. Louden DT, Rutman LE. Inotropic therapy for sepsis. Pediatr Emerg Care. 2018;34(2):132–5. https://doi.org/10.1097/PEC.0000000000001399.
60. Tamburro RF, Barfield RC, Shaffer ML, Rajasekaran S, Woodard P, Morrison RR, et al. Changes in outcomes (1996–2004) for pediatric oncology and hematopoietic stem cell transplant patients requiring invasive mechanical ventilation. Pediatr Crit Care Med. 2008;9(3):270–7. https://doi.org/10.1097/PCC.0b013e31816c7260.
61. Curley MAQ, Thompson JE. Oxygenation and ventilation. In: Curley M, Moloney-Harmon PA, editors. Critical care nursing of infants and children. Philadelphia: W. B. Saunders Company; 2001. p. 233–308.

62. Grant MJC, Curley MAQ. Pulmonary critical care problems. In: Curley M, Moloney-Harmon PA, editors. Critical care nursing of infants and children. Philadelphia: W. B. Saunders Company; 2001. p. 655–94.
63. Cocoros NM, Kleinman K, Priebe GP, Lee G, et al. Ventilator-associated events in neonates and children – a new paradigm. Crit Care Med. 2016;44:14–22. https://doi.org/10.1097/CCM.0000000000001372.
64. Klompas M, Branson R, Eichenwald E, Greene L, Howell M, Berenholtz S, et al. Strategies to prevent ventilator-associated pneumonia in acute care hospitals: 2014 update. Infect Control Hosp Epidemiol. 2014;35:915–36. https://doi.org/10.1086/677144.
65. The Acute Respiratory Distress Syndrome Network. Ventilation with lower tidal volumes as compared with traditional tidal volumes for acute lung injury and the acute respiratory distress syndrome. N Engl J Med. 2000;342:1301–8. https://doi.org/10.1056/NEJM200005043421801.
66. Pediatric Acute Lung Injury Consensus Conference. Pediatric acute respiratory distress syndrome: consensus recommendations from the. Pediatr Crit Care Med. 2015;16:428–39. https://doi.org/10.1097/PCC.0000000000000350.
67. Fuchs H, Rossmann N, Schmid MB, Hoenig M, Thome U, Mayer B, et al. Permissive hypercapnia for severe acute respiratory distress syndrome in immunocompromised children: a single center experience. PLoS One. 12(6):e0179974. https://doi.org/10.1371/journal.pone.0179974.
68. Kluge S, Baumann HJ, Nierhaus A, Kröger N, Meyer A, Kreymann G. Safety of percutaneous dilational tracheostomy in hematopoietic stem cell transplantation recipients requiring long-term mechanical ventilation. J Crit Care. 2008;23:394–8. https://doi.org/10.1016/j.jcrc.2007.05.001.
69. Gordin A, Netzer A, Joachims HZ, Golz A. Percutaneous tracheotomy in bone marrow transplant patients with severe thrombocytopenia. J Otolaryngol Head Neck Surg. 2005;133:377–80. https://doi.org/10.1016/j.otohns.2005.06.004.
70. Elbahlawan L, Rains KJ, Stokes DC. Respiratory care considerations in the childhood cancer patient. Respir Care [Internet]. 2017;62(6):765–75. Available from: http://rc.rcjournal.com/lookup/doi/10.4187/respcare.05223
71. Hertzog JH, Dalton HJ, Anderson BD, Shad AT, Gootenberg JE, Hauser GJ. Prospective evaluation of propofol anesthesia in the pediatric intensive care unit for elective oncology procedures in ambulatory and hospitalized children. Pediatrics. 2000;106(4):742–7.
72. Holdsworth MT, Raisch DW, Winter SS, Frost JD, Moro MA, Doran NH, Phillips J, Pankey JM, Mathew P. Pain and distress from bone marrow aspirations and lumbar punctures. Ann Pharmacother. 2003;37(1):17–22.
73. Spagrud LJ, von Baeyer CL, Ali K, Mpofu C, Fennell LP, Friesen K, Mitchell J. Pain, distress, and adult-child interaction during venipuncture in pediatric oncology: an examination of three types of venous access. J Pain Symptom Manag. 2008 Aug;36(2):173–84. https://doi.org/10.1016/j.jpainsymman.2007.10.009.
74. Zernikow B, Meyerhoff U, Michel E, Wiesel T, Hasan C, Janssen G, Kuhn N, Kontny U, Fengler R, Gortitz I, Andler W. Pain in pediatric oncology – childrens' and parents' perspectives. Eur J Pain. 2005;9:395–406. https://doi.org/10.1016/j.ejpain.2004.09.008.
75. Oakes LL. Caring practices: providing comfort. In: Curley M, Moloney-Harmon PA, editors. Critical care nursing of infants and children. Philadelphia: W. B. Saunders Company; 2001. p. 547–76.
76. Branowicki P, Houlahan KE, Conley S, Kline NE. Nursing care of patients with childhood cancer. In: Orkin SH, Fisher DE, Ginsburg D, Look AT, Lux SE, Nathan DG, editors. Nathan and Oski's hematology and oncology of infancy and childhood. Philadelphia: Elsevier Saunders; 2015. p. 2292–319.
77. Adlard K. Central venous access devices. In: Kline NE, editor. Essentials of pediatric hematology/oncology nursing: a core curriculum. 4th ed. Association of Pediatric Hematology/Oncology Nurses: Glenview; 2014.

78. Reigart JR, Chamberlain KH, Eldridge D, et al. Peripheral intravenous access in pediatric inpatients. Clin Pediatr. 2012;51(5):468–72. https://doi.org/10.1177/0009922811435164.
79. Kuensting LL, DeBoer S, Holleran R, Shultz BL, Steinmann RA, Venella J. Difficult venous access in children: taking control. J Emerg Nurs. 2009;35:419–24. https://doi.org/10.1016/j.jen.2009.01.014.
80. Higgerson RA, Lawson KA, Christie LM, Brown AM, McArthur JA, Totapally BR, Hanson SJ, National Association of Children's Hospitals and Related Institutions' Pediatric Intensive Care Unit FOCUS group. Incidence and risk factors associated with venous thrombotic events in pediatric intensive care unit patients. Pediatr Crit Care Med. 2011;12(6):628–34. https://doi.org/10.1097/PCC.0b013e318207124a.
81. Tullius BP, Athale U, van Ommen CH, Chan AKC, Palumbo JS, Balagtas JMS, for the Subcommittee on Hemostasis and Malignancy and the Subcommittee on Pediatric/Neonatal Thrombosis and Hemostasis. The identification of at-risk patients and prevention of venous thromboembolism in pediatric cancer: guidance from the SSC of the ISTH. J Thromb Haemost. 2018;16:175–80. https://doi.org/10.1111/jth.13895.
82. National Healthcare Safety Network (NHSN). Centers for Disease Control and Prevention. 2018. Bloodstream infection event (central lineassociated bloodstream infection and non-central line associated bloodstream infection). https://www.cdc.gov/nhsn/pdfs/pscmanual/4psc_clabscurrent.pdf
83. Centers for Disease Control and Prevention (CDC). National and state healthcare-associated infections progress report. 2016. Available at www.cdc.gov/HAI/pdfs/progress-report/hai-progress-report.pdf
84. Gaur AH, Bundy DG, Werner EJ, Hord JD, Miller MR, Li T, Lawlor JP, Billett AL. A prospective, holistic, multicenter approach to tracking and understanding bloodstream infections in pediatric hematology-oncology patients. Infect Control Hosp Epidemiol. 2017;38(6):690–6. https://doi.org/10.1017/ice.2017.57.
85. Bundy DG, Gaur AH, Billett AL, He B, Colantuoni EA, Miller MR, on behalf of Children's Hospital Association Hematology/Oncology CLABSI Collaborative. Preventing CLABSIs among pediatric hematology/oncology inpatients: national collaborative results. Pediatrics. 2014;134(6):e1678–85. https://doi.org/10.1542/peds.2014-0582.
86. The Joint Commission. Preventing central line–associated bloodstream infections: a global challenge, a global perspective. Oak Brook: Joint Commission Resources. 2012. http://www.PreventingCLABSIs.pdf. Accessed 1 Jan 2018.
87. Centers for Disease Control and Prevention (CDC). Operational guidance for acute care hospitals to report central line-associated bloodstream infection (CLABSI) data to CDC's NHSN for the purpose of fulfilling CMS's hospital inpatient quality reporting (IQR) requirements. 2014. Available at: http://www.cdc.gov/nhsn/PDFs/FINAL-ACH-CLABSI-Guidance.pdf. Accessed 14 Jan 2018.
88. Centers for Medicare and Medicaid Services (CMS). Hospital-acquired condition (HAC) reduction program. 2015. https://www.cms.gov/Medicare/Quality-Initiatives-Patient-Assessment-Instruments/Value-Based-Programs/HAC/Hospital-Acquired-Conditions.html. Accessed 15 Jan 2018.
89. Hanna HA, Raad I. Blood products: a significant risk factor for long-term catheter-related bloodstream infections in cancer patients. Infect Control Hosp Epidemiol. 2001;22:165–6.
90. Marschall J, Mermel L, Fakih M, Hadaway L, Kallen A, O'Grady N, et al. Strategies to prevent central line–associated bloodstream infections in acute care hospitals: 2014 update. Infect Control Hosp Epidemiol. 2014;35(7):753–71. https://doi.org/10.1086/676533.
91. Epstein L, See I, Edwards JR, Magill SS, Thompson ND. Mucosal barrier injury laboratory-confirmed bloodstream infections (MBI-LCBI): descriptive analysis of data reported to National Healthcare Safety Network (NHSN), 2013. Infect Control Hosp Epidemiol. 2016;37(1):2–7.
92. Metzger KE, Rucker Y, Callaghan M, et al. The burden of mucosal barrier injury laboratory-confirmed bloodstream infection among hematology, oncology, and stem cell trans-

plant patients. Infect Control Hosp Epidemiol. 2015;36:119–24. https://doi.org/10.1017/ice.2014.38.
93. Dandoy C, Haslam D, Davies S, et al. Healthcare burden, risk factors, and outcomes of mucosal barrier injury laboratory-confirmed bloodstream infections after stem cell transplantation. Biol Blood Marrow Transplant. 2016;22(9):1671–7. https://doi.org/10.1016/j.bbmt.2016.06.002.
94. Simon A, Furtwangler R, Graf N, et al. Surveillance of bloodstream infections in pediatric cancer centers: what have we learned and how do we move on? GMS Hyg Infect Control. 2016;11:1–47. https://doi.org/10.3205/dgkh000271.
95. See I, Iwamoto M, Allen-Bridson K, Horan T, Magill SS, Thompson ND. Mucosal barrier injury laboratory-confirmed bloodstream infection: results from a field test of a new National Healthcare Safety Network definition. Infect Control Hosp Epidemiol. 2013;34:769–76. https://doi.org/10.1086/671281.
96. Gaur AH, Miller MR, Gao C, et al. Evaluating application of the National Healthcare Safety Network central line-associated bloodstream infection surveillance definition: a survey of pediatric intensive care and hematology/oncology units. Infect Control Hosp Epidemiol. 2013;34:663–70. https://doi.org/10.1086/671005.
97. National Healthcare Safety Network (NHSN); Centers for Disease Control and Prevention (CDC). National Healthcare Safety Network (NHSN) patient safety component manual. 2018. Available from https://www.cdc.gov/nhsn/pdfs/pscmanual/pcsmanual_current.pdf. Accessed 1 Feb 2018.
98. Vaughan AM, Ross R, Gilman MM, Satchell L, Ditaranto S, Reilly AF, Kersun LS, Shanahan A, Coffin SE, Sammons JS. Mucosal barrier injury central-line–associated bloodstream infections: what is the impact of standard prevention bundles? Infect Control Hosp Epidemiol. 2017;38(11):1385–7. https://doi.org/10.1017/ice.2017.
99. Miller MR, Griswold M, Harris JM II, et al. Decreasing PICU catheter-associated bloodstream infections: NACHRI's quality transformation efforts. Pediatrics. 2010;125(2):206–13. https://doi.org/10.1542/peds.2009-1382.
100. Miller MR, Niedner MF, Huskins WC, et al. Reducing PICU central line-associated bloodstream infections: 3-year results. Pediatrics. 2011;128(5). Available at: www.pediatrics.org/cgi/content/full/128/5/e1077
101. Solutions for Patient Safety (SPS). SPS prevention bundle: central line associated blood stream infection (CLABSI). In: SPS prevention bundles. 2014. http://www.solutionsforpatientsafety.org/wp-content/uploads/SPS-Prevention-Bundles.pdf
102. O'Grady NP, Alexander M, Burns LA, Dellinger P, Garland J, Heard SO, Lipsett PA, Masur H, Mermel LA, Pearson ML, Raad II, Randolph A, Rupp ME, Saint S, and the Healthcare Infection Control Practices Advisory Committee (HICPAC). Guidelines for the prevention of intravascular catheter-related infections, 2011. Centers for Disease Control. 2011. https://www.cdc.gov/hai/pdfs/bsi-guidelines-2011.pdf
103. Siegel JD, Rhinehart E, Jackson M, Chiarello L, the Healthcare Infection Control Practices Advisory Committee. 2007. 2007 Guideline for isolation precautions: preventing transmission of infectious agents in healthcare settings. Accessed 25 Jan 2017 from http://www.cdc.gov/ncidod/dhqp/pdf/isolation2007.pdf
104. Zitella LJ, Friese CR, Hauser J, Gobel BH, Woolery M, O'Leary C, Andrews FA. Putting evidence into practice: prevention of infection. Clin J Oncol Nurs. 2006;10(6):739–50. https://doi.org/10.1188/06.cjon.739-750.
105. Stelfox H, Bates D, Redelmeier D. Safety of patients isolated for infection control. JAMA. 2003;290:1899–905.
106. Evans HL, Shaffer MM, Hughes MG, Smith RL, Chong TW, Raymond DP, et al. Contact isolation in surgical patients: a barrier to care? Surgery. 2003;134:180–8.
107. CDC. Guidelines for environmental control in health-care facilities. MMWR. 2003:52(No. RR--10).

108. Mize L, Harris N, Stokhuyzen A, Avery T, Cash J, Kasse M, Sanborn C, Leonardelli A, Rodgers C, Hockenberry M. Neutropenia precautions for children receiving chemotherapy or stem cell transplantation for cancer. J Pediatr Oncol Nurs. 2014;31:200–10. https://doi.org/10.1177/1043454214532027.
109. Saria M. Preventing and managing infections in neutropenic stem cell transplantation recipients: evidence-based review. Clin J Oncol Nurs. 2011;15(2):133–9. https://doi.org/10.1188/11.CJON.133-139.
110. Costello C. Skin changes. In: Kline N, editor. Essentials of pediatric hematology/oncology nursing: a core curriculum. 4th ed. Chicago: APHON; 2014. p. 234–6.
111. Curley M, Hasbani N, Quigley S, Stellar J, Pasek T, Wypij D, et al. Predicting pressure injury risk in pediatric patients: the Braden QD scale. J Pediatr. 2018;192:189–97. https://doi.org/10.1016/j.jpeds.2017.09.045.
112. Razmus I, Bergquist-Beringer S. Pressure injury prevalence and the rate of hospital-acquired pressure injury among pediatric patients in acute care. J Wound Ostomy Continence Nurs. 2017;44(2):110–7. https://doi.org/10.1097/WON.0000000000000306.
113. Friedman B, Berdahl T, Simpson LA, McCormick MC, Owens PL, Andrews R, et al. Annual report on health care for children and youth in the United States: focus on trends in hospital use and quality. Acad Pediatr. 2011;11:263–79. https://doi.org/10.1016/j.acap.2011.04.002.
114. Schindler C, Mikhailov T, Kuhn E, Christopher J, Conway P, Simpson V, et al. Protecting fragile skin: nursing interventions to decrease development of pressure ulcers in pediatric intensive care. Am J Crit Care. 2011;20(1):26–34. https://doi.org/10.4037/ajcc2011754.
115. Curley MAQ, Razmus IS, Roberts KE, Wypij D. Predicting pressure ulcer risk in pediatric patients: the Braden Q scale. Nurs Res. 2003;52(1):22–33.
116. Larson E, Nirenberg A. Evidence-based nursing practice to prevent infection in hospitalized neutropenic patients with cancer. Oncol Nurs Forum. 2004;31(4):717–23. https://doi.org/10.1188/04.ONF.717-725.
117. Ladas EJ, Sacks N, Brophy P, Rogers PC. Standards of nutritional care in pediatric oncology: results from a nationwide survey on the standards of practice in pediatric oncology: a Children's Oncology Group study. Pediatr Blood Cancer. 2006;46(3):339–44. http://doi.wiley.com/10.1002/pbc.20435
118. Hooke M, Baggott C, Robinson D, Woolery M, Maloney AM, Dulczak S, et al. Managing disease-and treatment-related complications in pediatric oncology. In: Baggott C, Fochtman D, Foley GV, Kelly KP, editors. Nursing care of children and adolescents with cancer and blood disorders. 4th ed. Glenview: Association of Pediatric Hematology/Oncology Nurses; 2011. p. 510–84.
119. CDC Centers for Disease Control and Prevention [Internet]. BMI Percentile calculator for child and teen 2018 [cited 2018 Feb 21]. Available from: https://nccd.cdc.gov/dnpabmi/calculator.aspx
120. Trimpe K, Shaw MR, Wilson M, Haberman MR. Review of the effectiveness of enteral feeding in pediatric oncology patients. J Pediatr Oncol Nurs. 2017;34(6):439–45. http://journals.sagepub.com/doi/10.1177/1043454217712982
121. DeSwarte-Wallace J, Firouzbakhsh S, Finklestein JZ. Using research to change practice: enteral feedings for pediatric oncology patients. J Pediatr Oncol Nurs. 2001;18(5):217–23.
122. Skolin I, Hursti UKK, Wahlin YB. Parents' perception of their child's food intake after the start of chemotherapy. J Pediatr Oncol Nurs. 2001;18(3):124–36.
123. Weinstein R. Red blood cell transfusion: a pocket guide for the clinician. 2016. Available from: RedCellsTxPocketGuideWEB2016.pdf
124. Andrews J, Galel S, Wong W, Glader B. Hematologic supportive care for children with cancer. In: Pizzo P, Poplack P, editors. Principles and practice of pediatric oncology. 7th ed. Philadelphia: Wolters Kluwer; 2016. p. 991–1007.
125. Carson JL, Guyatt G, Heddle NM, Grossman BJ, Cohn CS, Fung MK, et al. Clinical practice guidelines from the AABB: red blood cell transfusion thresholds and storage. JAMA. 2016;316(19):2025–35. https://doi.org/10.1001/jama.2016.9185.

126. Conte T. Blood product support. In: Kline N, editor. Essentials of pediatric hematology/oncology nursing: a core curriculum. 4th ed. Chicago: APHON; 2014. p. 289–94.
127. Burke ML, Salani D. Hematologic and oncologic emergencies requiring critical care. In: Hazinski MF, editor. Nursing care of the critically ill child. 3rd ed. St. Louis: Elsevier; 2013. p. 825–50.
128. Slichter SJ. Evidence-based platelet transfusion guidelines. Hematology. 2007;1:172–8. Available from: http://www.asheducationbook.org/cgi/doi/10.1182/asheducation-2007.1.172
129. Nester T, Shweta J, Poisson J. Hemotherapy decisions and their outcomes. In: Fung M, Grossman B, Hillyer C, Westhoff C, editors. Technical manual. 18th ed. Bethesda: AABB. p. 499–544.
130. Jackups R, Savage W. Gaps in research on adverse events to transfusion in pediatrics. Transfus Med Rev. 2016;30(4):209–12. https://doi.org/10.1016/j.tmrv.2016.06.001.
131. Spinella PC, Dressler A, Tucci M, Carroll CL, Rosen RS, Hume H, et al. Survey of transfusion policies at US and Canadian children's hospitals in 2008 and 2009. Transfusion. 2010;50(11):2328–35. https://doi.org/10.1111/j.1537-2995.2010.02708.x.
132. Josephson C, Meyer E. Neonatal and pediatric transfusion practice. In: Fung M, Grossman B, Hillyer C, Westhoff C, editors. Technical manual. 18th ed. Bethesda: AABB. p. 571–97.
133. Bryant R, Norville R. Management of blood component deficiencies. In: Baggott C, Fochtman D, Foley GV, Kelly KP, editors. Nursing care of children and adolescents with cancer and blood disorders. 4th ed. Glenview: Association of Pediatric Hematology/Oncology Nurses; 2011. p. 585–611.
134. Mazzei C, Popovsky M, Kopko P. Noninfectious complications of blood transfusion. In: Fung M, Grossman B, Hillyer C, Westhoff C, editors. Technical manual. 18th ed. Bethesda: AABB. p. 665–96.
135. Silliman CC. The two-event model of transfusion-related acute lung injury. Crit Care Med. 2006;34(5 SUPPL) https://doi.org/10.1097/01.CCM.0000214292.62276.8E.
136. Sanchez R, Toy P. Transfusion related acute lung injury: a pediatric perspective. Pediatr Blood Cancer. 2005;45(3):248–55. http://doi.wiley.com/10.1002/pbc.20395
137. American Association of Blood Banks. Standards for blood banks and transfusion services. 29th edition. Summary of significant changes. Available from: http://www.aabb.org/sa/standards/Documents/sigchngstds29.pdf
138. Neuss MN, Polovich M, McNiff K, Esper P, Gilmore TR, LeFebvre KB, et al. 2013 updated American Society of Clinical Oncology/Oncology Nursing Society chemotherapy administration safety standards including standards for the safe administration and management of oral chemotherapy. J Oncol Pract. 2013;9(2 Suppl):5s–13s. https://doi.org/10.1200/JOP.2013.000874.
139. Belderson KM, Billett AL. Chemotherapy safety standards: a pediatric perspective. J Pediatr Oncol Nurs. 2017;34:156–9. https://doi.org/10.1177/1043454217697670.
140. Neuss MN, Gilmore TR, Belderson KM, Billett AL, Conti-Kalchik T, Harvey BE, et al. 2016 updated American Society of Clinical Oncology/Oncology Nursing Society Chemotherapy Administration Safety Standards, Including Standards for Pediatric Oncology. J Oncol Pract. 2016;12(12):1262–71. Available from: http://ascopubs.org/doi/10.1200/JOP.2016.017905
141. Oncology Nursing Society. Education of the nurse who administers and cares for the individual receiving chemotherapy, targeted therapy, and immunotherapy. Position statement. 2017. Available from: https://www.ons.org/sites/default/files/Education_Nurse_Who_Administers_Chemo.pdf
142. James J. A new, evidence-based estimate of patient harms associated with hospital care. J Patient Saf. 2013;9(3):122–8. Available from: http://journals.lww.com/journalpatientsafety/Fulltext/2013/09000/A_New,_Evidence_based_Estimate_of_Patient_Harms.2.aspx
143. Mueller BU, Billett AL. Maximizing safety in cancer treatment. In: Pizzo P, Poplack P, editors. Principles and practice of pediatric oncology. 7th ed. Philadelphia: Wolters Kluwer; 2016. p. 452–61.

144. Institute for Safe Medication Practices (ISMP). ISMP's list of high-alert medications in acute care settings. 2014. Available from: http://www.ismp.org/Tools/highalertmedications.pdf
145. Nixon C, Rae ML. Administration considerations. In: Kline N, editor. The pediatric chemotherapy and biotherapy curriculum. 3rd ed. Chicago: APHON; 2011. p. 73–104.
146. Unger JM, Cook E, Tai E, Bleyer A. The role of clinical trial participation in cancer research: barriers, evidence, and strategies. Am Soc Clin Oncol Meet In: Am Soc Clin Oncol Educ book. 2016;35:185–98. Available from: http://meetinglibrary.asco.org/content/156686-176
147. Wong D, Baker C. Pain in children: comparison of assessment scales. Pediatr Nurs. 1988;14(1):9–17.
148. Whaley L, Wong D. Nursing care of infants and children. 4th ed. St Louis; 1991. p. 1148.
149. von Baeyer CL, Spagrud LJ, McCormick JC, Choo E, Neville K, Connelly MA. Three new datasets supporting use of the Numerical Rating Scale (NRS-11) for children's self-reports of pain intensity. Pain. 2009;143(3):223–7. https://doi.org/10.1016/j.pain.2009.03.002.
150. Shields BJ, Cohen DM, Harbeck-Weber C, Powers JD, Smith GA. Pediatric pain measurement using a visual analogue scale: a comparison of two teaching methods. Clin Pediatr. 2003;42:227–34.
151. World Health Organization (WHO). WHO guidelines on the pharmacological treatment of persisting pain in children with medical illness. Geneva: World Health Organization; 2012. https://doi.org/10.1017/CBO9781107415324.004.
152. Merkel F, Voepel SI, Lewis T, Shayevitz JR, Malviya S. FLACC Behavioral Pain Assessment Scale. Pediatr Nurs. 1997;23(3):293–7.
153. Manworren RC, Hynan LS. Clinical validation of FLACC: preverbal patient pain scale. Pediatr Nurs. 2003;29(2):140–6.
154. Voepel-Lewis T, Merkel S, Tait AR, Trzcinka A, Malviya S. The reliability and validity of the face, legs, activity, cry, consolability observational tool as a measure of pain in children with cognitive impairment. Anesth Analg. 2002;95:1224–9.
155. Voepel-Lewis T, Zanotti J, Dammeyer JA, Merkel S. Reliability and validity of the face, legs, activity, cry, consolability behavioral tool in assessing acute pain in critically ill patients. Am J Crit Care. 2010;19(1):55–61. https://doi.org/10.4037/ajcc2010624.
156. Fanurik D, Koh JL, Schmitz ML, Harrison RD, Conrad TM. Children with cognitive impairment: parent report of pain and coping. J Dev Behav Pediatr. 1999;20(4):228–34.
157. von Baeyer CL, Spagrud LJ. Systematic review of observational (behavioral) measures of pain for children and adolescents aged 3 to 18 years. Pain. 2007;127(1–2):140–50. https://doi.org/10.1016/j.pain.2006.08.014.
158. Dorfman TL, Sumamo E, Rempel GR, Scott SD, Hartling L. An evaluation of instruments for scoring physiological and behavioral cues of pain, non-pain related distress, and adequacy of analgesia and sedation in pediatric mechanically ventilated patients: a systematic review. Int J Nurs Stud. 2014;51(4):654–76. https://doi.org/10.1016/j.ijnurstu.2013.07.009.
159. Curley MAQ, Harris SK, Fraser K, Johnson R, Arnold JH. State behavioral scale: a sedation assessment instrument for infants and young children supported on mechanical ventilation. Pediatr Crit Care Med. 2006;7(2):107–14. https://doi.org/10.1097/01.PCC.0000200955.40962.38.
160. Ambuel B, Hamlett KW, Marx CM, Blumer JL. Assessing distress in pediatric intensive care environments: the COMFORT scale. J Pediatr Psychol. 1992;17(1):95–109.
161. Van Dijk M, De Boer JB, Koot HM, Tibboel D, Passchier J, Duivenvoorden HJ. The reliability and validity of the COMFORT scale as a postoperative pain instrument in 0 to 3-year-old infants. Pain. 2000;84:367–77.
162. Simone S, Sorce L. Analgesia, paralytics, sedation, and withdrawal. In: Reuter-Rice K, Bolick B, editors. Pediatric acute care: a guide for interprofessional practice. Burlington: Jones & Barlett Learning; 2015. p. 151–87.
163. Zernikow B, Meyerhoff U, Michel E, Wiesel T, Hasan C, Janssen G, Kuhn N, Kontny U, Fengler R, Görtitz I, Andler W. Pain in pediatric oncology – children's and parents' perspectives. Eur J Pain. 2005;9:395–406. https://doi.org/10.1016/j.ejpain.2004.09.008.

164. Jodarski K, Wilson K. Pain. In: Kline N, editor. Essentials of pediatric oncology nursing: a core curriculum. 2nd ed. APHON: Chicago; 2004. p. 155–9.
165. Dolan EA, Paice JA, Wile S. Managing cancer-related pain in critical care settings. AACN Adv Crit Care. 2011;22(4):365–78. https://doi.org/10.1097/NCI.0b013e318232c6b8.
166. Kudchadkar SR, Yaster M, Punjabi NM. Sedation, sleep promotion, and delirium screening practices in the care of mechanically ventilated children: a wake-up call for the pediatric critical care community. Crit Care Med. 2014;42(7):1592–600. https://doi.org/10.1097/CCM.0000000000000326.
167. Curley MA, Wypij D, Watson RS, Grant MJ, Asaro LA, Cheifetz IM, Dodson BL, Franck LS, Gedeit RG, Angus DC, et al. Protocolized sedation vs usual care in pediatric patients mechanically ventilated for acute respiratory failure: a randomized clinical trial. JAMA. 2015;313(4):379–89. https://doi.org/10.1001/jama.2014.18399.
168. Dreyfus L, Javouhey E, Denis A, Touzet S, Bordet F. Implementation and evaluation of a paediatric nurse-driven sedation protocol in a paediatric intensive care unit. Ann Intensive Care. 2017;7:36. https://doi.org/10.1186/s13613-017-0256-7.
169. Gaillard-Le Roux G, Liet JM, Bourgoin P, Legrand A, Roze JC, Joram N. Implementation of a nurse-driven sedation protocol in a PICU decreases daily doses of midazolam. Pediatr Crit Care Med. 2017;18:e9–e17. https://doi.org/10.1097/PCC.0000000000000998.
170. Jacob E. Pain. In: Kline N, editor. Essentials of pediatric hematology/oncology nursing: a core curriculum. 4th ed. APHON: Chicago; 2014. p. 244–52.
171. Kennedy RM, Luhmann J, Zempsky WT. Clinical implications of unmanaged needle-insertion pain and distress in children. Pediatrics. 2008;122(Supplement 3):S130–3. https://doi.org/10.1542/peds.2008-1055e.
172. Padula M. Renal and bladder complications. In: Kline N, editor. Essentials of pediatric hematology/oncology nursing: a core curriculum. 4th ed. Chicago: APHON; 2014. p. 232–4.
173. Czaja AS, Zimmerman JJ. The use of dexmedetomidine in critically ill children. Pediatr Crit Care Med. 2009;10(3):381–6. https://doi.org/10.1097/PCC.0b013e3181a3191f.
174. Grant MJC, Schneider JB, Asaro LA, et al. Dexmedetomidine use in critically ill children with acute respiratory failure. Pediatr Crit Care Med. 2016;17(12):1131–41. https://doi.org/10.1097/PCC.0000000000000941.
175. Phan H, Nahata MC. Clinical uses of dexmedetomidine in pediatric patients. Paediatr Drugs. 2008;10(1):49–69. http://www.ncbi.nlm.nih.gov/pubmed/18162008
176. Jouguelet-Lacoste J, La Colla L, Schilling D, Chelly JE. The use of intravenous infusion or single dose of low-dose ketamine for postoperative analgesia: a review of the current literature. Pain Med. 2015;16(2):383–403. https://doi.org/10.1111/pme.12619.
177. Fitzgibbon EJ, Hall P, Schroder C, Seely J, Viola R. Low dose ketamine as an analgesic adjuvant in difficult pain syndromes: a strategy for conversion from parenteral to oral ketamine. J Pain Symptom Manag. 2002;23(2):165–70. https://doi.org/10.1016/S0885-3924(01)00393-1.
178. Finkel JC, Pestieau SR, Quezado ZMN. Ketamine as an adjuvant for treatment of cancer pain in children and adolescents. J Pain. 2007;8(6):515–21. https://doi.org/10.1016/j.jpain.2007.02.429.
179. Zempsky WT, Loiselle KA, Corsi JM, Hagstrom JN. Use of low-dose ketamine infusion for pediatric patients with sickle cell disease-related pain: a case series. Clin J Pain. 2010;26:163–7. https://doi.org/10.1097/AJP.0b013e3181b511ab.
180. Neri CM, Pestieau SR, Darbari DS. Low-dose ketamine as a potential adjuvant therapy for painful vaso-occlusive crises in sickle cell disease. Paediatr Anaesth. 2013;23(8):684–9. https://doi.org/10.1111/pan.12172.
181. Feudtner C, Freedman J, Kang T, Womer JW, Dai D, Faerber J. Comparative effectiveness of senna to prevent problematic constipation in pediatric oncology patients receiving opioids: a multicenter study of clinically detailed administrative data. J Pain Symptom Manag. 2014;48(2):272–80. https://doi.org/10.1016/j.jpainsymman.2013.09.009.

182. O'Hanlon Curry J, Nixon C. Gastrointestinal complications. In: Kline N, editor. Essentials of pediatric hematology/oncology nursing: a core curriculum. 4th ed. Chicago: APHON; 2014. p. 221–32.
183. Rodrigues A, Wong C, Mattiussi A, Alexander S, Lau E, Dupuis LL. Methylnaltrexone for opioid-induced constipation in pediatric oncology patients. Pediatr Blood Cancer. 2013;60:1667–70. https://doi.org/10.1002/pbc.24615.
184. Flerlage JE, Baker JN. Methylnaltrexone for opioid-induced constipation in children and adolescents and young adults with progressive incurable cancer at the end of life. J Palliat Med. 2015;18(7):631–3. https://doi.org/10.1089/jpm.2014.0364.
185. Anghelescu D, Faughnan L, Hankins G, Ward D, Oakes L. Methadone use in children and young adults at a cancer center – a retrospective study. J Opioid Manag. 2011;7(5):353–61.
186. Anghelescu DL, Patel RM, Mahoney DP, et al. Methadone prolongs cardiac conduction in young patients with cancer-related pain. J Opioid Manag. 2016;12(2):131–8. https://doi.org/10.5055/jom.2016.0325.
187. Madden K, Park M, Liu D, Bruera E. The frequency of QTc prolongation among pediatric and young adult patients receiving methadone for cancer pain. Pediatr Blood Cancer. 2017;64(11) https://doi.org/10.1002/pbc.26614.
188. Haenecour AS, Seto W, Urbain CM, Stephens D, Laussen PC, Balit CR. Prolonged dexmedetomidine infusion and drug withdrawal in critically ill children. J Pediatr Pharmacol Ther. 2017;22(6):453–60. https://doi.org/10.5863/1551-6776-22.6.453.
189. Franck LS, Harris S, Soetenga D, Amling J, Curley M. The Withdrawal Assessment Tool-1 (WAT-1): an assessment instrument for monitoring opioid and benzodiazepine withdrawal symptoms in pediatric patients. Pediatr Crit Care Med. 2008;9(6):573–80. https://doi.org/10.1097/PCC.0b013e31818c8328.
190. Macpherson CF. Sedation for painful procedures. In: Kline N, editor. Essentials of pediatric hematology/oncology nursing: a core curriculum. 4th ed. Chicago: APHON; 2014. p. 267–8.
191. American Society of Anesthesiology. Committee on Quality Management and Departmental Administration. Continuum of depth of sedation: definition of general anesthesia and levels of sedation/analgesia. 2014. Accessed from http://www.asahq.org/quality-and-practice-management/standards-guidelines-and-related-resources/continuum-of-depth-of-sedation-definition-of-general-anesthesia-and-levels-of-sedation-analgesia
192. Cote CJ, Wilson S. Guidelines for monitoring and management of pediatric patients before, during, and after sedation for diagnostic and therapeutic procedures: update 2016. Pediatrics. 2016;138(1):e20161212–e20161212. https://doi.org/10.1542/peds.2016-1212.
193. American Society of Anesthesiologists Task Force on Moderate Procedural Sedation and Analgesia, the American Association of Oral and Maxillofacial Surgeons, American College of Radiology, American Dental Association, American Society of Dentist Anesthesiologists, and Society of Interventional Radiology. Practice guidelines for moderate procedural sedation and analgesia 2018. Anesthesiology. 2018;128:437–79. https://doi.org/10.1097/ALN.0000000000002043.
194. Dahan A, Aarts L, Smith TW. Incidence, reversal, and prevention of opioid-induced respiratory depression. Anesthesiology. 2010;112(1):226–38. https://doi.org/10.1097/ALN.0b013e3181c38c25.
195. Macpherson CF. Psychological preparation and support for painful procedures. In: Kline N, editor. Essentials of pediatric hematology/oncology nursing: a core curriculum. 4th ed. Chicago: APHON; 2014. p. 264–7.
196. Oakes L. Pain causes and treatment. In: Baggott C, Fochtman D, Foley G V, Kelly KP. Nursing care of children and adolescents with cancer and blood disorders. 4th ed. Chicago: Association of Pediatric Hematology/Oncology Nurses; 2011. p. 642–668.
197. Duncan J, Kobler K. Communication in pediatrics. In: Dahlin C, Coyne P, Ferrell B, editors. Advanced practice palliative care. 3rd ed. New York: Oxford; 2016. p. 597–608.

198. Brennan CW, Prince-Paul M, Wiencek CA. Providing a "good death" for oncology patients during the final hours of life in the intensive care unit. AACN Adv Crit Care. 2011;22(4):379–96. https://doi.org/10.1097/NCI.0b013e31823100dc.
199. Anghelescu D, Hamilton H, Faughnan L, Johnson L, Baker J. Pediatric palliative sedation therapy with propofol: recommendations based on experience in children with terminal cancer. J Palliat Med. 2012;15(10):1082–90. https://doi.org/10.1089/jpm.2011.05001.
200. Hooke MC, Grund E, Quammen H, Miller B, McCormick P, Bostrom B. Propofol use in pediatric patients with severe cancer pain at the end of life. J Pediatr Oncol Nurs. 2007;24(1):29–34. https://doi.org/10.1177/1043454206296026.
201. Rohaly-Davis J, Johnston K. A new collaborative practice: critical care and hematology/oncology--altering the misconceptions. Crit Care Nurs Q. 1996;18(4):61–5.
202. Demaret P, Pettersen G, Hubert P, Teira P, Emeriaud G. The critically-ill pediatric hemato-oncology patient: epidemiology, management, and strategy of transfer to the pediatric intensive care unit. Ann Intensive Care. 2012;2(1):1–20. https://doi.org/10.1186/2110-5820-2-14.
203. Pirschel C. Critical care for patients with cancer. Oncol Nurs Forum Voice. 2017;32(7):14–8.
204. American Academy of Pediatrics. Guidelines for developing admission and discharge policies for the pediatric intensive care unit. Pediatrics. 1999;27:843–5.
205. McArthur J, Pettersen G, Jouvet P, Christensen M, Tamburro R. The care of critically ill children after hematopoietic SCT: a North American survey. Bone Marrow Transplant. 2011;46(2):227–31. https://doi.org/10.1038/bmt.2010.89.
206. Hull CS. Oncology–critical care nursing collaboration. Clin J Oncol Nurs. 2007;11(6):925–8. https://doi.org/10.1188/07.CJON.925-927.
207. Little J. Management in the inpatient setting. In: Reuter-Rice K, Bolic B, editors. Pediatric acute care: a guide for interprofessional practice. Burlington: Jones & Barlett Learning; 2015. p. 97–124.
208. Piastra M, De Luca D, Pietrini D, et al. Noninvasive pressure-support ventilation in immunocompromised children with ARDS: a feasibility study. Intensive Care Med. 2009;35(8):1420–7. https://doi.org/10.1007/s00134-009-1558-5.
209. Cogo PE, Poole D, Codazzi D, et al. Outcome of children admitted to adult intensive care units in Italy between 2003 and 2007. Intensive Care Med. 2010;36:1403–9.
210. Kache S, Weiss IK, Moore TB. Changing outcomes for children requiring intensive care following hematopoietic stem cell transplantation. Pediatr Transplant. 2006;10(3):299–303. https://doi.org/10.1111/j.1399-3046.2005.00453.x.
211. Squadrone V, Massaia M, Bruno B, et al. Early CPAP prevents evolution of acute lung injury in patients with hematologic malignancy. Intensive Care Med. 2010;36:1666–74. https://doi.org/10.1007/s00134-010-1934-1.
212. Chapman SM, Grocott MPW, Franck LS. Systematic review of paediatric alert criteria for identifying hospitalised children at risk of critical deterioration. Intensive Care Med. 2010;36(4):600–11. https://doi.org/10.1007/s00134-009-1715-x.
213. Demmel KM, Williams L, Flesch L. Implementation of the pediatric early warning scoring system on a pediatric hematology/oncology unit. J Pediatr Oncol Nurs. 2010;27(4):229–40. https://doi.org/10.1177/1043454209358410.
214. Swartz C. Recognition of clinical deterioration: a clinical leadership opportunity for nurse executive. J Nurs Adm. 2013;43(7–8):377–81. https://doi.org/10.1097/NNA.0b013e31829d606a.
215. Kyriacos U, Jelsma J, Jordan S. Monitoring vital signs using early warning scoring systems: a review of the literature. J Nurs Manag. 2011;19(3):311–30. https://doi.org/10.1111/j.1365-2834.2011.01246.x.
216. Monaghan A. Detecting and managing deterioration in children. Pediatr Care. 2005;17(1):32–5. https://doi.org/10.7748/paed2005.02.17.1.32.c964.
217. Tucker KM, Brewer TL, Baker RB, Demeritt B, Vossmeyer MT. Prospective evaluation of a pediatric inpatient early warning scoring system. J Spec Pediatr Nurs. 2009;14(2):79–85. https://doi.org/10.1111/j.1744-6155.2008.00178.x.

218. Robson MAJ, Cooper CL, Medicus LA, Quintero MJ, Zuniga SA. Comparison of three acute care pediatric early warning scoring tools. J Pediatr Nurs. 2013;28(6):e33–41. https://doi.org/10.1016/j.pedn.2012.12.002.
219. McLellan MC, Gauvreau K, Connor JA. Validation of the children's hospital early warning system for critical deterioration recognition. J Pediatr Nurs 2017;32:52–58. Available from: https://doi.org/10.1016/j.pedn.2016.10.005.
220. Gawronski O, Ciofi degli Atti ML, Di Ciommo V, Cecchetti C, Bertaina A, Tiozzo E, Raponi M, the Stem Cell Transplant Unit Bedside PEWS Study Group. Accuracy of bedside paediatric early warning system (Bedside PEWS) in a pediatric stem cell transplant unit. J Pediatr Oncol Nurs. 2016;33(4):249–56. https://doi.org/10.1177/1043454215600154.
221. Dingley C, Daugherty K, Derieg MK, Persing R. Improving patient safety through provider communication strategy enhancements. In: Henriksen K, Battles JB, Keyes MA, Grady ML, editors. Advances in patient safety: new directions and alternative approaches. Vol. 3: performance and tools. Agency for Healthcare Research and Quality: Rockville; 2008. Available from: https://www.ncbi.nlm.nih.gov/books/NBK43663/?report=printable.
222. Lee S-H, Phan PH, Dorman T, Weaver SJ, Pronovost PJ. Handoffs, safety culture, and practices: evidence from the hospital survey on patient safety culture. BMC Health Serv Res. 2016;16(1):254. Available from: http://bmchealthservres.biomedcentral.com/articles/10.1186/s12913-016-1502-7
223. Starmer AJ, Spector ND, Srivastava R, Allen AD, Landrigan CP, Sectish TC. I-PASS, a mnemonic to standardize verbal handoffs. Pediatrics. 2012;129(2):201–4. Available from: http://pediatrics.aappublications.org/cgi/doi/10.1542/peds.2011-2966
224. American Association of Critical Care Nurses (AACN). AACN standards for establishing and sustaining healthy work environments: a journey to excellence, 2nd edition. 2016. Available from https://www.aacn.org/wd/hwe/docs/hwestandards.pdf
225. Stewart B, et al. Perceptions of collaboration and communication between the RN-MD relationship in an oncology ICU. Oncol Nurs Forum. 2008;35(3):488.
226. Kaplow R. Special nursing considerations. Crit Care Clin. 2001;17(3):769–89. https://doi.org/10.1016/S0749-0704(05)70207-4.
227. Leary B, Mott S. Perceptions of nurses caring for pediatric bone marrow transplant patients requiring intensive care level support. Biol Blood Marrow Transplant. 2016;22(3):S113. https://doi.org/10.1016/j.bbmt.2015.11.1110.
228. American Academy of Pediatrics (AAP). Patient- and family-centered care and the pediatrician's role. Pediatrics. 2012;129(2):394–404. Available from: http://pediatrics.aappublications.org/cgi/doi/10.1542/peds.2011-3084
229. Richards CA, Starks H, MR OC, Doorenbos AZ. Elements of family-centered care in the pediatric intensive care unit. J Hosp Palliat Nurs. 2017;19(3):238–46. https://doi.org/10.1097/NJH.0000000000000335.
230. Doorenbos A, Curtis JR. Palliative care in the pediatric ICU: challenges and opportunities for family-centered practice. Soc Work End Life Palliat Care. 2012;8(4):297–315. https://doi.org/10.1080/15524256.2012.732461.
231. Gallagher R, Gormley D. Perceptions of stress, burnout, and support systems in pediatric bone marrow transplantation nursing. Clin J Oncol Nurs. 2009;13(6) https://doi.org/10.1188/09.CJON.681-685.
232. Sabo BM. Compassionate presence: the meaning of hematopoietic stem cell transplant nursing. Eur J Oncol Nurs. 2011;15(2):103–11. https://doi.org/10.1016/j.ejon.2010.06.006.
233. Cook KA, Mott S, Lawrence P, Jablonski J, Grady MR, Norton D, et al. Coping while caring for the dying child: nurses' experiences in an acute care setting. J Pediatr Nurs 2012; 27(4):e11–e21. Available from: https://doi.org/10.1016/j.pedn.2011.05.010.
234. Conte TM. The lived experience of work-related loss and grief among pediatric oncology nurses. J Hosp Palliat Nurs [Internet]. 2014;16(1):40–6. https://doi.org/10.1097/NJH.0000000000000019.

235. Berger J, Polivka B, Smoot EA, Owens H. Compassion fatigue in pediatric nurses. J Pediatr Nurs. 2015;30(6):11–7. https://doi.org/10.1016/j.pedn.2015.02.005.
236. Leung D, Fillion L, Duval S, Brown J, Rodin G, Howell D. Meaning in bone marrow transplant nurses' work: experiences before and after a meaning-centered intervention. Cancer Nurs. 2012;35(5):374–81. https://doi.org/10.1097/NCC.0b013e318232e237.
237. Moody K, Kramer D, Santizo RO, Magro L, Wyshogrod D, Ambrosio J, et al. Helping the helpers: mindfulness training for burnout in pediatric oncology-a pilot program. J Pediatr Oncol Nurs. 2013;30(5):275–84. https://doi.org/10.1177/1043454213504497.
238. Morrison CF, Morris EJ. The practices and meanings of care for nurses working on a pediatric bone marrow transplant unit. J Pediatr Oncol Nurs. 2017;34(3):214–21. https://doi.org/10.1177/10434542166886.
239. Zander M, Hutton A. Paediatric oncology nursing: working and coping when kids have cancer – a thematic review. Neonatal, Paediatr Child Heal Nurs. 2009;12(3):15–27. http://ahs.idm.oclc.org/login?url=http://search.ebscohost.com/
240. Rushton CH, Batcheller J, Schroeder K, Donohue P. Burnout and resilience among nurses practicing in high-intensity settings. Am J Crit Care. 2015;5:412–20. https://doi.org/10.4037/ajcc2015291.
241. Stamm BH. The concise ProQOL manual. 2nd ed. Pocatello: ProQOL.org; 2010.
242. Yoder EA. Compassion fatigue in nurses. Appl Nurs Res. 2010;23(4):191–7. https://doi.org/10.1016/j.apnr.2008.09.003.
243. Joinson C. Coping with compassion fatigue. Nursing. 1992;22(4):116, 118–120.
244. Lombardo B, Eyre C. Compassion fatigue: a nurse's primer. Online J Issues Nurs. 2011;16:3.
245. Jameton A. Nursing practice: the ethical issues. Englewood Cliffs: Prentice-Hall; 1984. p. 6.
246. Jameton A. What moral distress in nursing history could suggest about the future of health care. AMA J Ethic. 2017;19(6):617–28. Available from: http://journalofethics.ama-assn.org/2017/06/mhst1-1706.html
247. Rushton CH. Defining and addressing moral distress tools for critical care nursing leaders. AACN Adv Crit Care. 2006;17(2):161–8. Available from: http://www.ncbi.nlm.nih.gov/pubmed/16767017
248. Dudzinski DM. Navigating moral distress using the moral distress map. J Med Ethics. 2016;42(5):321–4. https://doi.org/10.1136/medethics-2015-103156.
249. Leung D, Esplen MJ, Peter E, Howell D, Rodin G, Fitch M. How haematological cancer nurses experience the threat of patients' mortality. J Adv Nurs. 2012;68(10):2175–84. https://doi.org/10.1111/j.1365-2648.2011.05902.x.
250. Barnard D, Street A, Love AW. Relationships between stressors, work supports, and burnout among cancer nurses. Cancer Nurs. 2006;29(4):338–45.
251. Trousselard M, Dutheil F, Naughton G, Cosserant S, Amadon S, Dualé C, et al. Stress among nurses working in emergency, anesthesiology and intensive care units depends on qualification: a Job Demand-Control survey. Int Arch Occup Environ Health. 2016;89(2):221–9. https://doi.org/10.1007/s00420-015-1065-7.
252. Pavlish C, Brown-Saltzman K, So L, Wong J. SUPPORT: an evidence-based model for leaders addressing moral distress. J Nurs Adm. 2016;46(6):313–20.
253. Hiler CA, Hickman RL Jr, Reimer AP, Wilson K. Predictors of moral distress in a us sample of critical care nurses. Am J Crit Care. 2018;27(1):59–66. https://doi.org/10.4037/ajcc2018968login.aspx?direct=true&db=rzh&AN=105268666&site=ehost-live.
254. Aiken LH. Hospital nurse staffing and patient mortality, nurse burnout, and job dissatisfaction. JAMA. 2002;288(16):1987. Available from: http://jama.jamanetwork.com/article.aspx?doi=10.1001/jama.288.16.1987
255. Meadors P, Lamson A. Compassion fatigue and secondary traumatization: provider self care on intensive care units for children. J Pediatr Heal Care. 2008;22(1):24–34. https://doi.org/10.1016/j.pedhc.2007.01.006.

256. Wocial LD, Weaver MT. Development and psychometric testing of a new tool for detecting moral distress: the moral distress thermometer. J Adv Nurs. 2013;69(1):167–74. https://doi.org/10.1111/j.1365-2648.2012.06036.x.
257. Maslach C, Jackson SE, Leiter MP. Maslach burnout inventory manual. 3rd ed. Palo Alto: Consulting Psychologists Press; 1996.
258. Zomorodi M, Lynn MR. Instrument development measuring critical care nurses' attitudes and behaviors with end-of-life care. Nurs Res. 2010;59(4):234–40. https://doi.org/10.1097/NNR.0b013e3181dd25ef.
259. Rushton CH. Moral resilience: a capacity for navigating moral distress in critical care. AACN Adv Crit Care. 2016;27(1):111–9. https://doi.org/10.4037/aacnacc2016275.
260. AACN. The 4 A's to rise above moral distress. 2012. Available from http://www.emergingrn-leader.com/wp-content/uploads/2012/06/4As_to_Rise_Above_Moral_Distress.pdf
261. Kelly LA, Lefton C. Effect of meaningful recognition on critical care nurses' compassion fatigue. Am J Crit Care. 2017;26(6):438–44. https://doi.org/10.4037/ajcc2017471.
262. Johnson LM, Church CL, Metzger M, Baker JN. Ethics consultation in pediatrics: long-term experience from a pediatric oncology center. Am J Bioeth. 2015;15(5):3–17. https://doi.org/10.1080/15265161.2015.1021965.
263. Robinson EM, Lee SM, Zollfrank A, Jurchak M, Frost D, Grace P. Enhancing moral agency: clinical ethics residency for nurses. Hast Cent Rep. 2014;44(5):12–20. https://doi.org/10.1002/hast.353.
264. Hinds PS, Puckett P, Donohoe M, Milligan M, Payne K, Phipps S, Davis SE, Martin GA. The impact of a grief workshop for pediatric oncology nurses on their grief and perceived stress. J Pediatr Nurs. 1994;9(6):388–97.

Index

C. N. Duncan et al. (eds.), *Critical Care of the Pediatric Immunocompromised Hematology/Oncology Patient*, https://doi.org/10.1007/978-3-030-01322-6

www.ingramcontent.com/pod-product-compliance
Lightning Source LLC
Chambersburg PA
CBHW061649050126
37739CB00003B/77
9783030013219